Surgery for Gastric Cancer

Sung Hoon Noh • Woo Jin Hyung
Editors

Surgery for Gastric Cancer

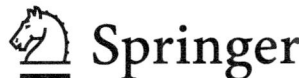 Springer

Editors
Sung Hoon Noh
Department of Surgery
Yonsei University College of Medicine
Seoul
South Korea

Woo Jin Hyung
Department of Surgery
Yonsei University College of Medicine
Seoul
South Korea

ISBN 978-3-662-45582-1   ISBN 978-3-662-45583-8   (eBook)
https://doi.org/10.1007/978-3-662-45583-8

Library of Congress Control Number: 2018968148

This Springer imprint is published by the registered company Springer-Verlag GmbH, DE part of Springer Nature.
The registered company address is: Heidelberger Platz 3, 14197 Berlin, Germany

Contents

Part I

History of Gastric Cancer Surgery

Keiichi Maruyama

We have many dramatic and exciting stories in the history of surgery [1–4]. I would like to recommend my colleagues to read such interesting books, for example, *Das Jahrhundert der Chirurgen* (*The Century of the Surgeon* (English edition)) [5] and *Das Weltreich der Chirurgen* (*The Triumph of Surgery* (English edition)) [6] written by Jurgen Thorwald.

Progress of Supportive Background for Gastric Cancer Surgery

Progress of the following supportive technologies was essential in the development of gastric cancer surgery.

Anesthesia

The dawn of surgery was broken by development of anesthesia [7, 8]. By the late 1830s, it was widely known that nitrous oxide and ether produced drunken condition, and they were used for

K. Maruyama (✉)
Department of Surgical Oncology,
University of Health and Welfare Sanno Medical Center,
Tokyo, Japan

Department of Surgical Oncology, National Cancer
Center Hospital, Tokyo, Japan
e-mail: keiichi-maruyama@rOl.itscom.net

amusement such as "ether frolics." An American dentist in Boston Horace Wells (1815–1848) (Fig. 1.1a) used nitrous oxide for a painless dental extraction in 1845 [9]. His business partner and fellow dentist William T. G Morton (1819–1868) (Fig. 1.1b, e) used dimethyl ether also for dental extractions. He expanded the use for general surgery. He demonstrated his method for neck tumor resection to the prominent surgeon John Collins Warren at the Massachusetts General Hospital on the 16th of October 1846 (Fig. 1.1e) [10]. The next year, a Scottish obstetrician James Young Simpson (1811–1870) (Fig. 1.1e) of Edinburgh used chloroform for general anesthesia [11]. Chloroform anesthesia was rapidly popularized after the application for Queen Victoria's labor in 1853. These developments released patients from terrible pain and fear during surgery.

Aseptic Method

A Hungarian obstetrician Ignaz Fulop Semmelweis (1818–1865) (Fig. 1.1d) noticed that a clean condition reduced maternal death. He reported in 1847 that the death rate went dramatically down by handwashing and rinsing of medical instruments and linens with chlorinated lime solution at the Vienna General Hospital [12]. Semmelweis's work was furthered by a Scottish surgeon Joseph Lister (1827–1912) (Fig. 1.2a). He used phenol (carbolic acid) to clean surgical gauze at the Glasgow Royal

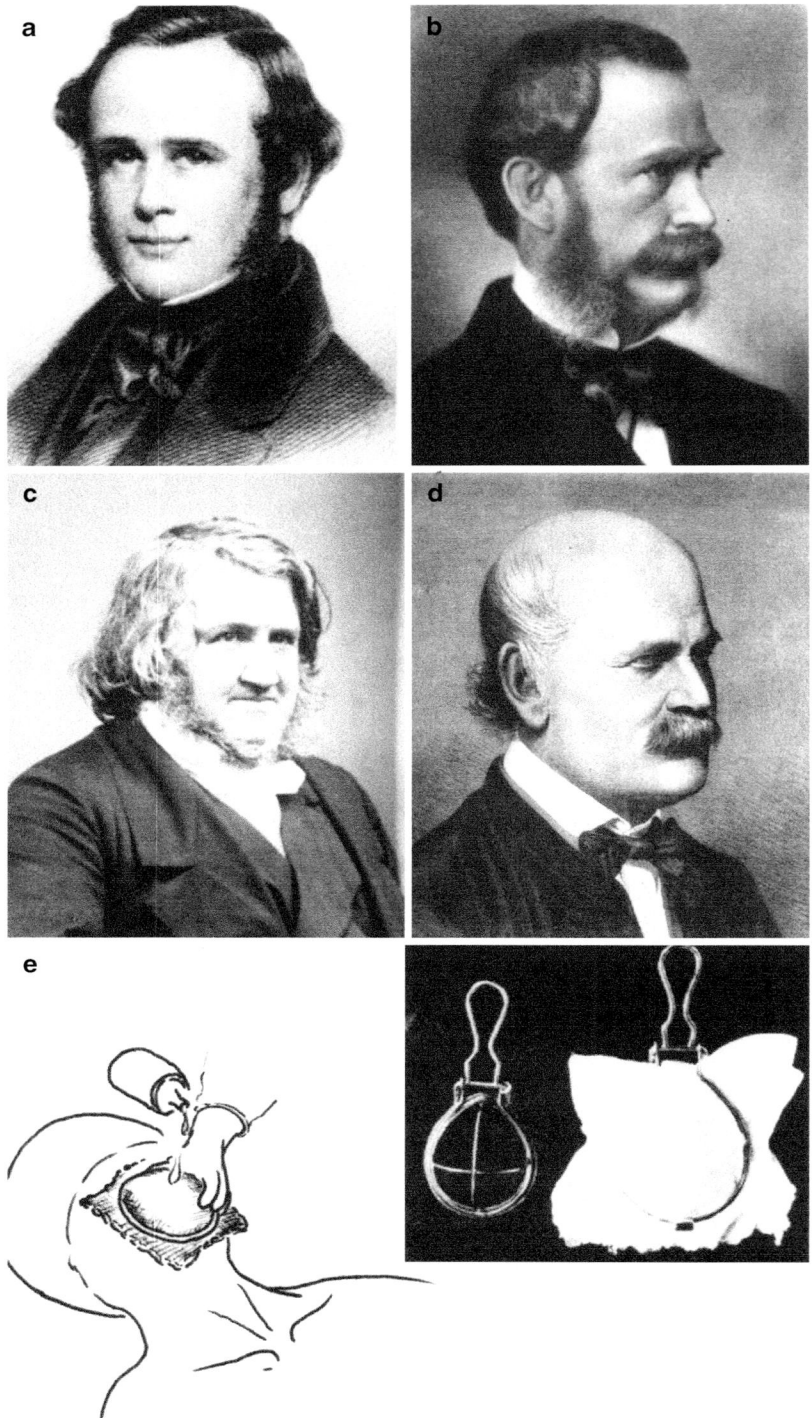

Fig. 1.1 (a–f) Historical leaders, pictures of ether anesthesia, and Lister's aseptic method. (a) Horace Wells: nitrous oxide anesthesia, (b) William T.G. Morton: ether anesthesia, (c) James Young Simpson: chloroform anesthesia, (d) Ignaz F. Semmelweis: chlorinated lime wash, (e) ether mask for inhalation anesthesia (ether solution was dropped on the mask with gauze), (f) Lister's aseptic method (carbolic acid solution was used for washing and spray)

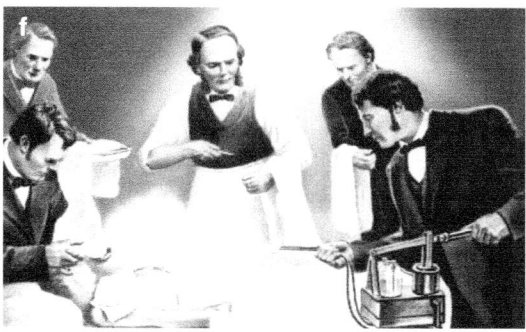

Fig. 1.1 (continued)

Infirmary of Edinburgh from 1866. And he introduced phenol vapor to clean his operating room (Fig. 1.1f) [13]. Ernst von Bergmann (1836–1907) (Fig. 1.2b), professor of surgery in the University of Berlin, and his coworker Curt Schimmelbusch (1860–1895) developed a heat sterilization method for surgical instruments in 1886 (Fig. 1.2g) [14]. We have a very romantic history in development of the surgical rubber glove. The world famous surgeon, William Stewart Halsted (1852–1922) (Fig.1.2c) of the Johns Hopkins Hospital, USA, used strictly Lister's method using carbolic acid. This antiseptic solution produced severe hand skin damage of the head nurse of the operation theater, Miss Caroline Hampton. He ordered special thin skin rubber gloves for her from the Goodyear Tire and Rubber Company in 1890 [15]. They got married in 1890. An Austrian surgeon Antonio Grossich (1849–1926) (Fig. 1.2d) introduced iodine tincture for rapid skin sterilization of the surgical field in 1908 [16]. These aseptic strategies were scientifically supported by the discovery of "microorganisms." Louis Pasteur (1822–1895) (Fig. 1.2e) of the Ecole Nationale Superieure des Beaux-Arts, Paris, confirmed that the microorganisms caused the fermentation and putrefaction in 1847 [17]. Robert H. H. Koch (1843–1910) (Fig. 1.2f), a Nobel Prize microbiologist in the University of Berlin, found the bacteria which caused various infectious diseases in 1878 [18]. These developments reduced dramatically fatal surgical infections.

Antibacterial Agents

The next significant progress appeared on antibacterial agents. Bayer chemists (German) Gerhard Domagk (1895–1964) (Fig. 1.3a) and Josef Klarer (1898–1953) synthesized "sulfonamide," a strong anti-gram-positive cocci substance, in 1935 [19]. A Scottish Nobel Prize scientist Alexander Fleming (1881–1955) (Fig. 1.3b) discovered penicillin at St Mary's Hospital, London, in 1928 [20]. He actually opened a new era in medicine. Penicillin was purified by Howard Walter Florey (1898–1968) and Ernst Boris Chain (1906–1979) of the University of Oxford in 1941 [21]. Penicillin showed miraculous effectiveness during the World War II. Nowadays, we have various antibacterial agents.

Intravenous Infusion Therapy

This treatment offered a non-oral route administration of fluid, minerals, calories, and drugs to the patient. Using the infusion therapy, the patient can stop drinking and eating after surgery. Thomas Latta (1796–1833), a surgeon in Leith, Scotland, developed this technology for patients with cholera in 1832 [22]. Stanley J. Dudrick of the University of Pennsylvania, USA, developed parenteral nutrition in 1968, and this method was widely used particularly through the central venous route [23].

Suture Materials and Surgical Instruments

In the 1850s, the popular suture materials were linen, cotton, catgut, and silk. They were now completely disappeared except silk. Various synthesized absorbable sutures with atraumatic needle are now in use. Mechanical anastomotic instruments showed remarkable development. The first reliable liner stapler was developed by a Hungarian surgeon Aladar von Petz (1888–1956) of the Trinity Hospital in Györ in 1921 (Fig. 1.3c) [24]. The first circular stapler was developed by Masaru Mine of the Kyoto Prefectural Medical University, Japan, in 1962 [25]. The improved models, SPTU and PKS-25 M, were provided by a Russian company (Fig. 1.3d). An American company, the United States Surgical Corporation, bought the license from Russia and supplied the

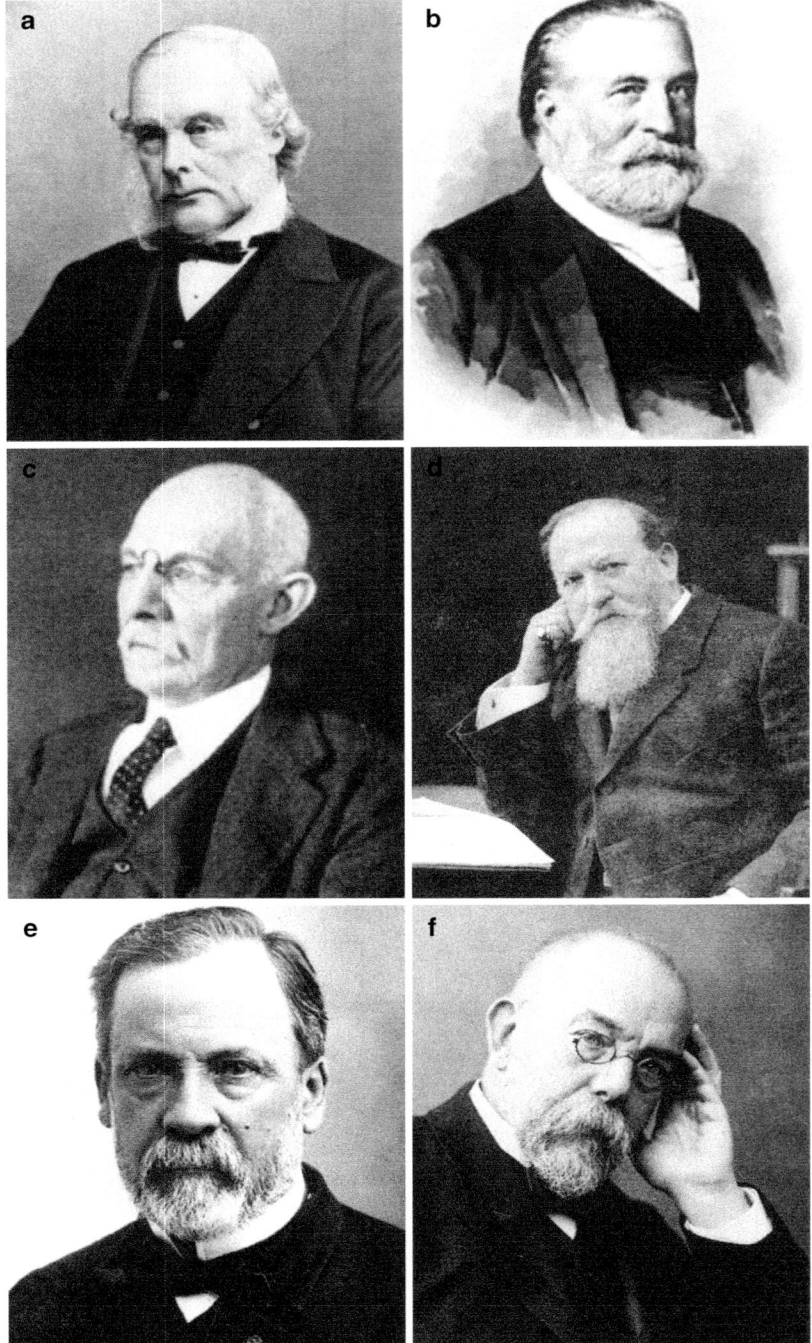

Fig. 1.2 (a–g) Historical leaders and Schimmelbusch sterilization apparatus. (a) Joseph Lister: carbolic acid antiseptic, (b) Ernst von Bergmann: heat sterilization, (c) William Stewart Halsted: surgical glove, (d) Antonio Grossich: iodine tincture, (e) Louis Pasteur: microorganisms, (f) Robert Koch: infectious bacteria, (g) Schimmelbusch heat sterilization system: for medical instruments

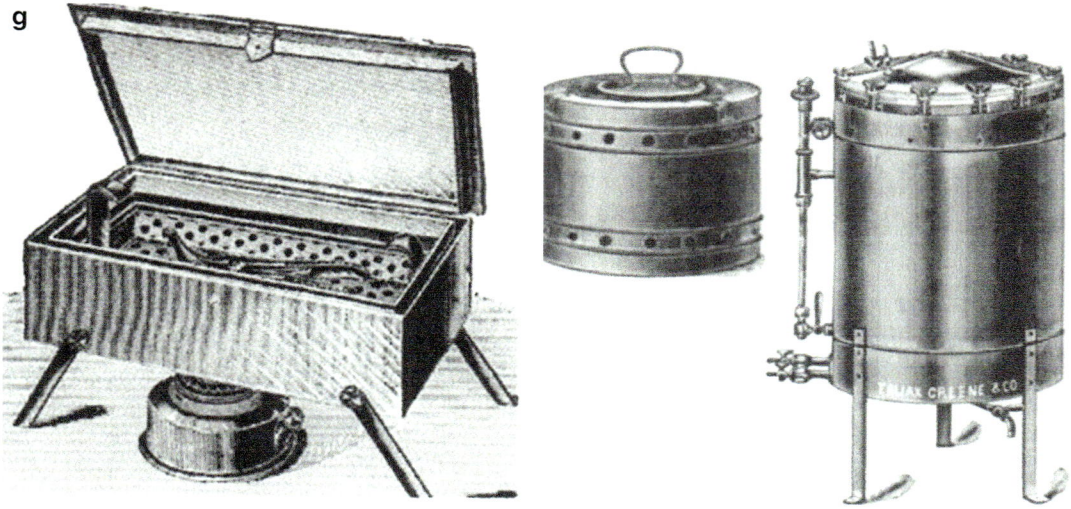

Fig. 1.2 (continued)

Fig. 1.3 (**a–e**) Historical leaders and various mechanical staplers. (**a**) Gerhard Domagk: antibiotic sulfonamide; (**b**) Alexander Fleming: antibiotic penicillin; (**c**) von Petz linear stapler; (**d**) Russian circular stapler, SPTU; (**e**) United States Surgical Corporation, EEA stapler

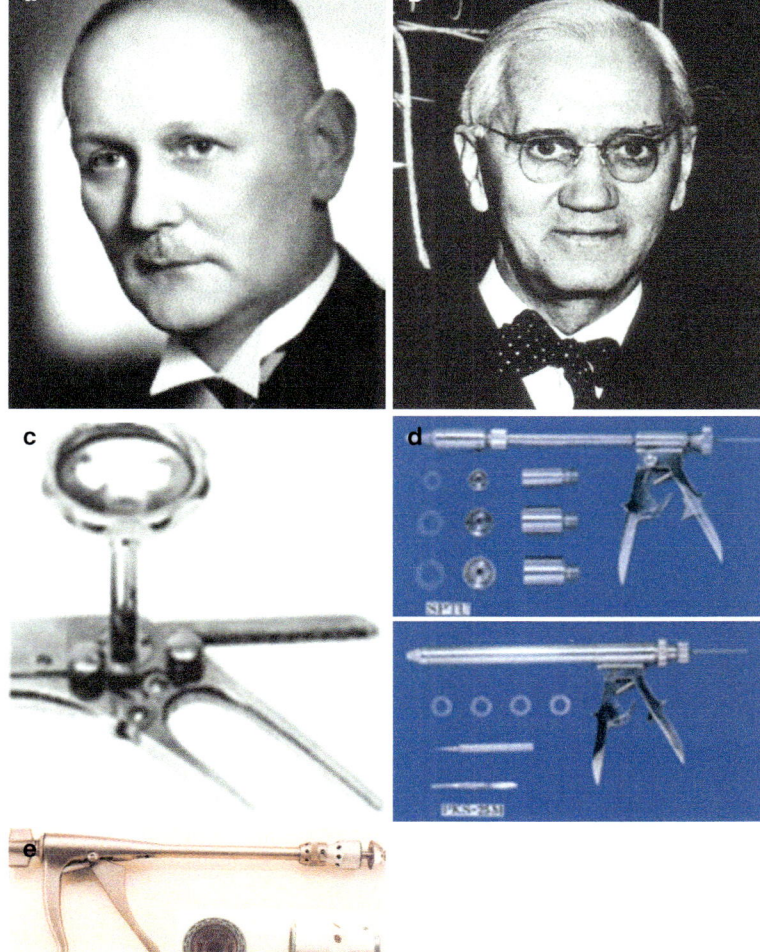

improved and disposable devices of TA, GIA, and EEA (Fig. 1.3e). Electrocautery was also improved, and we have now various devices for different procedures. The other progress was laparoscopic instruments and robot surgery machines. Minimally invasive surgery becomes popular supported by these progress.

Advancement in Pathological Knowledge

Pathology of gastric cancer showed a remarkable advancement. A German pathologist R. Borrmann in Bremen published a famous textbook about gastric cancer in 1926 [26]. He described the macroscopic-type so-called Borrmann's classification. Detailed and huge follow-up data informed us the characteristics of the disease. The data supported the establishment of rational treatments.

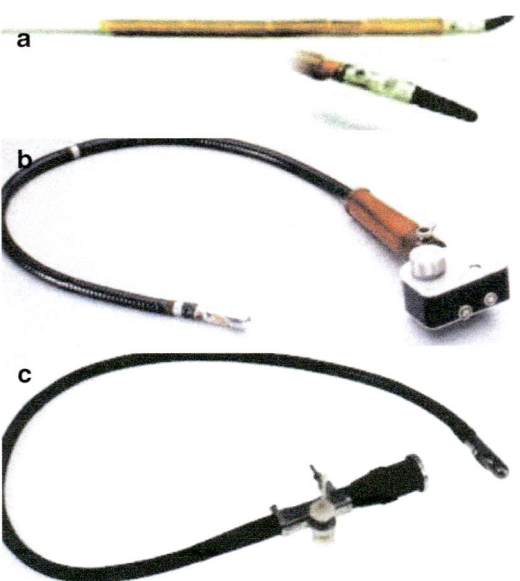

Fig. 1.4 (**a–c**) Development of gastroendoscope. (**a**) Schindler's prism flexible gastroscope, 1932; (**b**) Olympus gastrocamera, 1950; (**c**) Hirschowitz gastrofiberscope, 1964

Progress of Diagnostic Methods

Preoperative assessment of cancer extension and biological characteristics became significantly accurate by endoscopy (Fig. 1.4a, b, c), endoscopic biopsy, double-contrast XP study, CT, ultrasonography, tumor markers, etc. Nowadays surgeons can make the most appropriate treatment plan for each individual patient based on these information.

Challengers of Gastric Resection

Before the introduction of anesthesia and antiseptic method, a few successful gastric surgeries were reported. Most of them were removal of foreign body such as swallowed knife from the stomach [27, 28].

Three great pioneers performed the memorial gastric resections for pyloric cancer in the short period between 1879 and 1981. Jules-Émile Péan (1830–1898) (Fig. 1.5a) of St Louis Hospital, Paris, performed the first distal gastric resection (actually a pylorus resection) for a pyloroduode-

nal cancer with stenosis on 9 April 1879 [29]. The procedures lasted two hours and half under a 13-cm-long paraumbilical incision. The patient died on the fifth postoperative day but autopsy was denied. Pe'an did not leave the detailed medical record, and the cause of death was not clear. But mismatched blood transfusion or anastomotic leakage caused by catgut suture was speculated.

The Polish surgeon Ludwik Rydygier (1850–1920) (Fig. 1.5b) carried out the second gastric resection for a 64-year-old bugle soldier with pylorus stenosis on 16 November 1880. He was a research-oriented surgeon and he left the exact and detailed record [30, 31]. He made a series of animal experiments on gastric resection and reconstruction techniques. He applied Lister's carbolic acid sterilization for hands, instruments, and linens by washing and air spraying. He carried out the surgery at his private clinic with 25 beds in Kulm, Poland. Rydygier performed the surgery very carefully taking four hours and half under an upper midline incision using 60 stitches for gastroduodenal anastomosis (Fig. 1.5c). The

Fig. 1.5 (a–c)
Historical leaders and
Rydygier's operation.
(**a**) Jules-Émile
Péan: first gastric
resection, (**b**) Ludwik
Rydygier: second gastric
resection, (**c**) pyloric
resection procedure by
Rydygier in 1880 (the
tumor was located close
to the pylorus. It was
resected and a two-layer
gastroduodenal
anastomosis was made
at the lesser curvature
side). (From S. Sokół's
drawing [161])

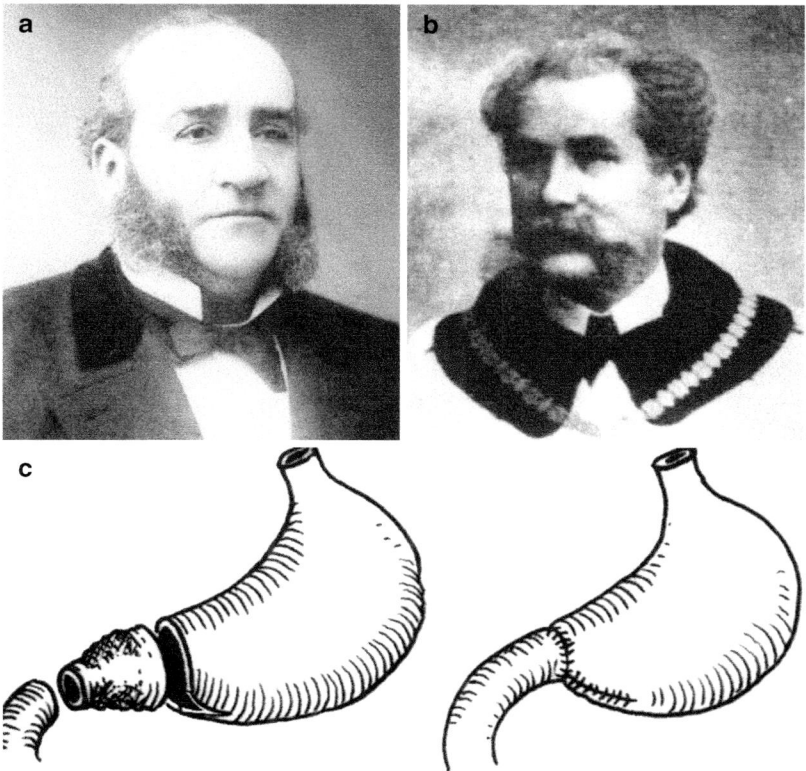

patient had smooth recovery after the surgery but suddenly died in the early morning of the first postoperative day. The cause of death would be collapse brought by the preoperative poor condition. The autopsy revealed no residual tumor and no infection. Anastomotic leakage was denied by water inflation test of the resected material.

The honor of the first successful gastric resection was given to Theodor Billroth (1829–1894) (Fig. 1.6a), professor of surgery at the University of Vienna and chairman of the Second Surgical Clinic of the Wien Allgemeines Krankenhaus (Vienna General Hospital) (Fig. 1.6c). He prepared his surgery very carefully. His two staffs, Carl Gussenbauer (1842–1903) and Alexander von Winiwarter (1848–1917), made animal experiments on the surgical techniques of gastric resection and anastomosis using dogs [32]. They also made detailed research on pyloric cancer behavior and possibility of curative resection using 542 autopsy records. Gussenbauer was the successor of Billroth at the University of Vienna,

and Winiwarter became a professor of surgery at the University of Liege, Belgium. Billroth sent his staffs to the Royal Infirmary of Edinburgh and King's College Hospital, London, for introducing Lister's aseptic method. On 29 January 1881, Billroth performed distal gastric resection on Therese Heller, a 43-year-old Vienna housewife having eight children.

Billroth wrote a letter to Professor L. Wittelshöfer, the publisher of the *Wiener Medizinische Wochenschrift* (*Vienna Medical Weekly*), by himself informing his historical gastric resection [33]. And his operation record was published by his colleague Anton Wölfler (1850–1917) (Fig. 1.6b) [34], and the record was studied in detail by Herbert Ziegler (Fig. 1.6d) [35]. On the day, his team applied Lister's aseptic procedures except carbolic acid vapor spray method. The surgical instruments; suture material, silk thread and linens were sterilized with carbolic acid solution. They did not use catgut. Before starting the operation, her stomach was irrigated

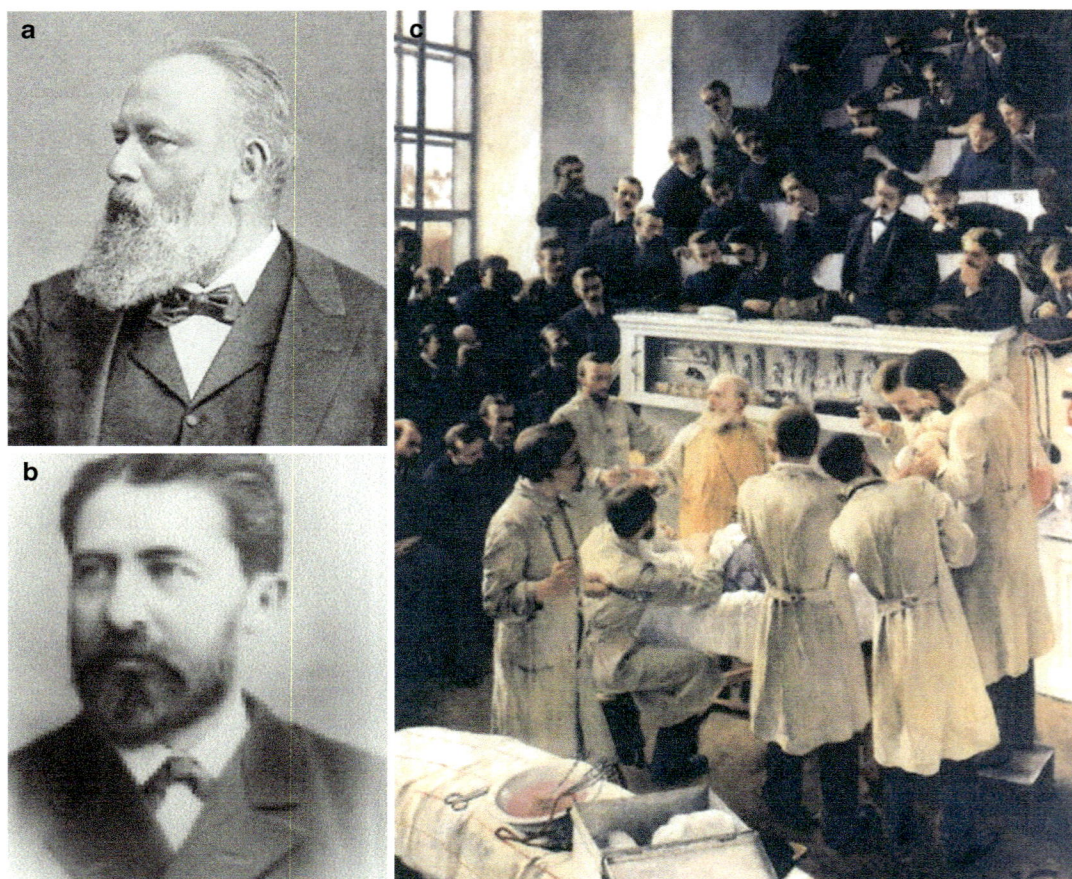

Fig. 1.6 (**a**–**f**) Historical leaders and Billroth's first successful gastrectomy. (**a**) Theodor Billroth: third gastric resection; (**b**) Anton Wolfler: gastroenterostomy; (**c**) painting depicting Billroth's operation in 1890 at Wien Allgemeines Krankenhaus by Albert F. Seligmann, Österreichische Galerie Belvedere Palace, Wien; (**d**) the first distal gastrectomy; (**e**) resected material of Therese Heller; (**f**) autopsy material, the duodenum left side (these pathological materials are exhibited at the Josephinum Medizinischen Museum Universität Wien)

with 1.5 liters of warm water consuming one hour. Under chloroform anesthesia, Billroth made an 11-cm-long right transverse incision, crossing the midline just over the palpable tumor. A few hazelnut-size swollen lymph nodes were found, and metastasis of medullary carcinoma was microscopically confirmed on one sample node. Billroth followed the surgical procedures established by dog experiments, and he spent only one hour and 30 minutes for his operation. The duodenum was divided 1.5 cm distal from the tumor mass, and the middle part of the stomach was divided. The divided stomach stump was narrowed by 21 stitches at the greater curvature side for adjusting the anastomotic size. Thirty-three interrupted sutures were applied for gastro-duodenal anastomosis not including the mucosal layer. He used carbolized silk for ligatures and sutures (Fig. 1.6d).

The patient took smooth recovery from the surgery. She could drink and eat well from the third postoperative day. The dressing was changed on the 6th postoperative day, and there was no sign of infection. The patient was discharged from the hospital on the 22nd postoperative day.

The patient died of recurrence on 24 May 1881, 4 months after the operation. A pathologist of the Vienna University, Dr. Zemann, made the

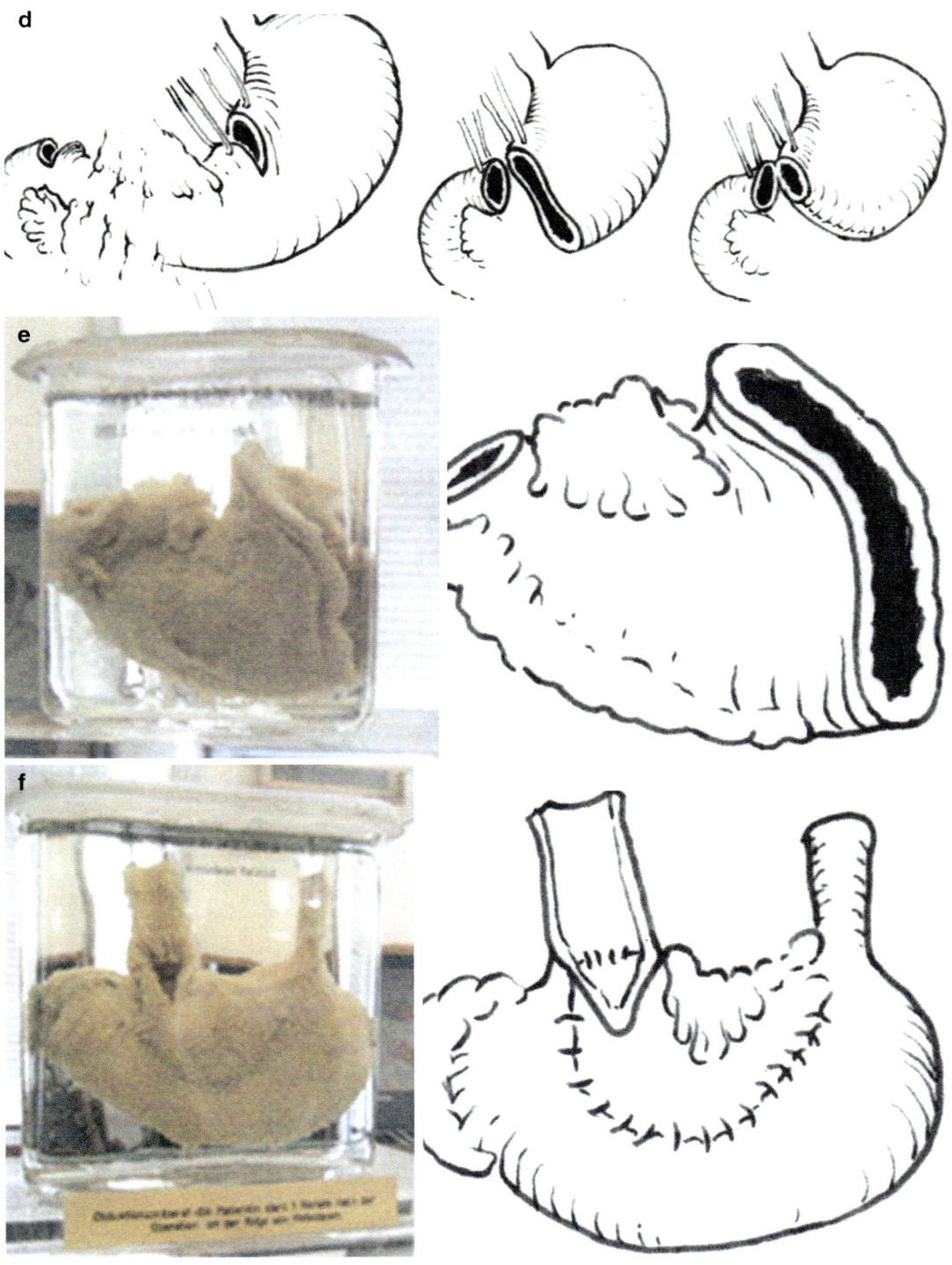

Fig. 1.6 (continued)

autopsy, and Ziegler made the detailed study [35]. We can see the resected specimen and the autopsy material in the Josephinum Medical Museum of the University of Vienna (Fig. 1.6e, f).

Within 2 months of Billroth's operation, 21 similar gastrectomies had been performed, several of them in Billroth's clinic. Survived cases were only three from them, one by Billroth and the other two by his colleagues, Wölfler and Vincenz Czerny (1842–1916) (Fig. 1.7a) [34]. Czerny was appointed professor at the University of Heidelberg where he founded the German Institute for Experimental Cancer Research in 1906. A Polish-German surgeon from Danzig, Hans

Haberkant, reported that the surgical mortality rate was 69% (72/109 patients) in Europe in 1879–1887. The mortality rate was improved to 43% (42/98 patients) in 1888–1894 [36]. This report informed us that gastric resection remained as a risky surgery even after the first successful operation.

Theodor Billroth placed the gastroduodenal anastomosis at the lesser curvature side (Fig. 1.8a) for his first and second patients, but he changed the anastomotic site at the greater curvature side (Fig. 1.8b) for the third patient [35]. Emil Theodor Kocher (1841–1917) (Fig. 1.7b), a Nobel Prize surgeon from the University of Bern, Switzerland, reported an unique procedure to prevent anastomotic leakage in 1892. He closed stomach stump and inserted the duodenal stump into the new incision of posterior wall of the remnant stomach (Fig. 1.8c) [37]. John M.T. Finney (1863–1942) (Fig. 1.9a) of the Johns Hopkins Hospital, USA, proposed a gastroduodenostomy method with whole gastric stump and lateral wall of the duodenum in 1924 (Fig. 1.8d) [38].

Various reconstruction methods with gastrojejunostomy were proposed after the first successful Billroth I operation (Fig. 1.10). They were named "Billroth II operation," with antecolic or retrocolic and iso- or antiperistaltic anastomosis, with or without Braun's enteroanastomosis, and with partial or whole cut end of the stomach [39]. In 1885 Billroth published his *Billroth II Operation* or the antecolic side-to-side gastrojejunostomy (Fig. 1.10a) [40, 41]. In 1888 this operation was modified by his Austrian staff Anton F. von Eiselsberg (1860–1939) (Fig. 1.9b). This procedure used retrocolic route with anastomosis between the stomach stump and side wall of the jejunum. Furthermore, this procedure was refined by Franz von Hofmeister (1867–1926) (Fig. 1.9c) of the University of Tübingen, Germany, based on a procedure by Eugen Alexander Pólya (1876–1944) (Fig. 1.9d) of Semmelweis University, Budapest (Fig. 1.10e) [42]. It was later refined by Hans Finsterer (1877–1955) (Fig. 1.11a) of the University of Vienna and became known as the "Hofmeister-Finsterer gastrectomy" (Fig. 1.10g) [43]. Here the stomach cut end of the lesser curvature side is

Fig. 1.7 (a–b) Historical leaders. (a) Vincenz Czerny: cancer surgery, (b) Emil Theodor Kocher: reconstruction

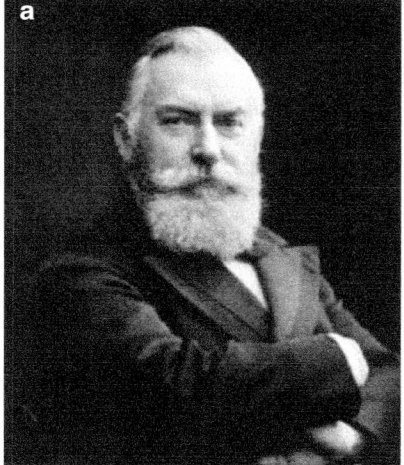
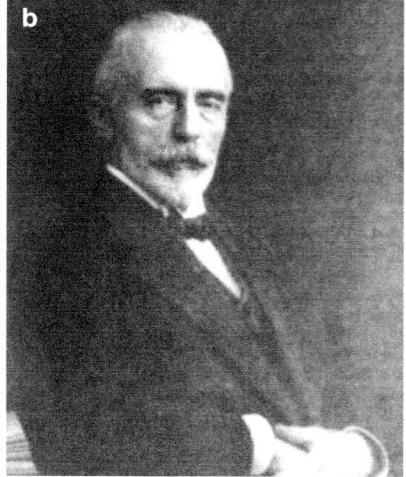

Fig. 1.8 (**a–d**) Various Billroth I type reconstructions. (**a**) Billroth T, 1881; (**b**) Billroth T, 1883; (**c**) Kocher E, 1891; (**d**) Finney JMT, 1924, and von Habere H, 1922

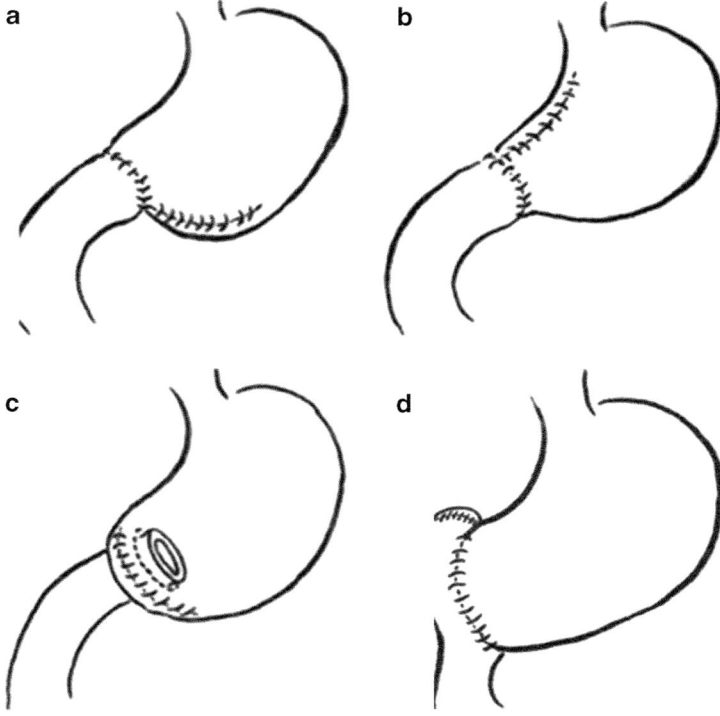

Fig. 1.9 (**a–d**) Historical leaders of the gastric cancer surgery. (**a**) John MT. Finney: reconstruction, (**b**) Anton F. von Eiselsberg: Billroth II operation, (**c**) Franz von Hofmeister: Billroth II reconstruction, (**d**) Eugen A. Pólya: Billroth II reconstruction

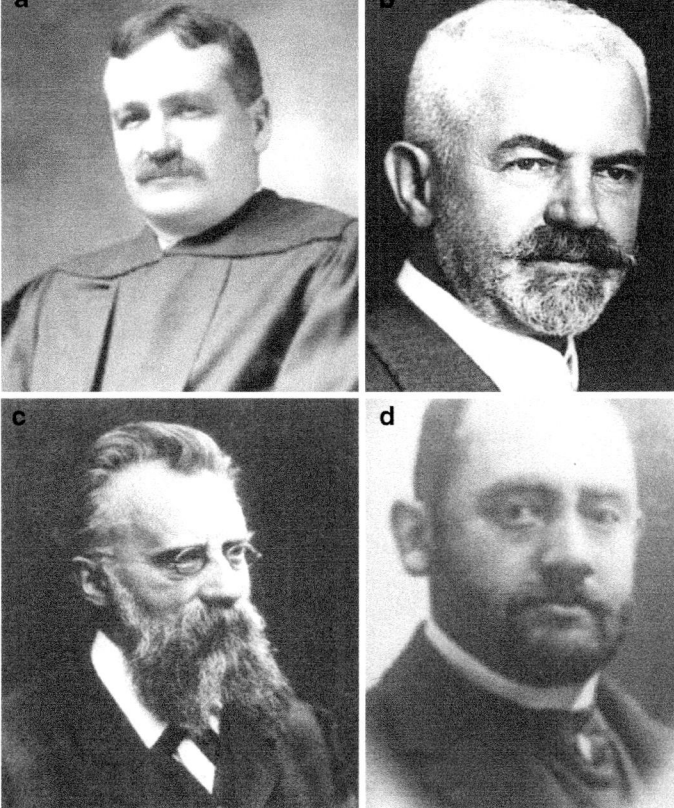

closed, and the remaining greater curvature side portion is anastomosed with the jejunum (Fig. 1.10f). This procedure was popularized by Finsterer based on his huge experiences of more than 10,000 gastric operations. Heinrich Ch. Braun (1847–1911) of the University of Königsberg, Germany, proposed side-to-side anastomosis between the afferent and efferent jejunal loop for better passage of duodenal juice in 1892 (Fig. 1.10g) [44]. Donald C. Balfour (1882–1963) of Mayo Clinic, USA, added Braun anastomosis to Po'lya, called Balfour-Pólya operation, in 1917 (Fig. 1.10g) [45, 46]. But several literatures described that this reconstruction

method was previously performed by Hofmeister. A pupil of Kocher, Ce'sar Roux (1857–1934) (Fig 1.11b) of the University of Lausanne, Switzerland, described the Roux-en-Y reconstruction in 1927 (Fig. 1.10h) [47], which can be applied not only for the distal gastric resection but also for the total gastrectomy.

In this period, many Japanese surgeons stayed in Germany, and they introduced the latest surgical technologies. In 1897, 16 years after Billroth's success, the first gastric cancer resection was done by Jihan Kondo (1866–1944) of Tokyo University Hospital [48]. A pupil of Mikulicz, Hayari Miyake (1866–1945) (Fig. 1.11c) of the

Fig. 1.10 (**a–h**) Various Billroth II type reconstructions. (**a**) Billroth T, Wölfler A, 1885; (**b**) Krönlein RU, 1888; (**c**) Mikulicz JR, 1897; (**d**) Moynihan B, 1923; (**e**) Polya EA, 1911; (**f**) Hofmeister-Finsterer, 1895; (**g**) Balfour DC, 1917; (**h**) Roux C, 1893–1898

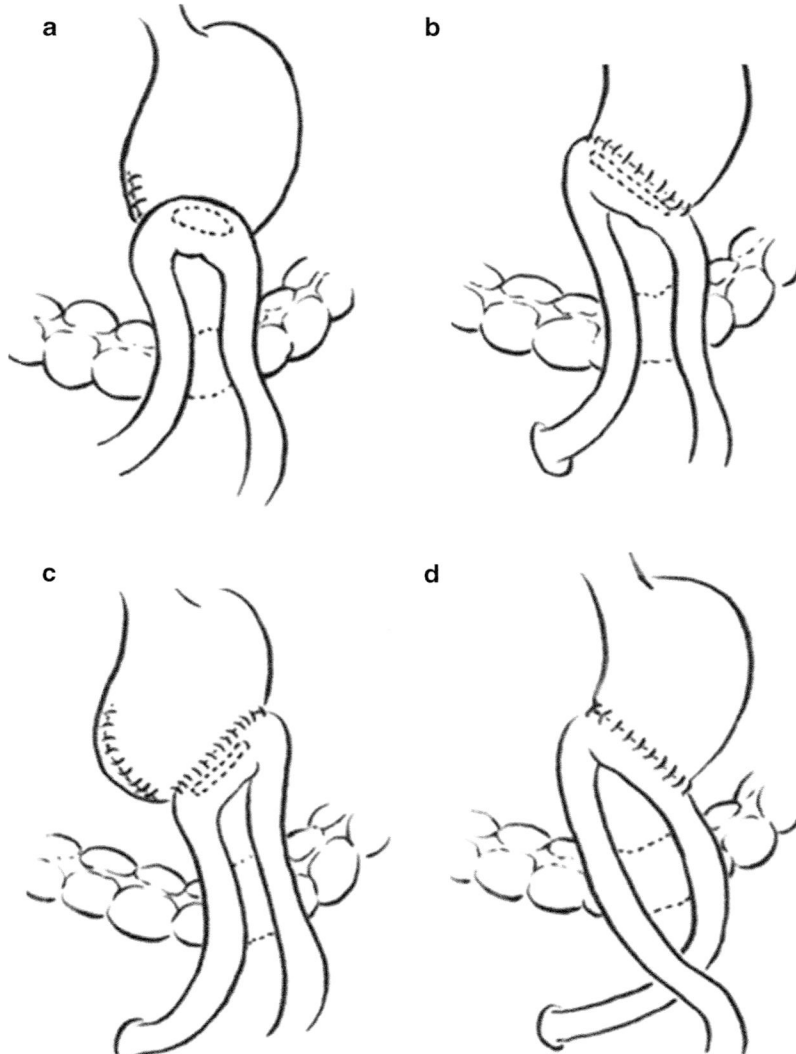

Fig. 1.10 (continued)

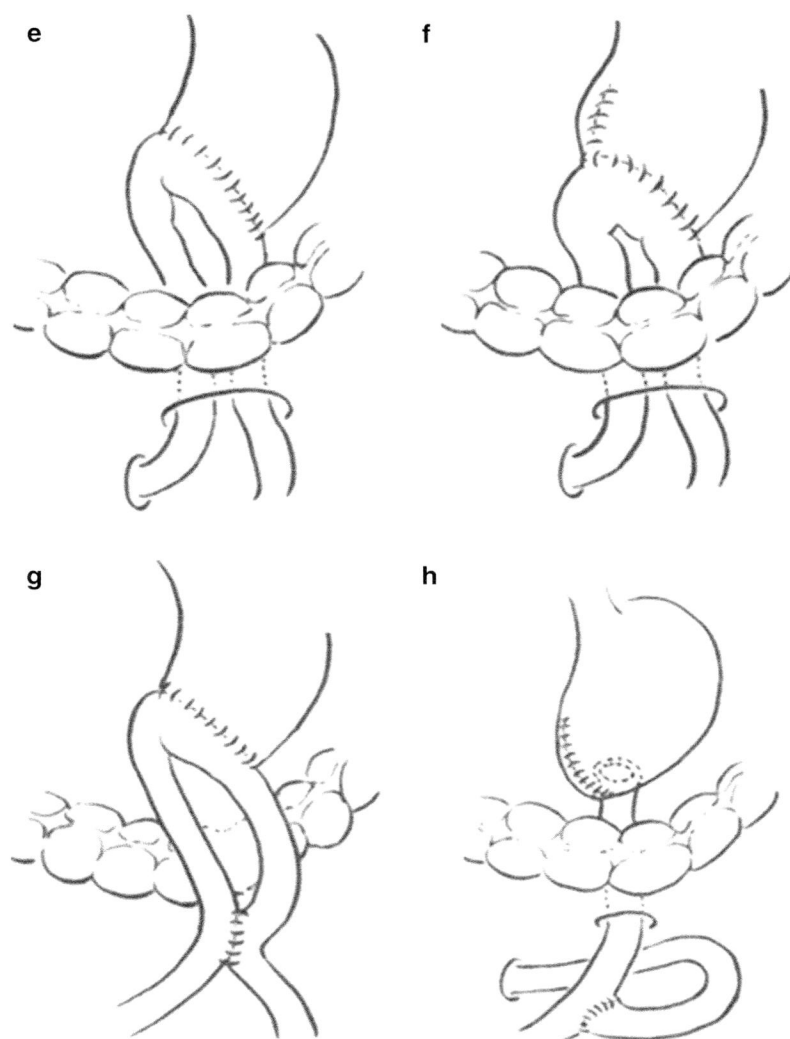

Kyushu University, Japan, reported that 58 patients died of postoperative complication from 177 patients (33%) treated in 1904–1914 in his department. He reported that the surgical death rate was improved to 14.2% (56/395 patients) in 1920–1927. The 3-year survival rate was 31.3% (108/345 patients) in his series [49].

Powerful Drive for Curability

Billroth's Polish-Austrian associate Johann F. von Mikulicz-Radecki (1850–1905) (Fig. 1.11d) of the Schlesischen Friedrich-Wilhelms Universität Breslau, Germany (now Wroclaw Poland), opened actually the door of scientific oncological surgery in 1898 [50–52]. He described that gastric cancer had four growth directions: (a) local extension, namely, the stomach wall infiltration and adjacent structure invasion, (b) extension through the lymphatic vessels to the regional nodes, (c) extension through the blood vessels to the liver, and (d) peritoneal dissemination. Mikulicz stressed that the cure could be obtained only when these targets were removed perfectly. To remove the direct wall expansion, total gastrectomy was proposed. Combined resection of neighboring organs was

Fig. 1.11 (a–d)
Historical leaders of the
gastric cancer surgery. (**a**)
Hans Finsterer: Billroth
II operation, (**b**) C'ésar
Roux: Roux-en-Y
anastomosis, (**c**) Hayari
Miyake: treatment
results, (**d**) Jan Mikulicz-
Radecki: surgical
oncology

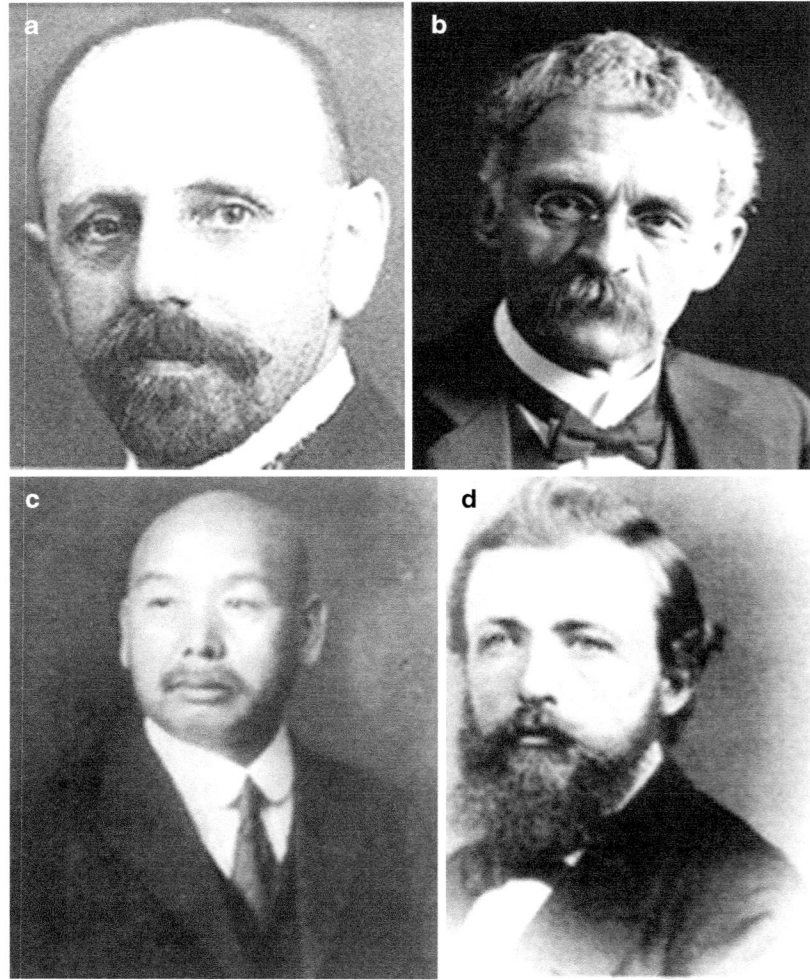

applied for invasion to the adjacent structures. Systematic lymph node dissection could remove the metastatic lymph nodes. However, cure from the liver and peritoneal metastases could not be achieved by surgical treatment. Followings are the progress of these surgical treatments.

Total Gastrectomy

In 1987, 6 years after Billroth's gastric resection, the first successful total gastrectomy for cancer was performed by a Billroth's staff, Carl B. Schlatter (1864–1934) (Fig. 1.13a) of the

University of Zurich, Switzerland [53, 54]. His reconstruction method was the Billroth II reconstruction with antecolic end-to-side esophagojejunostomy without Braun's anastomosis (Fig. 1.12a). The first total gastrectomy was successfully performed in Japan in 1902 by Otojiro Kitagawa (1864–1922) of the Nagoya Koseikan Hospital [55]. The surgical mortality rate was significantly high in this period. Various reconstruction methods were proposed with intention to prevent leakage of the esophagojejunal anastomosis and regurgitation esophagitis (Fig. 1.12).

Fig. 1.12 (**a–h**) Various reconstruction methods after total gastrectomy. (**a**) Schlatter C, 1897; (**b**) Schlöffer H, 1917; (**c**) Roux C, 1907; (**d**) Orr TG, 1943; (**e**) Graham RR, 1940; (**f**) Nishi M, 1972; (**g**) Siewert-Peiper, 1972; (**h**) Hunt CJ, 1952

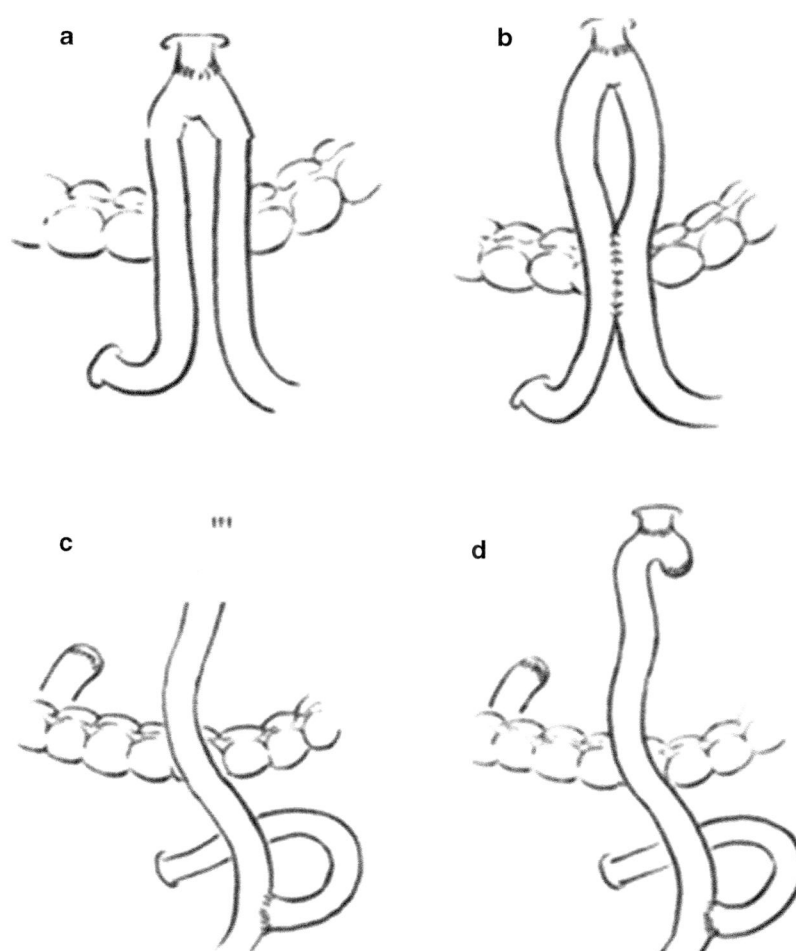

Fig. 1.12 (continued)

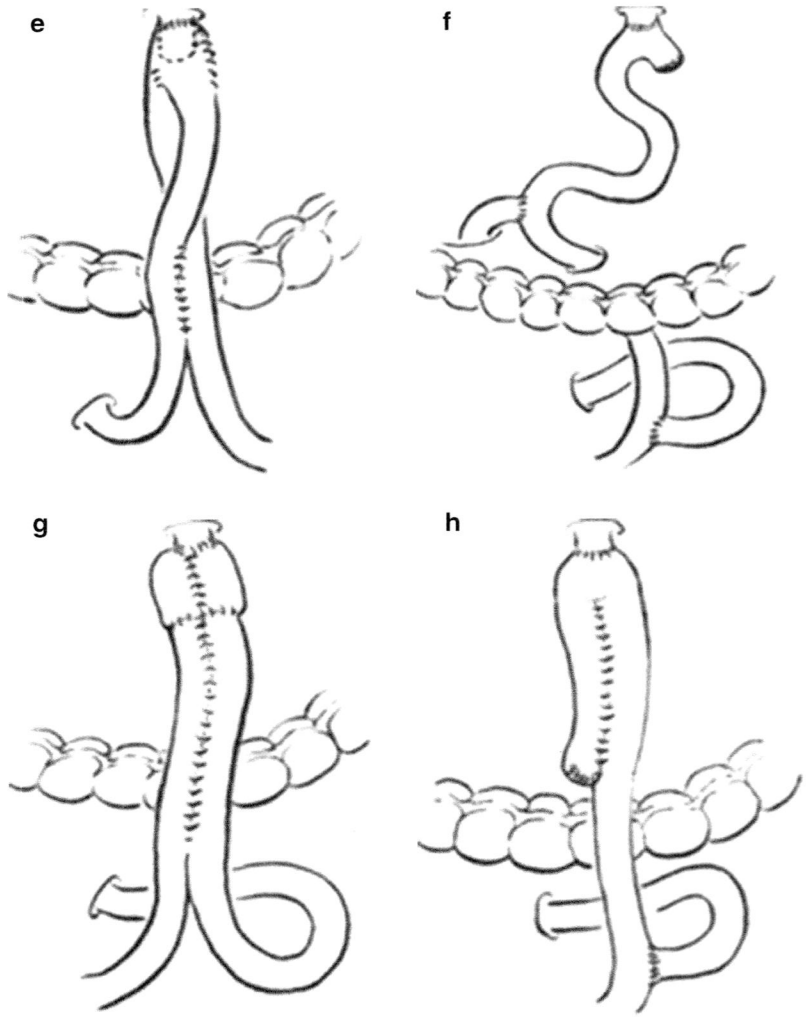

Hermann Schlöffer (1868–1937) (Fig. 1.13b) of the University of Prague added Braun's jejunoje-junostomy to Schlatter's reconstruction in 1917 (Fig. 1.12b) [56]. César Roux applied his "Roux-en-Y anastomosis" for the reconstruction after total gastrectomy in 1907 (Fig. 1.12c) [57]. Thomas G. Orr (1884–1955) (Fig. 1.13c) of the University of Kansas, USA, modified Roux-en-Y reconstruction by end-of-esophagus-to-side-of-jejunum anastomosis in 1943 (Fig. 1.12c)

[58]. This procedure became the most popular reconstruction method. Roscoe R. Graham (1890–1948) (Fig 1.13d) of the University of Toronto, Canada, developed a unique anasto-motic method in 1940, reinforcement of the esophagojejunostomy using the jejunal stump like a sandwich (Fig. 1.12e) [59, 60]. Mitsumasa Nishi (1925–1998) (Fig. 1.13e) of the Cancer Institute, Tokyo, proposed the so-called double-tract method in 1972 connecting the duodenal

stump to the side of the jejunum in Roux-en-Y reconstruction (Fig. 1.12f) [61]. We have now various reconstructions after total gastrectomy (Fig. 1.12) [62–64].

Reconstruction by the jejunal segment interposition between the esophagus and duodenum (Fig. 1.14a) was developed by Sadanobu Seo (1886–1946) (Fig. 1.13f) of the Chiba University, Japan, in 1941 [65] and by William Polk Longmire (1913–2003) (Fig. 1.13g) of the UCLA Medical Center, Los Angeles, in 1952 [66]. The other trend was building a reservoir in place of the resected stomach. Longmire created a single lumen tube from jejunal loop, like a long Braun anastomosis [67]. We have various interposition methods (Fig. 1.14) [68] including interposition of the ileocolic segment (Fig. 1.14d) [69].

By these efforts, the surgical mortality rate was remarkably improved and total gastrectomy became safer. This improvement led to a new opinion and trend; active application of total gastrectomy for obtaining the better curability particularly in the USA. Gordon

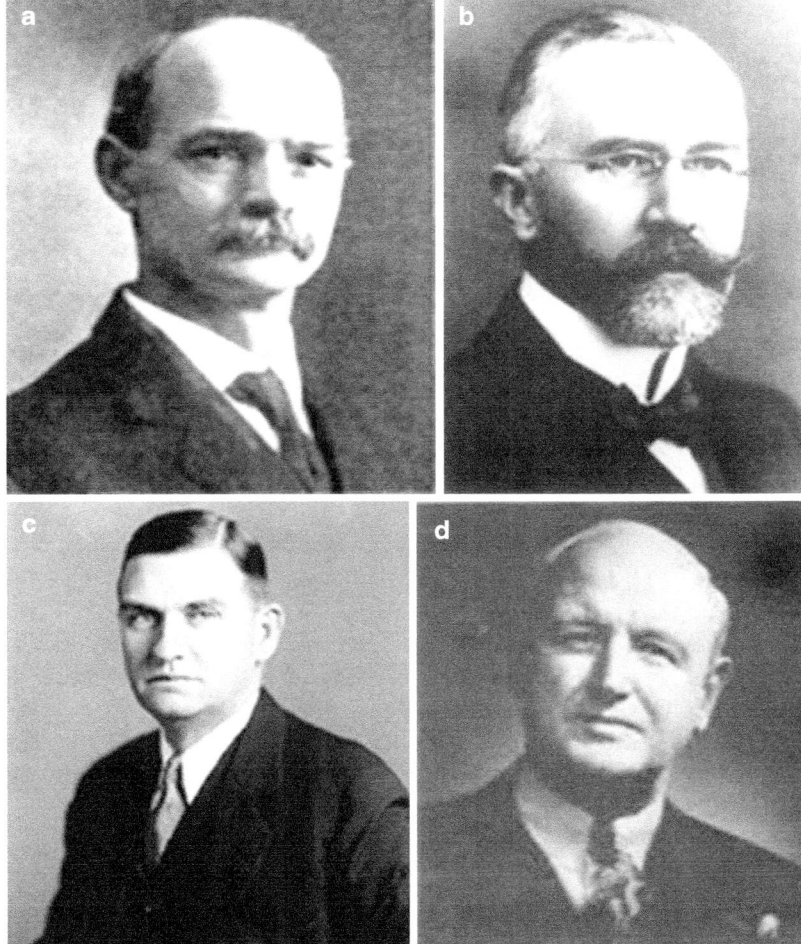

Fig. 1.13 (a–h) Historical leaders of the gastric cancer surgery. (a) Carl B. Schlatter: total gastrectomy, (b) Hermann Schlöffer: esophagojejunostomy, (c) Thomas G. Orr: Roux-en-Y anastomosis, (d) Roscoe R. Graham: anastomosis, (e) Mitsumasa Nishi: double-tract anastomosis, (f) Sadanobu Seo: jejunal interposition, (g) William P. Longmire: jejunal interposition, (h) Gordon McNeer: extended radical total gastrectomy

Fig. 1.13 (continued)

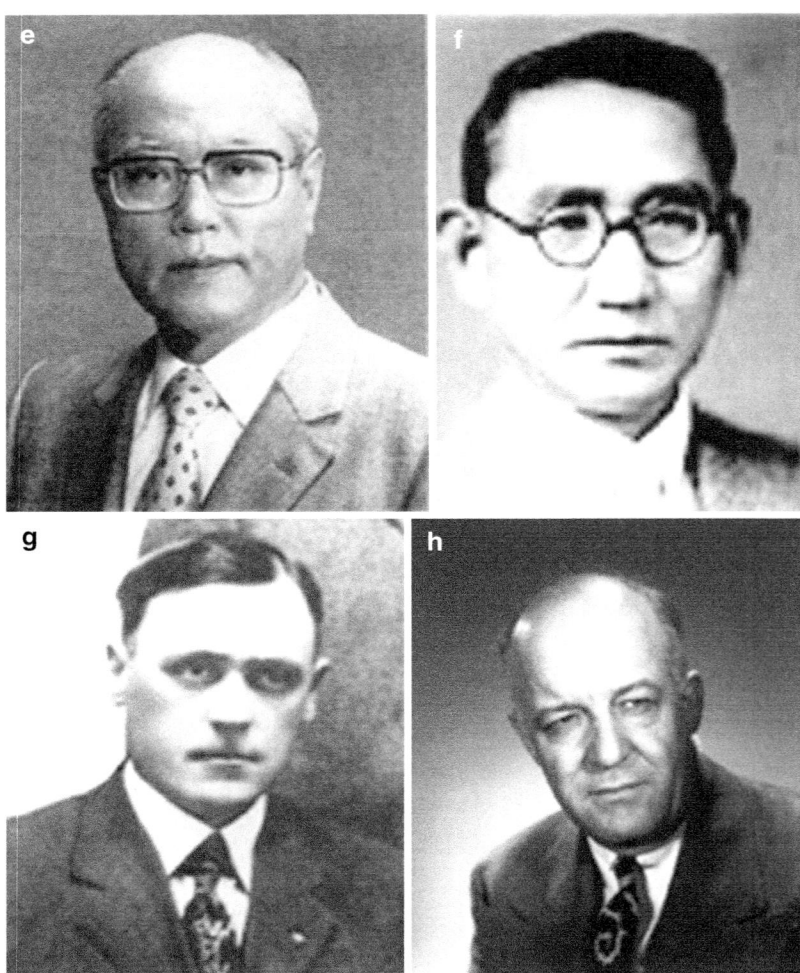

McNeer (1905–1967) (Fig. 1.14h) of the Memorial Sloan Kettering Cancer Center, New York, reported that aggressive surgery showed good survival rate in 1948 [70–73]. Frank H. Lahay (1880–1953) (Fig. 1.15a) of the Lahey Clinic, Boston, reported the indication and treatment results of total gastrectomy in 1944 [74]. This idea was accepted by Mayo Clinic [75] and many leading institutions in the USA. Some specialists recommended that total gastrectomy should be applied for any gastric cancer regardless of location and extension [76, 77]. However the total gastrectomy is now indicated in case when the proximal safe margin from the cardia cannot be achieved by distal gastrectomy.

Combined Resection of the Neighboring Organs

To remove the cancer invasion to the neighboring organs, these organs should be removed surgically. Invasion to the transverse colon and mesocolon and liver is not rare. Resection of these organs is not difficult and is widely per-

Fig. 1.14 (a–d) Various reconstruction methods with interposition after total gastrectomy. (**a**) Seo T, 1941, and Longmire WP, 1952; (**b**) Schreiber HJ, 1978; (**c**) Henley FA, 1952; (**d**) Longmire/Beal, 1952

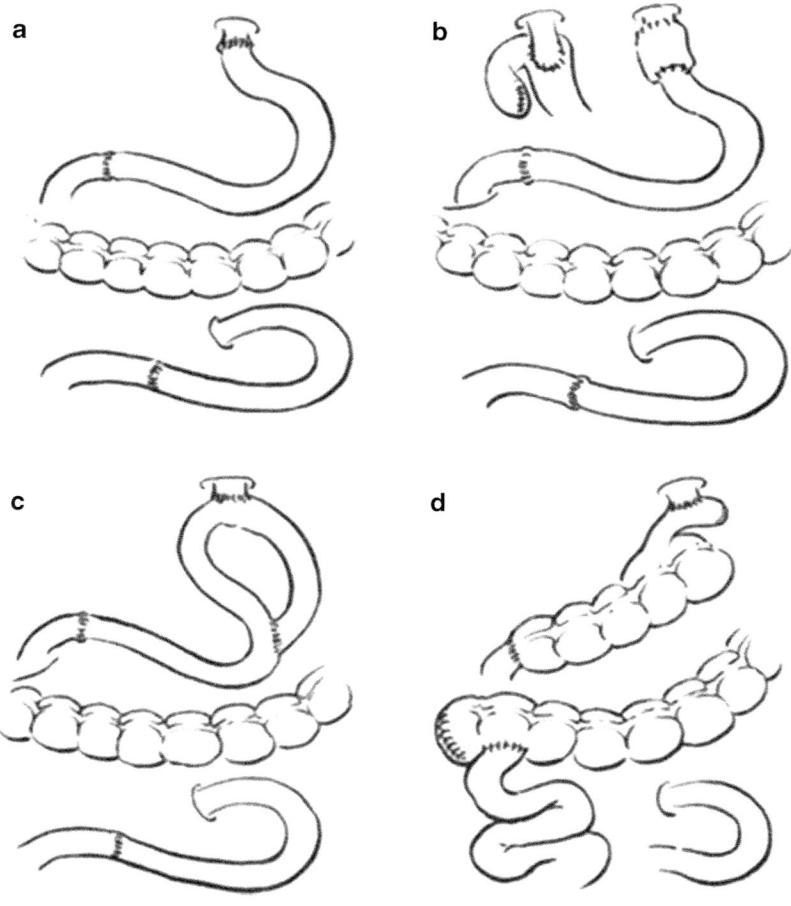

formed. Combined resection of distal part of the pancreas was firstly proposed by Mikulicz in 1898 [50]. This surgical technique system was successively established by Alexander Brunschwig (1901–1969) (Fig. 1.15b) of the Memorial Sloan Kettering Cancer Center, New York, in 1948 [78] and Jirou Suzuki (1911–1968) of Chiba University in 1954 (Fig. 1.16a) [79]. The surgical mortality rate of total gastrectomy with splenopancreatectomy was dramatically improved; 1.8% (1/57 patients) in 1955 by Tamaki Kajitani (1909–1991) (Fig. 1.15c) of the Cancer Institute Tokyo [80, 81], and 1.8% (2/113 patients) in 1956 by Komei Nakayama (1910–2005) (Fig. 1.15d) of the Tokyo Women's

Medical University [82]. This procedure became much more aggressive. Gordon McNeer demonstrated the combined resection technique of the spleen, distal pancreas, and transverse colon with total gastrectomy in 1948 [83]. Also Frank Lahay reported extensive combined resection of the left lobe of the liver, spleen, distal pancreas, and most part of the colon including the terminal ileum in 1944 (Fig. 1.16b) [84]. In 1991 Mitsumasa Nishi proposed the so-called left upper abdominal exenteration removing the stomach, spleen, pancreas tail, left adrenal grand, transverse colon, and if necessary diaphragm and lower esophagus [85, 86]. However combined resection of the distal pancreas is still

Fig. 1.15 (**a–d**)
Historical leaders of the
gastric cancer surgery. (**a**)
Frank H. Lahay: radical
total gastrectomy, (**b**)
Alexander
Brunschwig: distal
pancreatectomy, (**c**)
Tamaki Kajitani: distal
pancreatectomy, (**d**)
Komei Nakayama: distal
pancreatectomy

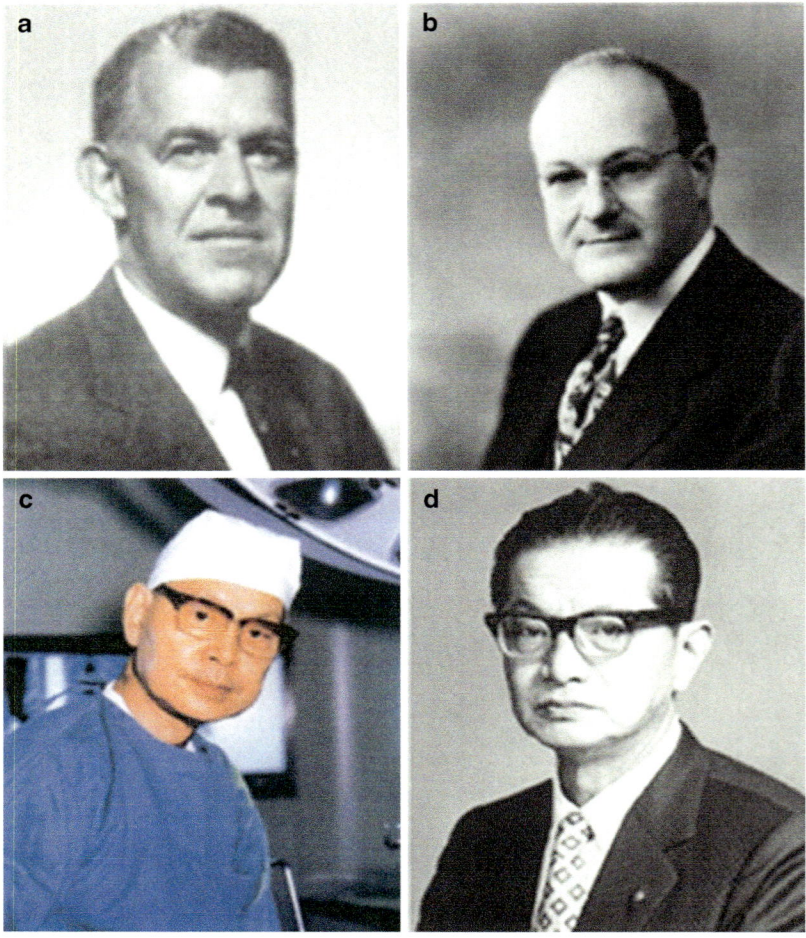

risky, because control of pancreatic juice leakage from the resection stump is difficult. It causes frequent acute pancreatitis, subphrenic abscess, anastomotic leakage, and rupture of the ligated artery stump. Furthermore, Brunschwig pointed out the postoperative diabetes mellitus occurred after resection of the tail of the pancreas [87]. Management of resection stump of the pancreas is still an important subject to be improved.

Lymph Node Dissection

The scientific study of the lymphatic system and cancer metastasis was started firstly by the Romanian anatomist Dimitrie Gerota (1867–1939) (Fig. 1.18a) of the University of Berlin in 1895. He developed the so-called Gerota method to visualize the lymphatic network [88]. For demonstrating lymphatic vessels, he produced a new contrast media: mixed fluid of Prussian blue oil, turpentine, and ether. He injected the fluid into the subserosal layer of the bowel [89]. Using the Gerota method, the famous Hungarian surgeon Polya (Fig. 1.9d) demonstrated lymphatic streams from the stomach using 19 miscarried fetus in 1903 [90]. A French anatomist Paul Poirier (1853–1907) (Fig. 1.18b) of the University of Paris and his coworker Adrien Charpy (1848–1911) of the University of Toulouse published a textbook of anatomy in 1902 [91]. The book included the detailed atlas of lymphatic streams and node stations from the stomach

a

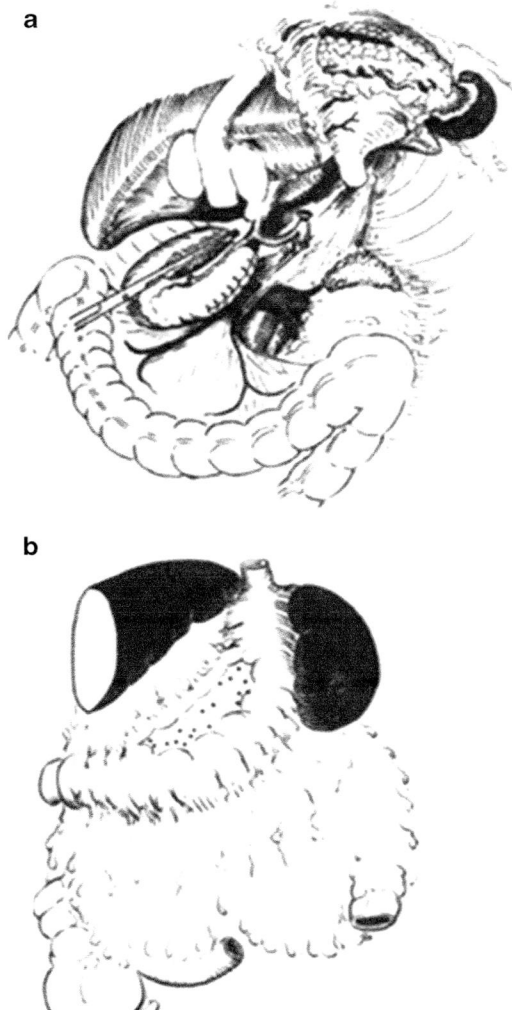

b

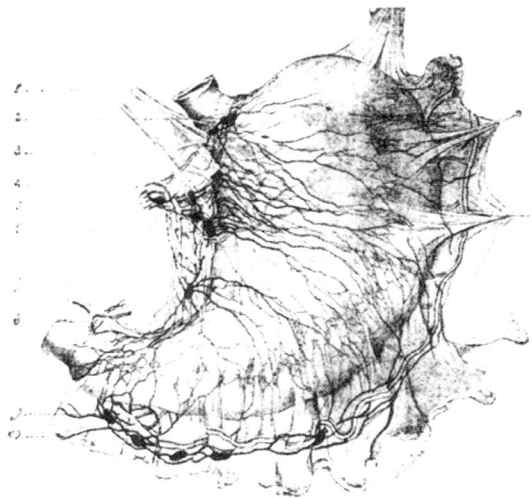

Fig. 1.17 Lymphatic streams of the stomach (demonstrated by Gerota's method, B. Cunéo and P. Poirier [162])

Fig. 1.16 Schema of splenopancreatectomy (**a**) and resected material of extended surgery by Lahay FH [84] (**b**). Lahay removed the whole stomach together with the abdominal esophagus, left lobe of the liver, distal pancreas, spleen, omentum, terminal ileum, cecum, and ascending/transverse/descending colon

(Fig. 1.17). They used both historical Sappey's mercury injection method [92] and Gerota's method. Anatomist John Kay Jamieson (1873–1948) (Fig. 1.18c) and surgeon Joseph Faulkner Dobson (1874–1934) of the University of Leeds, England, made a detailed study of lymphatic system of the stomach in 1907 [93]. They completed the classification of lymphatic streams and regional lymph node stations of the stomach.

The next progress was expansion of the regional node area beyond the upper border of the pancreas to deeper area. French anatomist Henri Rouviere (1876–1952) (Fig. 1.18d) of the University of Paris published an important textbook in 1932. He described historical achievements and his own study including the lymphatic system around the celiac artery and the abdominal aorta [94]. Japanese anatomist Inoue Y. of the University of Tokyo made a lymphographic study by an unique contrast media, India-ink, using 104 miscarried fetus in 1936 [95].

Along the idea of Mikulicz, big efforts were paid to develop the effective surgical procedures to remove the metastatic nodes. In 1944 Kajitani stressed the low reliability of macroscopic judgment whether a node is metastatic or not. He found 20 false-negative patients (12%) in his 162 series [96]. That means the extent of node dissection should have enough safe margin based on the lymphatic stream study. Many leading surgical oncologists in Japan (Fig. 1.19a) [61, 80, 82, 97, 98], Korea (Fig. 1.19b, c) [99], Germany (Fig. 1.19d, e) [100, 101], the UK (Fig. 1.19f) [102], and the USA (Fig. 1.19g) [103–105] stressed the importance of systematic lymph node dissection. They conducted multicenter trials in their country for evaluating the systematic lymphadenectomy. The Japanese Research

Fig. 1.18 (a–d)
Historical leaders of
the lymphatic system
study on the stomach.
(**a**) Dimitrie
Gerota: lymphatic
system, (**b**) Paul
Poirier: lymphatic
system, (**c**) John Kay
Jamieson: lymphatic
system, (**d**) Henri
Rouviere: lymphatic
system

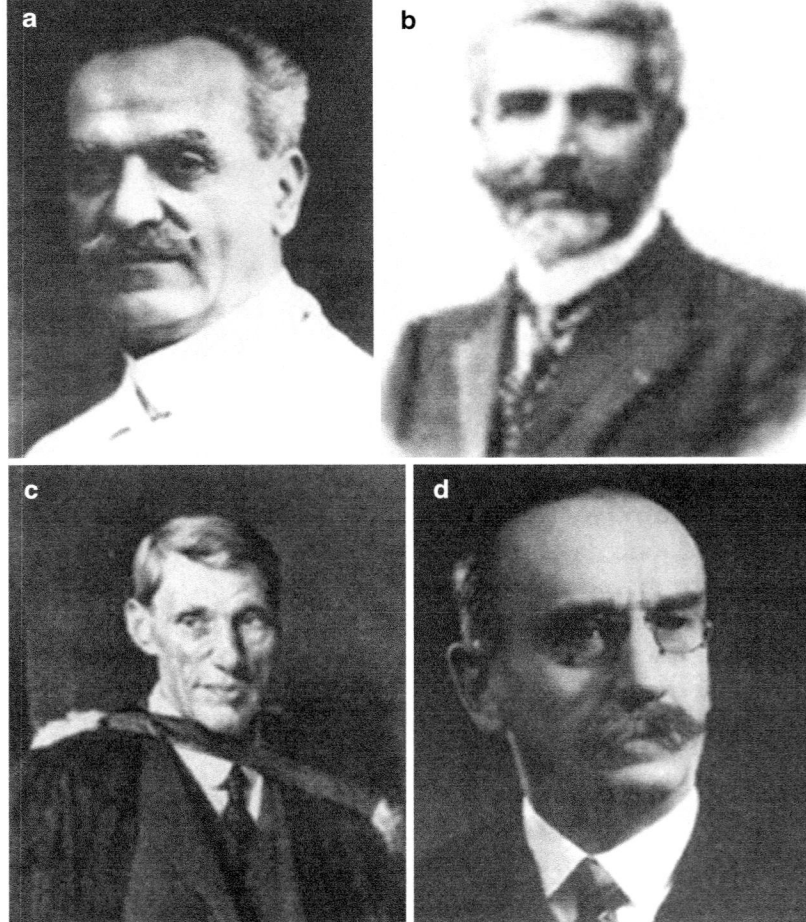

Society for Gastric Cancer was established and published the Japanese Manual in 1962 [106]. In the manual, 16 regional lymph node stations were anatomically defined (Fig. 1.21a) [107]. They were classified into N1, N2, N3, and N4 categories according to the occupation of main tumor based on the study of Inoue [95]. Complete removal of N1 and N2 nodes was called "D2 dissection." This procedure was strongly recommended, and it became the gold standard for gastric cancer surgery in Japan and Eastern countries. Systematic node dissection could reduce the local recurrence and lead to better survival. This is the significant effectiveness of this procedure. Japanese nationwide registry of gastric cancer reported that the 5-year survival rate was 37.5% in 1963–1966, which elevated to 70.1% in 2008 [107]. Improvement in survival was remarkable for Stage II, from 47.7% to 73.1%, and also for Stage III, from 26.4% to 44.5%. This improvement was brought by popularization of the D2 dissection.

For complete node removal around the distal pancreas and at the splenic hilum, pancreaticosplenectomy was considered essential (Fig. 1.16a). However this procedure had a high risk, and it produced various pancreas-related complications and elevated mortality rate.

Cornelis J. H. van de Velde (Fig. 1.19h) of the Leiden University, Netherlands, organized the Dutch multicenter clinical trial to compare the D1 and D2 node dissection. He reported miserable treatment results on *The Lancet* in 1995 [108]. The mortality rate was 10% for 331 D2 patients and 4% for 380 D1 patients. He concluded that "D2 dissection should not be used as standard treatment for Western patients." Many letters with strong oppositions were sent to *The Lancet*'s editor. They stressed that major reasons of the high mortality rate could be attributed to unexperienced surgeons, poorer patient condition, and particularly unnecessary pancreas resection [109]. To reduce the complications, "pancreas-preserving total gastrectomy" (Fig. 1.21b) was proposed by Keiichi Maruyama (Fig. 1.20a) of the National Cancer Center, Tokyo, in 1985 [110]. This procedure reduced the surgical death rate from 3.1% to 1.6% and the surgical complication rate from 39.4% to 19.6% with no dropdown of the survival. Furthermore it reduced the postoperative diabetes.

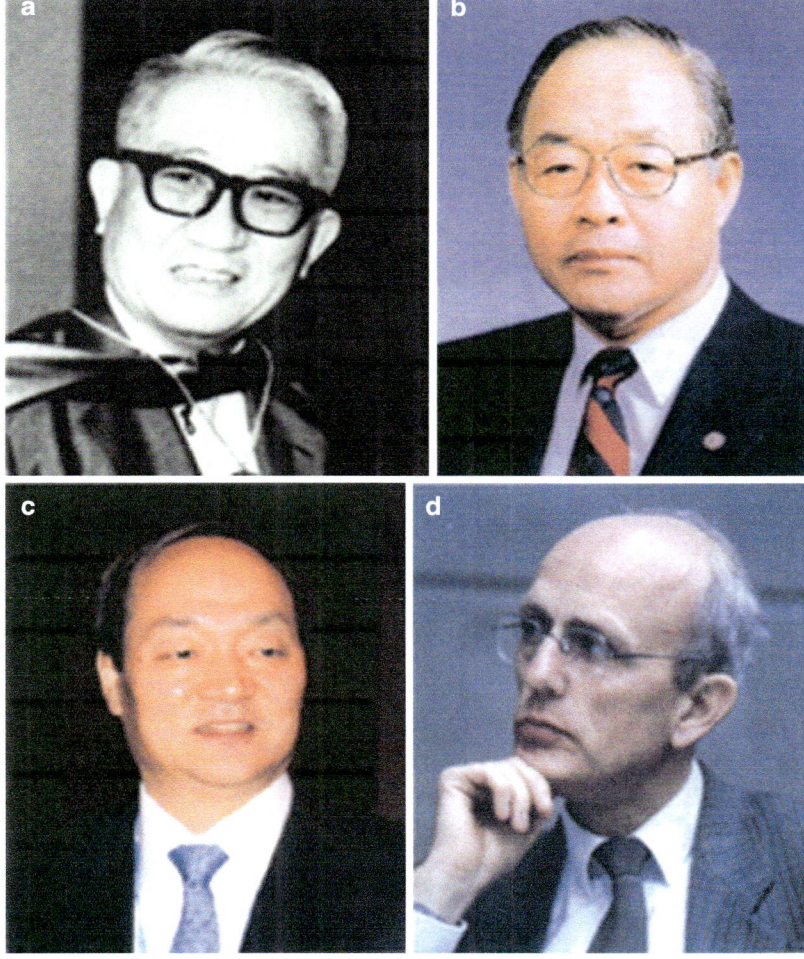

Fig. 1.19 (**a–h**) Historical leaders of the gastric cancer surgery. (**a**) Dennosuke Jinnai: lymphadenectomy; (**b**) Jin-Pok Kim: Korean GC Association; (**c**) Sung Hoon Noh: KGCA and IGCA; (**d**) Henning Rohde German: German TNM Study Group; (**e**) Jorg Rudiger Siewert: German GC Association; (**f**) Sir Alfred Cuschieri: British D2 trial, MRC; (**g**) Byrl James Kennedy: US SEER Program; (**h**) CJH van de Velde: Dutch D1/D2 Trial

Fig. 1.19 (continued)

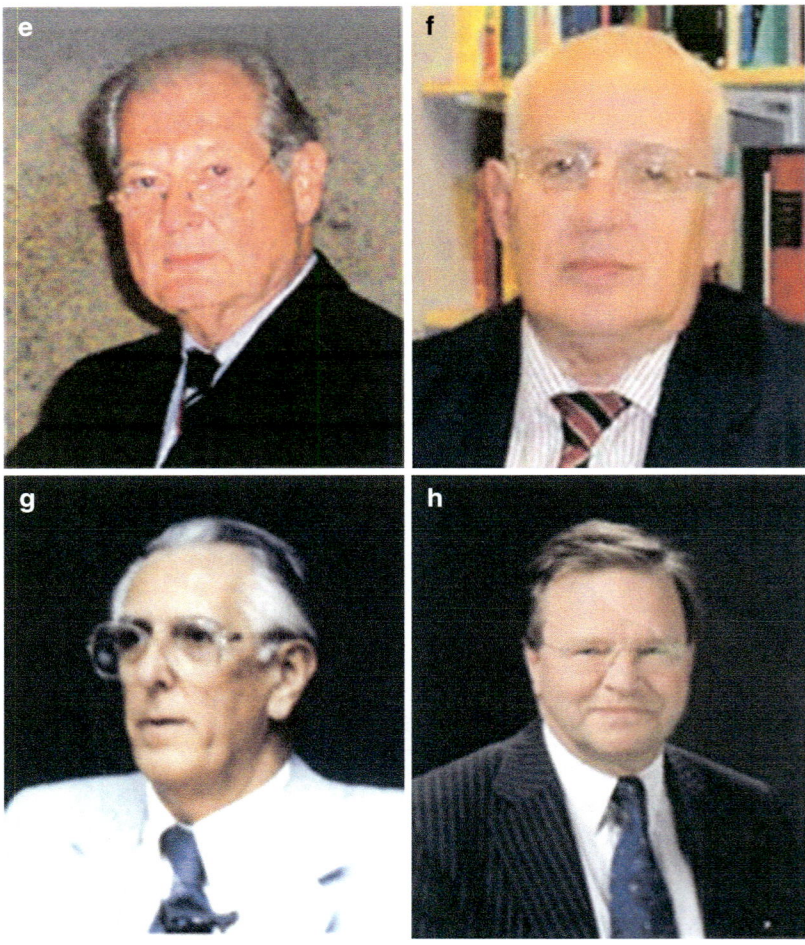

Fig. 1.20 (a–b)
Historical leaders of the
gastric cancer surgery.
(a) Keiichi
Maruyama: pancreas
preservation, (b) Paul
H. Sugarbaker: total
peritonectomy

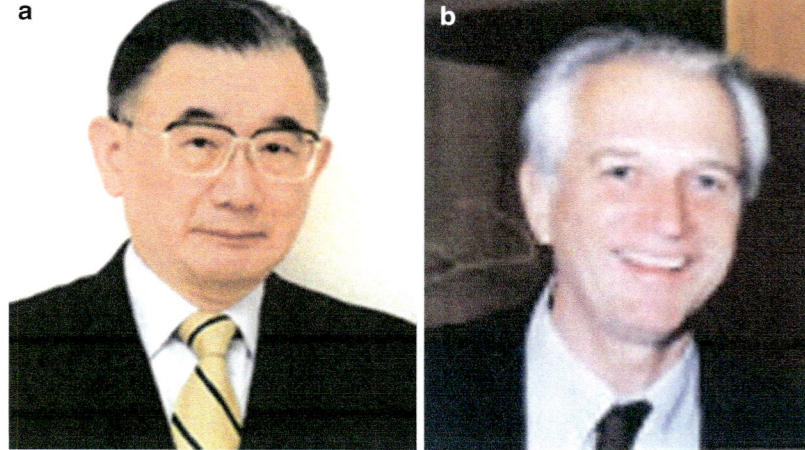

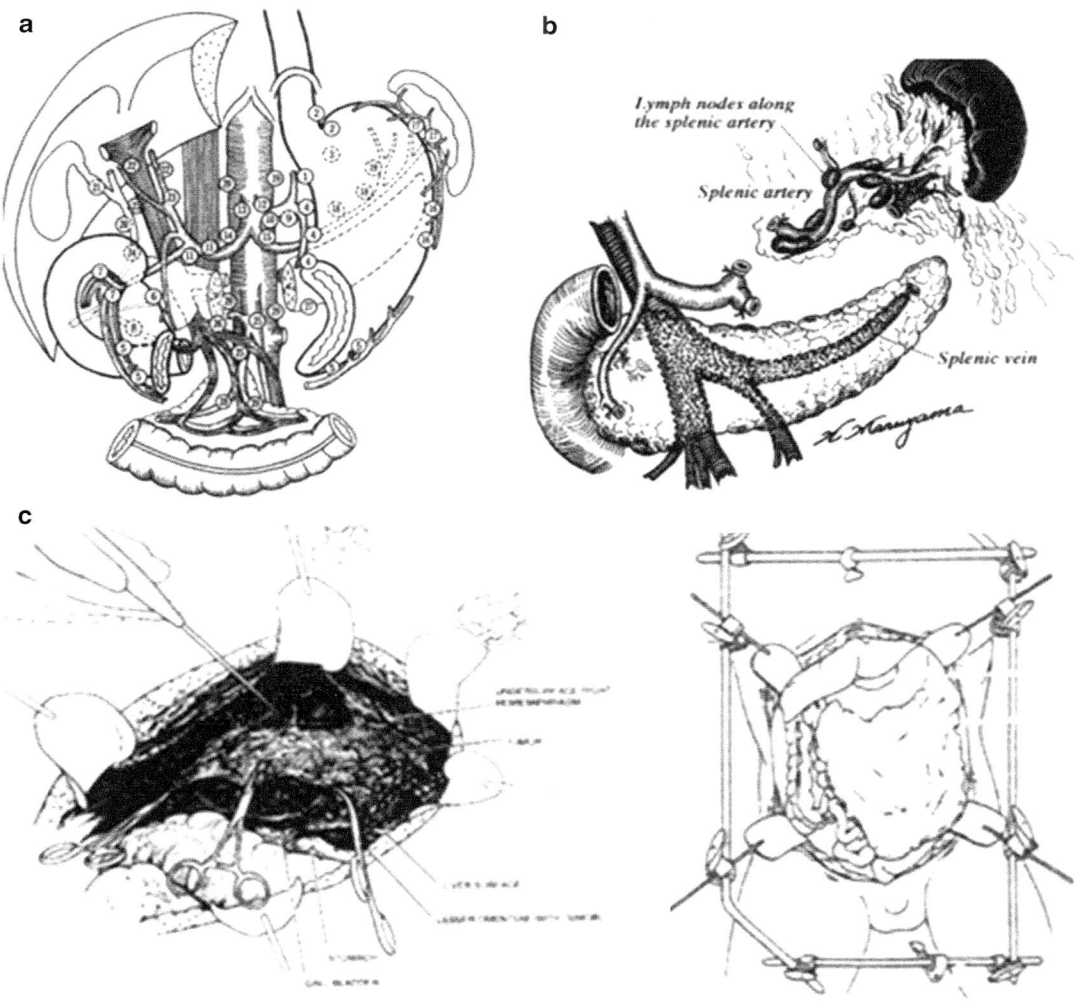

Fig. 1.21 (**a–c**) Classification of Japanese manual, pancreas preservation, and total peritonectomy. (**a**) Japanese classification of the regional lymph nodes of the stomach, (**b**) schema of the pancreas-preserving procedure [110], (**c**) Sugarbaker's procedure of total peritonectomy (left). Continuous intraperitoneal perfusion by heated fluid with anticancer agent (right)

Surgery for Peritoneal Metastasis

Mikulicz wrote that gastric cancer extension had four directions: direct invasion, lymphatic metastasis, vascular metastasis, and peritoneal dissemination [50]. Ernest W. Hey Groves of the Bristol General Hospital, England, described the role of the omentum resection for removing the peritoneal dissemination in 1910 [111]. This idea was taken over by a famous oncological surgeon, Hans Finsterer of the University of Vienna, and he developed the surgical technique [112, 113]. A Japanese surgeon Masao Muto (1898–1972) (Fig. 1.22a) of the Tohoku University published a detailed histological study on cancer metastasis of the omental bursa in 1958 [114].

He found histologically confirmed metastases in 78% of 643 resected omentum specimen using continuous section study. He suggested that the metastatic mechanisms were not only by seeding in the peritoneal cavity but also by lymphatic and vascular routes. Peritoneal metastasis does not occur in the T1 and T2 tumor, and the omentectomy is not indicated for these tumors. However the major role of bursectomy is now considered for accurate lymph node dissection around the pancreas, not for treatment of peritoneal metastasis.

Paul H. Sugarbaker (Fig. 1.20b) of the Washington Hospital Center, USA, published a unique strategy against peritoneal carcinomatosis in 1995 [115]. He developed a surgical procedure of total peritonectomy combined with intraperitoneal chemo-hyperthermia intended for cytoreduction (Fig. 1.21c). Yutaka Yonemura of the University of Kanazawa, Japan, applied this treatment for gastric cancer in 1999 [116]. He reported that this treatment showed better survival benefit than conventional chemotherapy and chemohyperthermic peritoneal perfusion. This treatment is now actively studied by Korean specialists [117].

New Trends: From Standardized Surgery to Individual Surgery

Since 1995 we had a new trend: a shift from "extended and standardized surgery for radical treatment" to "reasonable and individual surgery considering safety and quality of life (QOL)." Background of this shift were (1) remarkable increase of early-stage cancer, (2) demand for safe surgery and QOL, (3) progress of technology and instruments, and (4) storage of knowledge and experiences. This new trend produced a large variation in surgical treatments.

Function-Preserving Surgery

Japanese surgeon Tetsuo Maki (1908–2006) (Fig 1.22b) of the Tohoku University published an interesting surgical procedure, "Pyloruspreserving gastrectomy," in 1967 (Fig 1.23a) [118]. The intention of this procedure was to reduce dumping syndrome, postgastrectomy gallstone, and digestive function disturbances after distal gastrectomy for benign ulcer. His coworker Tsuneo Shiratori (1922–2012) (Fig 1.22c) of the Nara Medical University, Japan, expanded the indication for gastric cancer in 1991 [119]. It is now widely applied for a small-size gastric cancer located at the middle third of the stomach with no possibility of nodal metastasis around the pylorus.

Additionally nerve preservation was considered for early-stage cancer. The most important nerve is the cystic branch of the vagal nerve. It was frequently injured during the lymphadenectomy around the hepatoduodenal ligament. The injury caused contraction disturbance of the gall bladder and gallstone. Koichi Miwa (Fig. 1.22d) of the University of Kanazawa, Japan, recommended preservation of the pyloric and celiac nerves for the pylorus-preserving gastrectomy in 1996 (Fig. 1.23b) [120, 121].

Alexander Brunschwig of the Memorial SK Cancer Center, New York, pointed out the postoperative diabetes mellitus following resection of the distal pancreas [78]. For the patients with direct invasion to the pancreas, resection of the pancreas is essential. But the pancreas-preserving operation can be applied for the purpose of lymphadenectomy around the pancreas and at the splenic hilus [122].

Optimal Extent of Lymph Node Dissection

According to the new trends, the extent of node dissection should be reasonable and individualized based on the tumor extension. To get the optimal extent area, the following new strategies were proposed [122].

Keiichi Maruyama developed a computer system, so-called Maruyama's program, to estimate risk of metastasis at each regional lymph node station based on detailed database of 3785 patients in 1989 [123]. This program can be applicable even for Western patients showing very high sensitivity, specificity, and accuracy [124]. Elfriede Bollschweiler of the Technical

Fig. 1.22 (**a–d**)
Historical leaders of the
gastric cancer surgery.
(**a**) Masao
Muto: omentectomy, (**b**)
Tetsuo Maki: pylorus
preservation, (**c**) Tsuneo
Shiratori: pylorus
preservation, (**d**) Koichi
Miwa: nerve
preservation

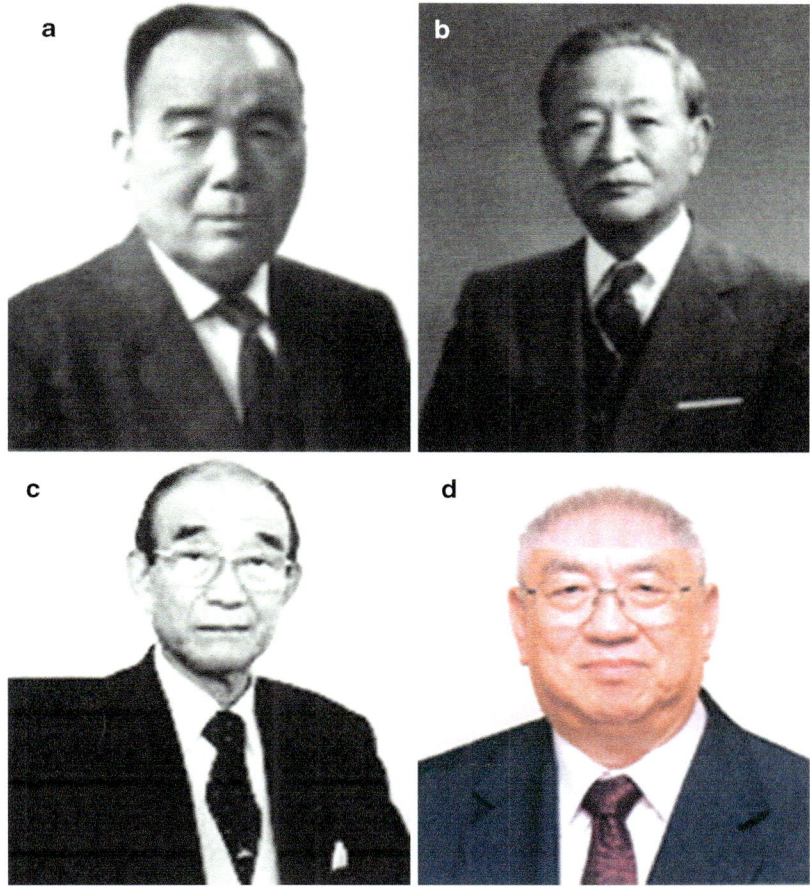

University of Munich produced the other computer system, "artificial neural network," for prediction of lymph node metastasis in 1996 [125]. She reported high reliability in the estimation of the node metastasis.

A unique method, "intraoperative lymphography by India-ink," was introduced to visualize the lymphatic streams and regional lymph nodes (Fig. 1.25) [122]. Toshio Takahashi (Fig. 1.24a) of the Kyoto Prefectural Medical University and his coworker Akio Hagiwara developed a fine activated carbon particle (190 nanometers in average diameter) in 1991 [126]. It had a strong affinity for lymphatic structures and became a useful contrast media, so colled "India ink." This staining became a useful guide for accurate node removal particularly for the para-aortic lymphadenectomy.

Lymphadenectomy areas were expanded to the hepatoduodenal ligament, the back surface of the pancreas head, the para-aortic area, and the mediastinum [127]. The survival benefit of "para-aortic lymphadenectomy" (Fig. 1.26) was not high [128–130]. Leading institutions reported that 5-year survival of the para-aortic node-positive patients was between 11% and 23% after para-aortic dissection. Mediastinal node metastasis was not rare for advanced proximal cancer with esophageal invasion. Most metastases were found in the lower paraesophageal lymph nodes (16.1%) and in the posterior mediastinal lymph nodes (3.2%). These nodes can be removed by the "transdiaphragmatic approach" proposed by Henrique Walter Pinotti (1929–2010) (Fig. 1.24b) of the University of São Paulo, Brazil, in 1983 [131]. Yuji Tachimori of the National Cancer Center, Tokyo, reported that the 30-day mortality of Pinotti's approach was 0% and the morbidity was 18% in his series [126, 132]. Next topic was

a

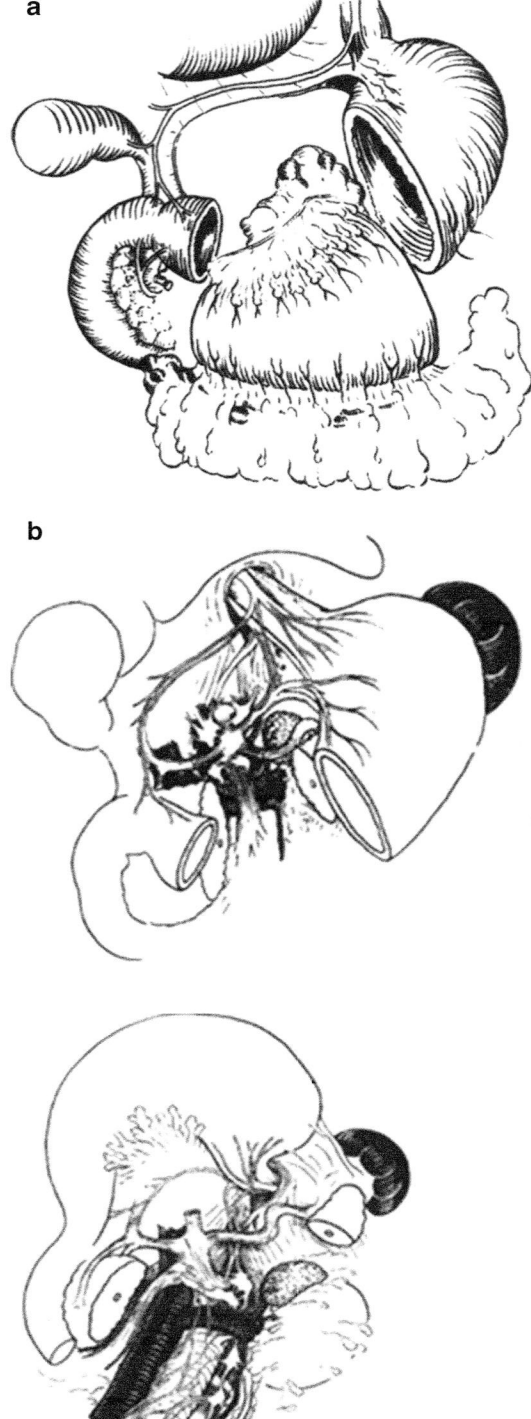

b

Fig. 1.23 (**a–b**) Pylorus-preserving gastrectomy and nerve branchings of the stomach. (**a**) Pylorus- and nerve-preserving gastrectomy, (**b**) nerve branchings (anterior view, back view)

"Sentinel Node Navigation Surgery" [132]. This idea is now accepted and clinically applied for breast cancer, melanoma, head and neck tumor, etc. Yuko Kitagawa (Fig. 1.28a) of the Keio University, Tokyo, published a detailed clinical study on this procedure for gastric cancer surgery in 2002 [133]. He applied a radioactive mm99 Tin colloid as the tracer. He reported high detection rate, sensitivity, and accuracy, 97%, 94%, and 99%, respectively, in 210 cT1 and cT2 patients. He found 3.9 hot nodes in average in his series. Kitagawa stressed that unnecessary lymph node dissection can be avoidable by the sentinel node navigation.

According to the instruction stated above, individual, reasonable, and effective lymph node dissection can be applied for each patient.

Minimally Invasive Surgery

Japanese endoscopist Masahiro Tada of the Yamaguchi University applied endoscopic polypectomy technique to remove small mucosal cancer in 1988 [134]. This idea was improved by endoscopist team of the National Cancer Center, Tokyo. They developed "endoscopic mucosal resection (EMR)" [135] and "endoscopic submucosal dissection (ESD)" (Fig. 1.27) [136]. Intention of the endoscopic resection is to avoid disadvantages and risk of open gastric resection and to get quick recovery. This treatment is indicated for early-stage cancer with definitely no node metastasis, namely, (a) mucosal cancer, (b) elevated or flat lesion, (c) differentiated adenocarcinoma, and (d) less than 3.0 cm in diameter. They developed a useful device "insulated ball tip electrosurgical knife (IT-knife)" for peeling the mucosal and submucosal layer from the muscle layer in 1996 [136, 137]. They reported no cancer death from their 1783 patients treated in 1989–2003 [138].

The laparoscopic surgery became popular all over the world, particularly in Japan [139–141], Korea [142, 143], Taiwan [144, 145], Germany [146], and Italy [147–149]. The intention is to get quick recovery, less pain, and cosmetic advantage. The indication was mostly for early-stage cancer but now expanded to advanced can-

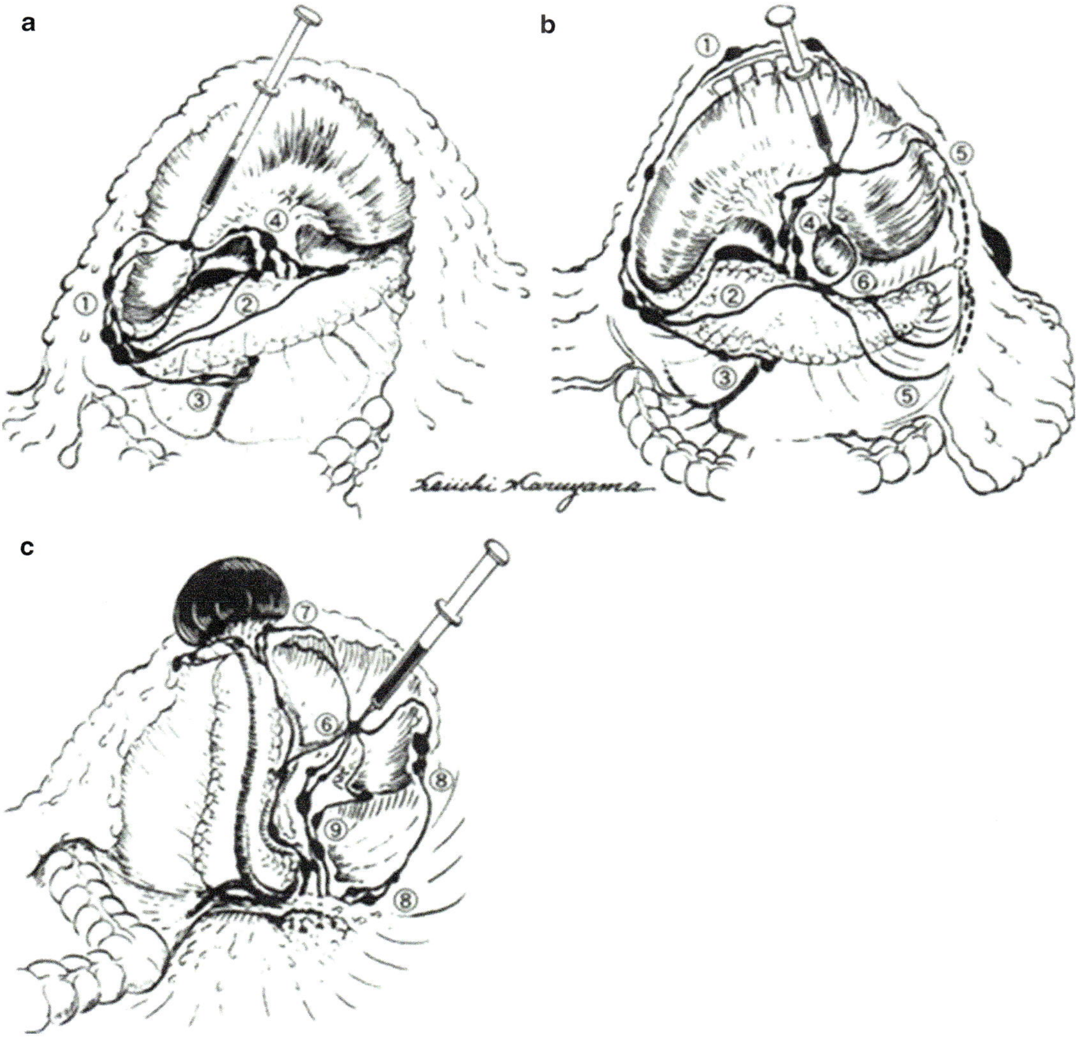

a

b

Keiichi Maruyama

c

Fig. 1.24 (**a–c**) Lymphatic channels from the distal third (**a**), middle third (**b**), and proximal third (**c**). (Demonstrated by intraoperative subserosal injection of the India ink (fine activated carbon particle solution))

Fig. 1.25 (**a–b**) Historical leaders. (**a**) Toshio Takahashi: activated carbon particle, (**b**) Henrique Walter Pinotti: transdiaphragmatic route

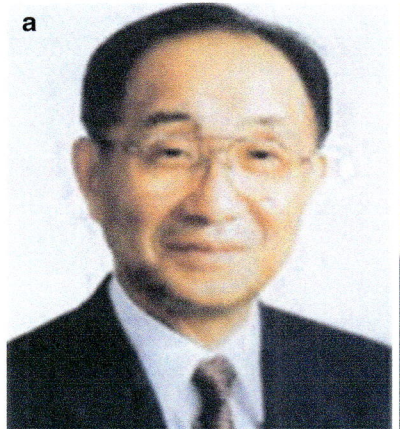

a

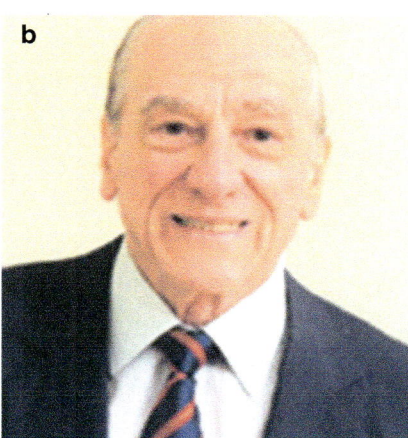

b

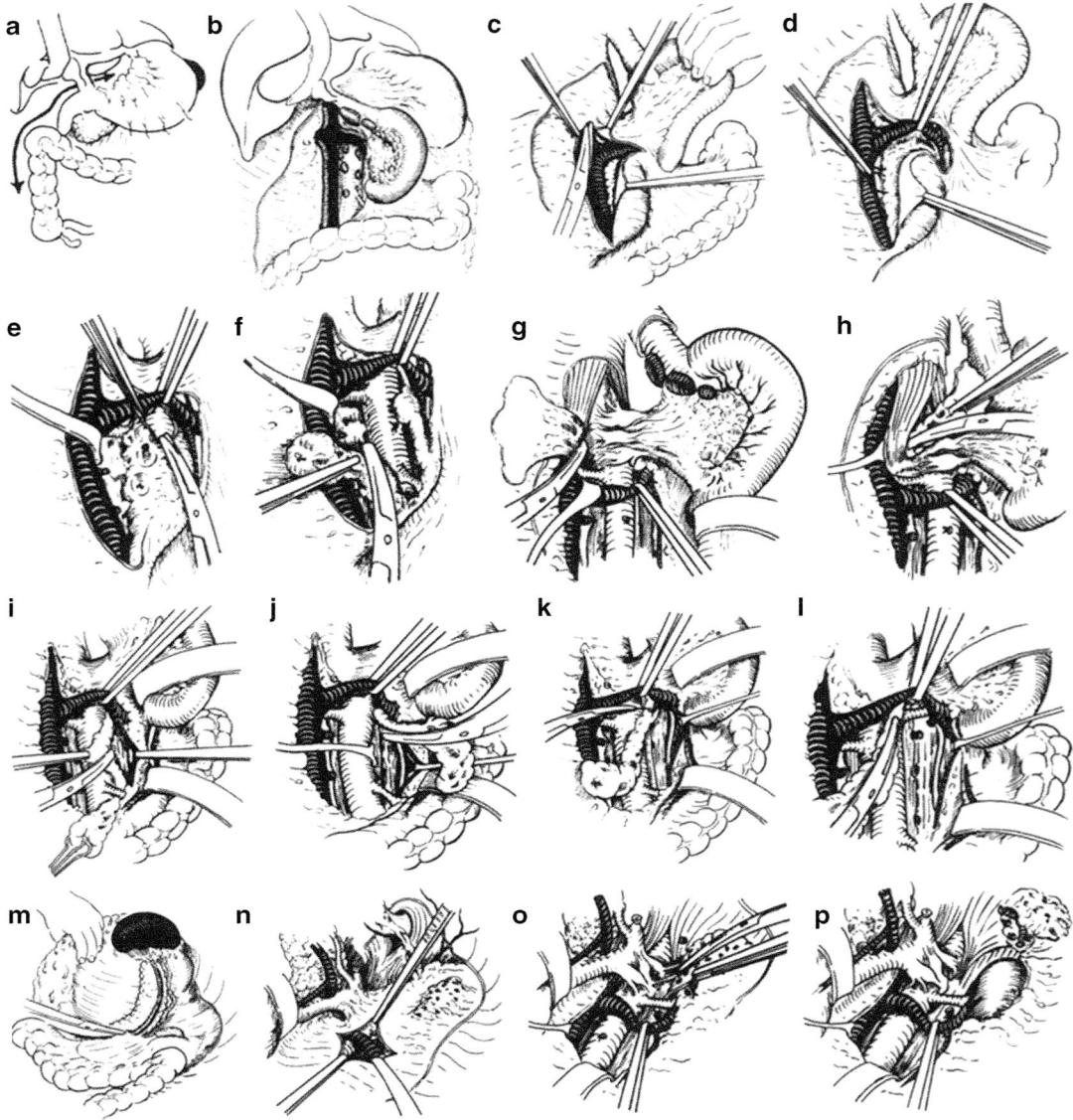

Fig. 1.26 (**a–p**) Techniques of the para-aortic lymph node dissection. Dissection of the lower right (**a–f**), the lower left (**g–h**), and the upper right (**i-l**) areas under extended pancreas head mobilization and upper left area (**m–p**) under mobilization of the spleen and distal pancreas

cer. Surgical technique, procedures, and instruments were remarkably developed in the last 20 years. And the quality of surgery is now evaluated as the same level of the open surgery. Masahiko Ohgami of the Keio University, Tokyo, proposed the "lesion lifting method" or wedge resection in 1987 [139]. Seigo Kitano (Fig. 1.28b) of the Oita University, Japan, developed "laparoscopic gastric resection with systematic LN dissection" in 1994 [141, 152]. Ichiro Uyama (Fig. 1.28c) of the Fujita Health University, Japan [141, 150, 151], and Cristiano G Hüscher (Fig. 1.28d) of the Azienda G Rummo Hospital, Benevento, Italy [147–149], developed

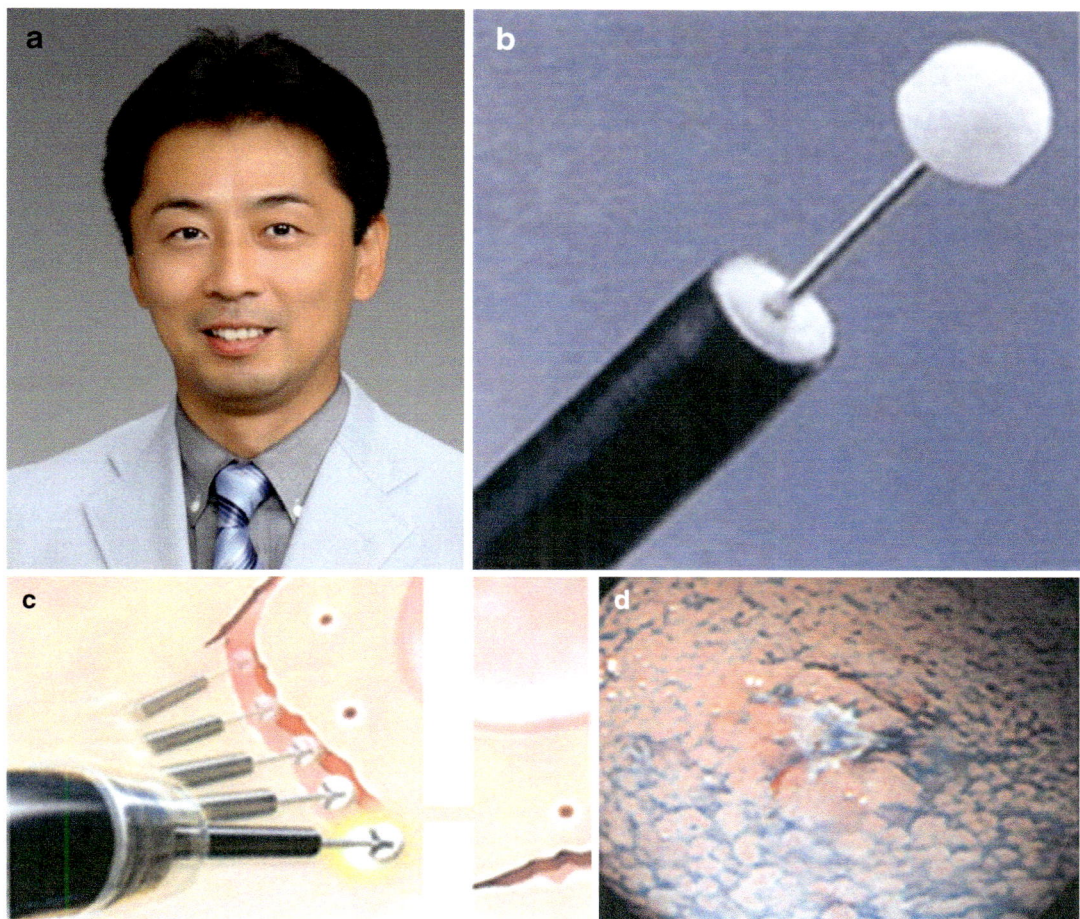

Fig. 1.27 (**a–h**) Endoscopic submucosal dissection (ESD). (**a**): EMR and ESD, (**b**) insulated ball tip knife (IT-knife), (**c**) cutting the mucosa by IT-knife avoiding perforation, (**e**) small-size mucosal cancer, (**f**) marking the cancer border by electric cautery, (**g**) mucosal cutting completed by IT-knife, (**h**) pealing up the mucosal and submucosal layers, (**g**) after the ESD exposing the muscular layer

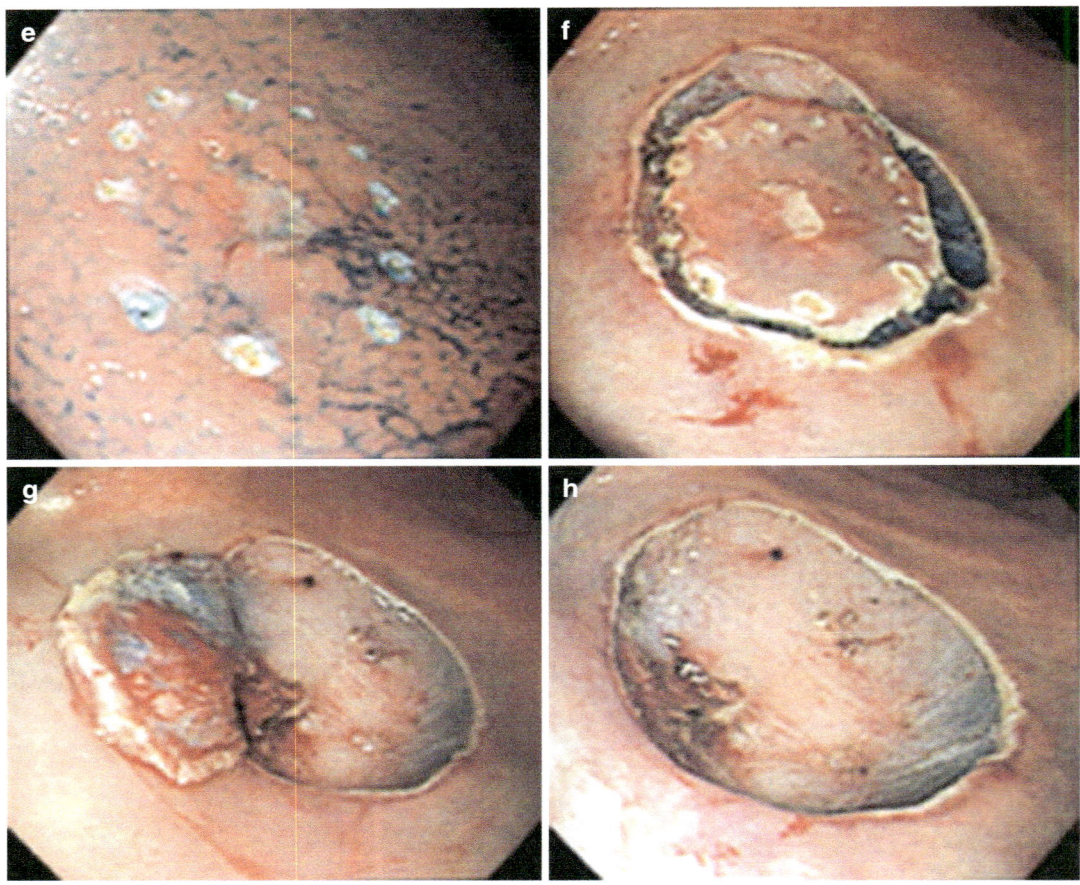

Fig. 1.27 (continued)

various new laparoscopic procedures. Japanese Laparoscopic Surgery Study Group reported the treatment results of 1294 patients with distal, proximal, and total gastrectomy in 2007. The postoperative morbidity was 14.8%, the mortality was 0.0%, and the recurrence was found in only six cases (0.6%).

We are now introducing "robot surgery system" for laparoscopic gastrectomy. Problems of this treatment were (a) expensive machine and devices and (b) a few institutions and experts. Therefore robotic gastrectomy can be done only at high-volume centers in the world. The leader of this field is now Korea. da Vinci robot surgery system was introduced to Yonsei University, Seoul, and the Seoul National University in the early period. From these institutions, Woo Jin Hyung (Fig. 1.28e) and Han-Kwang Yang (Fig. 1.28f) published their surgical techniques and treatment results [151, 152, 153]. Han-Kwang Yang is now trying the single-port laparoscopic surgery [154]. Japan and Italy actively introduced the robot machine and applied it for gastric cancer surgery [155–157].

National and International Study Groups for Gastric Cancer

The first edition of the UICC TNM classification *Livre de Poche* was published in 1968 [158] with cooperation of the American Joint Committee for Cancer Staging, the Canadian National Committee, the Japanese Joint Committee, and the Deutschsprachiges TNM Ausshuss. Intention of the manual is to offer "a common language" in recording their clinical findings and assessing the results of different treatment methods. After several revisions, the seventh edition is now in use worldwide [159].

Specialists of gastric cancer organized their national and international study groups and pub-

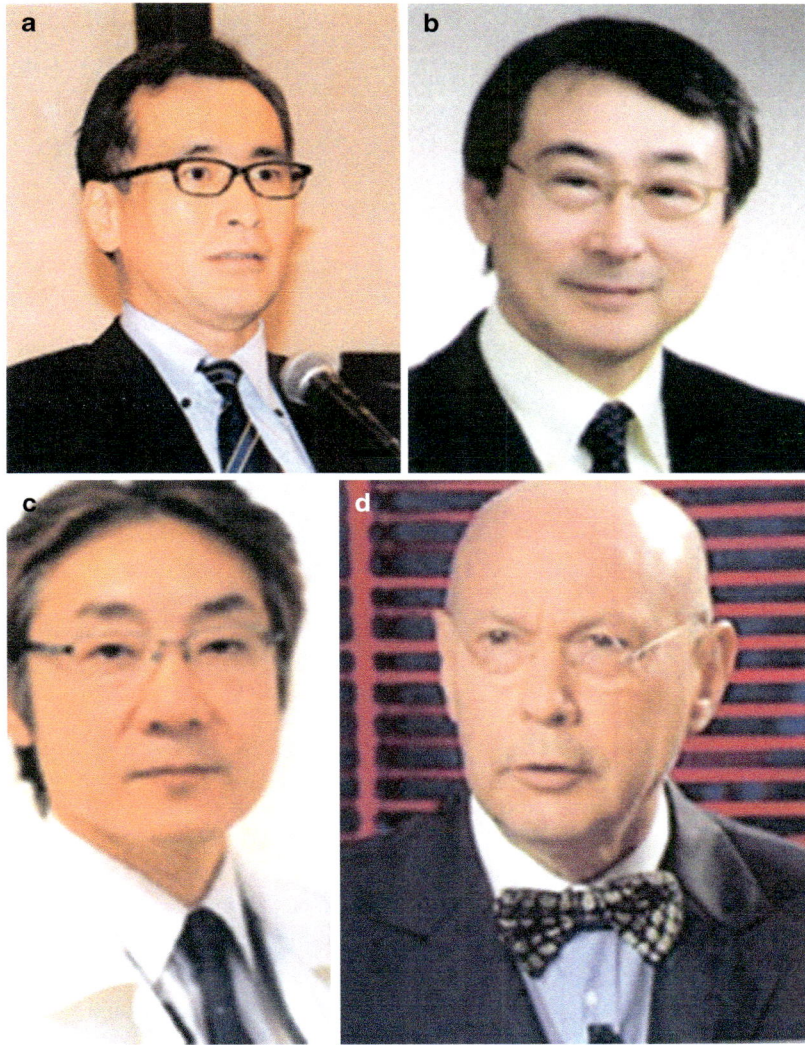

Fig. 1.28 (a–g) Historical leaders of the gastric cancer surgery and a robotic surgery system. (**a**) Yuko Kitagawa: sentinel node navigation, (**b**) Seigo Kitano: laparoscopic gastrectomy, (**c**) Ichiro Uyama: laparoscopic/robotic gastrectomy, (**d**) Cristiano G. Hilscher: laparoscopic gastrectomy, (**e**) Woo Jin Hyung: robotic gastrectomy, (**f**) Han-Kwang Yang: single-port laparoscopic, (**g**) da Vinci robotic surgery system

Fig. 1.28 (continued)

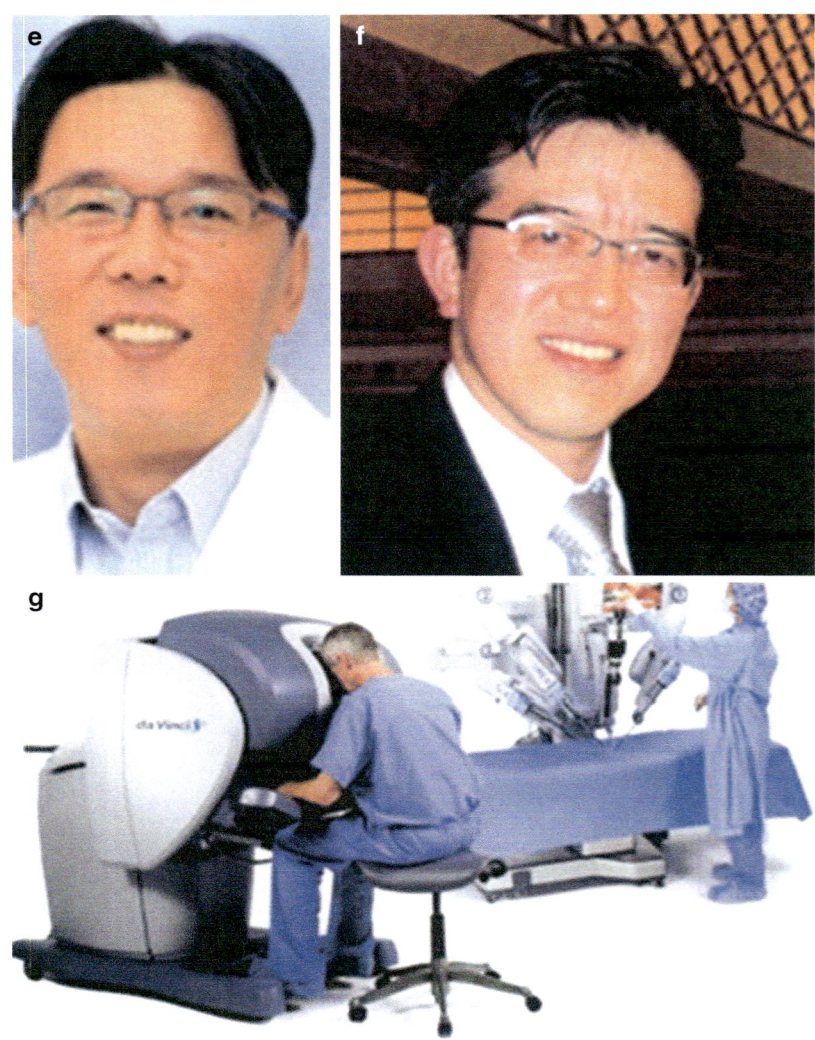

lished the manuals to record the findings of this disease. The most active national study groups are listed on Table 1.1. World Health Organization nominated the leading institutes as the WHO Collaborating Center for Gastric Cancer (WHO-CC) in 15 countries in 1970. The head quarter was placed at the National Cancer Center, Tokyo. The WHO-CC organized general meetings, seminars, and training courses and published the WHO classification and monographs. The roles were transferred to the International Gastric Cancer Association which was established in 1995. The first International Gastric Cancer Congress was held in Kyoto in 1995. The congress was held every 2 years in the cities of Asia, Europe, and America (Table 1.2). The association started to publish their journal *Gastric Cancer* in 1996 [160], and it got now very high citation.

Table 1.1 Active National Gastric Cancer Study Group

Japanese Gastric Cancer Association	1962	6000	Journal
Korean Gastric Cancer Association	1993		Journal
Taiwan Collaborative Oncology Group	1989	500	
Chinese Gastric Cancer Association	1976		
Italian Gastric Cancer Study Group	2001		
German Gastric Carcinoma Study Group	1982 and 1986		
Dutch Gastric Cancer Group	1989		
Polish Study Group on Gastric Cancer	1986		
Brazilian Gastric Cancer Association	1999		

Table 1.2 International Gastric Cancer Congress

1st	1995	Kyoto, Japan	Mitsumasa Nishi
2nd	1997	Munich, Germany	J. Rüdiger Siewert
3rd	1999	Seoul, Korea	Jin-Pok Kim
4th	2001	Rome, Italy	Eugenio Santoro
5th	2003	New York, USA	Murray Brennan
6th	2005	Yokohama, Japan	Masaki Kitajima
7th	2007	São Paulo, Brazil	J. Gama-Rodrigues
8th	2009	Krakow, Poland	Tadeusz Popiela
9th	2011	Seoul, Korea	Sung Hoon Noh
10th	2001	Verona, Italy	Giovanni de' Manzoni
11th	2015	São Paulo, Brazil	Bruno Zilberstein
12th	2017	Beijing, China	Jiafu Ji

Last Comment

The history of gastric cancer surgery is not long, only 135 years from Billroth's first gastric resection. In the period, the progress of surgery and supportive backgrounds were remarkable. From my viewpoint now, the major interest of most surgeons seems to be minimally invasive surgery and QOL for patients with early-stage cancer. However we have still a huge number of patients with advanced cancer or incurable cancer. I believe the oncological surgeons should pay their effort much more to cure the advanced cancer.

References

1. Wastell C, Nyhus LM, Donahue PE. Surgery of the esophagus, stomach, and small intestine. 5th ed. Boston/New York/Toronto/London: Little, Broum and Company; 1995.
2. Takahashi T, Arai K. History of gastric cancer surgery (in Japanese). Tokyo: Igakusyoin; 2011.
3. Shackelford RT, Zuidema GD. Surgery of the alimentary tract. 2nd ed. Philadelphia/London/Toronto/Sydney: Saunders; 1981.
4. Eiselsberg A. Die Geschichte des Magenoperationen (in German). Wien Med Wochenschr. 1936; 86: 3–4, 36–9, 68–70, 94–5, 122–3.
5. Thorwald J. Das Jahrhundert der Chirurgen (in German). Stuttgart: Steingriiben Verlag; 1956. The century of the surgeon (in English). London: Thames and Hudson; 1957.
6. Thorwald J. Das Weltreich der Chirurgen (in German). Stuttgart: Steingriiben Verlag; 1957. The triumph of surgery (in English). London: Thames and Hudson; 1960.
7. Edmond E. The wondrous story of anesthesia. 1st ed. New York: Springer; 2014.
8. Snow S. Blessed days of anaesthesia: how anaesthetics changed the world. Oxford: Oxford Press; 2008.
9. Wells H. Letter to the editor. Boston Medical and Surgical Journal. 1847;36:421.
10. Westhorpe R. William Morton and the first successful demonstration of anaesthesia. Anesth Intensive Care. 1996;24(5):529.
11. Simpson JY. On the use of chloroform in midwifery practice. Lancet. 1847;2:572.
12. Semmelweis IP. Die Aetiologie, der Begriff und die Prophylaxis des Kindbettfiebers (in German). Budapest/Wien/Leipzig: Hartleben; 1861.
13. Lister J. On the antiseptic principle in the practice of surgery. Br Med J. 1867;2:246.
14. Kaiser W, Völker A. Berolina iubilans: Berlin physicians as Halle doctoral candidates (VI). Curt Schimmelbusch (1860–1895), Halle doctoral candidate of 1886. Z Gesamte Inn Med. 1987;42(22):649–54.

15. Miller JM. William Stewart Halsted and the use of the surgical rubber glove. Surgery. 1982;92(3):541–3.
16. Petaros A, Skrobonja A. A century since the publication of Grossich's paper in Zentralblatt für Chirurgie--an innovation in the field of antisepsis. Zentralbl Chir. 2010;135(3):279–81.
17. Pasteur L. Recherche sur la putréfaction (in French). Comptes Rendus Hebdomadaires. 1863;56:1189–94.
18. Koch R. Untersuchungen über die Aetiologie de Wundinfektionskrankheiten (in German). Leipzig: F.C.W.Vogel; 1878.
19. Otten H. Domagk and the development of the sulphonamides. J Antimicrob Chemother. 1986;17(6):689–96.
20. Fleming A. On the antibacterial action of cultures of a penicillium, with special reference to their use in the isolation of B. influenzae. 1929. British J Exper Pathology. 1929;10(31):226–36.
21. Florey HW. Use of micro-organisms for therapeutic purposes. Br Med J. 1945;2(4427):635–42.
22. MacGillivray N. Dr Latta of Leith: pioneer in the treatment of cholera by intravenous saline infusion. J R Coll Physicians Edinb. 2006;36(1):80–5.
23. Dudrick SJ, Wilmore DW, Vars HM, Rhoads JE. Long-term total parenteral nutrition with growth, development, and positive nitrogen balance. Surgery. 1968;64(1):134–42.
24. von Petz A. Zur Technick der Magen Resektion: Ein neuer Magen-Darmnaht nähappart (in German). Zbl Chir. 1924;51:179–88.
25. Mine M, et al. A new anastomotic stapler for the esophagus, stomach, and bowel (in Japanese). Jpn J Medical Instrument. 1962;32:377.
26. Borrmann R. Geschwülste des Magens und Duodenums, in Henke F. Lubarsch 0 (ed), Handbuch der speziellen pathologischen Anatomie und Histologie (in German). Berlin: Splinger-Verlag; 1926.
27. Oswaldi Crollii. Basilica chymica. Frankfurt; 1609. pp. 64–5.
28. Becker D. Cultrivori prussiaci curatio singularis (in French). Leyden Maire. 1640;122:17.
29. Péan J. De 1'ablation des tumeurs de l'estomac par la gastrectomie (in French). Gaz des höpitaux. 1879;52:473–5.
30. Rydygier L. Dtsch Zeitschr Chir. 1881; Bd. XVI: S252.
31. Rydygier L. Die erste Magenresection beim Magengeschwürst (in German). Berlin Klin Wochenschr. 1882;19:39.
32. Gussenbauer C, Winiwarter A. Die partielle Magenresektion, Eine experimentelle operative Studie, nebst einer Zusammenstellung der im pathologisch-anatomischen Institute zu Wien in dem Zeitraume von 1817 bis 1875 beobacheteten Magencarcinome (in German). v Langenbeck Arch Chir. 1876;19:347–80.
33. Billroth T. Offenes Schreiben an Herren Dr. L. Wittelshöfer (in German). Wien Med Wochensch. 1881;31:161–5.
34. Wölfler A. Uber die von Herrn Professor Billroth Ausgeführten Resektionen des carcinomatösen Pylorus (in German). Vienna: Braumüller; 1881.

35. Ziegler H. Billroths erste Magenresektion. (in German). Krebsarzt. 1949;4(2):49–59.
36. Haberkant H. Über die bis jetzt erzielten, ummitelbaren und weiteren Erfolge der verschiedenen Operationen am Magen (in German). Arch Klin Chir. 1896;51:546–77.
37. Kocher TE. Über eine neue Methode der Magenresektion mit nachfolgender Gastroenterostomie (in German). Zentralbl Chir. 1891;26.
38. Finney JMT. A new method of gastroduodenostomy, end-to-side with illustration. Trans South Surg Ass. 1924;36:576–8.
39. Heberrington JL. In: Scott HW, Sawyers JL, editors. Historic aspects of gastric surgery. in Surgery of the stomach, duodenum and small intestine. Boston: Blackwell Scientific; 1991.
40. Billroth T. Über 124 vom November 1878 bis Juni 1890 im meiner Klinik und Privatpraxis ausgeführte Resektionen am Magen- und Darmcanal, GastroEnterostomien und Narbenlösungen wegen chronischer Krankheitsprocesse (in German). Wien Klin Wochenschr. 1891;34:625–8.
41. Wölfler A. Gastro-Enterostomie (in German). Zentralbl Chir, Leipzig. 1881;8:705–8.
42. Pólya EA. Zur Stumpfversorgung nach Magenresektion (in German). Zlb Chir. 1911;38:892–4.
43. Finsterer H. Zur Technik der Magenresektion (in German). Deutsch Z Chir. 1914;128:514–73.
44. Braun H. Über Gastro-Enterostomie und gleichzeitig ausgeführte Entero-Anastomose (in German). Langenbecks Arch Klin Chir. 1892;45:361–4.
45. Balfour DC. Curability of cancer of the stomach. Surg Gynecol Obstet. 1932;540:312–6.
46. Eusterman GB, Balfour DC. The stomach and duodenum. Philadelphia: Saundars; 1935.
47. Roux C. Da la gastro-entérostomie, Etude basée sur les opérations pratiques du 21 juin 1888 au ler septembre 1896 (in French). Rev Gynec Chir Abdom. 1897;1:67–122.
48. Kondo J. Experiences of gastric resection (in Japanese). Jpn J Surg. 1900;1:234–58.
49. Miyake H, Miyagi J, Taniguchi K. Gastric cancer (in Japanese). Tokyo: Kokuseido shoten; 1928.
50. Mikulicz JR. Beiträge zur Technik der Operation des Magencarcinoms (in German). Arch Klin Chir. 1898;57:524–32.
51. von Bergmann E, Bruns P, Mikulicz J. Handbuch der praktischen Chirurgie, Band III Teil 1. Chirurgie des Unterleibes (in German). Stuttgart: Ferdinand Enke; 1900.
52. Eiselsberg AF. Johannes v. Miklicz-Radecki (in German). Wien Klin Wochenschr. 1905;52:1297–300.
53. Schlatter C. Vollständiger Entfernung des Magens. Ösophagoenterostomie, beim Menschen (in German). Beitr Klin Chir. 1897;19:757.
54. Schlatter C. A unique case of complete removal of the stomach – successful oesophagus- enterostomy – recovery. Med Rec. 1897;52:909–14.
55. Kitagawa O. Two cases of successful total gastrectomy for gastric cancer (in Japanese). Tokyo Iji Shinnshi. 1902;1258:827.

56. Schlöffer H. Resektion des Ganzen Magens (in German). Deutsch Med Woch. 1917.

57. Roux C. L' esophago-jejune-gastrome. Nouvelle Opération Pour Retricissement Infranchissable de L'ésophage. Semaine Med. 1907;27:37.

58. Orr TG. A modified technique for total gastrectomy. Arch Surg. 1947;54(3):279–86.

59. Graham RR. A technique for total gastrectomy. Surgery. 1940;8:257–64.

60. Graham RR. Total gastrectomy for carcinoma of the stomach. Arch Surg. 1943;46:907–14.

61. Nishi M, Ohta K, Kajitani T. Double-tract reconstruction after total gastrectomy (in Japanese). Shujutsu. 1972;26(8):785.

62. Siewert JR, Peiper HJ, Jennewein HM, et al. Die Ösophago-Jejunoplication (in German). Chirurg. 1973;44(3):113–20.

63. Steinberg ME. A double jejunal lumen gastrojejunal anastomosis; pantaloons anastomosis. Surg Gynecol Obstet. 1949;88(4):453–64.

64. Hunt CJ. Construction of food pouch from segment of jejunum as substitute for stomach in total gastrectomy. AMA Arch Surg. 1952;64(5):601–8.

65. Seo S. Total gastrectomy with jejunal interposition (in Japanese). Jpn J Surg. 1941;42:1004–5.

66. Longmire WP Jr. Total gastrectomy for carcinoma of the stomach. Surg Gynecol Obstet. 1947;84(1):21–30.

67. Longmire WP Jr, Beal JM. Construction of a substitute gastric reservoir following total gastrectomy. Ann Surg. 1952;135(5):637–45.

68. Schreiber HW, Eichfuss HP, Schumpelick V. Magenersatz (in German). Chirurg. 1978;49(2):72–80.

69. Lee CM Jr. Transposition of a colon segment as a gastric reservoir after total gastrectomy. Surg Gynecol Obstet. 1951;92(4):456–65.

70. Pack GT, McNeer G. End results in the treatment of cancer of the stomach; analysis of 795 cases. Surgery. 1948;24(5):769–78.

71. McNeer G, Sunderland DA, Lawrence W Jr, et al. A more thorough operation for gastric cancer; anatomical basis and description of technique. Cancer. 1951;4(5):957–67.

72. Lawrence W Jr, McNeer G, Ortega LG, Sunderland DA. Early results of extended total gastrectomy for cancer. Cancer. 1956;9(6):1153–9.

73. McNeer G, Pack GT. Neoplasms of the stomach. Philadelphia/Toronto: Lippincott; 1967.

74. Lahay FH, Marshal SF. Indications for, and experiences with, total gastrectomy: based upon seventy-three cases of total gastrectomy. Ann Surg. 1944;119(3):300–17.

75. Walters W. Modern improvements in the treatment of malignant lesions of the stomach and their results. Surg Clin North Am. 1951;31(4):977–93.

76. Lahay FH. Total gastroectomy for all patients with operable cancer of the stomach, Editorial. Surg Gynec Obst. 1950;90:246–8.

77. Lahay FH, Mashall SF. Should total gastrectomy be employed in early carcinoma of the stomach; experience with 139 total gastrectomies. Ann Surg. 1950;132(3):540–65.

78. Brunschwig A. Pancreato-total gastrectomy and splenectomy for advanced carcinoma of the stomach. Cancer. 1948;1(3):427–30.

79. Suzuki J. Combined resection of spleen and distal part of pancreas (in Japanese). Jpn J Surg. 1954;55:836–52.

80. Kajitani T, Hoshino T. Combined resection of pancreas for gastric cancer (in Japanese). Gann no Rinsho. 1955;1:263–8.

81. Kajitani T, Hoshino T, et al. Role of combined resection of spleen and tail of pancreas for gastric cancer (in Japanese). Gann no Rinsho. 1960;6:522–9.

82. Nakayama K. Pancreaticosplenectomy combined with gastrectomy in cancer of the stomach. Surgery. 1956;40(2):297–310.

83. McNeer G, James A. Resection of stomach and adjacent organs in continuity for advanced cancer. Cancer. 1948;1(3):449–54.

84. Lahay FH. Total gastrectomy, splenectomy, resection of the left lobe of the liver, omentumectomy and colectomy on one patient in one operation. Ann Surg. 1944;119(2):222–4.

85. Nakashima T, Nishi M, et al. Long-term results of exenteration of left upper intraperitoneal organs for advanced gastric cancer (in Japanese). Rinsho Geka. 1991;46(9):1083–8.

86. Oyama S, Nakajima T, Nishi M, et al. Left upper abdominal evisceration for advanced gastric cancer (in Japanese). Gan To Kagaku Ryoho. 1994;21(11):1781–6.

87. Brunschwig A, Gentil F. Postoperative diabetes mellitus following resection of the body and tail of the pancreas for secondary invasion by gastric cancer. Ann Surg. 1949;130(5):921–8.

88. Gerota D. Zur Technik der Lymphgefässinjection, Eine neue Injectionsmasse für Lymphgefässe. Polychrome Injection (in German). Anat Anz. 1896;12:216–23.

89. Jamieson JK, Dobson JF. On the Injection of Lymphatics by Prussian Blue. J Anat Physiol. 1910;45(1):7–10.

90. Pólya E, von Navratil D. Untersuchung über die Lymphbahnen des Wurmfortsatzes und des Magens (in German). Zeitschr Klin Chir. 1903;69:421–56.

91. Poirer P, Charpy A. Traité d'Anatomie Humaine, tome 2e. Les Lymphatiques (in French). Paris: Masson et Cie; 1902.

92. Sappey C. Description et Iconographie, Anatomie, Physiologie, Pathologie des Vaisseaux Lymphatiques considérés chez l'homme et vertèbres, 2e partie (in French). Paris: Adrién Delahaye; 1874.

93. Jamieson JK, Dobson JF. The lymphatic system of the stomach. Lancet. 1907;20:1061–6.

94. Rouvière H. Anatomie des Lymphatiques de l'Homme (in French). Paris: Masson et Cie; 1932.

95. Inoue Y. Lymphatic system of the stomach, duodenum, pancreas, and diaphragm (in Japanese). Jpn J Anat. 1936;9:35–123.

96. Kajitani T. Lymph node metastasis of gastric cancer (in Japanese). Jpn J Surgery. 1944;45:15–6.

97. Jiannai D. Surgical treatment of stomach cancer: extensive excision of the lymph nodes, with special reference to radical surgery of stomach cancer (in Japanese). Gan No Rinsho. 1972;Suppl:245–1.

98. Maruyama K, Gunvén P, et al. Lymph node metastases of gastric cancer. General pattern in 1931 patients. Ann Surg. 1989;210(5):596–602.

99. Kim JP, Hur YS, Yang HK. Lymph node metastasis as a significant prognostic factor in early gastric cancer: analysis of 1,136 early gastric cancers. Ann Surg Oncol. 1995;2(4):308–13.

100. Keller E, Rohde H, et al. Lymph node staging in 872 patients with carcinoma of the stomach and the presumed benefit of lymphadenectomy. German Stomach Cancer TNM Study Group. J Am Coll Surg. 1994;178(1):38–46.

101. Siewert JR, Böttcher K, et al. Prognostic relevance of systematic lymph node dissection in gastric carcinoma. German Gastric Carcinoma Study Group. Br J Surg. 1993;80(8):1015–8.

102. Cushieri A, Weeden S, et al. Patient survival after D1 and D2 resections for gastric cancer: long-term results of the MRC randomized surgical trial. Surgical Co-operative Group. Br J Cancer. 1999;79(9–10):1522–30.

103. Sunderland DA, McNeer G, et al. The lymphatic spread of gastric cancer. Cancer. 1953;6(5):987–96.

104. Wanebo HJ, Kennedy BJ, et al. Gastric carcinoma: does lymph node dissection alter survival? J Am Coll Surg. 1996;183(6):616–24.

105. Brennan MF, Karpeh MS Jr. Surgery for gastric cancer: the American view. Semin Oncol. 1996;23(3):352–9.

106. Japanese Research Society for Gastric Cancer. Japanese rules for gastric cancer study, 1st ed (in Japanese). Tokyo/Osaka/Kyoto: Kanehara & Co. LTD; 1962.

107. Japanese Research Society for Gastric Cancer. Annual report of nationwide registry of gastric cancer patients Volume 1–54 (in Japanese). Tokyo: National Cancer Center Press; 1972–1998.

108. Bonenkamp JJ, Songun I, Sasako M, et al. Randomised comparison of morbidity after D1 and D2 dissection for gastric cancer in 996 Dutch patients. Lancet. 1995;345(8952):745–8.

109. Sue-Ling HM, Johnston D, McCulloch P, et al. D1 versus D2 dissection for gastric cancer. Lancet. 1995;345(8963):1515–6.

110. Maruyama K, Sasako M, Kinoshita T, et al. Pancreas-preserving total gastrectomy for proximal gastric cancer. World J Surg. 1995;19(4):532–6.

111. Groves EW. On the radical operation for cancer of the pylorus: with especial reference to the advantages of the two-stage operation and to the question of the removal of the associated lymphatics. Br Med J. 1910;12(2563):366.

112. Finsterer H. Zur Klinik und chirurgischen Behandlung des Magenkrebs (in German). Arch Klin Chir. 1930;159:30–118.

113. Finstere H. Die Chirurgie des Magenkarzinoms (in German). Wien Klin Wochenschr. 1931;44:341–6.

114. Muto M. Clinical significance of gastric cancer metastasis on the omental bursa: histological and prognostic studies (in Japanese). Jpn J Surg. 1958;59:884–5.

115. Sugarbaker PH. Peritonectomy procedures. Ann Surg. 1995;221(1):29–42.

116. Yonemura Y, Fujimura T, Fushida S, et al. A new surgical approach (peritonectomy) for the treatment of peritoneal dissemination. Hepato-Gastroenterology. 1999;46(25):601–9.

117. Jeung HC, Rha SY, Jang WI, et al. Treatment of advanced gastric cancer by palliative gastrectomy, cytoreductive therapy and postoperative intraperitoneal chemotherapy. Br J Surg. 2002;89(4):460–6.

118. Maki T, Shiratori T, Hatafuku T, et al. Pylorus-preserving gastrectomy as an improved operation for gastric ulcer. Surgery. 1967;61(6):838–45.

119. Nakatani K, Watanabe A, Shiratori T, et al. Pylorus preserving gastrectomy for early gastric cancer: preliminary report (in Japanese). Jpn J Surg. 1991;92(6):763.

120. Miwa K, Kinami S, Miyazaki I, et al. Vagus-saving D2 procedure for early gastric carcinoma (in Japanese). Jpn J Surg. 1996;97(4):286–90.

121. Nakabayashi T, Mochiki E, Kuwano H, et al. Pyloric motility after pylorus-preserving gastrectomy with or without the pyloric branch of the vagus nerve. World J Surg. 2002;26(5):577–83.

122. Maruyama K, Sasako M, Kinoshita T, et al. Surgical treatment for gastric cancer: the Japanese approach. Semin Oncol. 1996;23(3):360–8.

123. Maruyama K, Sasako M, Kinoshita T, et al. Reasonable lymph node dissection in radical gastrectomy for gastric cancer: introduction of computer information system and lymphography technique by India-ink (in Japanese). Jpn J Surgery. 1989;90(9):1318–21.

124. Bollschweiler E, Boettcher K, Siewert JR, et al. Preoperative assessment of lymph node metastases in patients with gastric cancer: evaluation of the Maruyama computer program. Br J Surg. 1992;79(2):156–60.

125. Droste K, Bollschweiler E, Siewert JR, et al. Prediction of lymph node metastasis in gastric cancer patients with neural networks. Cancer Lett. 1996;109(1–2):141–8.

126. Takahashi T, Hagiwara A, et al. Type-oriented therapy for gastric cancer effective for lymph node metastasis: management of lymph node metastasis using activated carbon particles adsorbing an anticancer agent. Semin Surg Oncol. 1991;7(6):378–83.

127. Kajitani T. Surgical technique of extended lymph node dissection for gastric cancer (in Japanese). Jpn J Surg. 1953;54:464–5.

128. Nishi M, Ohta K, Ishihara S, et al. Para-aortic lymph node metastasis (in Japanese). Shokaki Geka. 1991;14(12):165–76.

129. Yonemura Y, Miwa K, Miyazaki I, et al. Surgical treatment of advanced gastric cancer with metastasis in para-aortic lymph node. Int Surg. 1991;76(4):222–5.

130. Sano T, Sasako M. Okajima K, et al. Gastric cancer surgery: morbidity and mortality results from a prospective randomized controlled trial comparing D2 and extended para-aortic lymphadenectomy--Japan Clinical Oncology Group study 9501. J Clin Oncol. 2004;22(14):2767–73.

131. Pinotti HW. A new approach to the thoracic esophagus by the abdominal transdiaphragmatic route. Langenbecks Arch Chir. 1983;359(4):229–35.

132. Maruyama K, Sasako M, Kinoshita T, et al. Can sentinel node biopsy indicate rational extent of lymphadenectomy in gastric cancer surgery? Fundamental and new information on lymph-node dissection. Langenbeck's Arch Surg. 1999;384(2):149–57.

133. Kitagawa Y, Fujii H, Kitajima M, et al. Radio-guided sentinel node detection for gastric cancer. Br J Surg. 2002;89(5):604–8.

134. Tada M, Karita M, Takemoto T, et al. Endoscopic therapy of early gastric cancer by strip biopsy. (in Japanese). Gan To Kagaku Ryoho. 1988;15(4):1460–5.

135. Ono H, Gotoda T, Yoshida S, et al. Endoscopic mucosal resection for treatment of early gastric cancer. Gut. 2001;48(2):225–9.

136. Kondo H, Gotoda T, Yoshida S, et al. Percutaneous traction-assisted EMR by using an insulation-tipped electrosurgical knife for early stage gastric cancer. Gastrointest Endosc. 2004;59(2):284–8.

137. Gotoda T, Kondo H, Saito D, et al. A new endoscopic mucosal resection procedure using an insulation-tipped electrosurgical knife for rectal flat lesions: report of two cases. Gastrointest Endosc. 1999;50(4):560–3.

138. Oda I, Gotoda T, Saito D, et al. Treatment strategy after non-curative endoscopic resection of early gastric cancer. Br J Surg. 2008;95(12):1495–500.

139. Ohgami M, Kumai K, Kitajima M, et al. Laparoscopic surgery for early gastric cancer. Jpn J Surg. 1996;97(4):279–85.

140. Kitano S, Iso Y, Sugimachi K, et al. Laparoscopy-assisted Billroth I gastrectomy. Surg Laparosc Endosc. 1994;4(2):146–8.

141. Uyama I, Sugioka A, Fujita J, et al. Completely laparoscopic proximal gastrectomy with jejunal interposition and lymphadenectomy. J Am Coll Surg. 2000;191(1):114–9.

142. Choi SH, Yoon DS, Min JS, et al. Laparoscopy-assisted radical subtotal gastrectomy for early gastric carcinoma. Yonsei Med J. 1996;37(3):174–80.

143. Kim W, Kim HH. KLASS Group. Decreased morbidity of laparoscopic distal gastrectomy compared with open distal gastrectomy for Stage I gastric cancer: short-term outcomes from a multicenter randomized controlled trial (KLASS-01). Ann Surg. 2016;263(1):28–35.

144. Kuo WH, Lee WJ, Chen CN, et al. Laparoscopic subtotal gastrectomy with lymphadenectomy in a patient with early gastric cancer. J Formos Med Assoc. 1998;97(2):127–30.

145. Chang TC, Chen CC, Lin MT, et al. Gasless laparoscopy-assisted distal gastrectomy for early gastric cancer: analysis of initial results. J Laparoendosc Adv Surg Tech A. 2011;21(3):215–20.

146. Bärlehner E. Initial experience with laparoscopic gastrectomy in benign and malignant tumors (in German). Zentralbl Chir. 1999;124(4):346–50.

147. Hüscher CG, Anastasi A, Crafa F, et al. Laparoscopic gastric resections. Semin Laparosc Surg. 2000;7(1):26–54.

148. Hüscher CG, Mingoli A, Sgarzini G, Sansonetti A, et al. Laparoscopic versus open subtotal gastrectomy for distal gastric cancer: five-year results of a randomized prospective trial. Ann Surg. 2005;241(2):232–7.

149. Hüscher CG, Mingoli A, Ponzano C, et al. Totally laparoscopic total and subtotal gastrectomy with extended lymph node dissection for early and advanced gastric cancer: early and long-term results of a 100-patient series. Am J Surg. 2007;194(6):839–44.

150. Matsui H, Uyama I, Sugioka A, et al. Linear stapling forms improved anastomoses during esophagojejunostomy after a total gastrectomy. Am J Surg. 2002;184(1):58–60.

151. Inaba K, Uyama I, Satoh S, et al. Overlap method: novel intracorporeal esophagojejunostomy after laparoscopic total gastrectomy. J Am Coll Surg. 2010;211(6):25–9.

152. Song J, Hyung WJ, Noh SH, et al. Role of robotic gastrectomy using da Vinci system compared with laparoscopic gastrectomy: initial experience of 20 consecutive cases. Surg Endosc. 2009;23(6):1204–11.

153. Song J, Hyung WJ, Noh SH, et al. Robot-assisted gastrectomy with lymph node dissection for gastric cancer: lessons learned from an initial 100 consecutive procedures. Ann Surg. 2009;249(6):927–32.

154. Kim HI, Yang HK, Hyung WJ, et al. Multicenter prospective comparative study of robotic versus laparoscopic gastrectomy for gastric adenocarcinoma. Ann Surg. 2016;263(1):103–9.

155. Isogaki J, Haruta S, Uyama I, et al. Robot-assisted surgery for gastric cancer: experience at our institute. Pathobiology. 2011;78(6):328–33.

156. Kakeji Y, Baba H, Maehara Y, et al. Robotic laparoscopic distal gastrectomy: a comparison of the da Vinci and Zeus systems. Int J Med Robot. 2006;2(4):299–304.

157. Roviello F, Piagnerelli R, Marrelli D, et al. Assessing the feasibility of full robotic interaortocaval nodal dissection for locally advanced gastric cancer. Int J Med Robot. 2015;11(2):218–22.

158. UICC. TNM Classification of malignant tumours. 1st ed. Geneva: Imprimerie G de Buren SA; 1968.

159. UICC. TNM Classification of malignant tumours. 7th ed. New York/Chichester/Weinheim/Brisbane/Singapore/Torornto: Wiley-Liss; 2009.

160. International Gastric Cancer Association, First volume. Gastric Cancer. 1996;1(1).

161. Sokół S. Ludwik Rydygier. Warsaw: Polish Medical Publication; 1961. p. 102.

162. Cuneo B, Poirier P. Les lymphatique de l'estomac. J Anat Physiol. 1900;16:393–4.

Part II

Staging of Gastric Cancer

Staging of Gastric Cancer: Current Revision and Future Proposal

2

Jingyu Deng, Jiping Wang, and Han Liang

Gastric cancer (GC) is the fourth most common malignancy and ranks the third as cause of death (990,000 cases, 738,000 deaths) worldwide (ref. [1] WHO). Due to the lack of cost-effective screening test and the lack of specific symptoms, most gastric cancer cases were diagnosed at the advanced stages. It is very important to appropriately stage GC patients since it is associated with the choice of treatment modalities and patients' prognosis. The current staging modalities include endoscopy, CT, PET/CT, and laparoscopy. The primary goals of the staging are to evaluate whether a patient has regional or distant metastasis (M), whether the tumor involves local/regional lymph nodes (N), and whether the depth of tumor invasion into the different histology layers between mucosa and serosa (T). Combining the three components, Union for International Control Cancer (UICC)/ American Joint Committee on Cancer (AJCC) has defined the most commonly used GC staging system, tumor-node-metastasis (TNM) staging system [1]. As the improvement in cancer awareness, methods in cancer screening, advancement in che-

motherapy and target therapy, and patients' disease characteristics are constantly changing and so does the prognosis. Hence, the UICC/AJCC TNM staging system has been revised accordingly every few years since its induction into clinical practice since 1977. The seventh edition UICC/AJCC TNM classification for GC was modified after the Buffalo Meeting 2008 as the result of the consensus between the Eastern (Japanese and Korean) and Western GC classification. In 2010, the seventh edition (7th ed.) TNM classification for GC, comprising of the data from Japan and Korean, was published with minor revisions in T stage and major revisions in N stage compared to the previous editions of TNM classification [2].

The seventh edition UICC/AJCC TNM classification for GC

T1a	Tumor invades lamina propria
T1b	Tumor invades submucosa
T2	Tumor invades muscularis propria
T3	Tumor invades subserosa
T4a	Tumor penetrates serosa without invasion of adjacent structures
T4b	Tumor invades adjacent structures
N1	Metastasis in 1–2 regional lymph nodes
N2	Metastasis in 3–6 regional lymph nodes
N3a	Metastasis in 7–15 regional lymph nodes
N3b	Metastasis in more than 15 regional lymph nodes
M0	No distant metastasis
M1	Distant metastasis
pM1	Distant metastasis microscopically confirmed

J. Deng · H. Liang (✉)
Department of Gastroenterology, Tianjin Medical University Cancer Hospital, City Key Laboratory of Tianjin Cancer Center and National Clinical Research Center for Cancer, Tianjin, China

J. Wang
Hepatobiliary Cancer, Division of Surgery Oncology, Brigham and Women's Hospital, Harvard Medical School, Boston, MA, USA

© Springer-Verlag GmbH Germany, part of Springer Nature 2019
S. H. Noh, W. J. Hyung (eds.), *Surgery for Gastric Cancer*,
https://doi.org/10.1007/978-3-662-45583-8_2

Stage grouping of GC in accordance with the seventh edition UICC/AJCC TNM classification

Stage 0	Tis	N0	M0
Stage IA	T1	N0	M0
Stage IB	T2	N0	M0
	T1	N1	M0
Stage IIA	T3	N0	M0
	T2	N1	M0
	T1	N2	M0
Stage IIB	T4a	N0	M0
	T3	N1	M0
	T2	N2	M0
	T1	N3	M0
Stage IIIA	T4a	N1	M0
	T3	N2	M0
	T2	N3	M0
Stage IIIIB	T4b	N0 or N1	M0
	T4a	N2	M0
	T3	N3	M0
Stage IIIC	T4a	N3	M0
	T4b	N2 or N3	M0
Stage IV	Any T	Any N	M1

Revisions on the Current Edition TNM Classification for Gastric Cancer

Explicit Staging in Esophagogastric Junction Carcinoma

Carcinoma of the esophagogastric junction (EGJ) is defined by the WHO as "tumors cross the EGJ regardless of where the bulk of the tumors lies" [3]. The classification carcinoma of EGJ, defined by Siewert and Stein, was approved at the second International Gastric Cancer Congress in Munich in April 1997 [4]. In accordance with the anatomic cardia, EGJ cancer can be divided into three subtypes: type I, adenocarcinoma of the distal esophagus with the tumor center located between 1 and 5 cm above the anatomic EGJ; type II, true carcinoma of the cardia with the tumor center within 1 cm above and 2 cm below the EGJ; and type III, subcardial carcinoma with the tumor center between 2 and 5 cm below EGJ. This classification was approved at the consensus conference of the International Gastric Cancer Association (IGCA) and the International

Society for Diseases of the Esophagus (ISDE) and has been accepted and used worldwide before the seventh edition TNM classification was published [5].

According to the sixth edition TNM classification, EGJ carcinoma may classify into either esophageal cancer or GC on the basis of the judgment of the physicians. However, many investigators found that adenocarcinoma of the proximal stomach was similar, or even identical, to Barrett's esophagus-associated distal esophageal adenocarcinoma on the basis of comparable characteristics in epidemiology [6], clinical presentations [7], molecular pathobiology [8], and histopathology [9]. Subsequently, AJCC adopted the notion that all EGJ cancer should be required to comply with the rule for esophageal adenocarcinoma, which has been published in the seventh edition of the cancer staging manual [10]. The seventh edition TNM classification included the meticulous classification of EGJ carcinoma. However, an obvious issue of major concern was the following rule: "A tumor with the epicenter of within 2 to 5 cm below the EGJ and also extends into the esophagus is classified and staged using the esophageal scheme. Tumors with an epicenter in the stomach greater than 5 cm from the EGJ or those within 5 cm of the EGJ without extension in the esophagus are classified and staged using the gastric carcinoma scheme." In another word, EGJ carcinoma included in the esophageal chapter on the basis of the new TNM staging system according to the anatomical criteria "5 cm rule" proposed by Siewert was based on an obscure concept of the tumor epicenter. Some of the gastric fundus tumor might be considered as esophageal cancer [11]. As the result, the current revision did not resolve the well-known controversial issue: Should type III tumors be treated as GC invading the EGJ, considering the origin of the tumors? Some literatures have shown that esophagectomy has not improved the survival rate compared to an extensive gastrectomy for type II tumors arising from the same origin as type III tumors [5]. In fact, more and more clinicians think that the optimal treatment modalities should be selected based on the distance of tumor invasion to the stomach or esophagus rather than the location of the central region of the tumor [12].

Proposal of Positive Cytology as Distant Metastasis

Peritoneal washing cytology, as a preoperative staging tool, has been gradually adapted into clinical practice. Leake et al. [13] recently demonstrated that recurrence rates for patients positive for peritoneal cytology ranged from 11.1% to 100%, while those negative for intraperitoneal free cancer cells (IFCCs) had recurrence rates of 0–51%. Overall survival was significantly decreased for patients with positive peritoneal cytology by using a systematic review of the accuracy and utility of peritoneal cytology in patients with gastric cancer. Other reports in the literature indicate that a positive peritoneal cytology is an independent predictor of poor prognosis following curative surgery, with median survival of as poor as distant metastasis [14–16]. In addition, Yamamoto et al. [17] also validated that GC with peritoneal cytology (+) had a poor prognosis because it is associated with non-curative factors, peritoneal dissemination, and liver or LNs metastases. Mezhir et al. [16] recommended to abandon gastrectomy for patients with positive peritoneal cytology even in the absence of gross peritoneal disease due to the poor outcomes. Thus, both the Japanese Gastric Cancer Association (JGCA) and the seventh edition TNM classification classify positive peritoneal cytology as stage IV disease [18]. Conversely, few authors reported that peritoneal washing cytology using samples harvested in the abdominal cavity was not able to predict peritoneal recurrence or survival in GC patients [19]. Depending on the various methods for performing a peritoneal washing cytology, there is a large discrepancy in the frequency of a positive peritoneal cytology. The rate of positive cases was found more than 20% on a routine cytology, 35% on immunohistochemistry, and 50% on RT-PCR in cases of a serosa invasion-positive GC [20]. Inevitably, there is a large discrepancy in the positive rates and median survival time

of the positive cases among different institutions. Therefore, the prognosis and treatment of patients with no macroscopic peritoneal metastases but with peritoneal cytology-positive diseases remain as controversial issues. Further rigorous definition of the methods in detecting peritoneal washing tumor cell and studies in the staging and the appropriate comprehensive treatment of this group of patients are needed.

Minimum Number of Examined Lymph Nodes

The recommended minimum number of examined (dissected) LNs required for proper staging remains controversial, because this number varies considerably between institutions and countries. Before 1997, all staging systems (UICC, AJCC, and Japanese Committee on Cancer) used for this disease defined N stage by the location of LN metastases relative to the primary tumor (I do not understand this sentence). Subsequently, many studies revealed that the number of positive nodes best defined the prognostic influence of metastatic LNs in GC. In 1997, the UICC and AJCC redefined the pathologic nodal status based on the number of involved nodes rather than their location. In an effort to improve staging accuracy, it was recommended that a minimum of 15 lymph nodes should be examined to guarantee the accuracy of prognostic prediction of N stage, especially in the definition of N0 [21]. Karpeh et al. [22] demonstrated that the overall distribution of patients staged by the fifth edition AJCC classification did not change significantly if 15 or more LNs were examined, but median survival for N1, N2, and N3 by the fifth edition AJCC classification increased significantly when 15 or more LNs were examined. It must be emphasized that the extent of LN dissection and the thoroughness of the pathologist's examination of the specimen together determine the number of LNs ultimately retrieved [23]. It is clear that techniques such as fat clearing can increase the number of nodes and that an increase in the number of examined lymph nodes will increase the number of positive nodes, which will alter the stages [24]. Recently,

Smith et al. [25] reported that survival would improve by 7.6% (T1/2N0), 5.7% (T1/2N1), 11% (T3 N0), or 7% (T3 N1) if every 10 extra LNs were dissected in the Surveillance, Epidemiology, and End Results database between 1973 and 1999. Furthermore, they demonstrated that a cut-point analysis yielded the greatest survival difference at 10 LNs examined but continued to detect significantly superior survival differences for cut points at up to 40 LNs, always in favor of more LNs examined [25]. Son et al. [26] analyzed the survival rates of 10,010 patients who underwent curative gastrectomy from 1987 to 2007 and then showed that patients who had T1 tumor classification, N0 LN status, and stage I disease with an insufficient number of examined LNs ($\leq$15 nodes) after curative gastrectomy had a significantly worse prognosis than patients who had $\geq$16 examined LNs. In accordance with the fifth/sixth edition TNM classification, Nio et al. [27] analyzed 223 pN0 patients with GC and then found that patients with pN0 in pT1 stage should be required for a minimum of six examined nodes. Jiao et al. [28] reported that the number of examined LNs was the independent predictors of overall survival of patients with node-negative GC, and patients with $\leq$15 examined LNs were more likely to experience locoregional and peritoneal recurrence than those with no less than 16 examined LNs.

Therefore, the latest edition TNM classification specifies that "histological examination of a regional lymphadenectomy specimen should ordinarily include 16 or more LNs" to avoid understaging. However, only 1/3 of the gastric cancer patients have more than 15 lymph nodes examined (my Annals of Surgery paper). In fact, the new UICC/AJCC system confirmed the following sentence (added in previous editions) as regards the pN0 definition: "If the LNs are negative, but the number ordinarily examined is not met, classify as pN0." Therefore, this appears to mean that the figure of 16 is a recommendation, but no longer a requirement, for pN0 staging [11]. At the meantime, Wang et al. [29] clearly showed that for patients who have N0 disease and <16 LN examined, their survival is the same for patients who had N1 disease with >15 examined

LN. All those evidence indicated two paradox problems that the seventh edition system is facing: It is well known that inadequate (<16) examined lymph nodes will cause stage migration. On the other hand, most American patients have <16 LN examined.

Bilici et al. [30] recently reported that the superiority of classification based on the ratio between metastatic and examined nodes to determine N stage for prediction of overall survival of patients with radically resected GC could not be proved, even in patients with <16 examined LNs. This numeric change seems to arise from the figure of 16 introduced for N3b in the seventh edition TNM classification more than from the "numeric controversies" of literature.

Has the latest UICC TNM stipulated that GC should be staged independent of the number of examined LNs? As we know, the main reasons for examination of an insufficient number of LN s after curative gastrectomy are inaccurate LN dissection or retrieval. Besides, harvesting of a number of nodes "small" to differentiate N subcategories is not a guarantee for enough extent of lymphadenectomy. Therefore, it is worthwhile to discuss whether the requirement of appropriate threshold of examined LNs for accurate evaluation N stage of GC.

Proposed Lymph Node Ratio to Be Included in the Staging System

The ratio between metastatic and dissected (examined) LNs has been proposed as a simple, convenient, and reproducible system that can be used to better identify the subgroup of gastric, breast, pancreatic, and colon cancer patients with similar prognosis, thus minimizing the stage migration phenomenon that can be observed using the TNM classification [31–33]. Owing to decrease the stage migration, many investigators emphasized that ratio between metastatic and dissected LNs is a convenient, repeatable, and creditable variable for accurate prediction of the prognosis of GC patients, regardless of the number of dissected LNs and extent of lymphadenectomy [34, 35]. It is still controversial whether the ratio between metastatic and dissected LNs is superior to the number of metastatic LNs for predication of the overall survival of GC patients. Wang et al. [29] demonstrated that AJCC staging misclassified 57% of patients and TNrM staging misclassified only 12% when misclassification was defined as any subgroup in which median survival fell outside the 95% confidence interval of the GC patient group's overall median survival.

On the other hand, several authors reported the negative results of the ratio between metastatic and dissected LNs for prediction the prognosis of patients with adequate dissected nodes, especially in the group of patients with 15 or more dissected nodes [36, 37]. Actually, it is absolutely incorrect that the number of the examined nodes can instead be use as an indicator of the extent of node dissection. In addition, how to accurately define the cutoffs of ratio between metastatic and dissected LNs is unclear else. However, we demonstrated that the ratio between metastatic and dissected LNs was an important variable which was capable of the improvement of the survival discrimination of GC patients with positive LNs [37]. Therefore, the clinical values of the ratio between metastatic and dissected LNs need to be further discussed in elaborate analysis.

Prefix "y" for TNM Classification After Neoadjuvantly Treated Tumor

For locally advanced lesion, the standard treatment is perioperative chemotherapy in Europe [38–42]. So far, R0 resection is aimed for by gastrectomy with standard D2 lymphadenectomy [41]. However, even with D2 gastrectomy and adjuvant chemotherapy with S-1, the prognosis of tumor is not satisfactory [43]. Neoadjuvant chemotherapy, which is an exception to improve the radical resection condition, is under heated discussion about its definite role in improving cure rate for GC patients [44, 45]. Authors reported that only about 21% GC patients had complete or subtotal tumor regression, which may provide objective and highly valuable prognostic information in addition to posttherapeutic lymph node status [46]. In addition, response of the primary

tumor does not guarantee recurrence-free long-term survival, but histopathological complete responders have better prognosis compared to partial responders [47]. Although the percentage of major responder tumors after perioperative chemotherapy is low in GC [48], the pathological assessment may be affected by possible tumor regression. In the seventh edition TNM classification, a clinical TNM classification recorded following the neoadjuvant therapy should be identified by the prefix "y," as "ycTcNcM." Actually, the ypTNM classification is used to reflect the extent variation of tumor after neoadjuvant therapy. In analyzing the results, it can be differentiated between patients treated with primary surgery (cTNM, pTNM) and those treated by surgery following neoadjuvant treatment (ycTNM, ypTNM) [49].

Proposal of the Next Edition TNM Classification for Gastric Cancer

Amendment Both Extent and Number of Dissected Lymph Nodes as the Prerequisites for Staging the Lymph Node Metastasis

As compared with the sixth edition TNM classification system involving N stage, the seventh edition more reliably and accurately categorized the number of metastatic LNs for the purpose of predicting the overall survival of patients after curative surgery, regardless of the extent of lymphadenectomy or the number of examined LNs. However, the only treatment known to offer cure for GC is adequate surgery for potentially exhaustive removal of the primary tumor and the metastatic LNs. It is undoubtedly that the stage migration may be brought out by using the seventh edition TNM classification in GC patients who have undergone D1 lymphadenectomy or presented with less than 16 examined LNs, which can result in lower N stage classifications and falsely higher survival rate. The patients with the extragastric LN metastasis had the obviously lower 5-year survival rate than patients with the perigastric LN metastasis or without any LN metastasis [50]. It is worth noting that limited lymphadenectomy cannot provide the accurate extent of LN metastasis owing to the lack of dissection and examination of extragastric LNs, which is the key causation for the bias of prognosis evaluation. D2 lymphadenectomy and no less than 16 examined/dissected LNs, as the requisite guarantees for adequate quality of the surgery, can provide sufficient information concerning nodal metastases to allow the prediction of prognosis using the seventh edition of the TNM classification system involving N staging [51].

Occult Tumor Cells in Lymph Nodes as a Novel Subcategory of N Stage

Although many researchers demonstrated that the postoperative prognosis of node-negative GC patients was significantly better than that of node-positive GC patients, minority of node-negative GC patients had recurrence and poor survival [52–54]. Multivariate analysis showed that D1 lymphadenectomy, few dissected nodes, and serosal involvement were the risk factors of postoperative recurrence of node-negative GC patients [54]. Biffi et al. [55] reported that more extended LN resection offers protection, as node-negative GC patients who had ≤15 nodes removed had significantly worse disease-free survival and overall survival at multivariate analysis than patients in whom >15 nodes were removed. In addition, authors also demonstrated that the sufficient number of negative LNs harvested might improve the overall survival rate of GC patients after curative gastrectomy [56, 57].

Occult tumor cells in LN may result in the inaccuracy of pathological N category [58]. Latest research revealed that the majority of the retrieved studies (75%) evaluating the predictive role of occult tumor cells concluded that its presence was associated with a worse prognosis of GC patients by using the systematic analysis [59]. Therefore, increasing the number of examined LNs during surgery could reduce the chance of residual malignancy and improve the prognosis of

GC, even in negative-node patients [60]. Occult tumor cells that comprised micrometastases (MM; >0.2 mm and < or = 2.0 mm) and isolated tumor cells (ITC; < or = 0.2 mm) are the original hematoxylin and eosin-stained sections of all LNs from patients that are previously considered as tumor-negative by the local pathologist. The number of examined LNs and the percentage of occult tumor cell in positive LNs were identified to be independent risk factors for locoregional disease recurrence and distant disease recurrence, respectively [58]. Yonemura et al. [61] demonstrated that 5 of the 37 negative-node patients with isolated tumor cells (pN0(i+)) versus 1 of the 271 negative-node patients with no evidence of isolated tumor cells (pN0(i−)) died from recurrence by using immunohistochemical detection ($P = 0.014$). Lee et al. [62] found that LN micrometastases were identified by cytokeratin immunostaining in 196 GC patients classified as pN1, consisting of 20 cases with micrometastases (pN1mi(i+)), 34 cases with only micrometastases (pN1mi), and 142 cases with pN1 with one or more macrometastases (pN1). Although the association between occult tumor cells and patients' overall survival is still controversial, the high recurrence rate for patients has been detected by using immunohistochemical method with micrometastases [63].

Extracapsular Lymph Node Involvement in Gastric Cancer

Tumor penetration of the LN capsule in metastatic LNs is called as extracapsular LN involvement. For several nongastrointestinal malignancies, like breast, prostate, pharynx, larynx, and bladder cancer, the prognostic value of extracapsular LN involvement has already been demonstrated to be negatively associated with overall and disease-free survival of patients [64–70]. Recent systematic review showed that extracapsular LN involvement was a common phenomenon in patients with gastrointestinal malignancies and could identify a subgroup of patients with a significantly worse survival [71]. Tanaka and colleagues concluded that extracapsular LN involvement was a significant risk factor for peritoneal dissemination and liver metastasis in GC patients [72, 73], which was similar to the research results reported by Alakus in 2010 [74]. With the multivariate analysis, extracapsular LN involvement also was identified to be an independent risk factor influencing the outcome of patients with GC [75]. The further study showed that the presence of extracapsular LN involvement could affect the survival of GC patients with only single LN metastasis [75]. Additionally, Nakamura reported that extracapsular LN involvement was also identified to be useful in combination with N stage of the TNM classification, representing a promising indicator to refine the LN metastatic category in GC [76].

Other Variables' Assessment for Enhancement of the Efficiency of Stage of Gastric Cancer

Recent researchers showed some variables might be potential targets for improvement of the efficiency of the stage of GC, which need to be assessed in the future large-scale. Owing to peritoneal dissemination and distal metastases occurring in the comparatively late stages of disease, accurate diagnosis is critical for successful design of the therapeutic strategy of GC and for greatly enhancement of the efficacy of medical intervention [77]. To date, many potential biomarkers have been elucidated in GC by detecting serum protein antigens, oncogenic genes, or gene families through improving molecular biological technologies [78]. DNA methylation plays a significant role in the oncogenesis and the progress of human carcinogenesis. It has been validated the significant relationship between specific gene methylation and clinicopathological features in GC. The ability to detect small amounts of methylated DNA among tissues allows researchers to use DNA methylation as a molecular biomarker in GC in a variety of samples, including serum, plasma, and GC [79]. Gene amplification and protein overexpression of human epidermal growth factor receptor 2 (HER2) play an important role in the proliferation, apoptosis, adhesion, angiogenesis, and aggressiveness of many solid tumors, including GC [80]. More recent studies released that HER2 is a poor prognostic factor in GC patients [81–83], especially those with liver metastases and/or LN metastasis [84, 85].

Yamaguchi et al. [86] proposed that tumor size, given as the maximum diameter of tumor, could provide important information useful for evaluating the potential impact of GC double time screening programs in terms of the degree of improvement in prognosis. Surgeons usually pay more attention to tumor size than depth of tumor invasion because tumor size might have a direct impact upon patients' surgical management and outcome. Researchers demonstrated that there were obvious correlations between tumor size and other tumor-relative clinicopathological variables such as LN metastasis, depth of tumor invasion, and type of Lauren classification, which might result in the poor prognosis of GC patients [87–90].

In view of the impact of occult tumor cells on prognostic evaluation, the negative LNs, identified by the conventionally pathological examination, should be reconsidered for the reality of the negative results of these LNS. Recently, several results were reported to demonstrate that the number of negative LNs was a potential predictor of prognosis of GC. Deng et al. [91, 92] showed the detailed contents of researches of negative LNs in gastric cancer as follows: (1) negative lymph node count was significantly associated with the overall survival of patients, which could enhance the prognostic prediction accuracy of the ratio between positive and dissected LNs for the GC patients; (2) negative lymph node count is a key factor for improvement of the prognosis of GC patients who underwent the D2 lymphadenectomy; (3) ratio between negative and positive LNs was identified to be the optimal lymph node category for evaluation of the overall survival of gastric cancer, rather than N stage or ratio between positive and dissected LNs.

Lastly, a complete harmonization between the TNM classification of stomach tumors proposed by UICC/AJCC and JGCA would be of great importance. Does the No.14v really need to be excluded from the local lymph nodes in advanced GC?

References

1. Kim JP, Lee JH, Kim SJ, Yu HJ, Yang HK. Clinicopathologic characteristics and prognostic factors in 10.783 patients with gastric cancer. Gastric Cancer. 1998;1(2):125–33.
2. Sobin LH, Gospodarowicz MK, Wittekind C. UICC TNM classification of malignant tumors. 7th ed. Oxford: Wiley-Blackwell; 2010.
3. Huang Q, Fan X, Agoston AT, Feng A, Yu H, Lauwers G, Zhang L, Odze RD. Comparison of gastro-oesophageal junction carcinomas in Chinese versus American patients. Histopathology. 2011;59(2):188–97.
4. Siewert JR, Stein HJ. Carcinoma of the gastroesophageal junction-classification, pathology and extent of resection. Dis Esophagus. 1996;9:173–82.
5. Hasegawa S, Yoshikawa T. Adenocarcinoma of the esophagogastric junction: incidence, characteristics, and treatment strategies. Gastric Cancer. 2010;13(2):63–73.
6. Keeney S, Bauer TL. Epidemiology of adenocarcinoma of the esophagogastric junction. Surg Oncol Clin N Am. 2006;15(4):687–96.
7. Marsman WA, Tytgat GN, ten Kate FJ, van Lanschot JJ. Differences and similarities of adenocarcinomas of the esophagus and esophagogastric junction. J Surg Oncol. 2005;92(3):160–8.
8. Wijnhoven BP, Siersema PD, Hop WC, van Dekken H, Tilanus HW. Adenocarcinomas of the distal oesophagus and gastric cardia are one clinical entity. Rotterdam Oesophageal Tumour Study Group. Br J Surg. 1999;86(4):529–35.
9. Chandrasoma P, Wickramasinghe K, Ma Y, DeMeester T. Adenocarcinomas of the distal esophagus and "gastric cardia" are predominantly esophageal carcinomas. Am J Surg Pathol. 2007;31(4):569–75.
10. American Joint Committee on Cancer. AJCC Cancer Staging Manual. Chapter 10, Esophagus and esophagogastric junction. 7th ed. New York: Springer; 2009. p. 129–44.
11. Rausei S, Dionigi G, Boni L, Rovera F, Dionigi R. How does the 7th TNM edition fit in gastric cancer management? Ann Surg Oncol. 2011;18(5):1219–21.
12. Kwon SJ. Evaluation of the 7th UICC TNM staging system of gastric cancer. J Gastric Cancer. 2011;11(2):78–85.
13. Leake PA, Cardoso R, Seevaratnam R, Lourenco L, Helyer L, Mahar A, Rowsell C, Coburn NG. A systematic review of the accuracy and utility of peritoneal cytology in patients with gastric cancer. Gastric Cancer. 2012;15(Suppl 1):S27–37.
14. Bentrem D, Wilton A, Mazumdar M, Brennan M, Coit D. The value of peritoneal cytology as a preoperative predictor in patients with gastric carcinoma undergoing a curative resection. Ann Surg Oncol. 2005;12(5):347–53.
15. Burke EC, Karpeh MS Jr, Conlon KC, Brennan MF. Peritoneal lavage cytology in gastric cancer: an independent predictor of outcome. Ann Surg Oncol. 1998;5(5):411–5.
16. Mezhir JJ, Shah MA, Jacks LM, Brennan MF, Coit DG, Strong VE. Positive peritoneal cytology in patients with gastric cancer: natural history and outcome of 291 patients. Ann Surg Oncol. 2010;17(12):3173–80.
17. Yamamoto M, Matsuyama A, Kameyama T, Okamoto M, Okazaki J, Utsunomiya T, Tsutsui S, Fujiwara M, Ishida T. Prognostic re-evaluation of peritoneal lavage cytology in Japanese patients with gastric carcinoma. Hepato-Gastroenterology. 2009;56(89):261–5.
18. Japanese Gastric Cancer A. Japanese classification of gastric carcinoma: 3rd English edition. Gastric Cancer. 2011;14(2):101–12.
19. Kang KK, Hur H, Byun CS, Kim YB, Han SU, Cho YK. Conventional cytology is not beneficial for predicting peritoneal recurrence after curative surgery for gastric cancer: results of a prospective clinical study. J Gastric Cancer. 2014;14(1):23–31.
20. Kodera Y, Nakanishi H, Ito S, Nakao A. Clinical significance of isolated tumor cells and micrometastases in patients with gastric carcinoma. Gan To Kagaku Ryoho. 2007;34(6):817–23.
21. Sobin LH, Fleming ID. TNM classification of malignant tumors. Cancer. 1997;80(9):1803–4.
22. Karpeh MS, Leon L, Klimstra D, Brennan MF. Lymph node staging in gastric cancer: is location more important than Number? An analysis of 1,038 patients. Ann Surg. 2000;232(3):362–71.
23. Bunt AM, Hermans J, van de Velde CJ, Sasako M, Hoefsloot FA, Fleuren G, Bruijn JA. Lymph node retrieval in a randomized trial on Western-type versus Japanese-type surgery in gastric cancer. J Clin Oncol. 1996;14(8):2289–94.
24. Candela FC, Urmacher C, Brennan MF. Comparison of the conventional method of lymph node staging with a comprehensive fat-clearing method for gastric adenocarcinoma. Cancer. 1990;66(8):1828–32.
25. Smith DD, Schwarz RR, Schwarz RE. Impact of total lymph node count on staging and survival after gastrectomy for gastric cancer: data from a large US-population database. J Clin Oncol. 2005;23(28):7114–24.
26. Son T, Hyung WJ, Lee JH, Kim YM, Kim HI, An JY, Cheong JH, Noh SH. Clinical implication of an insufficient number of examined lymph nodes after curative resection for gastric cancer. Cancer. 2012;118(19):4687–93.
27. Nio Y, Yamasawa K, Yamaguchi K, Itakura M, Omori H, Koike M, Kitamura Y, Tsuji M, Endo S, Ogo Y, Yano S, Sumi S. Problems in the N-classification of the new 1997 UICC TNM stage classification for gastric cancer: an analysis of over 10 years' outcome of Japanese patients. Anticancer Res. 2003;23(1B):697–705.
28. Jiao XG, Deng JY, Zhang RP, Wu LL, Wang L, Liu HG, Hao XS, Liang H. Prognostic value of number of examined lymph nodes in patients with node-negative gastric cancer. World J Gastroenterol. 2014;20(13):3640–8.

29. Wang J, Dang P, Raut CP, Pandalai PK, Maduekwe UN, Rattner DW, Lauwers GY, Yoon SS. Comparison of a lymph node ratio-based staging system with the 7th AJCC system for gastric cancer: analysis of 18,043 patients from the SEER database. Ann Surg. 2012;255(3):478–85.

30. Bilici A, Ustaalioglu BB, Gumus M, Seker M, Yilmaz B, Kefeli U, Yildirim E, Sonmez B, Salepci T, Kement M, Mayadagli A. Is metastatic lymph node ratio superior to the number of metastatic lymph nodes to assess outcome and survival of gastric cancer? Onkologie. 2010;33(3):101–5.

31. van der Wal BC, Butzelaar RM, van der Meij S, Boermeester MA. Axillary lymph node ratio and total number of removed lymph nodes: predictors of survival in stage I and II breast cancer. Eur J Surg Oncol. 2002;28(5):481–9.

32. Pawlik TM, Gleisner AL, Cameron JL, Winter JM, Assumpcao L, Lillemoe KD, Wolfgang C, Hruban RH, Schulick RD, Yeo CJ, Choti MA. Prognostic relevance of lymph node ratio following pancreaticoduodenectomy for pancreatic cancer. Surgery. 2007;141(5):610–8.

33. Telian SH, Bilchik AJ. Significance of the lymph node ratio in stage III colon cancer. Ann Surg Oncol. 2008;15(6):1557–8.

34. Marchet A, Mocellin S, Ambrosi A, Morgagni P, Garcea D, Marrelli D, Roviello F, de Manzoni G, Minicozzi A, Natalini G, De Santis F, Baiocchi L, Coniglio A, Nitti D, Italian Research Group for Gastric Cancer (IRGGC). The ratio between metastatic and examined lymph nodes (N ratio) is an independent prognostic factor in gastric cancer regardless of the type of lymphadenectomy: results from an Italian multicentric study in 1853 patients. Ann Surg. 2007;245(4):543–52.

35. Kong SH, Lee HJ, Ahn HS, Kim JW, Kim WH, Lee KU, Yang HK. Stage migration effect on survival in gastric cancer surgery with extended lymphadenectomy: the reappraisal of positive lymph node ratio as a proper N-staging. Ann Surg. 2012;255(1):50–8.

36. Deng J, Liang H. Discussion the applicability of positive lymph node ratio as a proper N-staging for predication the prognosis of gastric cancer after curative surgery plus extended lymphadenectomy. Ann Surg. 2012;256(6):e35–6.

37. Deng J, Liang H, Sun D, Pan Y. The prognostic analysis of lymph node-positive gastric cancer patients following curative resection. J Surg Res. 2010;161(1):47–53.

38. Waddell T, Verheij M, Allum W, Cunningham D, Cervantes A, Arnold D, European Society for Medical Oncology (ESMO), European Society of Surgical Oncology (ESSO), European Society of Radiotherapy and Oncology (ESTRO). Gastric cancer: ESMO Clinical Practice Guidelines for diagnosis, treatment and follow-up. Ann Oncol. 2010;21(Suppl 5):v50–4.

39. Ychou M, Boige V, Pignon JP, Conroy T, Bouché O, Lebreton G, Ducourtieux M, Bedenne L, Fabre JM, Saint-Aubert B, Genève J, Lasser P, Rougier P. Perioperative chemotherapy compared with surgery alone for resectable gastroesophageal adenocarcinoma: an FNCLCC and FFCD multicenter phase III trial. J Clin Oncol. 2011;29(13):1715–21.

40. Yoshikawa T, Sasako M. Gastrointestinal cancer: Adjuvant chemotherapy after D2 gastrectomy for gastric cancer. Nat Rev Clin Oncol. 2012;9(4):192–4.

41. Japanese Gastric Cancer A. Japanese gastric cancer treatment guidelines 2010 (ver. 3). Gastric Cancer. 2011;14(2):113–23.

42. Bang YJ, Kim YW, Yang HK, Chung HC, Park YK, Lee KH, Lee KW, Kim YH, Noh SI, Cho JY, Mok YJ, Kim YH, Ji J, Yeh TS, Button P, Sirzén F, Noh SH, CLASSIC Trial Investigators. Adjuvant capecitabine and oxaliplatin for gastric cancer after D2 gastrectomy (CLASSIC): a phase 3 open-label, randomised controlled trial. Lancet. 2012;379(9813):315–21.

43. Sasako M, Sakuramoto S, Katai H, Kinoshita T, Furukawa H, Yamaguchi T, Nashimoto A, Fujii M, Nakajima T, Ohashi Y. Five-year outcomes of a randomized phase III trial comparing adjuvant chemotherapy with S-1 versus surgery alone in stage II or III gastric cancer. J Clin Oncol. 2011;29(33):4387–93.

44. Liao Y, Yang ZL, Peng JS, Xiang J, Wang JP. Neoadjuvant chemotherapy for gastric cancer: a meta-analysis of randomized, controlled trials. J Gastroenterol Hepatol. 2013;28(5):777–82.

45. Cunningham D, Allum WH, Stenning SP, Thompson JN, Van de Velde CJ, Nicolson M, Scarffe JH, Lofts FJ, Falk SJ, Iveson TJ, Smith DB, Langley RE, Verma M, Weeden S, Chua YJ, MAGIC Trial Participants. Perioperative chemotherapy versus surgery alone for resectable gastroesophageal cancer. N Engl J Med. 2006;355(1):11–20.

46. Becker K, Langer R, Reim D, Novotny A, Meyer zum Buschenfelde C, Engel J, Friess H, Hofler H. Significance of histopathological tumor regression after neoadjuvant chemotherapy in gastric adenocarcinomas: a summary of 480 cases. Ann Surg. 2011;253(5):934–9.

47. Ott K, Blank S, Becker K, Langer R, Weichert W, Roth W, Sisic L, Stange A, Jäger D, Büchler M, Siewert JR, Lordick F. Factors predicting prognosis and recurrence in patients with esophago-gastric adenocarcinoma and histopathological response with less than 10% residual tumor. Langenbeck's Arch Surg. 2013;398(2):239–49.

48. Mingol F, Gallego J, Orduña A, Martinez-Blasco A, Sola-Vera J, Moya P, Morcillo MA, Ruiz JA, Calpena R, Lacueva FJ. Tumor regression and survival after perioperative MAGIC-style chemotherapy in carcinoma of the stomach and gastroesophageal junction. BMC Surg. 2015;15:66.

49. Wittekind C. The development of the TNM classification of gastric cancer. Pathol Int. 2015;65(8):399–403.

50. Deng J, Zhang R, Pan Y, Wang B, Wu L, Hao X, Liang H. N stages of the seventh edition of TNM Classification are the most intensive variables for predictions of the overall survival of gastric cancer

patients who underwent limited lymphadenectomy. Tumour Biol. 2014;35(4):3269–81.

51. Reim D, Loos M, Vogl F, Novotny A, Schuster T, Langer R, Becker K, Höfler H, Siveke J, Bassermann F, Friess H, Schuhmacher C. Prognostic implications of the seventh edition of the international union against cancer classification for patients with gastric cancer: the Western experience of patients treated in a single-center European institution. J Clin Oncol. 2013;31(2):263–71.

52. Bruno L, Nesi G, Montinaro F, Carassale G, Boddi V, Bechi P, Cortesini C. Clinicopathologic characteristics and outcome indicators in node-negative gastric cancer. J Surg Oncol. 2000;74:30–2.

53. Hyung WJ, Lee JH, Choi SH, Min JS, Noh SH. Prognostic impact of lymphatic and/or blood vessel invasion in patients with node-negative advanced gastric cancer. Ann Surg Oncol. 2002;9(6):562–7.

54. Deng J, Liang H, Sun D, Zhang R, Zhan H, Wang X. Prognosis of gastric cancer patients with node-negative metastasis following curative resection: outcomes of the survival and recurrence. Can J Gastroenterol. 2008;22(10):835–9.

55. Biffi R, Botteri E, Cenciarelli S, Luca F, Pozzi S, Valvo M, Sonzogni A, Chiappa A, Leal Ghezzi T, Rotmensz N, Bagnardi V, Andreoni B. Impact on survival of the number of lymph nodes removed in patients with node-negative gastric cancer submitted to extended lymph node dissection. Eur J Surg Oncol. 2011;37(4):305–11.

56. Martinez-Ramos D, Calero A, Escrig-Sos J, Mingol F, Daroca-Jose JM, Sauri M, Arroyo A, Salvador-Sanchis JL, de Juan M, Calpena R, Lacueva FJ. Prognosis for gastric carcinomas with an insufficient number of examined negative lymph nodes. Eur J Surg Oncol. 2014;40(3):358–65.

57. Deng J, Liang H, Wang D, Sun D, Ding X, Pan Y, Liu X. Enhancement the prediction of postoperative survival in gastric cancer by combining the negative lymph node count with ratio between positive and examined lymph nodes. Ann Surg Oncol. 2010;17(4):1043–51.

58. Doekhie FS, Mesker WE, van Krieken JH, Kok NF, Hartgrink HH, Kranenbarg EK, Putter H, Kuppen PJ, Tanke HJ, Tollenaar RA, van de Velde CJ. Clinical relevance of occult tumor cells in lymph nodes from gastric cancer patients. Am J Surg Pathol. 2005;29(9):1135–44.

59. Tavares A, Monteiro-Soares M, Viveiros F, Maciel Barbosa J, Dinis-Ribeiro M. Occult tumor cells in lymph nodes of patients with gastric cancer: A systematic review on their prevalence and predictive role. Oncology. 2015 Jul 7. [Epub ahead of print].

60. Wu Song, Yujie Yuan, Liang Wang, Weiling He, Xinhua Zhang, Chuangqi Chen, Changhua Zhang, Shirong Cai, Yulong He. The prognostic value of lymph nodes dissection number on survival of patients with lymph node-negative gastric cancer. Gastroenterol Res Pract. 2014;2014:603194.

61. Yonemura Y, Endo Y, Hayashi I, Kawamura T, Yun HY, Bandou E. Proliferative activity of micrometastases in the lymph nodes of patients with gastric cancer. Br J Surg. 2007;94(6):731–6.

62. Lee HS, Kim MA, Yang HK, Lee BL, Kim WH. Prognostic implication of isolated tumor cells and micrometastases in regional lymph nodes of gastric cancer. World J Gastroenterol. 2005;11(38):5920–5.

63. Jeuck TL, Wittekind C. Gastric carcinoma: stage migration by immunohistochemically detected lymph node micrometastases. Gastric Cancer. 2015;18(1):100–8.

64. Brasilino de Carvalho M. Quantitative analysis of the extent of extracapsular invasion and its prognostic significance: a prospective study of 170 cases of carcinoma of the larynx and hypopharynx. Head Neck. 1998;20(1):16–21.

65. Fisher BJ, Perera FE, Cooke AL, Opeitum A, Dar AR, Venkatesan VM, Stitt L, Radwan JS. Extracapsular axillary node extension in patients receiving adjuvant systemic therapy: an indication for radiotherapy? Int J Radiat Oncol Biol Phys. 1997;38(3):551–9.

66. Fleischmann A, Thalmann GN, Markwalder R, Studer UE. Prognostic implications of extracapsular extension of pelvic lymph node metastases in urothelial carcinoma of the bladder. Am J Surg Pathol. 2005;29(1):89–95.

67. Griebling TL, Ozkutlu D, See WA, Cohen MB. Prognostic implications of extracapsular extension of lymph node metastases in prostate cancer. Mod Pathol. 1997;10(8):804–9.

68. Myers JN, Greenberg JS, Mo V, Roberts D. Extracapsular spread. A significant predictor of treatment failure in patients with squamous cell carcinoma of the tongue. Cancer. 2001;92(12):3030–306.

69. Ishida T, Tateishi M, Kaneko S, Sugimachi K. Surgical treatment of patients with nonsmall-cell lung cancer and mediastinal lymph node involvement. J Surg Oncol. 1990;43(3):161–6.

70. van der Velden J, van Lindert AC, Lammes FB, Lammes FB, ten Kate FJ, Sie-Go DM, Oosting H, Heintz AP. Extracapsular growth of lymph node metastases in squamous cell carcinoma of the vulva. The impact on recurrence and survival. Cancer. 1995;75(12):2885–90.

71. Wind J, Lagarde SM, Ten Kate FJ, Ubbink DT, Bemelman WA, van Lanschot JJ. A systematic review on the significance of extracapsular lymph node involvement in gastrointestinal malignancies. Eur J Surg Oncol. 2007;33(4):401–8.

72. Tanaka T, Kumagai K, Shimizu K, Masuo K, Yamagata K. Peritoneal metastasis in gastric cancer with particular reference to lymphatic advancement; extranodal invasion is a significant risk factor for peritoneal metastasis. J Surg Oncol. 2000;75(3):165–71.

73. Kumagai K, Tanaka T, Yamagata K, Yokoyama N, Shimizu K. Liver metastasis in gastric cancer with particular reference to lymphatic advancement. Gastric Cancer. 2001;4(3):150–5.

74. Alakus H, Hölscher AH, Grass G, Hartmann E, Schulte C, Drebber U, Baldus SE, Bollschweiler E, Metzger R, Mönig SP. Extracapsular lymph node spread: a new prognostic factor in gastric cancer. Cancer. 2010;116(2):309–15.

75. Okamoto T, Tsuburaya A, Kameda Y, Yoshikawa T, Cho H, Tsuchida K, Hasegawa S, Noguchi Y. Prognostic value of extracapsular invasion and fibrotic focus in single lymph node metastasis of gastric cancer. Gastric Cancer. 2008;11(3):160–7.

76. Nakamura K, Ozaki N, Yamada T, Hata T, Sugimoto S, Hikino H, Kanazawa A, Tokuka A, Nagaoka S. Evaluation of prognostic significance in extracapsular spread of lymph node metastasis in patients with gastric cancer. Surgery. 2005;137(5):511–7.

77. Cho JY. Molecular diagnosis for personalized target therapy in gastric cancer. J Gastric Cancer. 2013;13(3):129–35.

78. Wu HH, Lin WC, Tsai KW. Advances in molecular biomarkers for gastric cancer: miRNAs as emerging novel cancer markers. Expert Rev Mol Med. 2014;16:e1.

79. Tahara T, Arisawa T. DNA methylation as a molecular biomarker in gastric cancer. Epigenomics. 2015;7(3):475–86.

80. Kaur A, Dasanu CA. Targeting the HER2 pathway for the therapy of lower esophageal and gastric adenocarcinoma. Expert Opin Pharmacother. 2011;12(16):2493–503.

81. Ananiev J, Gulubova M, Manolova I, Tchernev G. Prognostic significance of HER2/neu expression in gastric cancer. Wien Klin Wochenschr. 2011;123(13–14):450–4.

82. Jørgensen JT, Hersom M. HER2 as a prognostic marker in gastric cancer – a systematic analysis of data from the literature. J Cancer. 2012;3:137–44.

83. Bouché O, Penault-Llorca F. HER2 and gastric cancer: a novel therapeutic target for trastuzumab. Bull Cancer. 2010;97(12):1429–40.

84. He C, Bian XY, Ni XZ, Shen DP, Shen YY, Liu H, Shen ZY, Liu Q. Correlation of human epidermal growth factor receptor 2 expression with clinicopathological characteristics and prognosis in gastric cancer. World J Gastroenterol. 2013;19(14):2171–8.

85. Dang HZ, Yu Y, Jiao SC. Prognosis of HER2 overexpressing gastric cancer patients with liver metastasis. World J Gastroenterol. 2012;18(19):2402–7.

86. Yamaguchi N, Yanagawa T, Yoshimura T, Kohrogi N, Tanaka K, Nakamura Y, Okubo T. Use of tumor diameter to estimate the growth kinetics of cancer and sensitivity of screening tests. Environ Health Perspect. 1990;87:63–7.

87. Wang X, Wan F, Pan J, Yu GZ, Chen Y, Wang JJ. Tumor size: a non-neglectable independent prognostic factor for gastric cancer. J Surg Oncol. 2008;97(3):236–40.

88. Liu X, Xu Y, Long Z, Zhu H, Wang Y. Prognostic significance of tumor size in T3 gastric cancer. Ann Surg Oncol. 2009;16(7):1875–82.

89. Jun KH, Jung H, Baek JM, Chin HM, Park WB. Does tumor size have an impact on gastric cancer? A single institute experience. Langenbeck's Arch Surg. 2009;394(4):631–5.

90. Bilici A, Uygun K, Seker M, Ustaalioglu BB, Aliustaoglu M, Temiz S, Aksu G, Gezen C, Yavuzer D, Kaya S, Salepci T, Mayadagli A, Gumus M. The effect of tumor size on overall survival in patients with pT3 gastric cancer: experiences from 3 centers. Onkologie. 2010;33(12):676–82.

91. Deng J, Liang H, Sun D, Pan Y, Liu Y, Wang DC. Extended lymphadenectomy improvement of overall survival of GC patients with perigastric node metastasis. Langenbeck Arch Surg. 2011;396(5):615–23.

92. Deng J, Zhang R, Wu LL, Zhang L, Wang X, Liu Y, Hao X, Liang H. Superiority of the ratio between negative and positive lymph nodes for predicting the prognosis for patients with gastric cancer. Ann Surg Oncol. 2015;22(4):1258–66.

Part III

Diagnosis of Gastric Cancer

Endoscopic Diagnosis: Esophagogastroduodenoscopy (EGD) and Endoscopic Ultrasound (EUS)

3

Sang Kil Lee and Hyunsoo Chung

EGD

EGD is currently the procedure of choice for the diagnosis of gastric cancer regardless of stage. Gastric cancer typically presents as a mass lesion but may present as a non-healing gastric ulcer or as a diffuse infiltrative form known as linitis plastica [1]. The standard for the diagnosis of gastric cancer is endoscopic biopsy. Generally, the mass or abnormal mucosa is targeted for biopsy, although in the case of a malignant gastric ulcer, at least six to eight biopsies of the heaped-up edges of the ulcer and base should be performed [2]. However, a recent study suggested that three to four biopsy samples are usually sufficient to diagnose advanced gastric cancer in gastric ulcers with 95% sensitivity [3]. EGD has largely replaced upper GI series as the initial test of choice for the diagnosis of gastric cancer. From the survey in 2006 in Korea, Koreans prefer endoscopy as a gastric cancer screening method, compared to UGI (67% vs 33%) [4, 5]. If gastric cancer cannot be excluded, repeated biopsy should be performed, especially in patients aged over 60. A Japanese study reported that gastric cancer was detected at repeated EGD in 17.2% of patients with gas-

tric adenoma and in 2.2% of those with gastric ulcer in the initial examination [6].

Early Gastric Cancer (EGC)

EGC is defined as carcinoma limited to gastric mucosa and/or submucosa regardless of lymph node status [7]. The Paris endoscopic classification of superficial neoplastic lesions is currently being used for morphologic classification of EGC [8, 9] (Fig. 3.1). The three types include superficial polypoid (type 0-I), superficial flat/depressed (types 0-IIa-c), and superficial excavated (type 0-III) lesions.

Type 0 lesions are classified in three distinct groups:

- Type 0-I, polypoid (Fig. 3.2)
- *Type 0-I includes two variants: pedunculated (0-Ip) and sessile (0-Is).*
- Type 0-II, non-polypoid and non-excavated (Fig. 3.3)
- *Type 0-II includes three variants: slightly elevated (0-IIa), completely flat (0-IIb), and slightly depressed without ulcer (0-IIc).*
- Type 0-III, non-polypoid with a frank ulcer (Fig. 3.4)

The distinction between a depressed (0-IIc) and an excavated or ulcerated lesion (0-III) is readily made in the operative specimen. In the

S. K. Lee (✉) · H. Chung
Internal Medicine, Yonsei University College of Medicine, Seoul, Republic of Korea
e-mail: SKLEE@yuhs.ac

© Springer-Verlag GmbH Germany, part of Springer Nature 2019
S. H. Noh, W. J. Hyung (eds.), *Surgery for Gastric Cancer*,
https://doi.org/10.1007/978-3-662-45583-8_3

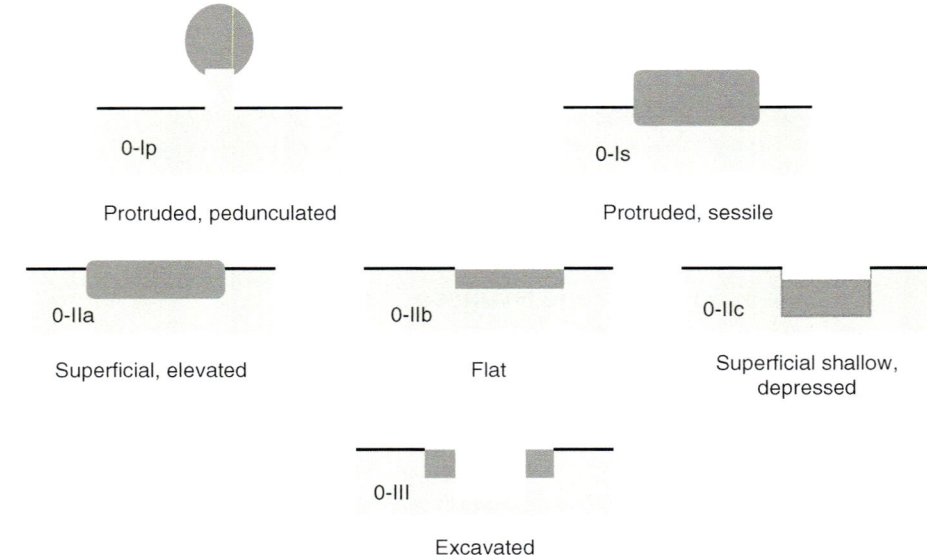

0-Ip

Protruded, pedunculated

0-Is

Protruded, sessile

0-IIa

Superficial, elevated

0-IIb

Flat

0-IIc

Superficial shallow, depressed

0-III

Excavated

Fig. 3.1 Schematic depiction of the major variants of type 0 neoplastic lesions of the stomach: polypoid (Ip and Is), non-polypoid (IIa, IIb, and IIc), and non-polypoid and excavated (III). (From Ref. [8])

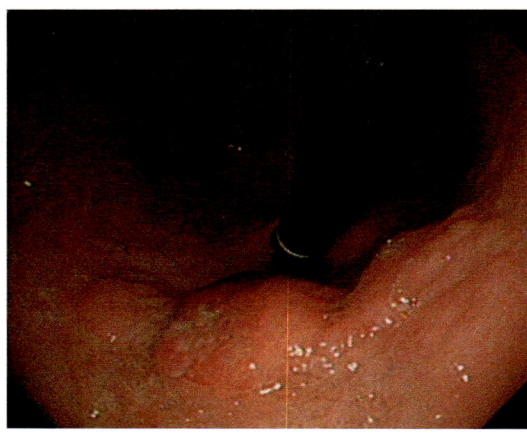

Fig. 3.2 Type 0-I, polypoid

excavated lesion, there is a sharp discontinuity in the epithelial layer, and the muscularis mucosae are interrupted. The most commonly observed subtype is 0-IIc. Mixed types associate two distinct types of morphology. Superficial tumors with two or more components should have all components recorded in order of the surface area occupied [10]. For instance, a depressed lesion with elevated borders or a central elevation is classified as type 0-IIc + IIa. An elevated lesion with a central depression at its top is classified as type 0-IIa + IIc. 0-IIa + IIc lesions have a poorer prognosis, with a risk of large invasion in the submucosa than all other types of lesions.

Tips for Early Detection of Gastric Cancer

To detect EGC, there are some important points on preparation and observation. First of all, removal of mucus is essential in the detection of superficial cancers because the surface of gastric mucosa is covered by thick mucus. This will make cleaning of mucus easier with a small amount of water mixed with dimethicone. Oral mucolytic (pronase) and anti-foring agents defoamers can improve the quality of examination by rinsing away mucus or bubbles. Enough obervation time is important for detection of early gastric cancer as withdrawal time of colonoscopy is important for polyp detection. Regardless of the appearance of the lesion, careful examination of color and shape, demarcation of rising borders, and surface pattern are important. Elevated lesions can be easily detected even for beginners. Differentiating neoplastic lesion such as adenocarcinoma and

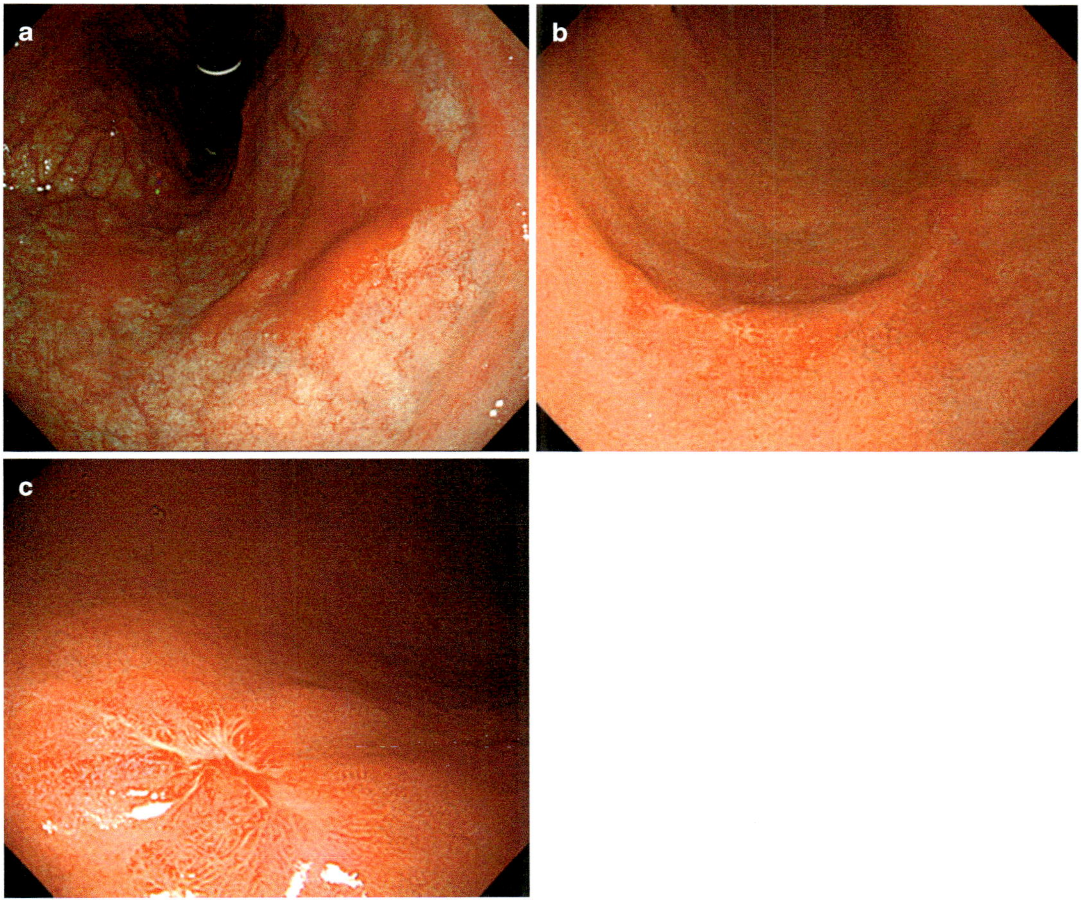

Fig. 3.3 Type 0-II, non-polypoid and non-excavated: (**a**) Ia, (**b**) IIb, (**c**) IIc

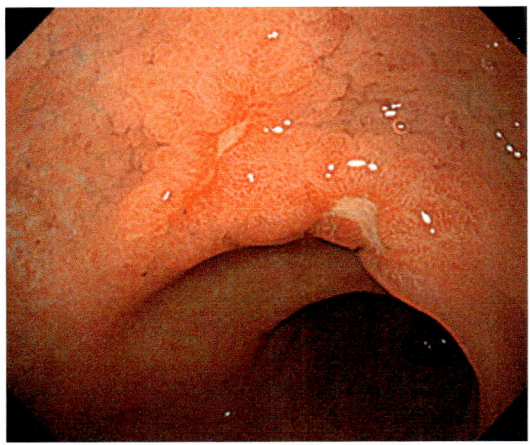

Fig. 3.4 Type 0-III, non-polypoid with a frank ulcer

tubular adenoma, from nonneoplastic lesions (hyperplastic polyp, fundic gland polyp, subepithelial lesions, or intestinal metaplasia), is important. If lesion shows red-colored, flat-elevated appearance with irregular surface patterns and irregular borders, biopsy should be taken to differentiated adenocarcinoma. Tubular adenoma shows well-demarcated flat-elevated lesions with regular nodular surface. Subepithelial lesions can be also seen as elevated lesions, but border of the lesion is generally smooth because the overlying mucosa is nonneoplastic. When depressed lesion is detected, it is important to differentiate erosion and focal atrophy from adenocarcinoma. Generally, well-differentiated adenocarcinoma is reddish in color, whereas undifferentiated adenocarcinoma is whitish because it destroys vessels while growing.

When lesion shows irregular but well-demarcated depressions, the risk of adenocarcinoma is high. Erosion or focal atrophy shows regular, smooth shapes with unclear demarcation.

Advanced Gastric Cancer (AGC)

T2–4 tumors usually manifest as advanced types. The gross appearance of advanced gastric carcinomas can be exophytic, ulcerated, infiltrative, or combined. Based on Borrmann's classification, the gross appearance of advanced gastric carcinomas can be divided into type I (mass) for polypoid tumors, sharply demarcated from the surrounding mucosa; type II (ulcerative) for ulcerated tumors with raised margins surrounded by a thickened gastric wall with clear margins; type III (infiltrative ulcerative) for ulcerated tumors with raised margins, surrounded by a thickened gastric wall; and type IV (diffuse infiltrative) for tumors without marked ulceration or raised margins, diffusely infiltrating growth which is also referred to as linitis plastica when most of gastric wall is involved by infiltrating tumor cells [11] (Fig. 3.5). Tumors that cannot be classified into any of the above types can be classified as type V (unclassifiable). Particularly, in type IV gastric cancer, caution should be exercised when taking biopsy and interpreting pathologic reports, because risk of false-negative result of biopsy specimen can be higher than any other types. Repeated deep biopsy at a focused lesion is recommended if there is no mucosal ulceration or defect in the stomach.

EUS

EUS plays an important role in the diagnosis and staging of gastric cancer. EUS allows the visualization of the five layers of the gastric wall. The superficial gastric mucosa is represented by an echogenic first layer and the deeper mucosa by a hypoechogenic second layer; the submucosa is represented by an echogenic third layer, the muscularis propria as a hypoechogenic fourth layer, and the serosa as an echogenic fifth layer.

EUS is especially useful in the locoregional staging for gastric cancer. The therapeutic extent in 30% of surgical candidates has changed by the use of EUS in the preoperative stage of gastric cancer, resulting in more limited surgical resections, especially in stages T1 and T3 [12]. The overall accuracy of EUS in determining T stage ranges from 71% to 92%. A recent systematic review by analyzing the data on 7747 people from 66 articles published from 1988 through 2012, with gastric cancer, who were staged with endoscopic ultrasonography (EUS), also support the usefulness of EUS for the locoregional staging (Fig. 3.6). It showed that sensitivity and specificity of EUS in discriminating T1–T2 (superficial) versus T3–T4 (advanced) gastric carcinomas were 0.86 (95% CI 0.81–0.90) and 0.90 (95% CI 0.87–0.93). For the diagnostic

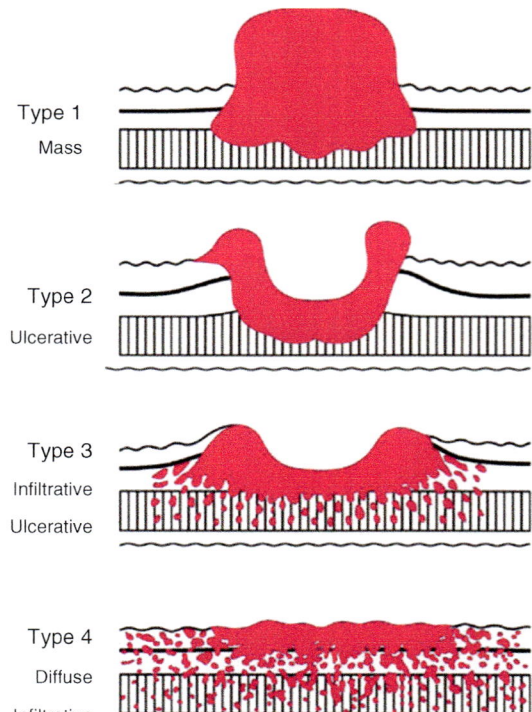

Fig. 3.5 Macroscopic type of AGC (Borrmann type): (**a**) Type 1, (**b**) Type 2, (**c**) Type 3, (**d**) Type 4

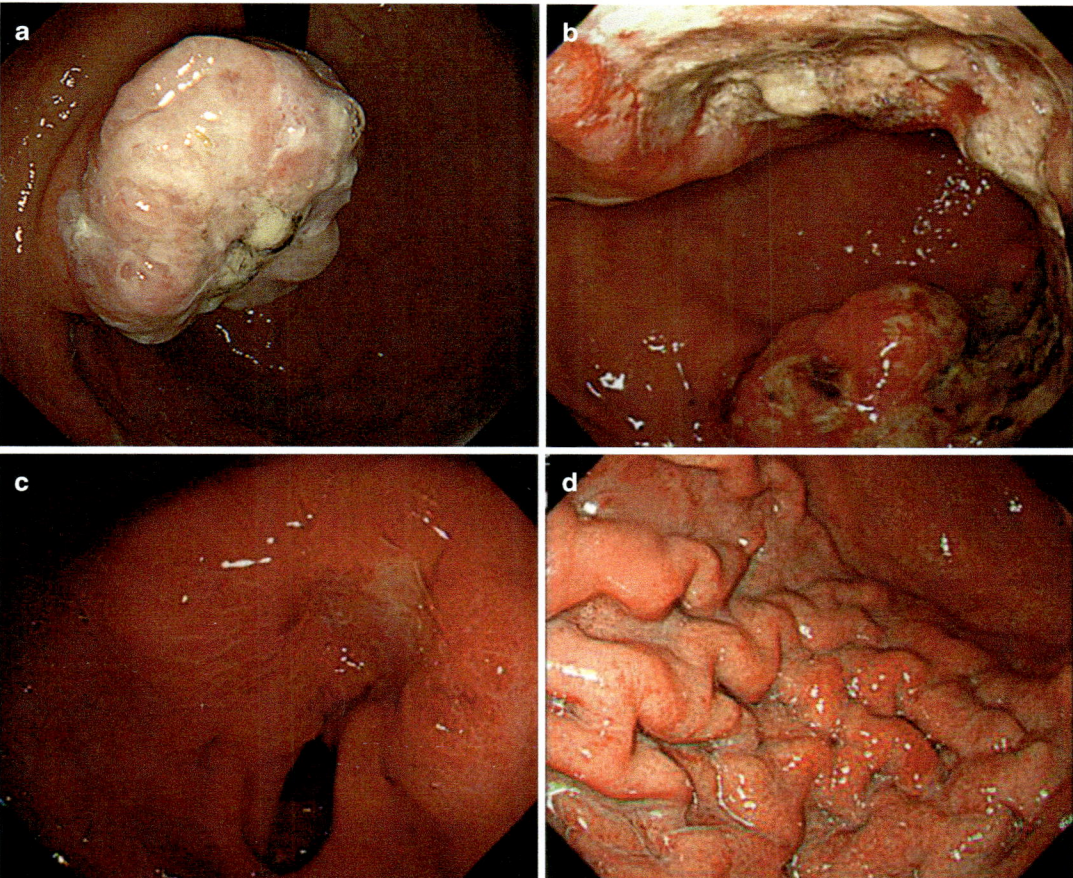

Fig. 3.5 (continued)

capacity to distinguish T1 (early gastric cancer, EGC) versus T2 (muscle-infiltrating) tumors, the sensitivity and specificity of EUS were 0.85 (95% CI 0.78–0.91) and 0.90 (95% CI 0.85–0.93), respectively. In addition, for the capacity to distinguish between T1a (mucosal) versus T1b (submucosal) cancers, sensitivity and specificity were 0.87 (95% CI 0.81–0.92) and 0.75 (95% CI 0.62–0.84), respectively [13]. In this systematic review, in the nodal staging, sensitivity and specificity were 0.83 (95% CI 0.79–0.87) and 0.67 (95% CI 0.61–0.72), respectively. Lower specificity for N staging may lie in the fact that many small lymph nodes can also harbor metastases, artifact of ultrasound can interfere full and thorough evaluation of regional lymph node station, and the scope cannot introduce the full

length of the stomach in some advanced cases. Overall, EUS accuracy can be considered clinically useful to guide physicians in the locoregional staging of patients with gastric cancer. However, the results must be taken with caution because between-study heterogeneity was not negligible, and thus all the results presented here must be taken with caution. Especially, accuracy for EUS T staging can be different according to the expertise of endoscopists, shape, and size of the lesion. In addition, overstaging is more common than understaging for the lesion with ulceration because overstaging could be attributed to peritumoral fibrosis, ulceration, and inflammation. EUS also can identify and sample by fine-needle aspiration and/or biopsy (FNA/FNB) submucosal or infiltrative lesions, such as gastric

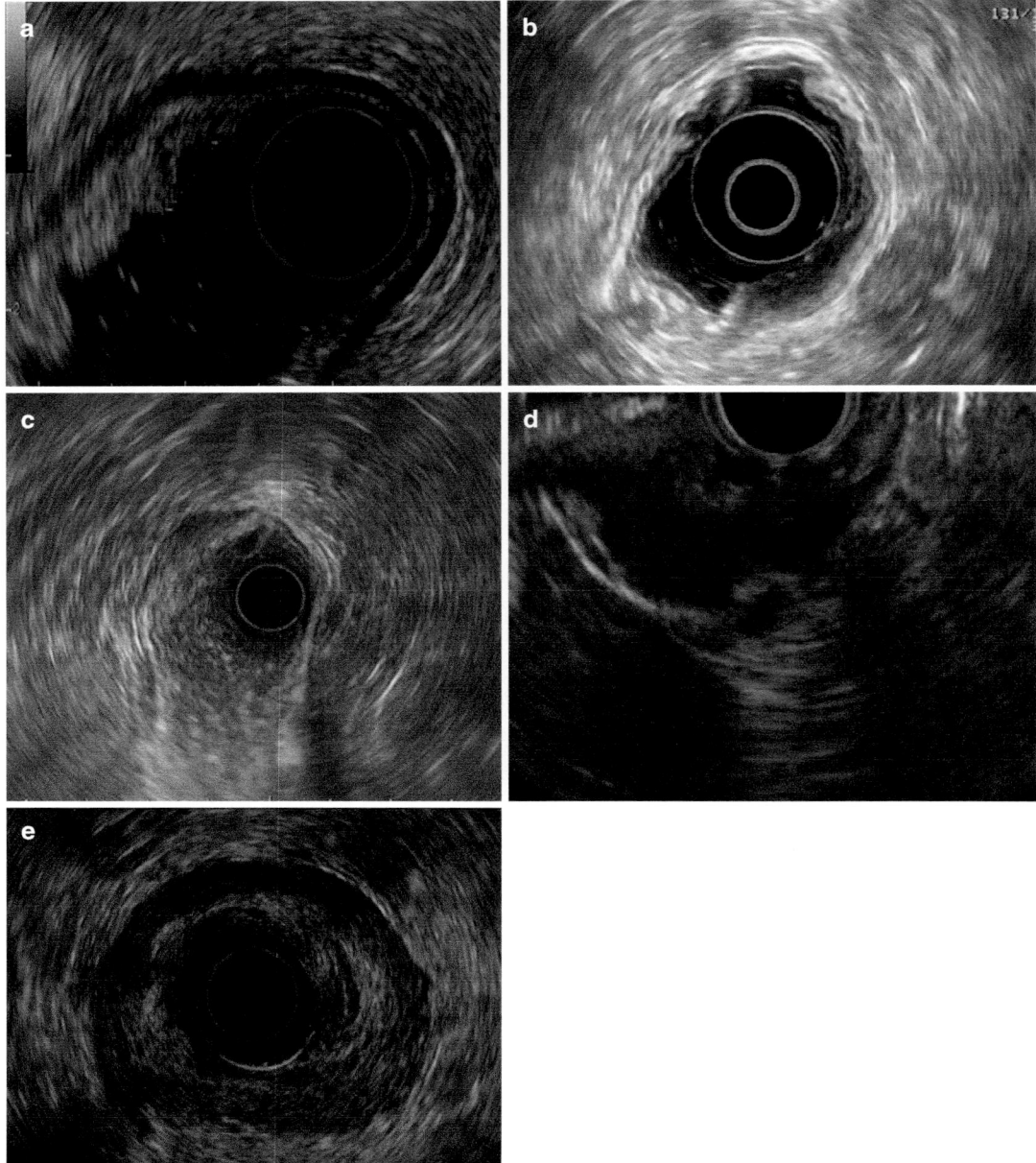

Fig. 3.6 EUS finding of each T stage. (**a**) T1a, invasion to mucosa; (**b**) T1b, invasion to submucosa; (**c**) T2, invasion to proper muscle; (**d**) T3, invasion to subserosa; (**e**) T4, invasion to serosa or adjacent structures

lymphomas, stromal tumors, and linitis plastica that are usually observed as thickened gastric fold on CT scan or endoscopy.

References

1. Committee ASoP, Evans JA, Chandrasekhara V, et al. The role of endoscopy in the management of premalignant and malignant conditions of the stomach. Gastrointest Endosc. 2015;82:1–8.
2. Graham DY, Schwartz JT, Cain GD, et al. Prospective evaluation of biopsy number in the diagnosis of esophageal and gastric carcinoma. Gastroenterology. 1982;82:228–31.
3. Choi Y, Choi HS, Jeon WK, et al. Optimal number of endoscopic biopsies in diagnosis of advanced gastric and colorectal cancer. J Korean Med Sci. 2012;27:36–9.
4. Jun JK, Choi KS, Lee HY, et al. Effectiveness of the Korean National Cancer Screening Program in reducing gastric cancer mortality. Gastroenterology. 2017;152:1319–1328 e7.
5. Choi KS, Kwak MS, Lee HY, et al. Screening for gastric cancer in Korea: population-based preferences for endoscopy versus upper gastrointestinal series. Cancer Epidemiol Biomark Prev. 2009;18:1390–8.
6. Hosokawa O, Watanabe K, Hatorri M, et al. Detection of gastric cancer by repeat endoscopy within a short time after negative examination. Endoscopy. 2001;33:301–5.
7. Saragoni L, Morgagni P, Gardini A, et al. Early gastric cancer: diagnosis, staging, and clinical impact. Evaluation of 530 patients. New elements for an updated definition and classification. Gastric Cancer. 2013;16:549–54.
8. The Paris endoscopic classification of superficial neoplastic lesions: esophagus, stomach, and colon: November 30 to December 1, 2002. Gastrointest Endosc. 2003;58:S3–43.
9. Endoscopic Classification Review G. Update on the Paris classification of superficial neoplastic lesions in the digestive tract. Endoscopy. 2005;37:570–8.
10. Japanese Gastric Cancer A. Japanese classification of gastric carcinoma: 3rd English edition. Gastric Cancer. 2011;14:101–12.
11. Hu B, El Hajj N, Sittler S, et al. Gastric cancer: classification, histology and application of molecular pathology. J Gastrointest Oncol. 2012;3:251–61.
12. Dinis-Ribeiro M, Kuipers EJ. Identification of gastric atrophic changes: from histopathology to endoscopy. Endoscopy. 2015;47:533–7.
13. Mocellin S, Pasquali S. Diagnostic accuracy of endoscopic ultrasonography (EUS) for the preoperative locoregional staging of primary gastric cancer. Cochrane Database Syst Rev. 2015:CD009944.

Radiologic Diagnosis (CT, MRI, & PET-CT)

4

Nieun Seo, Joon Seok Lim, and Arthur Cho

CT

Introduction

In patients with gastric cancer, CT has been routinely performed for preoperative evaluation and accurate tumor staging. In particular, technical development in CT such as multidetector-row helical CT (MDCT), three-dimensional (3D) reformation, and CT angiography provides dedicated tumor staging, extraluminal information, surgical mapping, and preoperative evaluation of perigastric vascular anatomy.

Tumor Staging

T Staging
Accurate T staging is the most essential part in determining proper treatment plans. Although the gastric wall consists of the five histologic layers (mucosa, submucosa, muscularis propria, subserosa, and serosa), the normal gastric wall is seen as a two- or three-layered structure at the contrast-enhanced CT, that is, (1) prominent enhancing

inner mucosa, (2) low-attenuation submucosa, and (3) slightly higher attenuation outer muscular-serosal layers [1]. Gastric cancer appears as thickening of gastric wall with increased enhancement and destruction of normal layered pattern. On CT, gastric cancer can manifest as focal wall thickening with or without ulceration, polypoid mass, or diffuse infiltrative lesion [2]. Particularly, signet ring cell subtype of gastric cancer usually demonstrates scirrhous tumor of the stomach, leading to the destruction of gastric folds and diffuse thickening of gastric wall (linitis plastica) (Fig. 4.1) [3].

Conventionally, the extent of mural invasion of gastric cancer on CT has been categorized as follows (Fig. 4.2) [4]: In T1 and T2 lesions,

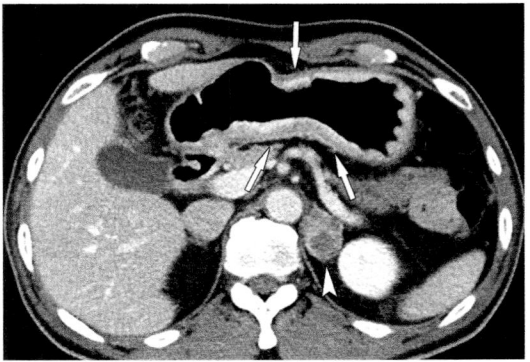

Fig. 4.1 Signet ring cell carcinoma in a 53-year-old man with stomach cancer. Axial CT image shows diffuse thickening of gastric wall due to linitis plastica. As a left adrenal mass (arrowhead) did not show interval change during follow-up, it is thought to be an adenoma

N. Seo · J. S. Lim (✉)
Department of Diagnostic Radiology, Yonsei University Health System, Seoul, Republic of Korea
e-mail: jslim1@yuhs.ac

A. Cho
Department of Nuclear Medicine, Yonsei University Health System, Seoul, Republic of Korea

© Springer-Verlag GmbH Germany, part of Springer Nature 2019
S. H. Noh, W. J. Hyung (eds.), *Surgery for Gastric Cancer*,
https://doi.org/10.1007/978-3-662-45583-8_4

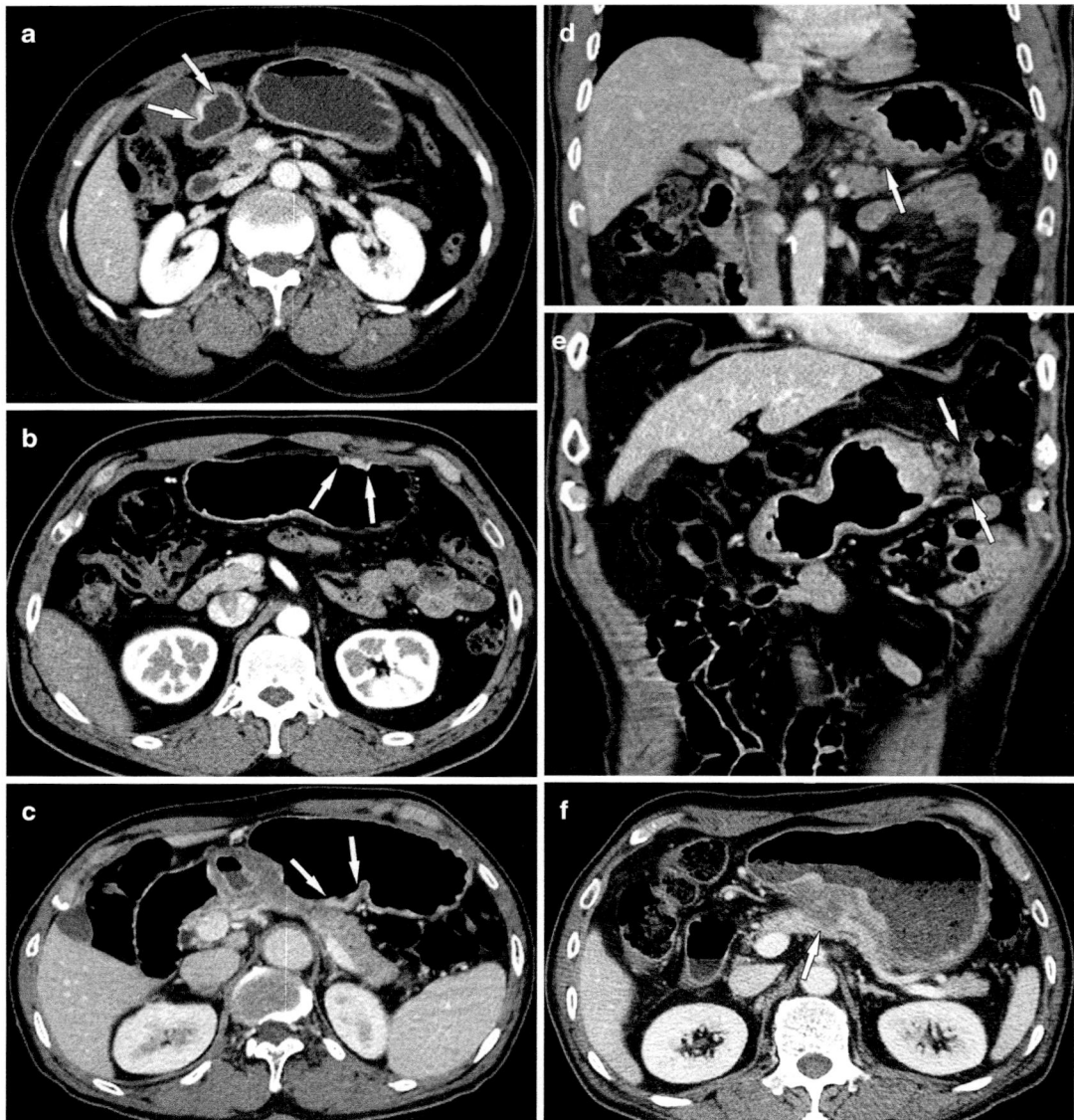

Fig. 4.2 Stage T1–T4 gastric cancers. (**a**) Axial CT image shows a stage T1 cancer (pathological T1b cancer) with focal nontransmural enhancement in the proximal antrum (arrows). (**b**) Axial CT image shows a stage T2 cancer (arrows), an ulcerofungating lesion at midbody without perigastric extension. (**c**) Axial CT image shows a stage T3 cancer (arrows), with minimal infiltration of the perigastric fat tissue in gastric angle. (**d**) Coronal reformatted image shows a stage T4a cancer (arrow), enhancing wall thickening of upper body with gross infiltration of the perigastric fat tissue. (**e**) Coronal reformatted image shows a stage T4b cancer (arrows), infiltrating the distal transverse colon. (**f**) Axial CT image demonstrates a stage T4b cancer (arrow), an advanced cancer with gross extension to the pancreatic body

invasion is limited to the gastric mural wall, and the outer border is smooth with clear perigastric fat. In T3 and T4a lesions, the outer border of gastric wall is obscured, and strand-like increased attenuation in the perigastric fat could be seen. In T4b lesions, direct extension of gastric cancer into adjacent organs or structures is visualized on CT.

Recently, the up-to-date MDCT technique using thin section thickness, optimal contrast enhancement, and MPR with 3D imaging provides the more detailed information for T staging.

T1a cancers often show increased enhancement of the inner mucosal layer without wall thickening, but they are not generally detected on 2D axial images. T1b cancers more frequently appear as well-enhancing mucosal thickening than T1a cancers do [5]. 3D endoluminal images can improve depiction of T1 gastric cancers (Fig. 4.3). In differentiation between T1b and T2 cancers, T1b cancers show visualized outer low-attenuation stripe of gastric wall, while T2 cancers show destruction of the outer low-attenuation stripe but clear outer surface of gastric wall [5]. In

T3 cancers with subserosal invasion, distinction between the enhancing gastric lesion and the outer layer is nearly impossible, and a smooth outer margin or a few small linear strandings in the perigastic tissue can be detected [6]. T4a cancers have serosal involvement and can show irregular or nodular outer margin of gastric wall with a dense band-like infiltration in perigastric fat [6]. T4b cancers demonstrate direct invasion of gastric tumor into a contiguous organ or structure and show obliteration of the fat plane between gastric cancer and contiguous organs. As the indications of laparoscopic gastrectomy include T1–3N0M0 disease, differentiation of T1–3 (within subsero-

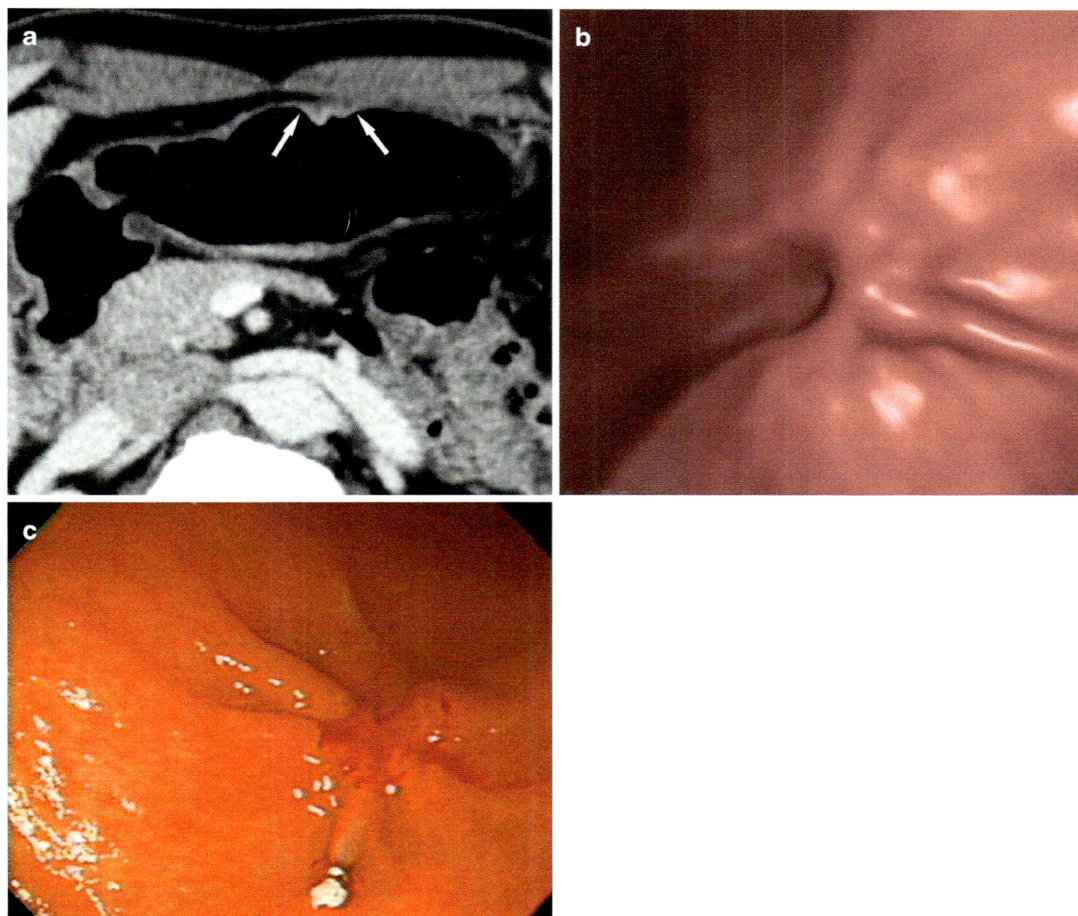

Fig. 4.3 Multidetector-row CT (MDCT) with three-dimensional (3D) imaging of T1b cancer. (**a**) Axial CT image depicts focal enhancement of a nontransmural lesion in proximal antrum (arrows). (**b**) Virtual gastros-copy shows an ulcerative lesion with clubbing or radiating fold at the corresponding site. (**c**) Endoscopy shows a discrete ulcer with abnormal surrounding folds at antrum. A hemoclip was applied to proximal margin of the lesion

sal extension) and T4 cancers (beyond subserosal extension) is especially important when considering whether laparoscopic gastrectomy could be indicated or not. Adding MPR images to axial CT images has been reported to improve the diagnostic performance for distinguishing T3 and T4a from T4b gastric cancer and predicting adjacent organ invasion [7]. However, differentiation between T3 and T4a cancers on CT imaging is nearly impossible because the discrimination between subserosal and serosal layers on visual assessment is impractical due to the limited spatial resolution of CT. Moreover, individual variations in the amount of subserosal adipose tissue make it more difficult to differentiate between T3 and T4a stage cancers [8].

Then, what about diagnostic performance of CT for T staging in gastric cancers? According to a meta-analysis which was published in 2006, the diagnostic accuracy of overall T staging on CT ranged from 77.1% to 88.9% [9]. The sensitivity and specificity for evaluating serosal exposure were 82.8–100% and 80–96.8%, respectively [9]. Another meta-analysis which was published in 2012 demonstrated that the overall pooled accuracy of T staging on CT was 71.5%, and CT scanners with more than four detectors and MPR images could improve diagnostic accuracy [10]. The detection rate of early gastric cancer (EGC) has been shown in various results from study to study. Kim et al. [6] reported that the detection rate of EGC was 76.3% on 2D images and 92.1% on 3D images, respectively. However, Lee et al. [5] reported disappointing results that the detection rate of EGC on 2D and 3D imaging was only 45% and 59%, respectively. 3D imaging including virtual gastroscopy improves the detection rate of EGC [11, 12], while combined MPR images and axial images improve the T staging accuracy, especially in advanced gastric cancer (AGC) [6].

N Staging

The N stage in the AJCC classification system is determined according to the number of metastatic lymph nodes [13]. Positive lymph nodes on CT are suspected on the basis of size, configuration, and enhancement pattern of lymph nodes. Reported CT criteria of metastatic lymph nodes include the

following: (1) lymph node more than 8–10 mm in diameter along the short axis, (2) nearly round shape (short-to-long axis ratios of more than 0.7), (3) central necrosis, (4) strong or heterogeneous enhancement, and (5) aggregated three or more perilesional lymph nodes regardless of their size [3, 14–16]. However, the diagnostic accuracy for preoperative diagnosis of metastatic lymph nodes is still unsatisfactory, ranged between 51% and 76% [1, 17–19]. A meta-analysis by Kwee et al. [9] demonstrated the wide ranges of sensitivity (62.5–91.9%) and specificity (50.0–87.9%) of MDCT for N staging, and these results indicate the lack of worldwide consensus for determining metastatic lymph nodes. CT has a major limitation in that it cannot detect cancer involvement of normal-size lymph nodes (microscopic metastasis) and rarely distinguish between reactive hyperplasia and metastatic enlargement. Even after the use of MPR images and 3D imaging in addition to axial CT images, accuracy of nodal staging has not significantly improved [11, 16].

Although the anatomical nodal location is not incorporated in the AJCC N staging, it is still important because the D classification, a description of the extent of lymphadenectomy, is based on the level of lymph node dissection (D1–D4). The D2 dissection is the standard surgical procedure for potentially curable T2–T4 gastric cancers and cT1N+ tumors (Figs. 4.4, 4.5 and 4.6) [20].

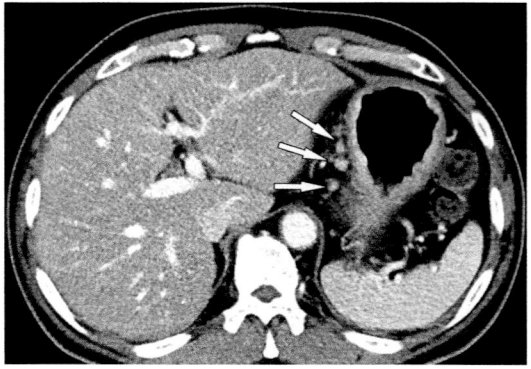

Fig. 4.4 Station 3 lymph node metastases in a 54-year-old man with stomach cancer. Axial CT image demonstrates several clustered round lymph nodes at lesser curvature along the branches of the left gastric artery (arrows)

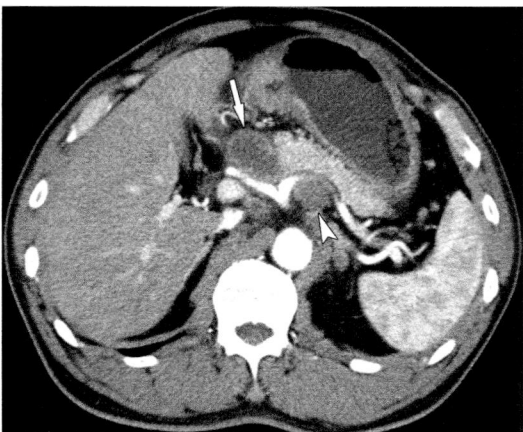

Fig. 4.5 Station 8 and 11 lymph node metastases in a 61-year-old man with stomach cancer. Axial CT image shows an enlarged necrotic lymph node in station 8 (arrow) adjacent to common hepatic artery and an enlarged lymph node in station 11 (arrowhead) along proximal splenic artery

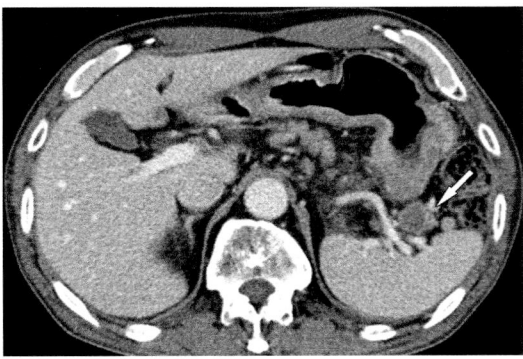

Fig. 4.6 Station 10 lymph node metastasis in a 74-year-old man with stomach cancer. Axial CT image depicts an enlarged necrotic lymph node in station 10 (arrow) at the splenic hilum

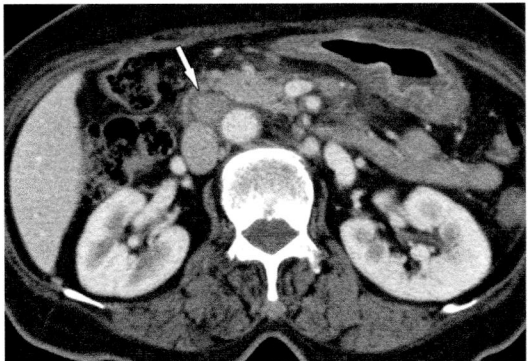

Fig. 4.7 Station 13 lymph node metastasis in a 79-year-old woman with stomach cancer. Axial CT image demonstrates a station 13 lymph node metastasis (arrow) on the posterior aspect of the pancreas head

Therefore, nodal enlargements of Nos. 12–16 on CT, which are not removed by routine D2 dissection, may significantly affect the decision of lymph node dissection extent. In addition, the regional lymph nodes of Nos. 12–16 (portal, retropancreatic, mesenteric, para-aortic locations) are classified as distant nodal group (M1), according to the AJCC classification (Figs. 4.7 and 4.8). Therefore, detailed anatomical descriptions of lymph node involvement remain an important part of preoperative nodal staging on CT.

Recently, several researchers have been made attempts to improve the accuracy of N staging and to facilitate preoperative sentinel lymph node map-

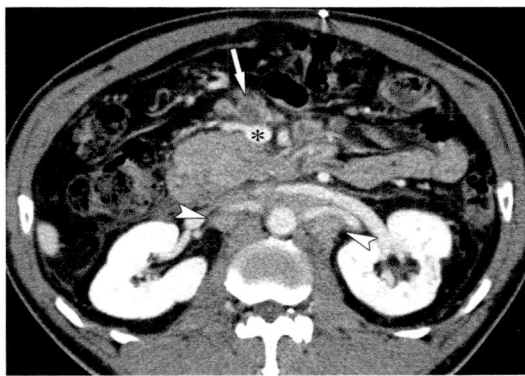

Fig. 4.8 Station 14 and 16 lymph node metastases in a 49-year-old man with stomach cancer. Axial CT image shows station 14 metastases (arrow) along the superior mesenteric vein (asterisk) and conglomerated station 16 lymph node metastases (arrowheads) along the abdominal aorta

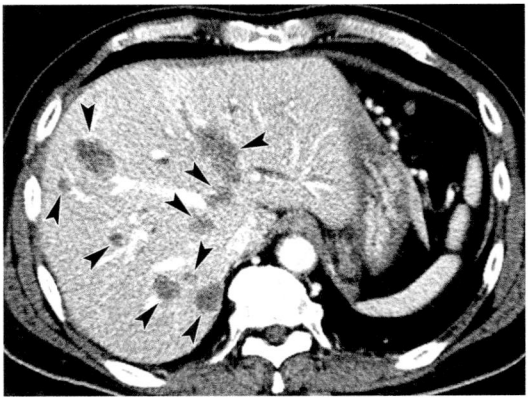

Fig. 4.9 Multiple hepatic metastases in a 49-year-old man with stomach cancer. Portal venous phase CT scan shows multiple metastatic nodules in both hepatic lobes (black arrowheads)

ping using CT lymphography. The feasibility of mapping the sentinel lymph node using ethiodized oil was reported in porcine stomachs and in patients with EGC [21]. CT lymphography using fluorescent iodized emulsion or nanoscale iodized oil emulsion could be also a promising tool for sentinel lymph node mapping, and it should be more validated in clinical model [22, 23].

M Staging

The pathway of distant metastases of gastric cancer can be categorized into three groups, that is, hematogenous metastases, lymphatic metastases, and peritoneal metastases. Solid organ metastasis is infrequently detected in gastric cancers at the time of initial diagnosis, but its detection is important for proper management. The liver is the most common organ of hematogenous metastasis, and it is explained by that the stomach is drained by portal vein [24, 25]. As hepatic metastases of gastric cancer are usually hypovascular, they are commonly detected during the portal venous phase of CT scan (Fig. 4.9). Hepatic metastases can also appear as target or rim-enhancing lesions on CT, because metastases have a tendency to outgrow their blood supply, causing central necrosis [26]. Other less affected organs of hematogenous metastasis include the lungs, adrenal glands, skeletal system, and ovaries (Figs. 4.10 and 4.11) [4]. Ovarian metastases

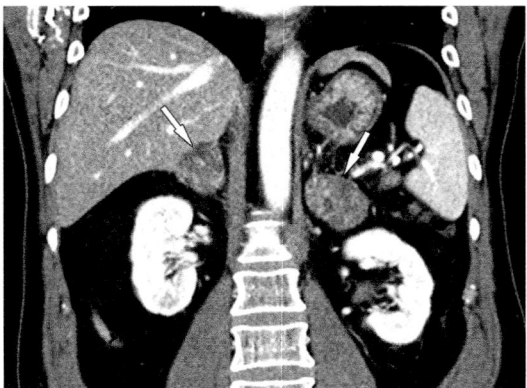

Fig. 4.10 Adrenal metastases in a 48-year-old man with stomach cancer. Coronal reformatted image shows heterogeneous enhancing metastatic masses in both adrenal glands (arrows)

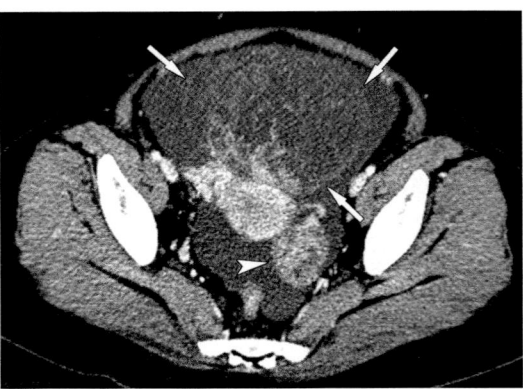

Fig. 4.11 Ovarian metastases in a 40-year-old woman with stomach cancer. Axial CT image shows a mixed cystic-solid mass in the right ovary (arrows) and a predominantly solid mass in the left ovary (arrowhead), suggesting ovarian metastases (Krukenberg tumor)

manifest as solid and cystic adnexal masses with heterogeneous contrast enhancement, and they often involve bilateral ovaries (Fig. 4.11) [25]. In the staging of gastric cancer, metastasis in distant lymph nodes, such as retropancreatic, mesenteric, para-aortic, retroperitoneal, and extra-abdominal area, is regarded as distant metastasis rather than nodal metastasis (Figs. 4.7 and 4.8). The presence of peritoneal metastasis implicates that the disease is incurable and the patient has a poor prognosis. Preoperative imaging diagnosis of peritoneal metastasis is important, because it allows the surgeon to preclude an unnecessary laparotomy. Reported CT findings of peritoneal carcinomatosis encompass ascites, omental cake, nodular or infiltrative soft tissue lesions on the peritoneal surface and bowel wall, irregular parietal peritoneal thickening with enhancement, intraperitoneal fat haziness, and small bowel wall thickening or irregularity (Figs. 4.12, 4.13 and 4.14) [27–29]. Ascites is one of the most common findings of peritoneal metastasis, and the presence of ascites on CT in AGC patients has been reported to predict peritoneal metastasis with 51% sensitivity and 97% specificity [30].

According to the study by Pan et al., the overall diagnostic accuracy of MDCT for M staging in patients with gastric cancer was over 90% [31]. However, the diagnostic accuracy of CT for diagnosing peritoneal metastasis is disappoint-

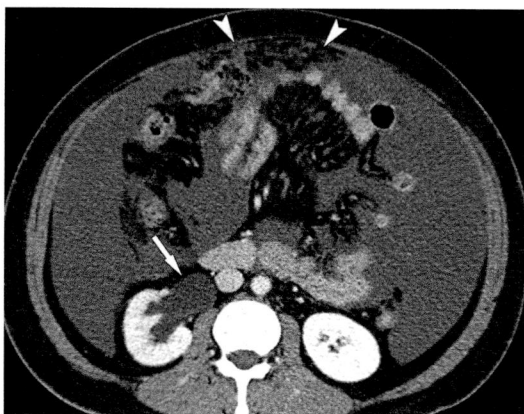

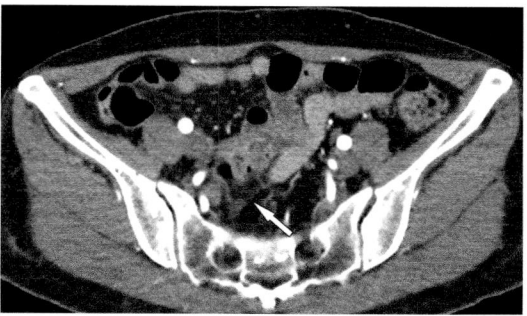

Fig. 4.14 Peritoneal metastasis in a 57-year-old woman with stomach cancer. Axial CT image demonstrates scanty ascites and minimal peritoneal infiltration (arrow). The diagnosis of peritoneal metastasis is not definite on CT. The following diagnostic laparoscopy confirmed that the patients had peritoneal metastasis

Fig. 4.12 Peritoneal metastasis in a 40-year-old woman with stomach cancer. Axial CT image demonstrates a large volume of ascites and nodular infiltration in the omentum (arrowheads). CT scan also shows right hydronephrosis (arrow) due to periureteral metastasis (not shown)

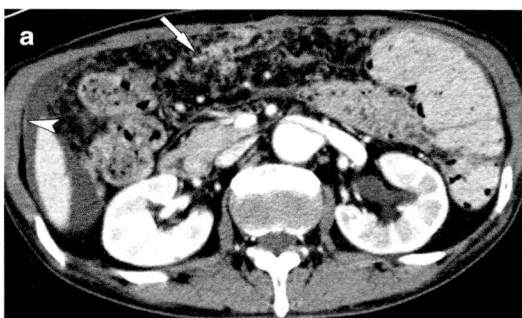

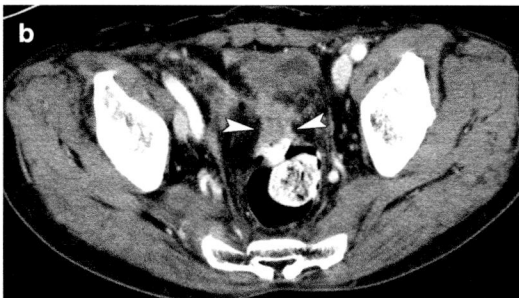

Fig. 4.13 Peritoneal metastasis in a 59-year-old man with stomach cancer. (**a**) Axial CT image shows enhanced peritoneal thickening (arrowhead), ascites, and omental cake (arrow). Left hydronephrosis is also seen. (**b**) Axial CT image in the same patient shows an infiltrative soft tissue mass (arrowheads) at the rectovesical space

ing. A systemic review including 22 CT studies reported that the sensitivity of CT for detecting peritoneal metastasis was only 33% [32]. With use of low threshold (at least one finding of peritoneal metastasis was equivocally present) as positive finding, one study reported that sensitivity and specificity of MDCT for detecting peritoneal metastasis were 50.9% and 96.2%, respectively [27]. Therefore, in patients with suspicious but not definite findings of peritoneal metastasis on CT, diagnostic laparoscopy is justified in the cases of larger tumor volume and advanced T stage (Fig. 4.14) [27].

Preoperative Evaluation of Perigastric Vascular Anatomy

As laparoscopic gastrectomy is technically demanding and requires a more comprehensive understanding of local anatomy than open gastrectomy, preoperative knowledge of the perigastric vascular anatomy may be valuable for laparoscopic gastrectomy [33]. For safe ligation of the arterial origins and veins, and for dissection of the lymph nodes under laparoscopic guidance, 3D CT angiography (CTA) has been considered to be helpful (Fig. 4.15) [34–36]. One study reported that dual-phase (arterial and

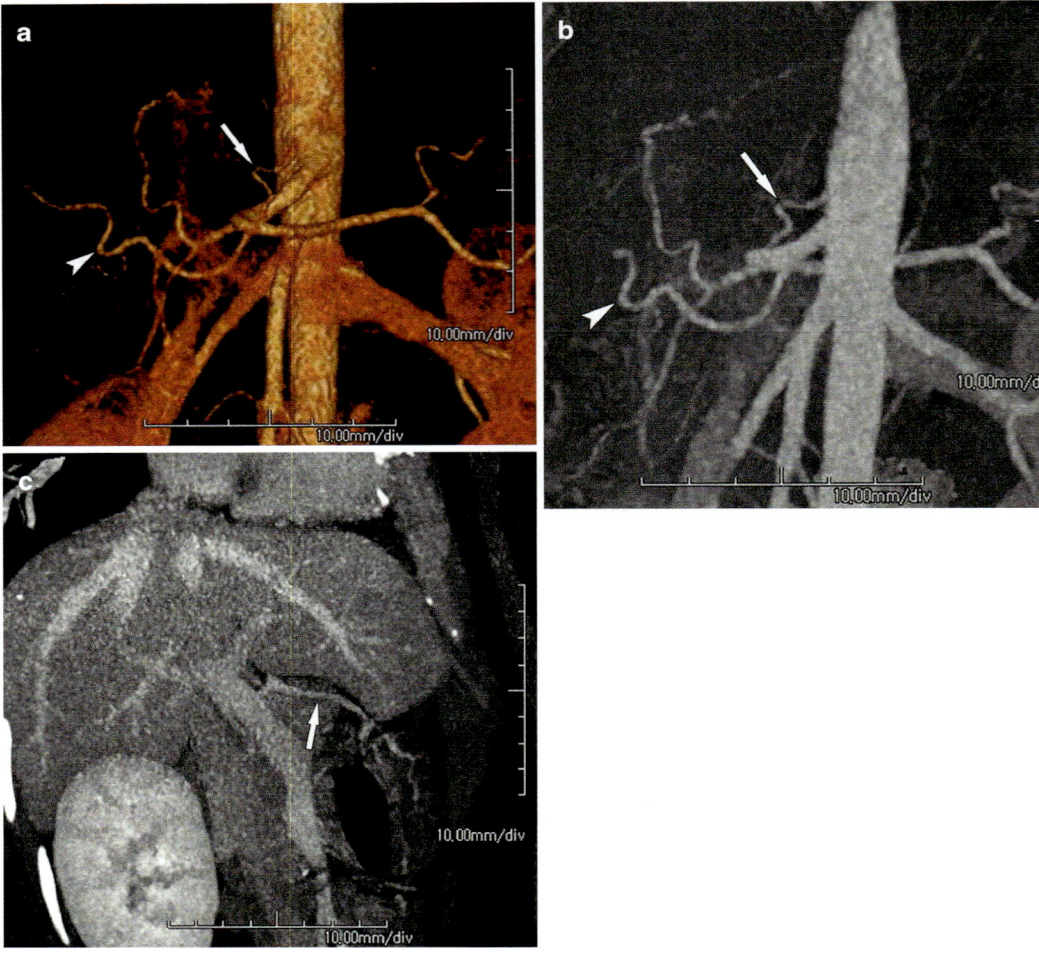

Fig. 4.15 Preoperative assessment of perigastric vascular anatomy on 3D CT imaging. (**a**) Volume-rendered 3D CT image and (**b**) maximum intensity projection image show the replaced right hepatic artery (arrowhead) from the celiac axis and the isolated left gastric artery (arrow) from the aorta. (**c**) Maximum intensity projection image shows the left gastric vein into the main portal vein (arrow)

venous phase) 3D CTA correctly identified the celiac trunk, left and right gastric artery, left gastric coronary vein, gastrocolic trunk, right gastroepiploic vein, and accessory right colic vein [35]. As 3D CTA shows the stomach, the main arteries, and veins integrated in one image, it provides a vascular "road map" for surgical guidance [36]. Preoperative consideration of vascular anatomy such as right and left gastric arteries and the left gastric vein was helpful for accomplishing a secure lymphadenectomy and for avoiding accidental hemorrhage and ischemic liver damage [36].

Differential Diagnosis

Gastric adenocarcinoma is the most common gastric malignancy, occupying over 95% of malignancy of the stomach, and non-mucinous subtypes account for most of the gastric cancers. Mucinous subtype of gastric cancers is known to have poorer prognosis than non-mucinous subtypes, and it shows different CT findings from non-mucinous subtype. In addition, various other malignant and benign gastric diseases can potentially mimic gastric cancers. MDCT has a primary role in characterizing and differentiating several gastric conditions because it provides an excellent evaluation of the gastric lumen, gastric wall, adjacent structures, and other distant organs.

Mucinous Adenocarcinoma

Mucinous carcinoma is a rare subtype of gastric cancers, which is observed in approximately 3–5% of all gastric cancers [37–39]. Mucinous carcinoma is defined as "an adenocarcinoma in which a substantial amount of extracellular mucin (more than 50% of the tumor) is retained within tumor" by the World Health Organization classification [40]. As the patients with mucinous carcinoma showed worse overall survival rate than that in patients with non-mucinous cancer [37, 38, 41], it is clinically meaningful to distinguish mucinous from non-mucinous gastric cancer on the CT imaging. Mucinous carcinoma tends to show segmental or diffuse low-attenuation wall thickening of middle or outer layer of the stomach with layered pattern of contrast enhancement, while non-mucinous carcinoma shows thickened high-attenuating inner layer with homogeneous enhancement (Fig. 4.16) [42]. Poorly enhancing thickened gastric wall of mucinous carcinoma on CT corresponds to the mucin pool in the submucosa or deeper layer [42]. Some cases with mucinous carcinoma demonstrated miliary punctate calcification in infiltrative lesions (Fig. 4.16) [42–44].

Lymphoma

Gastric lymphoma accounts for 1–5% of malignant gastric tumors [45]. Primary gastric lymphomas represent approximately 35% of gastrointestinal lymphomas and are mainly non-Hodgkin lymphomas of B-cell origin [46]. Lymphoma of mucosa-associated lymphoid tissue (MALT) is a distinct type of extranodal lymphoma, and there is evidence of strong association between *Helicobacter pylori (H. pylori)* gastritis and the development of MALT lymphoma (Fig. 4.17) [47]. MALT has relatively indolent clinical course and a better prognosis than gastric adenocarcinoma, with overall 5-year survival rates of 50–60% [48]. The typical CT findings of gastric lymphoma include segmental or diffuse marked gastric wall thickening (>1 cm) with homogeneous and less prominent enhancement than gastric cancers (Figs. 4.17 and 4.18) [2, 3]. Transpyloric extension of tumor occurs in approximately 30% of patients with lymphoma [49]. Preservation of the fat plane between the gastric lesion and adjacent organs and bulky retroperitoneal lymphadenopathy below the level of the renal hilum more likely indicate lymphoma than adenocarcinoma [45, 50]. In spite of diffuse lymphomatous infiltration, distensibility of the stomach is usually preserved without significant luminal narrowing [3].

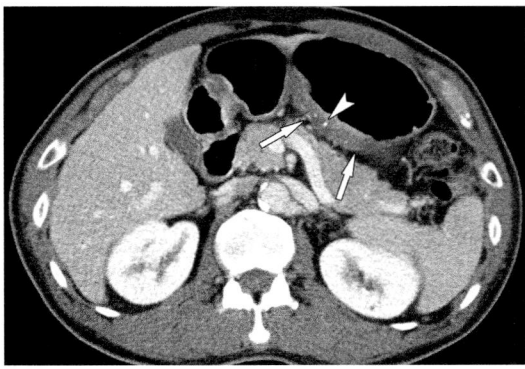

Fig. 4.16 Mucinous carcinoma in a 57-year-old man with stomach cancer. Axial CT image demonstrates low-attenuation wall thickening (arrows) with punctate calcifications (arrowhead) of the gastric body

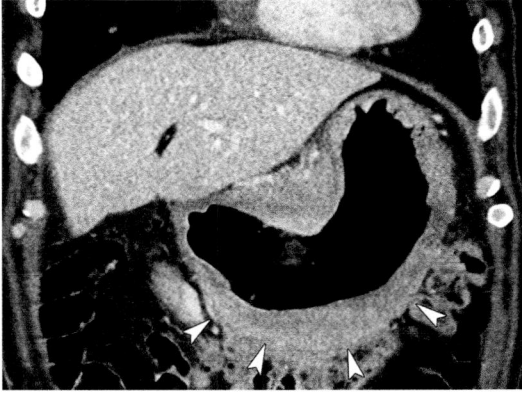

Fig. 4.17 Gastric lymphoma in a 56-year-old man. Coronal reformatted image shows diffuse wall thickening with homogeneous enhancement of near entire gastric wall (arrowheads). The gastric lesion was histologically proved as mucosa-associated lymphoid tissue (MALT) lymphoma

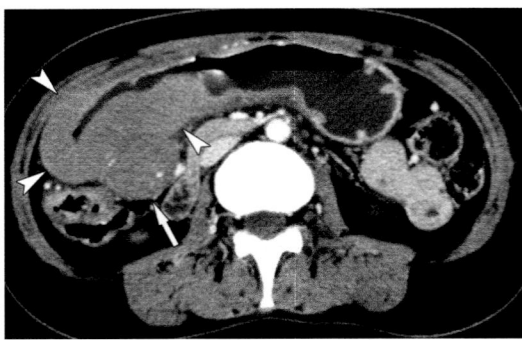

Fig. 4.18 Gastric lymphoma in a 36-year-old woman. Axial CT image shows marked diffuse circular wall thickening with homogeneous enhancement of lower body and antrum (arrowheads). Bulky lymphadenopathy is also noted along lesser curvature of the stomach (arrow)

Helicobacter Gastritis

H. pylori infection is prevalent worldwide and affects more than 90% of the population in developing countries and 50% of the population in developed countries [51]. *H. pylori* infection of the stomach and duodenum is a well-known cause of active, chronic gastritis. The antrum is the most commonly involved site for *H. pylori* gastritis. The most common CT features of *H. pylori* gastritis is prominent circumferential wall thickening of gastric antrum [52]. Thickening of the posterior gastric wall along the greater curvature was also observed [52]. In cases of acute severe inflammation of *H. pylori* gastritis, their CT findings may simulate those of gastric malignancy [52, 53]. Findings of absent lymphadenopathy, preservation of fat planes, and absent invasion of adjacent organs favor *H. pylori* gastritis rather than gastric cancer [52].

MR Imaging

Despite the intrinsic advantage of magnetic resonance imaging (MRI) such as better soft tissue contrast, multiplanar imaging acquisition, and the absence of radiation hazard, MRI for the staging of gastric cancer has not been preferred than CT because of its higher cost, prolonged scanning time, and motion artifact by respiration, pulsation, and peristalsis [54]. MRI has been mainly used in the limited clinical situation when patients are hypersensitive to iodinated CT contrast agents.

However, recent advances in fast MR imaging technique using parallel acquisition imaging and gradient sequence gained attention as a promising modality. Several studies for evaluating MR accuracy on T and N staging have been performed. The overall results of the studies suggest that there is no significant difference in T and N staging accuracy between MRI and CT [55–58] (Fig. 4.1). The reported MR accuracy for staging gastric cancer was in the range of 73–88% of accuracy for T staging and 52–55% of accuracy for N staging [9, 57, 59, 60]. The diagnostic criteria of MR imaging for nodal metastasis are similar to that of CT imaging. Both of them diagnose the nodal metastasis on the basis of the size and shape of lymph nodes. Therefore, CT and MR imaging has the same issues related with microscopic metastasis in small-sized lymph nodes and enlarged reactive lymph nodes, which result in relatively lower diagnostic accuracy.

Recently, there have been several technical developments in MR imaging. Diffusion-weighted imaging (DWI) has shown substantial promise for diagnosing nodal metastasis in the variable oncologic field. DWI derives its contrast from differences in the cellular density between tissues [61]. As malignant lesions are usually more cellular or have higher signal intensities than benign lesions, DWI has been expected to be a useful method for diagnosing nodal metastasis (Fig. 4.19). However, the studies on diagnostic performance of DWI for nodal metastasis are extremely rare. Joo et al. reported that MRI with DWI showed a higher accuracy than CT or MRI without DWI, but there was no statistical significant difference [62]. MR imaging with lymph node-specific contrast agents was attempted for improving the diagnostic accuracy of nodal metastasis in gastric cancer. Ferumoxtran-10 consists of ultrasmall superparamagnetic iron oxide particles which can be obtained by normal lymph nodes. Tatsumi et al. reported that ferumoxtran-10-enhanced MRI showed the promising diagnostic accuracy of nodal metastasis in gastric cancer patients [63]. However, feru-

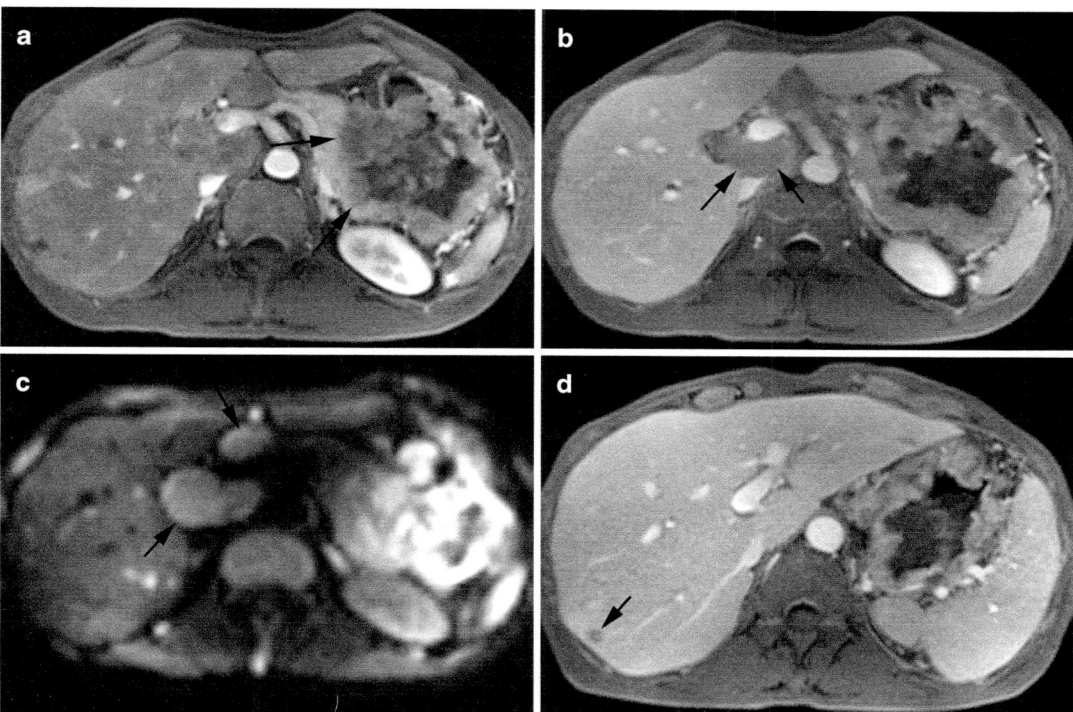

Fig. 4.19 A large ulceroinfiltrative mass demonstrates direct pancreatic body invasion on dynamic enhancement T1-weighted axial image (**a**; arrows). An enlarged metastatic lymph node is seen at the posterior side of the main portal vein, which suggests station 12p (**b**; arrows). Diffusion-weighted image shows the increased signal intensity at the metastatic lymph nodes (**c**; arrows). A small solid hepatic metastasis is also seen in the posterior segment of the right lobe of the liver (**d**; arrow)

moxtran-10 has not yet been approved by the US Food and Drug Administration because of relatively high false positive issue, leading to unnecessary surgical intervention or avoidance of surgical treatment [64]. The development of second-generation lymph node selective contrast agents is expected for accurate lymph node staging of gastric cancer.

PET-CT

Introduction

18Fluoro-deoxy-2-glucose (FDG) is the most widely used positron emission tomography (PET) radiotracer in cancer imaging. FDG, a radiotracer analogue of glucose, is injected into the body, and imaging acquisition with positron emission tomography-computed tomography (PET/CT) will reveal FDG distribution that reflects glucose usage in the body. FDG in cancer imaging is based on the hypothesis initially proposed by Warburg, where cancer cells exhibit higher rates of glycolysis in the presence of oxygen [65].

Due to the increased availability of cyclotrons, FDG PET/CT has become more widely used in the routine workup in certain cancers for staging, therapy response, and recur evaluation. Recent guidelines have suggested that FDG PET/CT be used in the diagnostic workup in selected gastric cancers. National Comprehensive Cancer Network (NCCN) staging guidelines have suggested that PET/CT be included in the staging of gastric cancer patients with lesions greater than T1 and no evidence of distant metastasis [66]. The European Society for Medical Oncology (ESMO) guidelines have also included FDG PET/CT, in that it may improve staging by detection of involved lymph nodes or metastatic disease, but may be uninformative in mucinous tumors [67].

Diagnosis and TNM Staging with FDG PET/CT

The anatomical resolution of contrast-enhanced CT has been an established protocol in the TNM staging evaluation of gastric cancer. FDG PET/CT has the advantage of evaluating the whole body for unsuspected metastasis, as well as noninvasively evaluating the metabolism of the tumor, which has been shown to be correlated with prognosis in many cancers. However, there are a few limitations, as FDG PET/CT has insufficient spatial resolution (approximately 5–7 mm) to fully evaluate local T staging in gastric cancers. Another limitation in evaluating the malignant infiltration extent in the stomach is the physiologic FDG uptake in the collapsed stomach. The stomach has variable FDG uptake, which can impede in fully evaluating tumor extent in the stomach wall and is a reason for lowered sensitivity in detecting incidental gastric cancers. This physiologic stomach uptake can be reduced by expanding the stomach with fluid, which can reduce physiologic stomach uptake, allowing clearer visualization and delineation of gastric cancer. Yun et al. have showed in their study that stomach distention with water results in 90% visualization of gastric cancers [68]. The imaging protocol consists of having the patient drink water after the routine whole-body scan and then acquiring an additional PET/CT of the stomach region. Using this method, a recent study has shown that the normal gastric wall uptake can be significantly reduced from SUVmax of 3.1 ± 0.8 to 1.6 ± 0.6 and helped in the resolution of 36% of indeterminate lesions [69].

Another variable that has to be considered during TNM evaluation of gastric cancers with FDG PET/CT is the difference in FDG avidity according to histopathology and tumor grade. Tumors of low cellularity, such as signet ring cell (SRC) type or extracellular mucin adenocarcinoma, show lower FDG uptake compared to intestinal-type adenocarcinomas (Fig. 4.20) [70–72]. Stahl et al. have shown significantly more tumors of intestinal growth type were detected (83%) than non-intestinal-type carcinoma (41%)

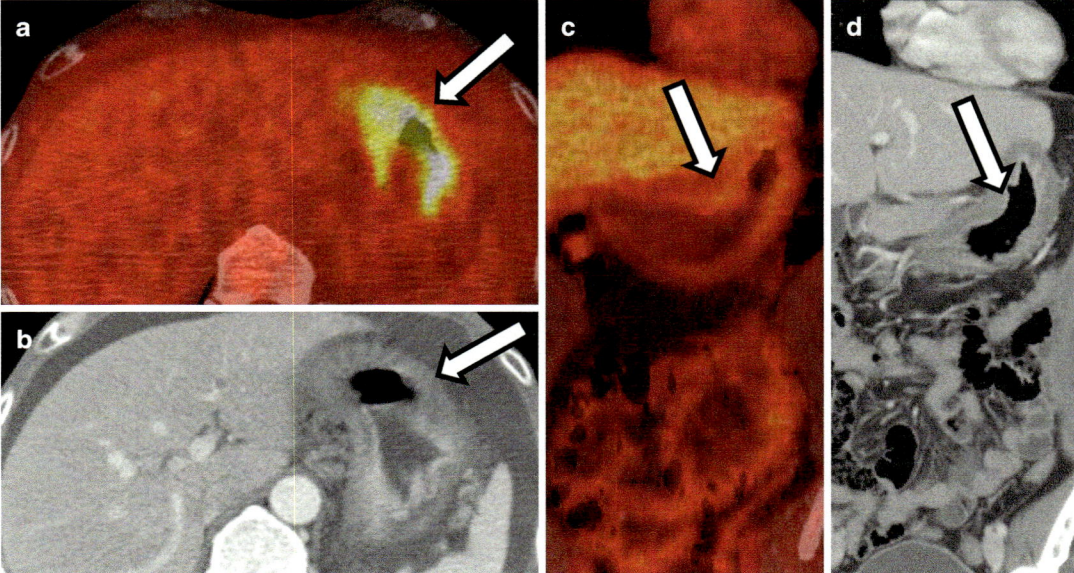

Fig. 4.20 Variability of FDG uptake according to histologic subtype. (**a**, **b**) PET/CT and CT images of intestinal-type gastric cancer with intense FDG uptake. (**c**, **d**) Mild FDG uptake is seen in the signet ring cell-type gastric cancer

[71]. They suggested that the extracellular or intracellular mucus deposition, which leads to lower cellular density, is the likely cause of decreased FDG uptake in non-intestinal-type carcinomas. However, SRC has also been shown to have lower GLUT1 expression (2%) compared to other adenocarcinomas such as papillary adenocarcinomas (44%), tubular adenocarcinomas (32%), or poorly differentiated adenocarcinomas (28%) [73].

Diagnosis

Multiple studies have evaluated the clinical role of FDG PET/CT in gastric cancer. A recent analysis evaluated studies using National Oncologic PET Registry and has shown that PET/CT had a 37% change in intended treatment, and imaging-adjusted impact was 14.5% [74]. The NCCN data has also shown that PET/CT has higher accuracy in gastric cancer staging (84%), compared to CT alone (64%) [75]. In the detection and preoperative staging of gastric cancer, stand-alone PET is not an adequate diagnostic procedure, but may be useful in conjunction with CT [4, 76]. FDG PET/CT has better sensitivity for advanced gastric cancer (98%) compared to early gastric cancer (63%) in detection of gastric cancer [77]. However, previously mentioned biologic factors affect FDG avidity, which may decrease detection sensitivity. For example, higher mean standardized uptake value (SUVmean 7.7) is seen in intestinal-type gastric adenocarcinoma, compared to mucinous and signet ring cell carcinoma (SUVmean 4.2) [77], which may account for the lowered sensitivity of 61% for diffuse-type and 77% for intestinal-type gastric cancer [76].

Tumor size has repeatedly been shown to be an important factor in primary lesion detection [70, 77–79]. Tumor depth is an important factor for visualization of stomach cancer. Mochiki et al. have shown that only 40% were detected in T1 tumors, 88% for T2 tumors, 90% for T3 tumors, and 100% for T4 tumors [80]. Overall, specificity for detection rates was reported to be over 90% [70, 77, 80, 81]. Lesions larger than 3.5 cm and deeper invasion have been reported to have higher detection rates [82]. In a systematic review by Kaneko et al., larger tumor size

(>3 cm), non-signet ring cell carcinoma type pathology, and GLUT1 expression were significant predictors of FDG avidity. Using a PET scoring system using these factors, they have shown that FDG avid tumors can be detected with sensitivity of 85% and specificity of 71%, which can be useful in selecting which patients that should undergo PET/CT for staging [83].

Finally, adjustment of imaging protocols has been shown to be helpful in improving initial diagnosis. Stomach distention method described earlier can reduce false positive from 30% to 8% [84]. Additional delayed imaging 2 hours after initial PET/CT may also be helpful in differentiating benign from malignant lesions [85]. Also, knowledge of physiologic uptake is also helpful to reduce false positive rates. Focal FDG uptake in the gastroesophageal junction may be physiologic in the absence of abnormal findings on CT. Linear uptake in the GE junction extending linearly into the distal esophagus is also likely a benign finding such as gastroesophageal reflux disease [86]. Other known benign lesions that show increased FDG uptake are mucosal inflammation, such as superficial gastritis and erosive gastritis [87].

Lymph Node Staging

The limited spatial resolution and variable FDG uptake according to histopathology limits the evaluation of T stage with PET/CT. FDG PET/CT is more clinically useful in the N staging of gastric cancers. Overall, FDG PET/CT has low sensitivity, but high specificity in detection of LN metastasis, as shown in a recent meta-analysis where sensitivity was 54.7% and specificity was 92.2% [88]. Especially in N1 disease, PET/CT shows significantly lower sensitivity compared to conventional CT (PET/CT, 46.4% and 41%; CT, 89.3% and 75%, respectively) [89, 90]. This may be due to smaller size of perigastric LNs and relatively intense FDG uptake in the adjacent primary gastric cancer (Fig. 4.21) [89]. However, because surgically resectable AGCs undergo at least D1 dissection during gastrectomy, determination of D1 LN metastasis may be less clinically significant [91]. A previous study by Chen et al. has shown that FDG PET/CT has lower sensitiv-

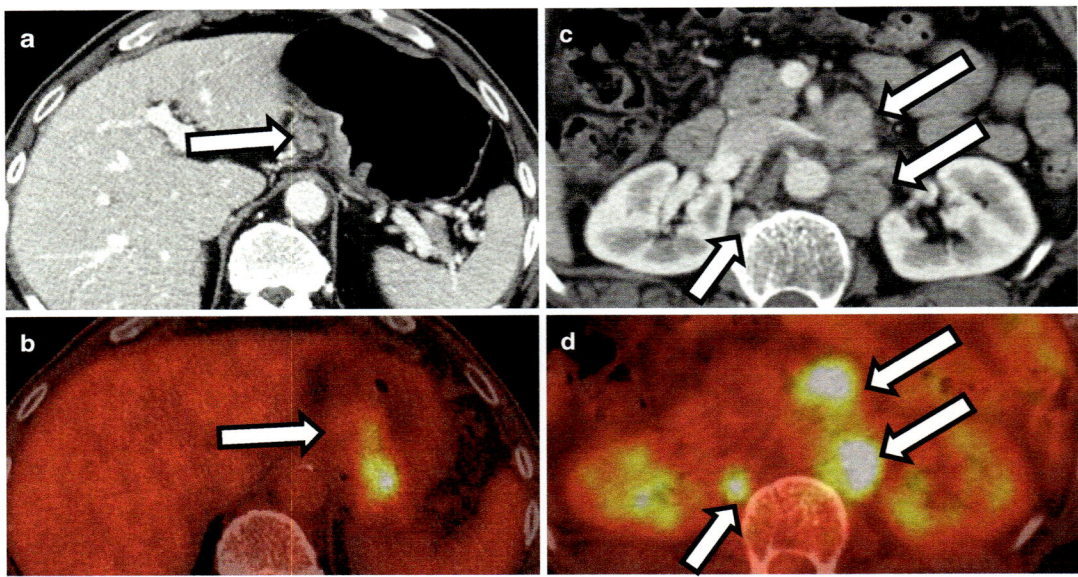

Fig. 4.21 FDG avidity of lymph node (LN) metastasis in gastric cancer. (**a, b**) Minimal FDG uptake is seen in the perigastric LNs. (**c, d**) Intense FDG uptake in the retroperitoneal LNs

ity than CT in detecting local LN metastasis (56% vs 78%), but showed higher specificity (92% vs 62%) [77]. Yun et al. have shown a sensitivity of 34% for N1/N2 disease and 50% for N3 disease for FDG PET/CT. In contrast, CT showed higher sensitivity for detection of N1 disease (58%) [92]. Evaluation of accuracy has shown concordant findings, in that accuracy for distant LN metastasis was significantly higher for PET than CT (85% vs 62%) [93]. Other studies have also showed similar findings of low sensitivity (31–58.3%) but high specificity (95–97%) in detection of LN metastasis [92, 94, 95]. Shimada et al. have compiled studies about the diagnostic ability of FDG PET/CT in detecting LN metastasis and have shown consistent findings of high specificity (89–100%), but low sensitivity (21–40%), with an overall accuracy between 46% and 85% [81].

Factors affecting FDG uptake in LN metastasis are similar to factors influencing FDG uptake in the primary lesion. Therefore, evaluation of initial FDG uptake in the primary lesion is important not only for staging but also in the subsequent follow-up PET/CT, as knowledge of FDG avidity of the primary lesion may be helpful in

determining metabolically significant uptake in LN metastasis. Evaluation of FDG intensity in the primary gastric cancer not only helps in detecting LN metastasis but is useful in the prediction of LN metastasis [77, 80, 89, 90, 96, 97]. The mean SUV in the primary tumor was higher in group 3 LN metastasis (6.2 ± 0.7) compared to patients without LN metastasis (3.5 ± 0.3). In another study, average maximum SUV of primary gastric cancer was higher in patients with LN metastasis (7.5–8.7) compared to patients without LN metastasis (3.6) [77, 80]. In an extensively analyzed study evaluating LN metastasis according to primary tumor histopathology, Kim et al. have shown that signet ring cell-type pathology was associated with lowest sensitivity (15%), in contrast to other cell types with modest sensitivity (30–71%) [90]. Another recent study showed that FDG uptake in LN metastasis was correlated with higher GLUT-1 expression and Ki-67 index in LN metastases [96].

Metastasis

FDG PET/CT has been helpful in the evaluation of metastasis. Due to the high incidence of liver, bone, peritoneal, and lung metastasis, determining patients with metastasis is important to reduce futile surgeries and improve patient prognosis. Because FDG uptake is heavily influenced by the histologic subtype in the primary lesion, it is helpful to consider predominate dissemination patterns according to histologic subtype. Diffuse-type gastric cancer more frequently disseminates peritoneal metastasis and lymph node metastasis and forms Krukenberg tumors. In contrast, intestinal type frequently involves liver as well as lymph node metastasis [98–100]. The metastasis pattern of diffuse-type gastric cancer, as well as the relatively low cellularity or small size of peritoneal seeding nodules, is the likely reason why FDG PET/CT has been shown to have low sensitivity for carcinomatosis [101]. However, like LN metastasis, FDG PET/CT has been shown to have high specificity in detecting carcinomatosis. In a meta-analysis of 4 FDG PET/CT studies and 15 CT studies on peritoneal metastasis, Wang et al. showed a pooled sensitivity of 0.33 (95% CI: 0.16–0.56) and 0.28 (95% CI: 0.17–0.44) for CT and PET/CT, respectively. Pooled specificity for CT and FDG was 0.99 (95%

CI: 0.98–1.00) and 0.97 (95% CI: 0.83–1.00) [32]. They also showed that CT and PET had similar sensitivity (0.74 and 0.70, respectively) and specificity (0.99 and 0.96, respectively), but CT had much higher diagnostic odds ratio (the ratio of odds of positive test results in diseased group relative to odds of positive results in non-diseased group) of 251.1, which is an indicator of test accuracy. In contrast, FDG PET was 56.46 [32]. A potential false positive for peritoneal carcinomatosis is peritoneal tuberculosis, which may show intense FDG uptake (Fig. 4.22).

In a review of previous studies evaluating diagnostic ability of PET/CT in metastasis evaluation, FDG PET/CT shows high specificity of 74–99%, but variable low sensitivity (35–74%), with an overall accuracy of 73–96% in detecting distant metastasis [81, 102–105]. A recent study evaluating FDG avidity in metastasis is strongly influenced by the FDG uptake avidity in the primary lesion [106]. The FDG avid tumor group had a 82.1% sensitivity in detecting recurrence, and FDG non-avid group had a 47.4% in detect-

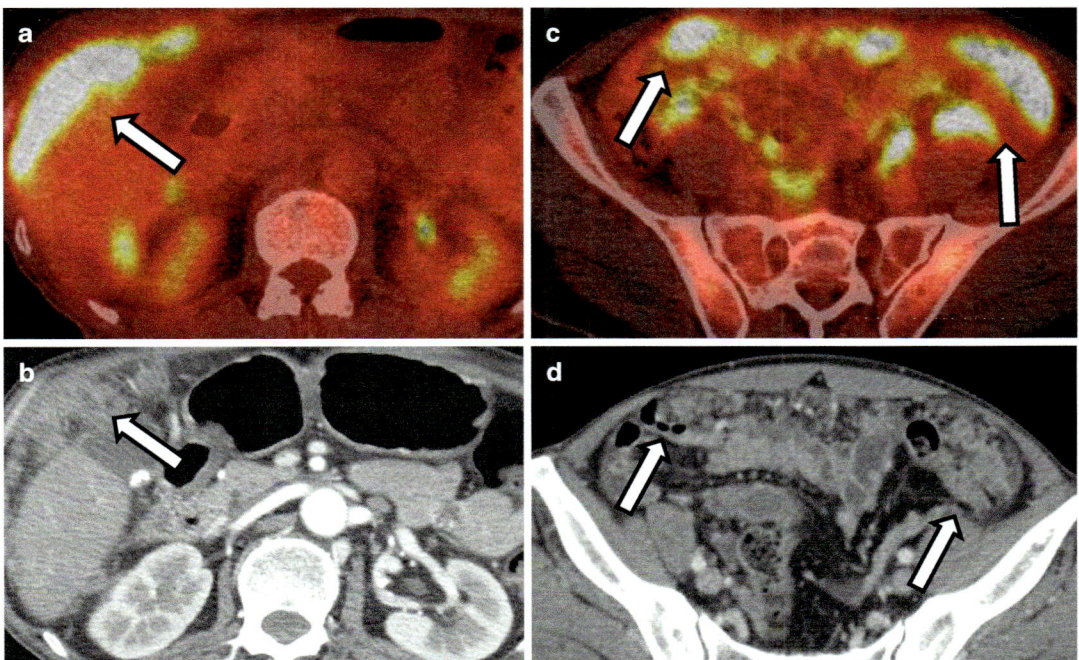

Fig. 4.22 Intense FDG uptake in both carcinomatosis and tuberculosis peritonitis. (**a, b**) Tuberculosis peritonitis showing intense FDG uptake. (**c, d**) AGC patient with peritoneal carcinomatosis. Intense FDG uptake is seen in the carcinomatosis

ing recurrence not in the remnant stomach or anastomosis site. They have also shown in their study that although intestinal-type cancer showed significantly increased PET sensitivity, there was no significant correlation between signet ring cell type and PET sensitivity. In another recent study, FDG avidity in the primary gastric malignancy is related to shorter time to recurrence [107]. These studies show the importance of performing FDG PET/CT in the staging of gastric cancers, as FDG avidity in metastatic foci is correlated with FDG uptake in the initial primary gastric cancer and cannot be predicted based solely on histopathology. Also, knowledge of FDG avidity in the primary lesion may be helpful in the recurrence evaluation interval during follow-up.

References

1. Minami M, Kawauchi N, Itai Y, Niki T, Sasaki Y. Gastric tumors: radiologic-pathologic correlation and accuracy of T staging with dynamic CT. Radiology. 1992;185(1):173–8. https://doi.org/10.1148/radiology.185.1.1523303.
2. Virmani V, Khandelwal A, Sethi V, Fraser-Hill M, Fasih N, Kielar A. Neoplastic stomach lesions and their mimickers: spectrum of imaging manifestations. Cancer Imag. 2012;12:269–78. https://doi.org/10.1102/1470-7330.2012.0031.
3. Ba-Ssalamah A, Prokop M, Uffmann M, Pokieser P, Teleky B, Lechner G. Dedicated multidetector CT of the stomach: spectrum of diseases. Radiographics. 2003;23(3):625–44. https://doi.org/10.1148/rg.2330 25127.
4. Lim JS, Yun MJ, Kim MJ, Hyung WJ, Park MS, Choi JY, Kim TS, Lee JD, Noh SH, Kim KW. CT and PET in stomach cancer: preoperative staging and monitoring of response to therapy. Radiographics. 2006;26(1):143–56. https://doi.org/10.1148/rg.2610 55078.
5. Lee IJ, Lee JM, Kim SH, Shin CI, Lee JY, Kim SH, Han JK, Choi BI. Diagnostic performance of 64-channel multidetector CT in the evaluation of gastric cancer: differentiation of mucosal cancer (T1a) from submucosal involvement (T1b and T2). Radiology. 2010;255(3):805–14. https://doi.org/10.1148/radiol. 10091313.
6. Kim JW, Shin SS, Heo SH, Choi YD, Lim HS, Park YK, Park CH, Jeong YY, Kang HK. Diagnostic performance of 64-section CT using CT gastrography in preoperative T staging of gastric cancer according to 7th edition of AJCC cancer staging manual. Eur Radiol. 2012;22(3):654–62. https://doi.org/10.1007/s00330-011-2283-3.
7. Kim YH, Lee KH, Park SH, Kim HH, Hahn S, Park do J, Lee HS. Staging of T3 and T4 gastric carcinoma with multidetector CT: added value of multiplanar reformations for prediction of adjacent organ invasion. Radiology. 2009;250(3):767–75. https://doi.org/10.1148/radiol.2502071872.
8. Lee MH, Choi D, Park MJ, Lee MW. Gastric cancer: imaging and staging with MDCT based on the 7th AJCC guidelines. Abdom Imaging. 2012;37(4):531–40. https://doi.org/10.1007/s00261-011-9780-3.
9. Kwee RM, Kwee TC. Imaging in local staging of gastric cancer: a systematic review. J Clin Oncol. 2007;25(15):2107–16. https://doi.org/10.1200/jco.2006.09.5224.
10. Seevaratnam R, Cardoso R, McGregor C, Lourenco L, Mahar A, Sutradhar R, Law C, Paszat L, Coburn N. How useful is preoperative imaging for tumor, node, metastasis (TNM) staging of gastric cancer? A meta-analysis. Gastric Cancer. 2012;15(Suppl 1):S3–18. https://doi.org/10.1007/s10120-011-0069-6.
11. Kim HJ, Kim AY, Oh ST, Kim JS, Kim KW, Kim PN, Lee MG, Ha HK. Gastric cancer staging at multi-detector row CT gastrography: comparison of transverse and volumetric CT scanning. Radiology. 2005;236(3):879–85. https://doi.org/10.1148/radiol.2363041101.
12. Kim JH, Eun HW, Choi JH, Hong SS, Kang W, Auh YH. Diagnostic performance of virtual gastroscopy using MDCT in early gastric cancer compared with 2D axial CT: focusing on interobserver variation. AJR Am J Roentgenol. 2007;189(2):299–305. https://doi.org/10.2214/ajr.07.2201.
13. AJCC Cancer Staging Handbook. 7th ed. Philadelphia: Spinger-Verlag; 2010.
14. D'Elia F, Zingarelli A, Palli D, Grani M. Hydrodynamic CT preoperative staging of gastric cancer: correlation with pathological findings. A prospective study of 107 cases. Eur Radiol. 2000;10(12):1877–85. https://doi.org/10.1007/s003300000537.
15. Fukuya T, Honda H, Hayashi T, Kaneko K, Tateshi Y, Ro T, Maehara Y, Tanaka M, Tsuneyoshi M, Masuda K. Lymph-node metastases: efficacy for detection with helical CT in patients with gastric cancer. Radiology. 1995;197(3):705–11. https://doi.org/10.1148/radiology.197.3.7480743.
16. Chen CY, Hsu JS, Wu DC, Kang WY, Hsieh JS, Jaw TS, Wu MT, Liu GC. Gastric cancer: preoperative local staging with 3D multi-detector row CT – correlation with surgical and histopathologic results. Radiology. 2007;242(2):472–82. https://doi.org/10.1148/radiol.2422051557.
17. Kim AY, Kim HJ, Ha HK. Gastric cancer by multidetector row CT: preoperative staging. Abdom Imaging. 2005;30(4):465–72. https://doi.org/10.1007/s00261-004-0273-5.
18. Kim HS, Han HY, Choi JA, Park CM, Cha IH, Chung KB, Mok YJ. Preoperative evaluation of gastric cancer: value of spiral CT during gastric arteriography (CTGA). Abdom Imaging. 2001;26(2):123–30.

19. Cho JS, Kim JK, Rho SM, Lee HY, Jeong HY, Lee CS. Preoperative assessment of gastric carcinoma: value of two-phase dynamic CT with mechanical iv. injection of contrast material. AJR Am J Roentgenol. 1994;163(1):69–75. https://doi.org/10.2214/ajr.163.1.8010251.

20. Association JGC. Japanese gastric cancer treatment guidelines 2010 (ver. 3). Gastric Cancer. 2011;14(2):113–23. https://doi.org/10.1007/s10120-011-0042-4.

21. Kim YH, Lee YJ, Park JH, Lee KH, Lee HS, Park YS, Park do J, Kim HH. Early gastric cancer: feasibility of CT lymphography with ethiodized oil for sentinel node mapping. Radiology. 2013;267(2):414–21. https://doi.org/10.1148/radiol.12121527.

22. Kim H, Lee SK, Kim YM, Lee EH, Lim SJ, Kim SH, Yang J, Lim JS, Hyung WJ. Fluorescent iodized emulsion for pre- and intraoperative sentinel lymph node imaging: validation in a preclinical model. Radiology. 2015;275(1):196–204. https://doi.org/10.1148/radiol.14141159.

23. Lim JS, Choi J, Song J, Chung YE, Lim SJ, Lee SK, Hyung WJ. Nanoscale iodized oil emulsion: a useful tracer for pretreatment sentinel node detection using CT lymphography in a normal canine gastric model. Surg Endosc. 2012;26(8):2267–74. https://doi.org/10.1007/s00464-012-2170-2.

24. Miller FH, Kochman ML, Talamonti MS, Ghahremani GG, Gore RM. Gastric cancer. Radiologic staging. Radiol Clin N Am. 1997;35(2):331–49.

25. Gore RM. Gastric cancer. Clinical and pathologic features. Radiol Clin N Am. 1997;35(2):295–310.

26. Cotran RS, Kumar V, Robbins SL. Robbins pathologic basis of disease, vol. 962. 4th ed. Philadelphia: Saunders; 1989.

27. Kim SJ, Kim HH, Kim YH, Hwang SH, Lee HS, Park do J, Kim SY, Lee KH. Peritoneal metastasis: detection with 16- or 64-detector row CT in patients undergoing surgery for gastric cancer. Radiology. 2009;253(2):407–15. https://doi.org/10.1148/radiol.2532082272.

28. Chang DK, Kim JW, Kim BK, Lee KL, Song CS, Han JK, Song IS. Clinical significance of CT-defined minimal ascites in patients with gastric cancer. World J Gastroenterol. 2005;11(42):6587–92.

29. Walkey MM, Friedman AC, Sohotra P, Radecki PD. CT manifestations of peritoneal carcinomatosis. AJR Am J Roentgenol. 1988;150(5):1035–41. https://doi.org/10.2214/ajr.150.5.1035.

30. Yajima K, Kanda T, Ohashi M, Wakai T, Nakagawa S, Sasamoto R, Hatakeyama K. Clinical and diagnostic significance of preoperative computed tomography findings of ascites in patients with advanced gastric cancer. Am J Surg. 2006;192(2):185–90. https://doi.org/10.1016/j.amjsurg.2006.05.007.

31. Pan Z, Zhang H, Yan C, Du L, Ding B, Song Q, Ling H, Huang B, Chen K. Determining gastric cancer resectability by dynamic MDCT. Eur Radiol. 2010;20(3):613–20. https://doi.org/10.1007/s00330-009-1576-2.

32. Wang Z, Chen JQ. Imaging in assessing hepatic and peritoneal metastases of gastric cancer: a systematic review. BMC Gastroenterol. 2011;11:19. https://doi.org/10.1186/1471-230x-11-19.

33. Botet JF, Lightdale CJ, Zauber AG, Gerdes H, Winawer SJ, Urmacher C, Brennan MF. Preoperative staging of gastric cancer: comparison of endoscopic US and dynamic CT. Radiology. 1991;181(2):426–32. https://doi.org/10.1148/radiology.181.2.1924784.

34. Takiguchi S, Sekimoto M, Fujiwara Y, Yasuda T, Yano M, Hori M, Murakami T, Nakamura H, Monden M. Laparoscopic lymph node dissection for gastric cancer with intraoperative navigation using three-dimensional angio computed tomography images reconstructed as laparoscopic view. Surg Endosc. 2004;18(1):106–10. https://doi.org/10.1007/s00464-003-8116-y.

35. Matsuki M, Tanikake M, Kani H, Tatsugami F, Kanazawa S, Kanamoto T, Inada Y, Yoshikawa S, Narabayashi I, Lee SW, Nomura E, Okuda J, Tanigawa N. Dual-phase 3D CT angiography during a single breath-hold using 16-MDCT: assessment of vascular anatomy before laparoscopic gastrectomy. AJR Am J Roentgenol. 2006;186(4):1079–85. https://doi.org/10.2214/ajr.04.0733.

36. Lee SW, Shinohara H, Matsuki M, Okuda J, Nomura E, Mabuchi H, Nishiguchi K, Takaori K, Narabayashi I, Tanigawa N. Preoperative simulation of vascular anatomy by three-dimensional computed tomography imaging in laparoscopic gastric cancer surgery. J Am Coll Surg. 2003;197(6):927–36. https://doi.org/10.1016/j.jamcollsurg.2003.07.021.

37. Adachi Y, Mori M, Kido A, Shimono R, Maehara Y, Sugimachi K. A clinicopathologic study of mucinous gastric carcinoma. Cancer. 1992;69(4):866–71.

38. Wu CY, Yeh HZ, Shih RT, Chen GH. A clinicopathologic study of mucinous gastric carcinoma including multivariate analysis. Cancer. 1998;83(7):1312–8.

39. Songur Y, Okai T, Watanabe H, Fujii T, Motoo Y, Sawabu N. Preoperative diagnosis of mucinous gastric adenocarcinoma by endoscopic ultrasonography. Am J Gastroenterol. 1996;91(8):1586–90.

40. Watanabe H, Jass JR, Sobin LH. Histological typing of esophageal and gastric tumours. WHO international histological classification of tumors. 2nd ed. Berlin: Spriner-Verlag; 1990.

41. Hyung WJ, Noh SH, Shin DW, Yoo CH, Kim CB, Min JS, Lee KS. Clinicopathologic characteristics of mucinous gastric adenocarcinoma. Yonsei Med J. 1999;40(2):99–106.

42. Park MS, Yu JS, Kim MJ, Yoon SW, Kim SH, Noh TW, Lee KH, Lee JT, Yoo HS, Kim KW. Mucinous versus nonmucinous gastric carcinoma: differentiation with helical CT. Radiology. 2002;223(2):540–6. https://doi.org/10.1148/radiol.2232010905.

43. Nishimura K, Togashi K, Tohdo G, Dodo Y, Tanada S, Nakano Y, Torizuka K. Computed tomography of calcified gastric carcinoma. J Comput Assist Tomogr. 1984;8(5):1010–1.

44. Libson E, Bloom RA, Blank P, Emerson DS. Calcified mucinous adenocarcinoma of the stomach – the CT appearances. Comput Radiol. 1985;9(4):255–8.

45. Gossios K, Katsimbri P, Tsianos E. CT features of gastric lymphoma. Eur Radiol. 2000;10(3):425–30. https://doi.org/10.1007/s003300050069.

46. Lewin KJ, Ranchod M, Dorfman RF. Lymphomas of the gastrointestinal tract: a study of 117 cases presenting with gastrointestinal disease. Cancer. 1978;42(2):693–707.

47. Wotherspoon AC, Ortiz-Hidalgo C, Falzon MR, Isaacson PG. Helicobacter pylori-associated gastritis and primary B-cell gastric lymphoma. Lancet (London, England). 1991;338(8776):1175–6.

48. Isaacson PG, Spencer J, Finn T. Primary B-cell gastric lymphoma. Hum Pathol. 1986;17(1):72–82.

49. Cho KC, Baker SR, Alterman DD, Fusco JM, Cho S. Transpyloric spread of gastric tumors: comparison of adenocarcinoma and lymphoma. AJR Am J Roentgenol. 1996;167(2):467–9. https://doi.org/10.2214/ajr.167.2.8686627.

50. Buy JN, Moss AA. Computed tomography of gastric lymphoma. AJR Am J Roentgenol. 1982;138(5):859–65. https://doi.org/10.2214/ajr.138.5.859.

51. Kul S, Sert B, Sari A, Arslan M, Kosucu P, Ahmetoglu A, Dinc H. Effect of subclinical Helicobacter pylori infection on gastric wall thickness: multislice CT evaluation. Diagn Interv Radiol (Ankara, Turkey). 2008;14(3):138–42.

52. Urban BA, Fishman EK, Hruban RH. Helicobacter pylori gastritis mimicking gastric carcinoma at CT evaluation. Radiology. 1991;179(3):689–91. https://doi.org/10.1148/radiology.179.3.1888360.

53. Frommer DJ, Carrick J, Lee A, Hazell SL. Acute presentation of Campylobacter pylori gastritis. Am J Gastroenterol. 1988;83(10):1168–71.

54. Hallinan JT, Venkatesh SK. Gastric carcinoma: imaging diagnosis, staging and assessment of treatment response. Cancer Imaging. 2013;13:212–27. https://doi.org/10.1102/1470-7330.2013.0023.

55. Maccioni F, Marcelli G, Al Ansari N, Zippi M, De Marco V, Kagarmanova A, Vestri A, Marcheggiano-Clarke L, Marini M. Preoperative T and N staging of gastric cancer: magnetic resonance imaging (MRI) versus multi detector computed tomography (MDCT). Clin Ter. 2010;161(2):e57–62.

56. Anzidei M, Napoli A, Zaccagna F, Di Paolo P, Zini C, Cavallo Marincola B, Geiger D, Catalano C, Passariello R. Diagnostic performance of 64-MDCT and 1.5-T MRI with high-resolution sequences in the T staging of gastric cancer: a comparative analysis with histopathology. Radiol Med. 2009;114(7):1065–79. https://doi.org/10.1007/s11547-009-0455-x.

57. Sohn KM, Lee JM, Lee SY, Ahn BY, Park SM, Kim KM. Comparing MR imaging and CT in the staging of gastric carcinoma. AJR Am J Roentgenol. 2000;174(6):1551–7. https://doi.org/10.2214/ajr.174.6.1741551.

58. Kim AY, Han JK, Seong CK, Kim TK, Choi BI. MRI in staging advanced gastric cancer: is it useful compared with spiral CT? J Comput Assist Tomogr. 2000;24(3):389–94.

59. Wang CK, Kuo YT, Liu GC, Tsai KB, Huang YS. Dynamic contrast-enhanced subtraction and delayed MRI of gastric tumors: radiologic-pathologic correlation. J Comput Assist Tomogr. 2000;24(6):872–7.

60. Kang BC, Kim JH, Kim KW, Lee DY, Baek SY, Lee SW, Jung WH. Value of the dynamic and delayed MR sequence with Gd-DTPA in the T-staging of stomach cancer: correlation with the histopathology. Abdom Imaging. 2000;25(1):14–24.

61. Kwee TC, Takahara T, Ochiai R, Nievelstein RA, Luijten PR. Diffusion-weighted whole-body imaging with background body signal suppression (DWIBS): features and potential applications in oncology. Eur Radiol. 2008;18(9):1937–52. https://doi.org/10.1007/s00330-008-0968-z.

62. Joo I, Lee JM, Kim JH, Shin CI, Han JK, Choi BI. Prospective comparison of 3T MRI with diffusion-weighted imaging and MDCT for the preoperative TNM staging of gastric cancer. J Magn Reson Imaging. 2015;41(3):814–21. https://doi.org/10.1002/jmri.24586.

63. Tatsumi Y, Tanigawa N, Nishimura H, Nomura E, Mabuchi H, Matsuki M, Narabayashi I. Preoperative diagnosis of lymph node metastases in gastric cancer by magnetic resonance imaging with ferumoxtran-10. Gastric Cancer. 2006;9(2):120–8. https://doi.org/10.1007/s10120-006-0365-8.

64. Wang YX. Superparamagnetic iron oxide based MRI contrast agents: Current status of clinical application. Quant Imaging Med Surg. 2011;1(1):35–40. https://doi.org/10.3978/j.issn.2223-4292.2011.08.03.

65. Warburg O, Wind F, Negelein E. The metabolism of tumors in the body. J Gen Physiol. 1927;8(6):519–30.

66. Ajani JA, Bentrem DJ, Besh S, D'Amico TA, Das P, Denlinger C, Fakih MG, Fuchs CS, Gerdes H, Glasgow RE. Gastric cancer, version 2.2013. J Natl Compr Cancer Netw. 2013;11(5):531–46.

67. Waddell T, Verheij M, Allum W, Cunningham D, Cervantes A, Arnold D, European Society for Medical O, European Society of Surgical O, European Society of R, Oncology. Gastric cancer: ESMO-ESSO-ESTRO clinical practice guidelines for diagnosis, treatment and follow-up. Eur J Surg Oncol. 2014;40(5):584–91. https://doi.org/10.1016/j.ejso.2013.09.020.

68. Yun M, Choi HS, Yoo E, Bong JK, Ryu YH, Lee JD. The role of gastric distention in differentiating recurrent tumor from physiologic uptake in the remnant stomach on 18F-FDG PET. J Nucl Med. 2005;46(6):953–7.

69. Le Roux PY, Duong CP, Cabalag CS, Parameswaran BK, Callahan J, Hicks RJ. Incremental diagnostic utility of gastric distension FDG PET/CT. Eur J Nucl Med Mol Imaging. 2015. https://doi.org/10.1007/s00259-015-3211-6.

70. Mukai K, Ishida Y, Okajima K, Isozaki H, Morimoto T, Nishiyama S. Usefulness of preoperative FDG-PET for detection of gastric cancer. Gastric

Cancer. 2006;9(3):192–6. https://doi.org/10.1007/s10120-006-0374-7.

71. Stahl A, Ott K, Weber WA, Becker K, Link T, Siewert JR, Schwaiger M, Fink U. FDG PET imaging of locally advanced gastric carcinomas: correlation with endoscopic and histopathological findings. Eur J Nucl Med Mol Imaging. 2003;30(2):288–95. https://doi.org/10.1007/s00259-002-1029-5.

72. Smyth E, Schoder H, Strong VE, Capanu M, Kelsen DP, Coit DG, Shah MA. A prospective evaluation of the utility of 2-deoxy-2-[(18) F]fluoro-D-glucose positron emission tomography and computed tomography in staging locally advanced gastric cancer. Cancer. 2012;118(22):5481–8. https://doi.org/10.1002/cncr.27550.

73. Kawamura T, Kusakabe T, Sugino T, Watanabe K, Fukuda T, Nashimoto A, Honma K, Suzuki T. Expression of glucose transporter-1 in human gastric carcinoma: association with tumor aggressiveness, metastasis, and patient survival. Cancer. 2001;92(3):634–41.

74. Hillner BE, Siegel BA, Shields AF, Liu D, Gareen IF, Hunt E, Coleman RE. Relationship between cancer type and impact of PET and PET/CT on intended management: findings of the national oncologic PET registry. J Nucl Med. 2008;49(12):1928–35. https://doi.org/10.2967/jnumed.108.056713.

75. Podoloff DA, Ball DW, Ben-Josef E, Benson AB 3rd, Cohen SJ, Coleman RE, Delbeke D, Ho M, Ilson DH, Kalemkerian GP, Lee RJ, Loeffler JS, Macapinlac HA, Morgan RJ Jr, Siegel BA, Singhal S, Tyler DS, Wong RJ. NCCN task force: clinical utility of PET in a variety of tumor types. J Natl Compr Cancer Netw. 2009;7(Suppl 2):S1–26.

76. Dassen AE, Lips DJ, Hoekstra CJ, Pruijt JF, Bosscha K. FDG-PET has no definite role in preoperative imaging in gastric cancer. Eur J Surg Oncol. 2009;35(5):449–55. https://doi.org/10.1016/j.ejso.2008.11.010.

77. Chen J, Cheong JH, Yun MJ, Kim J, Lim JS, Hyung WJ, Noh SH. Improvement in preoperative staging of gastric adenocarcinoma with positron emission tomography. Cancer. 2005;103(11):2383–90. https://doi.org/10.1002/cncr.21074.

78. Namikawa T, Okabayshi T, Nogami M, Ogawa Y, Kobayashi M, Hanazaki K. Assessment of (18) F-fluorodeoxyglucose positron emission tomography combined with computed tomography in the preoperative management of patients with gastric cancer. Int J Clin Oncol. 2014;19(4):649–55. https://doi.org/10.1007/s10147-013-0598-6.

79. Takebayashi R, Izuishi K, Yamamoto Y, Kameyama R, Mori H, Masaki T, Suzuki Y. [18F]Fluorodeoxyglucose accumulation as a biological marker of hypoxic status but not glucose transport ability in gastric cancer. J Exp Clin Cancer Res. 2013;32:34. https://doi.org/10.1186/1756-9966-32-34.

80. Mochiki E, Kuwano H, Katoh H, Asao T, Oriuchi N, Endo K. Evaluation of 18F-2-deoxy-2-fluoro-D-glucose positron emission tomography for gastric cancer. World J Surg. 2004;28(3):247–53. https://doi.org/10.1007/s00268-003-7191-5.

81. Shimada H, Okazumi S, Koyama M, Murakami K. Japanese Gastric Cancer Association Task Force for Research Promotion: clinical utility of (1)(8) F-fluoro-2-deoxyglucose positron emission tomography in gastric cancer. A systematic review of the literature. Gastric Cancer. 2011;14(1):13–21. https://doi.org/10.1007/s10120-011-0017-5.

82. Graziosi L, Evoli LP, Cavazzoni E, Donini A. The role of 18 FDG-PET in gastric cancer. Transl Gastrointest Cancer. 2012;1(2):186–8.

83. Kaneko Y, Murray WK, Link E, Hicks RJ, Duong C. Improving patient selection for 18F-FDG PET scanning in the staging of gastric cancer. J Nucl Med. 2015;56(4):523–9. https://doi.org/10.2967/jnumed.114.150946.

84. Malibari N, Hickeson M, Lisbona R. PET/computed Tomography in the diagnosis and staging of gastric cancers. PET Clin. 2015;10(3):311–26. https://doi.org/10.1016/j.cpet.2015.03.008.

85. Lan XL, Zhang YX, Wu ZJ, Jia Q, Wei H, Gao ZR. The value of dual time point (18)F-FDG PET imaging for the differentiation between malignant and benign lesions. Clin Radiol. 2008;63(7):756–64. https://doi.org/10.1016/j.crad.2008.01.003.

86. Salaun PY, Grewal RK, Dodamane I, Yeung HW, Larson SM, Strauss HW. An analysis of the 18F-FDG uptake pattern in the stomach. J Nucl Med. 2005;46(1):48–51.

87. Takahashi H, Ukawa K, Ohkawa N, Kato K, Hayashi Y, Yoshimoto K, Ishiyama A, Ueki N, Kuraoka K, Tsuchida T, Yamamoto Y, Chino A, Uragami N, Fujisaki J, Igarashi M, Fujita R, Koyama M, Yamashita T. Significance of (18)F-2-deoxy-2-fluoro-glucose accumulation in the stomach on positron emission tomography. Ann Nucl Med. 2009;23(4):391–7. https://doi.org/10.1007/s12149-009-0255-3.

88. Kwee RM, Kwee TC. Imaging in assessing lymph node status in gastric cancer. Gastric Cancer. 2009;12(1):6–22. https://doi.org/10.1007/s10120-008-0492-5.

89. Kim EY, Lee WJ, Choi D, Lee SJ, Choi JY, Kim BT, Kim HS. The value of PET/CT for preoperative staging of advanced gastric cancer: comparison with contrast-enhanced CT. Eur J Radiol. 2011;79(2):183–8. https://doi.org/10.1016/j.ejrad.2010.02.005.

90. Kim SK, Kang KW, Lee JS, Kim HK, Chang HJ, Choi JY, Lee JH, Ryu KW, Kim YW, Bae JM. Assessment of lymph node metastases using 18F-FDG PET in patients with advanced gastric cancer. Eur J Nucl Med Mol Imaging. 2006;33(2):148–55. https://doi.org/10.1007/s00259-005-1887-8.

91. Yun M. Imaging of gastric cancer metabolism using 18 F-FDG PET/CT. J Gastric Cancer. 2014;14(1):1–6. https://doi.org/10.5230/jgc.2014.14.1.1.

92. Yun M, Lim JS, Noh SH, Hyung WJ, Cheong JH, Bong JK, Cho A, Lee JD. Lymph node staging of gastric cancer using (18)F-FDG PET: a comparison study with CT. J Nucl Med. 2005;46(10):1582–8.

93. Lerut T, Flamen P, Ectors N, Van Cutsem E, Peeters M, Hiele M, De Wever W, Coosemans W, Decker G, De Leyn P, Deneffe G, Van Raemdonck D, Mortelmans L. Histopathologic validation of lymph node staging with FDG-PET scan in cancer of the esophagus and gastroesophageal junction: a prospective study based on primary surgery with extensive lymphadenectomy. Ann Surg. 2000;232(6):743–52.

94. Yang QM, Kawamura T, Itoh H, Bando E, Nemoto M, Akamoto S, Furukawa H, Yonemura Y. Is PET-CT suitable for predicting lymph node status for gastric cancer? Hepato-Gastroenterology. 2008;55(82–83):782–5.

95. Altini C, Niccoli Asabella A, Di Palo A, Fanelli M, Ferrari C, Moschetta M, Rubini G. 18F-FDG PET/CT role in staging of gastric carcinomas: comparison with conventional contrast enhancement computed tomography. Medicine (Baltimore). 2015;94(20):e864. https://doi.org/10.1097/MD.0000000000000864.

96. Kim YH, Choi JY, Do IG, Kim S, Kim BT. Factors affecting 18F-FDG uptake by metastatic lymph nodes in gastric cancer. J Comput Assist Tomogr. 2013;37(5):815–9. https://doi.org/10.1097/RCT.0b013e3182972989.

97. Oh HH, Lee SE, Choi IS, Choi WJ, Yoon DS, Min HS, Ra YM, Moon JI, Kang YH. The peak-standardized uptake value (P-SUV) by preoperative positron emission tomography-computed tomography (PET-CT) is a useful indicator of lymph node metastasis in gastric cancer. J Surg Oncol. 2011;104(5):530–3. https://doi.org/10.1002/jso.21985.

98. Duarte I, Llanos O. Patterns of metastases in intestinal and diffuse types of carcinoma of the stomach. Hum Pathol. 1981;12(3):237–42.

99. Esaki Y, Hirayama R, Hirokawa K. A comparison of patterns of metastasis in gastric cancer by histologic type and age. Cancer. 1990;65(9):2086–90.

100. Noda S, Soejima K, Inokuchi K. Clinicopathological analysis of the intestinal type and diffuse type of gastric carcinoma. Jpn J Surg. 1980;10(4):277–83.

101. Lim JS, Kim MJ, Yun MJ, Oh YT, Kim JH, Hwang HS, Park MS, Cha SW, Lee JD, Noh SH, Yoo HS, Kim KW. Comparison of CT and 18F-FDG pet for detecting peritoneal metastasis on the preoperative evaluation for gastric carcinoma. Korean J Radiol. 2006;7(4):249–56.

102. Yoshioka T, Yamaguchi K, Kubota K, Saginoya T, Yamazaki T, Ido T, Yamaura G, Takahashi H, Fukuda H, Kanamaru R. Evaluation of 18F-FDG PET in patients with advanced, metastatic, or recurrent gastric cancer. J Nucl Med. 2003;44(5):690–9.

103. Lim JS, Kim M-J, Oh YT, Kim JH, Hwang HS, Park M-S, Cha S-W, Lee JD, Noh SH, Yoo HS. Comparison of CT and 18F-FDG pet for detecting peritoneal metastasis on the preoperative evaluation for gastric carcinoma. Korean J Radiol. 2006;7(4):249–56.

104. Turlakow A, Yeung HW, Salmon AS, Macapinlac HA, Larson SM. Peritoneal carcinomatosis: role of 18F-FDG PET. J Nucl Med. 2003;44(9):1407–12.

105. Yang Q-M, Bando E, Kawamura T, Tsukiyama G, Nemoto M, Yonemura Y, Furukawa H. The diagnostic value of PET-CT for peritoneal dissemination of abdominal malignancies. Gan To Kagaku Ryoho. 2006;33(12):1817–21.

106. Kim SJ, Cho YS, Moon SH, Bae JM, Kim S, Choe YS, Kim BT, Lee KH. Primary Tumor FDG Avidity affects the performance of FDG PET/CT for detecting gastric cancer recurrence. J Nucl Med. 2015. doi:https://doi.org/10.2967/jnumed.115.163295.

107. Lee JW, Jo K, Cho A, Noh SH, Lee JD, Yun M. Relationship between 18F-FDG uptake on PET and recurrence patterns after curative surgical resection in patients with advanced gastric cancer. J Nucl Med. 2015;56(10):1494–500. https://doi.org/10.2967/jnumed.115.160580.

Part IV

Treatment of Gastric Cancer

Endoscopic Treatment for Early Gastric Cancer

5

Takuji Gotoda

Abbreviations

CI	confidence interval
EGC	early gastric cancer
EMR	endoscopic mucosal resection
EMRC	EMR with cap-fitted panendoscope method
EMRL	EMR using multiband ligation
ESD	endoscopic submucosal dissection
IT knife	insulated-tip diathermic knife
LNM	lymph node metastasis
QOL	quality of life

Introduction

In the history of gastric cancer treatment, many of the cases with gastric cancer discovered in the 1970s were in the advanced stage. As represented by the Appleby operation, extended radical surgery was globally accepted as a mainstream approach to gastric cancer, even in the early gastric cancer (EGC). With the widespread adoption of nationwide screening [1] in Japan and South Korea and the advancement of endoscope technology in the 1980s, the number of patients diagnosed with early gastric cancer has increased. Nowadays endoscopic

T. Gotoda (✉)
Division of Gastroenterology and Hepatology, Department of Medicine, Nihon University School of Medicine, Tokyo, Japan

mucosal resection (EMR) and endoscopic submucosal dissection (ESD) offer less invasive options to patients. These options present important trade-offs such as less morbidity but also a higher risk of metachronous recurrence. Patients' preferences and particularly fear of recurrence are important elements in choosing the optimal therapy.

Endoscopic resection to treat cancer is perhaps the most gratifying endoscopy to perform because of its minimally invasive curative potentials. Here, this is a review for endoscopic resection of EGC, which is clinically used for the treatment of EGC in Japan and Korea and is increasingly used globally [2–6]. Endoscopic resection allows complete pathological staging of the cancer, which is critical for risk stratification of metastatic potential [7]. Patients who are stratified to have no or lower risk for lymph node metastasis (LNM) than the risk of mortality from surgery are ideal candidates for endoscopic resection [8]. The optimal staging method of early gastrointestinal cancer is to evaluate the pathology of an en bloc resected material [9, 10]. In addition to allow pathological staging, en bloc resection with R0 (negative vertical and horizontal margins) is to protect the patient from the risk of local recurrence.

History of Endoscopic Resection

The first endoscopic resection of early cancer was reported in colorectal polypectomy using high-frequency electric surgical unit [11]. Indeed the first endoscopic polypectomy used to treat pedunculated or semipedunculated EGC was first described in Japan in 1974 [12].

The "strip biopsy" technique, an early method of endoscopic mucosal resection (EMR) technique, was devised in 1984 as an application of endoscopic snare polypectomy [13]. To obtain the resected material with less tissue damage causing adequate pathological staging, a technique called ERHSE (endoscopic resection with local injection of hypertonic saline epinephrine solution), which is known as a model of ESD, was developed by Hirao and colleagues in 1988 [14].

EMR with cap-fitted panendoscope method (EMRC) was developed in 1992 for the resection of early esophageal cancer and directly applicable for the resection of EGC [15, 16]. The technique of EMR using ligation, which subsequently was extended to EMR using multiband ligation (EMRL), utilizes band ligation to create a "pseudopolyp" by suctioning the lesion into the banding cap and deploying a band underneath it [17, 18]. The EMRC and EMRL techniques have the advantage of being relatively simple. However, these techniques cannot be used to remove lesions en bloc larger than 2 cm [19, 20]. Piecemeal resections in lesions larger than 2 cm lead to a high risk for local cancer recurrence and inadequate pathological staging [21, 22].

Insulated-tip diathermic knife (IT knife) was devised in the late 1990s at the National Cancer Center Hospital, Japan, in order to resolve problems observed from the use of EMR techniques for the resection of EGC. IT knife has a ceramic ball tip, thus preventing it from puncturing the wall during the application of cautery and causing perforation. The knife can also be used to dissect the submucosa – leading to the name of the technique: endoscopic submucosal dissection (ESD) technique [23–25]. Subsequent studies have proven that ESD, using standard single-channel endoscope, can be used for resection of large lesions "en bloc," allowing a precise pathological staging (Fig. 5.1 a, b, c). Complete en bloc resection regardless of tumor size, location, and/or submucosal fibrosis can be now possible [26]. Other ESD knives and techniques have since been developed and studied in detail (Fig. 5.2) [27–31]. Very recently, ESD has been tried to improve an easier procedure [32, 33].

Treatment Strategy for Endoscopic Resection

Principle

EGC is defined when the cancer invasion is confined to the mucosa or submucosa (T1 cancer), irrespective of the presence of LNM [34]. Because the presence of LNM is a strong predictor on patients' prognosis [35, 36], gastrectomy with lymph node dissection had been the gold standard for treatment of EGC in Japan [37]. Such an extensive surgery however carries a significant risk of morbidity and mortality and is associated with long-term reduction of patients' quality of life [38].

Extensive long-term outcomes data from the National Cancer Center Hospital and others in Japan have shown that the 5-year cancer-specific

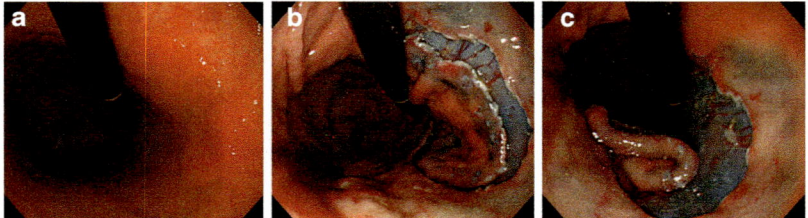

Fig. 5.1 (a) A large elevated lesion located on the lesser curvature of the middle gastric body, (b) circumferentially mucosal cutting at the periphery of the marking dots using IT knife-2 or Dual knife with PulseCut slow (40 W), (c) dissecting submucosal layer after additional submucosal injection

Fig. 5.2 (**a**) IT knife-2 (KD-611L, Olympus Medical Systems), (**b**) Hook knife (KD-620LR, Olympus Medical Systems), (**c**) Dual knife (KD-650L, Olympus Medical Systems), (**d**) Flash knife BT (Fujinon Optical Co., Ltd.), (**e**) Safe knife (DK2518DV1, Fujinon Optical Co., Ltd.), (**f**) Mucosectom (DP-2518, PENTAX)

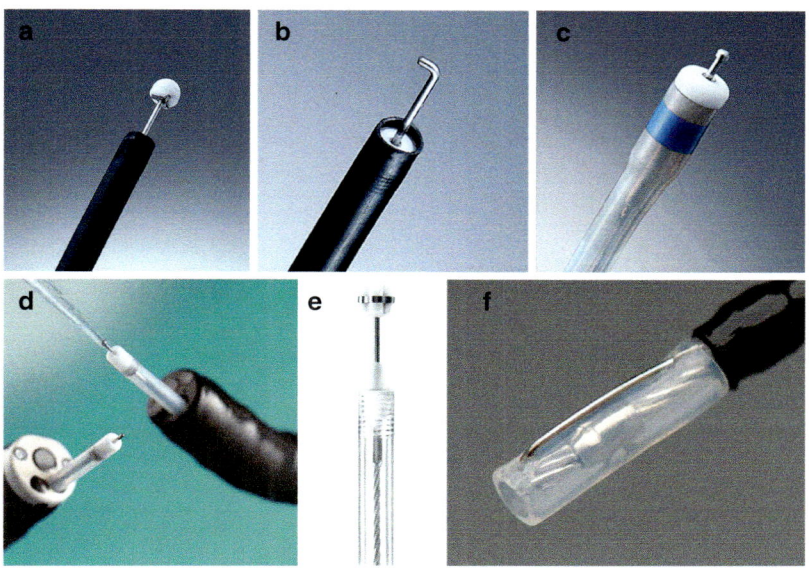

survival rates of EGC limited to the mucosa or the superficial submucosa were 99% and 96%, respectively [39]. In patients with intramucosal cancer, the incidence of LNM can be as high as 3%. In comparison, the risk increases to as high as 20% when the cancer involves the deep submucosa [40]. With stratification, subgroups of patients with EGC and minimal risk of LNM could be identified [41]. Patients who meet these very specific endoscopic and pathological criteria are therefore the most ideal candidates to have their cancer endoscopically resected.

The major advantage of endoscopic resection is the ability to provide an accurate pathological staging without precluding future surgical therapy [42, 43]. After endoscopic resection, pathological assessment of the depth of cancer invasion, degree of cancer differentiation, and involvement of lymphatics or vessels allows the prediction of the risk of LNM [44]. The risk of developing LNM or distant metastasis is then weighted against the risk of surgery [45].

Indication Criteria

The traditional criteria for endoscopic resection of EGC were founded on the technical limitation of traditional EMR for removing gastric lesions larger than 2 cm in diameter en bloc [41, 46]. The empirical indications for EMR were therefore [47] (1) papillary or tubular (differentiated) adenocarcinoma, (2) less than 2 cm in diameter, (3) without ulceration within tumor, and (4) no lymph-vascular involvement.

The subsequent advent of ESD dramatically changed the range of lesions indicated for endoscopic resection (Table 5.1). With an objective of expanding the indications, the risks of LNM in early gastric cancer were assessed in 5265 cases of surgical resection performed at two major oncology centers in Tokyo [48]. LNM was observed in 65 of 3016 cases of MGC (2.2%) and in 402 of 2249 cases of submucosal invasive carcinoma (17.9%). Furthermore, LNM was observed in none of the 1230 intramucosal cancers with lesions 30 mm or less in size with or without ulceration, with differentiated histology, and without lymphatic vessel invasion (95% confidence interval (CI): 0–0.3%). In intramucosal cancer without ulcerated lesions, LNM was observed in none of the 929 cases with differentiated histology and without lymphatic vessel invasion (95% CI: 0–0.4%). In cases with undifferentiated histology, analysis of subsequently accumulated cases revealed that LNM was observed in none of the 310 cases of intramucosal cancer, 20 mm or less in size, without either

Table 5.1 Early gastric cancer with no risk of lymph node metastasis

Criteria	Incidence (no. with metastasis/total number)	95% CI
Intramucosal cancer	0/1230; 0%	0–0.3
Differentiated (well and/or moderately differentiated and/or papillary adenocarcinoma) type		
No lymph-vascular involvement		
Irrespective of ulcer findings		
Tumor less than 3 cm in size		
Intramucosal cancer	0/929; 0%	0–0.4
Differentiated type		
No lymph-vascular involvement		
Without ulcer findings		
Irrespective of tumor size		
Intramucosal cancer	0/310; 0%	0–0.96
Undifferentiated (poorly differentiated adenocarcinoma and/or signet-ring cell carcinoma) type		
No lymph-vascular involvement		
Without ulcer findings		
Tumor less than 2 cm in size		
Minute submucosal penetration (sm1)	0/145; 0%	0–2.5
Differentiated type		
No lymph-vascular involvement		
Tumor less than 3 cm in size		

Modification by Refs. [41, 47]

lymphatic vessel invasion or ulcerated lesions (95% CI: 0–0.96%) [49].

The new findings from the study conducted by Choi and colleagues are described below. Their retrospective cohort study revealed that LNM was observed in 0.4% of the cases satisfying the expanded indications and even 0.3% of cases satisfying the absolute indications [50]. Their results are sufficient to indicate the importance of informing and helping patients before treatment to understand that, despite endoscopic resection, there is a low but not negligible risk of recurrence or metastasis because malignant tumors are treated.

Similarly to intramucosal cancer, there was a significant correlation between tumor size larger than 30 mm and lymph-vascular involvement with an increased risk of LNM. In addition, those cancers penetrating deeply into the submucosa were the most likely to be associated with regional LNM. The relationship between tumor characteristics such as size, depth of submucosal invasion, presence of ulceration, differentiation, and lymphatic or vascular permeation is shown. For well-differentiated tumors, subgroup analysis based on the pairing of individual factors such as of tumor size, depth of submucosal penetration, and lymph-vascular involvement failed to yield a subgroup entirely free of nodal metastasis. However, the subgroup of 145 lesions with size less than 3 cm, well-differentiated histology, lack of lymph-vascular involvement, and less than 500 μm submucosal penetration was entirely free of nodal metastasis (95% CI: 0–2.5%).

Pathological Staging

Proper pathological assessment of endoscopically resected specimens is crucial for an accurate diagnosis and patient's stratification for the risk of LNM. The Paris classification of superficial neoplasia of the gastrointestinal tract allows a straightforward endoscopic diagnosis of early lesions including an estimation of tumor depth and likelihood of risk of LNM [51]. These classifications provide a common terminology in order to speak the same language and compare results to that reported in the literature.

The importance of meticulous pathological staging after endoscopic resection is strongly emphasized. Pathological reports of the resected specimen must include pathological type, tumor depth, size, location, and macroscopic appearance. The presence of ulceration and lymph-vascular involvement, if any, and the status of the margin of resections should be reported. Without sufficient specimen, tumor staging cannot be accurately assessed, patient's prognosis cannot be estimated, and potential needs for additional therapy, which may be curative, cannot be obtained [52, 53].

Clinical Management After Endoscopic Resection

All patients with curative resection who met the traditional criteria were followed up by annual upper gastrointestinal endoscopy in order to detect local recurrence and/or metachronous gastric cancers [54]. Patients with curative resection who met the expanded criteria were additionally followed up by alternative abdominal CT and endoscopic ultrasound (EUS) every 6 months for 3 years in order to detect lymph node and distant metastases and annual upper gastrointestinal endoscopy.

Especially, in the expanded criteria with submucosal invasion, lesions with minute submucosal invasion – less than 500 μm submucosal invasion of differentiated EGC measuring less than 3 cm, without lymphatic-vascular involvement, no nodal metastasis was found (95% CI: 0–2.5%). However, this result is based on a retrospective examination of surgical resection cases in which patients suitable for such expanded criteria were determined to have a low risk of lymph node metastasis. This means there is a possibility of lymph node metastasis up to the upper limit of 95% CI whenever the lesions fulfill the expanded criteria on the histological assessment [55–57].

Long-term outcomes after EMR for small differentiated mucosal EGC less than 2 cm in diameter have been reported to be comparable to those following gastrectomy [58, 59]. Gotoda and colleagues have reported that patients who underwent treatment following the expanded criteria have similar long-term survival and outcomes as patients treated according to the traditional criteria [60]. The 5-year survival rate was 92% in patients with traditional criteria group and 93% in the expanded criteria group. There was no significant difference in overall survival between both groups. The multivariable hazard ratio for the patients of the expanded criteria group versus those of the traditional criteria group was 1.10 (95% CI: 0.67–1.81). Very recently several Korean investigators reported that ESD in the extended indication group had similarly acceptable clinical outcomes with a relatively high complete resection rate and a low local recurrence rate [61, 62]. ESD has been now widely acceptable technique and clinically applied in Korea. ESD might be better than EMR in terms of en bloc resection, complete resection, and long-term outcome [63].

Considering the risk of LNM and predicting prognosis, there are several scenarios after pathological evaluation. It is important to note that a non-curative endoscopic resection because of positive lateral margin is completely different to a non-curative endoscopic resection that did not fulfill the pathological factors highly associated with LNM such as deep submucosal invasion or positive lymph-vascular involvement. Non-curative resection generally requires radical surgical resection with lymph node dissection as the standard treatment due to the possibility of LNM for patient's prognosis (Fig. 5.3 a, b). Additional surgery following non-curative endoscopic resection improved overall and disease-free survival compared with nonsurgical observation even in elderly patients (>75 years) with non-curative endoscopic resection for EGC [64].

In cancer treatment, completely curing the illness is extremely important. However, if the quality of life (QOL) is impaired by procedures that are superior only in terms of reducing marginal risks, patients may have difficulties in daily life and social rehabilitation after treatment [65]. With the risks of surgical procedures and impaired postoperative QOL taken into account, there may be situations allowing more expanded indications for endoscopic resection, leading to approximately 10% of the incidence of metastasis and recurrence or, in other words, death from gastric cancer.

Fig. 5.3 (**a**) A large elevated lesion located on the anterior wall of the angle treated by ESD as non-curative resection with deep submucosal invasion, (**b**) multiple liver metastases were shown 6 months after ESD

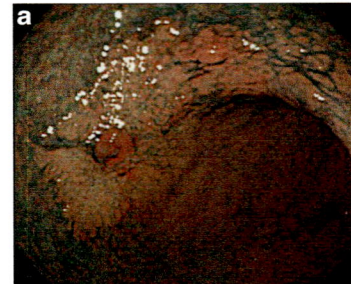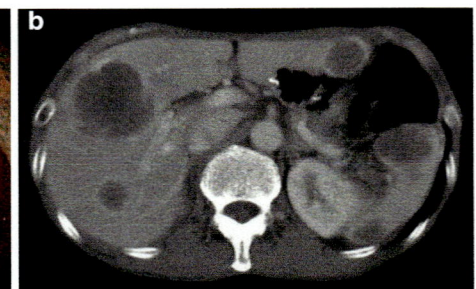

The stomach and small intestine are collectively referred to as the "second brain," as they are extremely vital for digestive and absorptive functions of the body. The stomach not only serves as a storage compartment but also plays a role in the external secretion of gastric acid essential for digestion and absorption of food, as well as in internal secretion, including gastrin and ghrelin. Gastrectomy results in a decrease or lack of digestive enzyme and hormonal secretion, causing increased stress on the small intestine. Consequently, it triggers postoperative aftereffects far worse than those associated with colectomy, including not only the well-known dumping syndrome but also chronic bowel movement disturbance, indigestion, and defective absorption. Therefore, if there is no difference of curability among different treatment methods, long-term QOL should be considered seriously when we select a treatment method.

Permanent cure of cancer is immensely important. However, if the focus is placed entirely on permanent cure and the patient's postoperative QOL is undermined as a result, it may pose difficulties in the patient's daily life or reintegration into society. In actual clinical practice, many factors should be considered, such as patient age and complications, as well as views on life and the philosophical outlook of patients and their families. Medical care will always be provided with consideration of the following points: whether ESD is really minimally invasive; whether "complete" treatment attempted by physicians, such as gastrectomy, is beneficial for patients; and whether treatment that is not the best but more tolerable to the patients is an option.

References

1. Gotoda T, Ishikawa H, Ohnishi H, et al. Randomized controlled trial comparing gastric cancer screening by gastrointestinal X-ray with serology for Helicobacter pylori and pepsinogens followed by gastrointestinal endoscopy. Gastric Cancer. 2015;18(3):605–11.
2. Rembacken BJ, Gotoda T, Fujii T, et al. Endoscopic mucosal resection. Endoscopy. 2001;33:709–18.
3. Soetikno R, Gotoda T, Nakanishi Y, et al. Endoscopic mucosal resection. Gastrointest Endosc. 2003;57:567–79.
4. Gotoda T. Endoscopic resection of early gastric cancer. Gastric Cancer. 2007;10:1–11.
5. Gotoda T, Yamamoto H, Soetikno R. Endoscopic Submucosal Dissection for early gastric cancer. J Gastroenterol. 2006;41:929–42.
6. Jung HY. Endoscopic resection for early gastric cancer: current status in Korea. Dig Endosc. 2012;24:159–65.
7. Hull M, Mino-Kenudson M, Nishioka NS, et al. Endoscopic mucosal resection: an improved diagnostic procedure for early gastroesophageal epithelial neoplasms. Am J Surg Pathol. 2006;30:114–8.
8. Ludwig K, Klautke G, Bernhard J, et al. Minimally invasive and local treatment for mucosal early gastric cancer. Surg Endosc. 2005;19:1362–6.
9. Ahmad NA, Kochman ML, Long WB, et al. Efficacy, safety, and clinical outcomes of endoscopic mucosal resection: a study of 101 cases. Gastrointest Endosc. 2002;55:390–6.
10. Katsube T, Konno S, Hamaguchi K, et al. The efficacy of endoscopic mucosal resection in the diagnosis and treatment of group III gastric lesions. Anticancer Res. 2005;25:3513–6.
11. Deyhle P, Largiader F, Jenny P. A method for endoscopic electroresection of sessile colonic polyps. Endoscopy. 1973;5:38–40.
12. Oguro Y. Endoscopic gastric polypectomy with high frequency currents. Stom Intest (in English abstract). 1974;9:309–16.
13. Tada M, Shimada M, Murakami F, et al. Development of strip-off biopsy. Gastroenterol Endosc (in English abstract). 1984;26:833–9.

14. Hirao M, Masuda K, Asanuma T, et al. Endoscopic resection of early gastric cancer and other tumors with local injection of hypertonic saline-epinephrine. Gastrointest Endosc. 1988;34:264–9.

15. Inoue H, Endo M, Takeshita K, et al. A new simplified technique of endoscopic esophageal mucosal resection using a cap-fitted panendoscope (EMRC). Surg Endosc. 1992;6:264–5.

16. Inoue H, Takeshita K, Hori H, et al. Endoscopic mucosal resection with a cap-fitted panendoscope for esophagus, stomach, and colon mucosal lesions. Gastrointest Endosc. 1993;39:58–62.

17. Akiyama M, Ota M, Nakajima H, et al. Endoscopic mucosal resection of gastric neoplasms using a ligating device. Gastrointest Endosc. 1997;45: 182–6.

18. Soehendra N, Seewald S, Groth S, et al. Use of modified multiband ligator facilitates circumferential EMR in Barrett's esophagus (with video). Gastrointest Endosc. 2006;63:847–52.

19. Korenaga D, Haraguchi M, Tsujitani S, et al. Clinicopathological features of mucosal carcinoma of the stomach with lymph node metastasis in eleven patients. Br J Surg. 1986;73:431–3.

20. Ell C, May A, Gossner L, et al. Endoscopic mucosectomy of early cancer and high-grade dysplasia in Barrett's esophagus. Gastroenterology. 2000;118:670–7.

21. Tanabe S, Koizumi W, Mitomi H, et al. Clinical outcome of endoscopic aspiration mucosectomy for early stage gastric cancer. Gastrointest Endosc. 2002;56:708–13.

22. Kim JJ, Lee JH, Jung HY, et al. EMR for early gastric cancer in Korea: a multicenter retrospective study. Gastrointest Endosc. 2007;66:693–700.

23. Ono H, Kondo H, Gotoda T, et al. Endoscopic mucosal resection for treatment of early gastric cancer. Gut. 2001;48:225–9.

24. Hosokawa K, Yoshida S. Recent advances in endoscopic mucosal resection for early gastric cancer. Jpn J Cancer Chemother (in English abstract). 1998;25:483.

25. Gotoda T, Kondo H, Ono H, et al. A new endoscopic mucosal resection (EMR) procedure using an insulation-tipped diathermic (IT) knife for rectal flat lesions. Gastrointest Endosc. 1999;50:560–3.

26. Yokoi C, Gotoda T, Oda I, et al. Endoscopic submucosal dissection (ESD) allows curative resection of local recurrent early gastric cancer after prior endoscopic mucosal resection. Gastrointest Endosc. 2006;64:212–8.

27. Oyama T, Kikuchi Y. Aggressive endoscopic mucosal resection in the upper GI tract – hook knife EMR method. Min Invas Ther Allied Technol. 2002;11:291–5.

28. Yahagi N, Fujishiro M, Kakushima N, et al. Endoscopic submucosal dissection for early gastric cancer using the tip of an electrosurgical snare (thin Type). Dig Endosc. 2004;16:34–8.

29. Ono H, Hasuike N, Inui T, et al. Usefulness of a novel electrosurgical knife, the insulation-tipped diathermic knife-2, for endoscopic submucosal dissection of early gastric cancer. Gastric Cancer. 2008;11:47–52.

30. Takeuchi Y, Uedo N, Ishihara R, et al. Efficacy of an endo-knife with a water jet function (Flushknife) for endoscopic submucosal dissection of superficial colorectal neoplasms. Am J Gastroenterol. 2010;105:314–22.

31. Toyonaga T, Man-I M, Fujita T, et al. The performance of a novel ball-tipped Flush knife for endoscopic submucosal dissection: a case–control study. Aliment Pharmacol Ther. 2010;32:908–15.

32. Suzuki S, Gotoda T, Kobayashi Y, et al. Usefulness of a traction method using dental floss and a hemoclip for gastric endoscopic submucosal dissection: a propensity score matching analysis (with videos). Gastrointest Endosc. 2016;83:337–46.

33. Yoshida M, Takizawa K, Ono H, et al. Efficacy of endoscopic submucosal dissection with dental floss clip traction for gastric epithelial neoplasia: a pilot study (with video). Surg Endosc. 2016;30(7):3100–6.

34. Japanese Gastric Cancer Association. Japanese classification of gastric carcinoma -3rd English edition. Gastric Cancer. 2011;14:101–12.

35. Itoh H, Oohata Y, Nakamura K, et al. Complete ten-year postgastrectomy follow-up of early gastric cancer. Am J Surg. 1989;158:14–6.

36. Ohta H, Noguchi Y, Takagi K, et al. Early gastric carcinoma with special reference to macroscopic classification. Cancer. 1987;60:1099–106.

37. Sano T, Sasako M, Kinoshita T, et al. Recurrence of early gastric cancer – follow-up of 1475 patients and review of Japanese literature. Cancer. 1993;72:3174–8.

38. Sasako M. Risk factors for surgical treatment in the Dutch gastric cancer trial. Br J Surg. 1997;84: 1567–71.

39. Sasako M, Kinoshita T, Maruyama K. Prognosis of early gastric cancer. Stom Intest (in English abstract). 1993;28:139–46.

40. Sano T, Kobori O, Muto T. Lymph node metastasis from early gastric cancer: endoscopic resection of tumour. Br J Surg. 1992;79:241–4.

41. Tsujitani S, Oka S, Saito H, et al. Less invasive surgery for early gastric cancer based on the low probability of lymph node metastasis. Surgery. 1999;125: 148–54.

42. Yanai H, Matsubara Y, Okamoto T, et al. Clinical impact of strip biopsy for early gastric cancer. Gastrointest Endosc. 2004;60:771–7.

43. Farrell JJ, Lauwers GY, Brugge WR. Endoscopic mucosal resection using a cap-fitted endoscope improves tissue resection and pathology interpretation: an animal study. Gastric Cancer. 2006;9: 3–8.

44. Gotoda T, Sasako M, Shimoda T, et al. An evaluation of the necessity of gastrectomy with lymph node dis-

section for patients with submucosal Invasive gastric cancer. Br J Surg. 2001;88:444–9.

45. Etoh T, Katai H, Fukagawa T, et al. Treatment of early gastric cancer in the elderly patient: results of EMR and gastrectomy at a national referral center in Japan. Gastrointest Endosc. 2005;62:868–71.

46. Yamao T, Shirao K, Ono H, et al. Risk factors for lymph node metastasis from intramucosal gastric carcinoma. Cancer. 1996;77:602–6.

47. Japanese Gastric Cancer Association. Japanese gastric cancer treatment guidelines 2010 (ver.3). Gastric Cancer. 2011;14:113–23.

48. Gotoda T, Yanagisawa A, Sasako M, Ono H, Nakanishi Y, Shimoda T, et al. Incidence of lymph node metastasis from early gastric cancer: estimation with a large number of cases at two large centers. Gastric Cancer. 2000;3(4):219–25.

49. Hirasawa T, Gotoda T, Miyata S, Kato Y, Shimoda T, Taniguchi H, et al. Incidence of lymph node metastasis and the feasibility of endoscopic resection for undifferentiated-type early gastric cancer. Gastric Cancer. 2009;12(3):148–52.

50. Choi KK, Bae JM, Kim SM, Sohn TS, Noh JH, Lee JH, et al. The risk of lymph node metastases in 3,951 surgically resected mucosal gastric cancers: implications for endoscopic resection. Gastrointest Endosc. 2015;3. [Epub ahead of print].

51. The Paris endoscopic classification of superficial neoplastic lesions: esophagus, stomach, and colon: November 30 to December 1, 2002. Gastrointest Endosc. 2003;58(6 Suppl):S3–43.

52. Nagano H, Ohyama S, Fukunaga T, et al. Indications for gastrectomy after incomplete EMR for early gastric cancer. Gastric Cancer. 2005;8:149–54.

53. Yano H, Kimura Y, Iwazawa T, et al. Laparoscopic management for local recurrence of early gastric cancer after endoscopic mucosal resection. Surg Endosc. 2005;19:981–5.

54. Nakajima T, Oda I, Gotoda T, et al. Metachronous gastric cancers after endoscopic resection: how effective is annual endoscopic surveillance? Gastric Cancer. 2006;9:93–8.

55. Nagano H, Fukunaga T, Hiki N, et al. Two rare cases of node-positive differentiated gastric cancer despite their infiltration to sm1, their small size, and lack of lymphatic invasion into the submucosal layer. Gastric Cancer. 2008;11:53–7.

56. Oya H, Gotoda T, Kinjo T, et al. A case of lymph node metastasis following a curative endoscopic submucosal dissection of an early gastric cancer. Gastric Cancer. 2012;15:221–5.

57. Chung JW, Jung HY, Choi KD, et al. Extended indication of endoscopic resection for mucosal early gastric cancer: analysis of a single center experience. J Gastroenterol Hepatol. 2011;26:884–7.

58. Uedo N, Iishi H, Tatsuta M, Ishihara R, Higashino K, Takeuchi Y, et al. Longterm outcome after endoscopic mucosal resection for early gastric cancer. Gastric Cancer. 2006;9:88–92.

59. Choi KS, Jung HY, Choi KD, et al. EMR versus gastrectomy for intramucosal gastric cancer: comparison of long-term outcomes. Gastrointest Endosc. 2011;73:942–8.

60. Gotoda T, Iwasaki M, Kusano C, et al. Endoscopic resection of early gastric cancer treated by guideline and expanded National Cancer Centre criteria. Br J Surg. 2010;97:868–71.

61. Chung IK, Lee JH, Lee SH, et al. Therapeutic outcomes in 1000 cases of endoscopic submucosal dissection for early gastric neoplasms: Korean ESD Study Group multicenter study. Gastrointest Endosc. 2009;69:1228–35.

62. Lee H, Yun WK, Min BH, et al. A feasibility study on the expanded indication for endoscopic submucosal dissection of early gastric cancer. Surg Endosc. 2011;25:1985–93.

63. Ahn JY, Jung HY, Choi KD, et al. Endoscopic and oncologic outcomes after endoscopic resection for early gastric cancer: 1370 cases of absolute and extended indications. Gastrointest Endosc. 2011;74:485–93.

64. Kusano C, Iwasaki M, Kaltenbach T, et al. Should elderly patients undergo additional surgery after noncurative endoscopic resection for early gastric cancer? long-term comparative outcomes. Am J Gastroenterol. 2011;106:1064–9.

65. Gotoda T, Yang HK. The desired balance between treatment and curability in treatment planning for early gastric cancer. Gastrointest Endosc. 2015;82(2):308–10.

Part V

Open Surgery for Gastric Cancer

Open Surgery for Gastric Cancer: Distal Subtotal Gastrectomy with D2 Lymph Node Dissection

Ji Yeong An,[s] Yoon Young Choi,[s]
and Sung Hoon Noh

Introduction

Gastric cancer is a major cancer worldwide but particularly in East Asia, where two-thirds of the cases were reported. This area includes Korea, Japan, and China [1]. Gastrectomy with lymph node dissection has been a standard treatment for gastric cancer [2]. The rationale behind this treatment option is twofold. Small tumors should be excised as they will progress to large tumors and invade other organs. Second, surgical resection of the primary tumors should effectively reduce the risk of metastatic relapse [3]. Outcomes of surgical resection for early stage of gastric cancer are quite good, with a greater than 90% 5-year overall survival, even without adjuvant chemotherapy or radiotherapy [4]. These statistics highlight the important role of surgeons in the treatment of gastric cancer.

D2 Lymph Node Dissection

The necessity for radical surgery following diagnosis of gastric cancer is not under question, but practitioners were often less sure about the ideal number of lymph nodes to remove. The stomach is supplied with blood mainly from five vessels: the right and left gastric arteries, the right and left gastroepiploic arteries, and the short gastric artery. It also has an abundant, complex lymphatic network. Consequently, cancer can spread in many directions from the stomach, and it can be difficult to predict metastases that may originate from the lymphatic system. Lymph node dissection has been the subject of the long debate in the medical community and

[s]Ji Yeong An and Yoon Young Choi are contributed equally to this manuscript

Electronic Supplementary Material The online version of this chapter (https://doi.org/10.1007/978-3-662-45583-8_6) contains supplementary material, which is available to authorized users.

J. Y. An
Department of Surgery, Yonsei University Health System, Yonsei University College of Medicine, Seoul, Republic of Korea

Department of Surgery, Samsung Medical Center, Sungkyunkwan University School of Medicine, Seoul, Republic of Korea

Y. Y. Choi
Department of Surgery, Yonsei University Health System, Yonsei University College of Medicine, Seoul, Republic of Korea

S. H. Noh (✉)
Department of Surgery, Yonsei University Health System, Yonsei University College of Medicine, Seoul, Republic of Korea

Brain Korea 21 PLUS Project for Medical Science, Yonsei University Health System, Yonsei University College of Medicine, Seoul, Republic of Korea
e-mail: sunghoonn@yuhs.ac

was addressed in randomized controlled trials [5–8]. The results of these trials have led to the recommendation by medical professionals in both the western and eastern hemispheres that the D2 lymph nodes be dissected in patients with advanced gastric cancer [2, 9, 10]. At present, distal subtotal gastrectomy and D2 lymph node dissection are the recommended basic procedure for gastric cancer.

The definition of the D2 lymph nodes has been modified by Japanese Gastric Cancer Association [11]. In this chapter, the procedures for D2 lymph node dissection are mainly based on the current Japanese treatment guidelines [2].

Oncologic Principles for Gastric Cancer Surgery

There are fundamental differences between surgery performed in patients with cancer and in patients with other benign conditions. Protocols based on oncological principles must be followed throughout surgical procedures on cancer patients to prevent contamination with, or dissemination of, the cancer cells. The fundamental goal of cancer surgery is complete surgical resection of tumor, en bloc lymph node dissection, and careful hemostasis. If this goal is not achieved, cancer cells can be disseminated through broken lymphatics and vessels. The extent of gastric resection should be decided upon based on the location of tumor in the stomach and the safety resection margin so that microscopic tumors are not left in remaining stomach. The "no-touch" technique should be used during the entire procedure. The no-touch technique entails wrapping the primary tumor. This is especially important in cases of serosa-positive gastric cancer, in which it is of utmost importance to prevent iatrogenic peritoneal seeding through the surgeon's hands. Unnecessary manipulation and dissection should be avoided as mitogenic factors for wound healing could be produced in response to the surgery; these could stimulate the proliferation of undetected micrometastatic tumors that remained after surgery [3].

Omentectomy and Bursectomy

Omentectomy and bursectomy are procedures that can be performed during gastric cancer surgery.

The omentum, part of the visceral peritoneum, controls the inflammation in the abdominal cavity [12]. Total omentectomy is recommended during surgery for advanced gastric cancer because the omentum can act as a gateway for metastasis [2, 13]. It is not a time-consuming procedure in open surgery (as it would be in laparoscopic surgery.) It is, in fact, easier to perform total omentectomy than partial omentectomy in open surgery as it is easy to access the avascular plane.

Bursectomy, removing the anterior membrane of the transverse mesocolon and the capsule of the pancreas, has been widely performed for advanced gastric cancer in Korea and Japan [14]. The rationale behind this procedure is that microscopic cancer cells could exist in the membranes that cover the posterior stomach cavity if the tumor invades the serosa layer of the stomach and removing this membrane may reduce the risk of cancer relapse in the peritoneal cavity [15]. The efficacy of bursectomies was assessed in a randomized, controlled trial that compared the long-term outcomes of D2 dissection alone or with bursectomy. In this study, bursectomies were the independent prognostic factors [16]. Bursectomies can be performed with minimal complication [17] and can provide an avascular plane in conjunction with omentectomy. Considering all the data, it appears that bursectomies should be recommended during surgeries for advanced gastric cancer, especially for serosa-positive gastric cancer located in posterior wall of the stomach.

Surgical Procedure for Distal Subtotal Gastrectomy with D2 Lymph Node Dissection

The specifics for this procedure are identified and explained below.

Indication

The procedure is indicated when distal stomach adenocarcinoma has been diagnosed.

Contraindication

The procedure is contraindicated in these circumstances:

- When it is not possible to secure the distal resection margin due to stomach pylorus invasion
- When there are enlarged lymph nodes around the head of the pancreas and the right gastroepiploic vessels, so that the cancer is unresectable

Preoperative preparation

Routine nasogastric tube insertion pre-/postoperatively is not recommended. However, when there is preoperative gastric outlet obstruction due to advanced gastric cancer, the gastric contents need to be removed through a nasogastric tube and gastric lavage before operation to avoid contamination of the surgical site by the gastric contents. In addition, if there is an electrolyte imbalance or malnutrition before operation, it should be corrected before the operation is performed. For early gastric cancer, preoperative endoscopic clipping on the proximal part of tumor is useful to detect the location of tumor and determine the secure resection margin for the operation.

Anesthesia

General anesthesia via an endotracheal tube is used routinely. After endotracheal tube insertion, prophylactic antibiotics should be injected.

Position of Patient During Surgery

The patient should be positioned in supine on the flat table with the legs fastened to the table with a belt. Usually, the patient is situated the right side of the table, and the operator stands on patient's right.

Incision, Exposure, and Preparation of Main Procedures

Although either upper midline or subcostal incisions are acceptable for distal subtotal gastrectomy, a midline incision extending from the xiphoid process to the umbilicus is the most common (Fig. 6.1a). An incision below the umbilicus is not usually necessary; however, the original incision can be extended to achieve a better operative field. After making the skin incision by knife, the linea alba should be divided, with careful hemostasis, using an electrocautery device such as Bovie. The open abdominal wall can be protected with a wound protector device to reduce the risk of cancer cell and bacterial contamination. During surgery, applying the wound retractor can provide better operative field (Fig. 6.1b). In cases in which peritoneal metastasis is suspected, it is useful to perform staging laparoscopy through a potential incision site before laparotomy. The surgeon should initially make small midline incisions, sufficient to permit the insertion of one hand so that the resectability of the stomach can be determined from the pancreas invasion and rectal shelf. The incisions can be expanded later, during the regular gastrectomy.

Exposure and dissection of the area of the #4sb lymph node is easier if the spleen is moved aside. This can be done by lifting the spleen up gently with the left hand and inserting one or two rolled surgical tapes behind it (Fig. 6.2). The tape roll(s) should be counted and removed before closing the abdominal wall. Sometimes dissecting the spleno-phrenic or splenorenal ligament is necessary for this procedure, and care should be taken not to injure the parenchyma of the spleen. If there are severe adhesions around the spleen from previous abdominal surgery, it would be better not to perform this procedure.

Fig. 6.1 Incision for open surgery of gastric cancer. (**a**) 15 cm of incision from xiphoid process to umbilicus for open surgery. (**b**) The open abdominal wall is protected by wound protector device

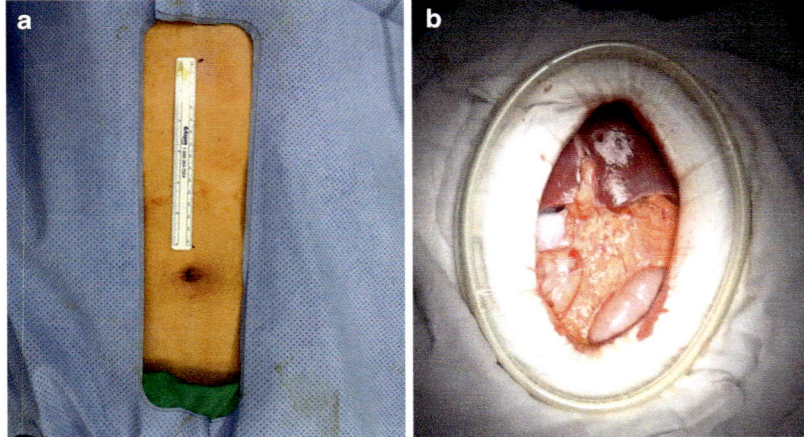

Fig. 6.2 The process of lifting the spleen up for achieving good operative field for #4sb lymph node dissection. The spleen is gently lifted up, and the rolled surgical tapes are inserted behind the spleen

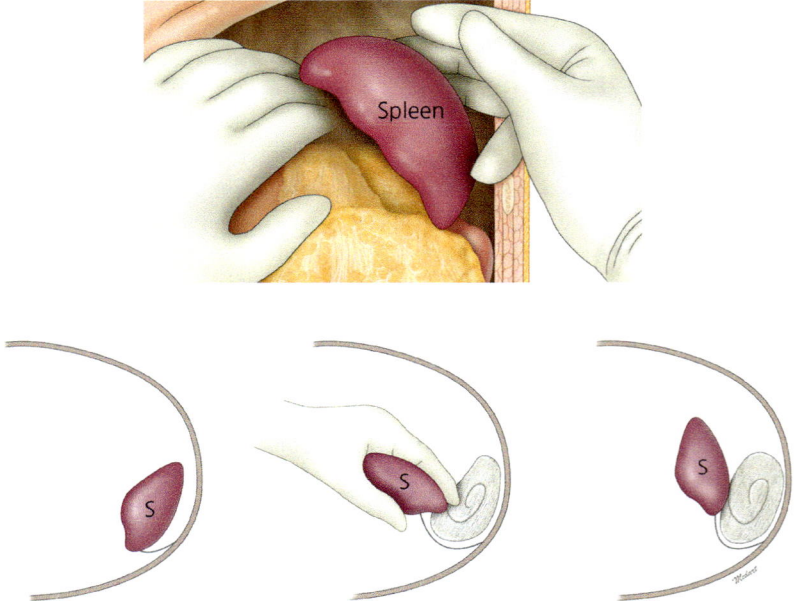

The dilated stomach and colon hinder surgery, and this problem should be addressed before the main procedure. Decompression of the dilated stomach and colon by applying suction with an 18G-needle is one way to accomplish this (Fig. 6.3). The location of the puncture site in the stomach should not be near the tumor site or the proximal part of the stomach that will remain after gastrectomy.

Details of Procedure for D2 Lymph Node Dissection

Total Omentectomy and Bursectomy

Total omentectomy and bursectomy are recommended for advanced gastric cancer, especially when the tumor is located in the posterior wall of stomach (Fig. 6.4a). The first assistant should grasp the transverse colon firmly with both

Fig. 6.3 Decompressing the dilated stomach and colon can provide good operative field during surgery. (**a**) The dilated stomach was punctured by 18G-needle with suction. (**b**) The stomach is decompressed. (**c**) The dilated colon was punctured by 18G-needle with suction. (**d**) The colon is decompressed

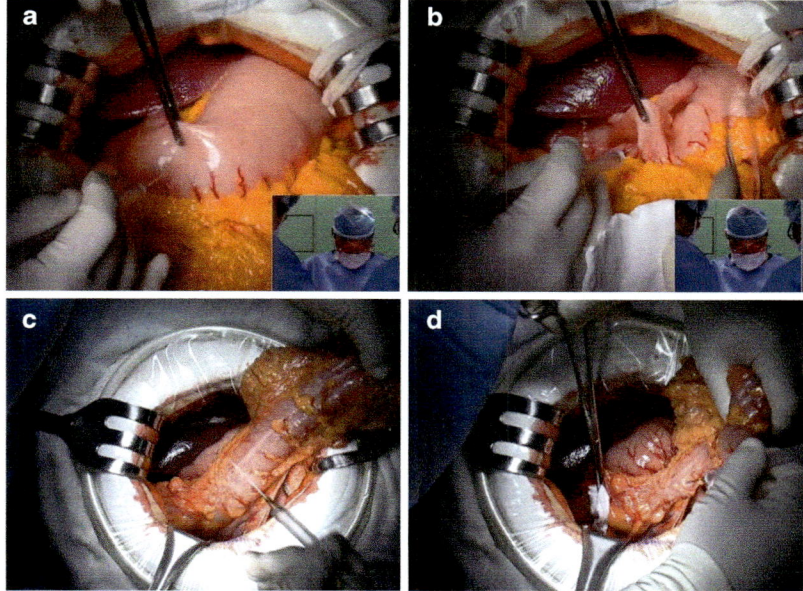

hands and spread it out so that the anatomy can be observed. The omentum should be wrapped and held gently upward and toward the patient's head by the second assistant (Fig. 6.4b). If this procedure is performed through the appropriate anatomical plane, the operation should proceed without bleeding (Fig. 6.4c).

Dissection of Lymph Node #6

This dissection should begin by dividing the greater omentum and dissecting it to the duodenum, head of the pancreas, and pylorus. The superior mesenteric vein is located below the inferior border of the pancreas. The adipose tissue surrounding this vein should not be dissected as it is part of the dissection of lymph node #14v, not part of a routine D2 lymph node dissection. Dissecting the peripancreatic fascia from the inferior border of the pancreas to the duodenum through the head of the pancreas will expose the right gastroepiploic vein and artery. The ideal level for transecting the right gastroepiploic vein is above the anterior superior pancreaticoduodenal vein (Fig. 6.5). The right gastroepiploic vein should be dissected and ligated, at the level of its root, from the gastroduodenal artery and between

the duodenum and pancreas. Sufficient exposure of the gastroduodenal ligament is helpful in the subsequent dissection of lymph node #5.

Dissection of Lymph Nodes #4d and #4sb

The greater omentum should be divided and dissected toward the lower pole of the spleen along the region of the anterior taenia of the transverse colon (Fig. 6.6). As the dissection progresses, the left side of the gastrocolic ligament and splenocolic ligament should be dissected. Once the gastrosplenic ligament has been dissected, the left gastroepiploic artery (LGEA) and vein can be identified and should be ligated in the root. Sometimes infarction in the lower spleen occurs when the LGEA is ligated in its root; however, this seems to have little clinical consequence. Careful dissection from the root of LGEA to its branches should permit identification of a branch artery directed to the lower pole of the spleen. Preserving this artery can prevent the infarction of the lower spleen. After ligating the LGEA, adipose tissue between it and the short gastric artery should be dissected. For gastric resection, the terminal branches of the LGEA to the stomach

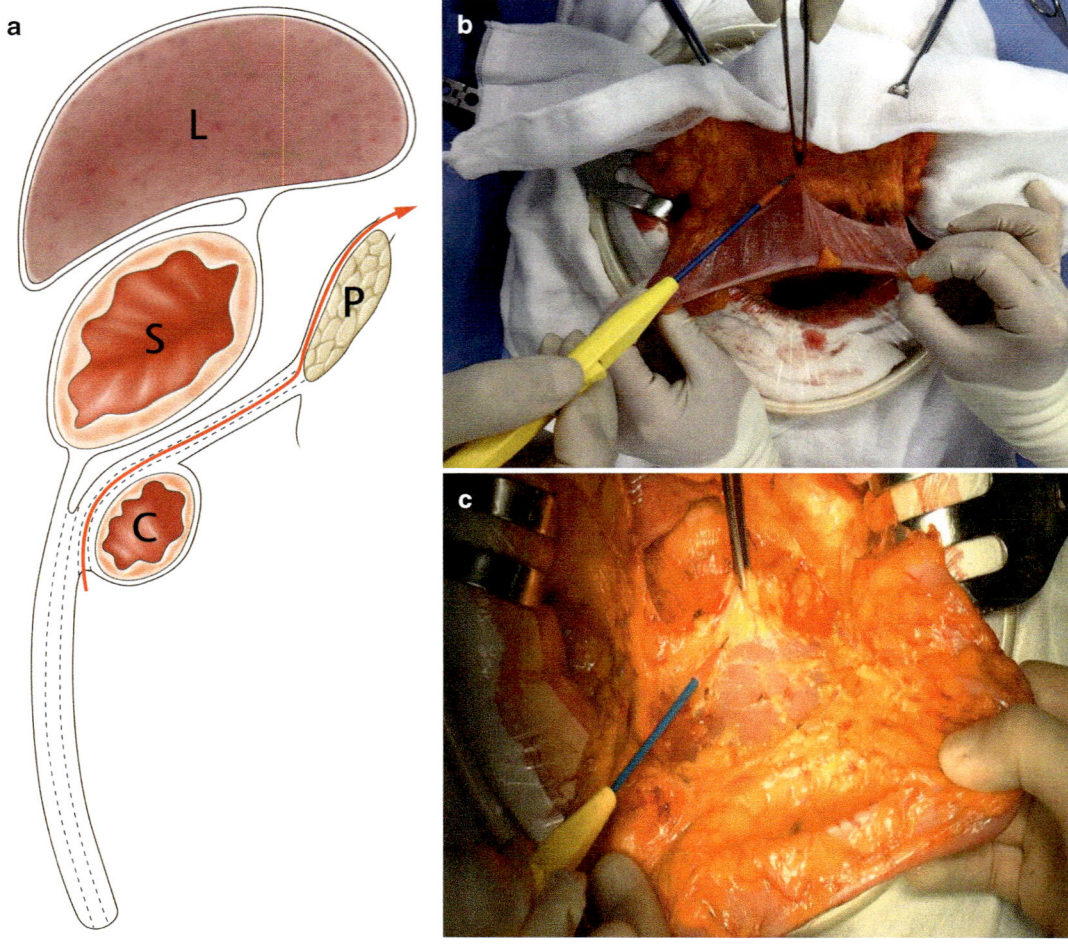

Fig. 6.4 Illustrations for omento-bursectomy for gastric cancer surgery. (**a**) The anatomy around the stomach with the plane for bursectomy (red line). (**b**) First assistant grasps the transverse colon with both hands and spread it out. Second assistant wraps omentum and holds it upward and toward the patients' head for omentectomy. (**c**) Dissecting anterior leaf of transverse mesocolon for bursectomy can be done through avascular anatomical plane. (*L* liver, *S* stomach, *P* pancreas, *C* colon)

in its greater curvature side should be dissected and ligated. This procedure can be performed by electric devices, clip, or tie ligation, but it also can be performed by an electrocautery device only (see video clip).

Next, a clean surgical tape should be applied anterior to the head of the pancreas and posterior to the stomach. Wrapping the stomach with a surgical towel will prevent the surgeon from touching the tumor during the next step (Fig. 6.7a–c). Clean surgical tape should next be inserted into the right subhepatic space, and the liver should be covered with surgical tape. The liver should be retracted by having the first assistant pulls the stomach toward the feet and the second assistant retracts it.

Dissection of Lymph Node #5 and Duodenal Transection

The lesser sac should be incised and opened and the visceral peritoneum of hepatoduodenal ligament dissected (Fig. 6.8). If the aberrant left hepatic artery from the left gastric artery is encountered, it should be incised vertically in the right side of

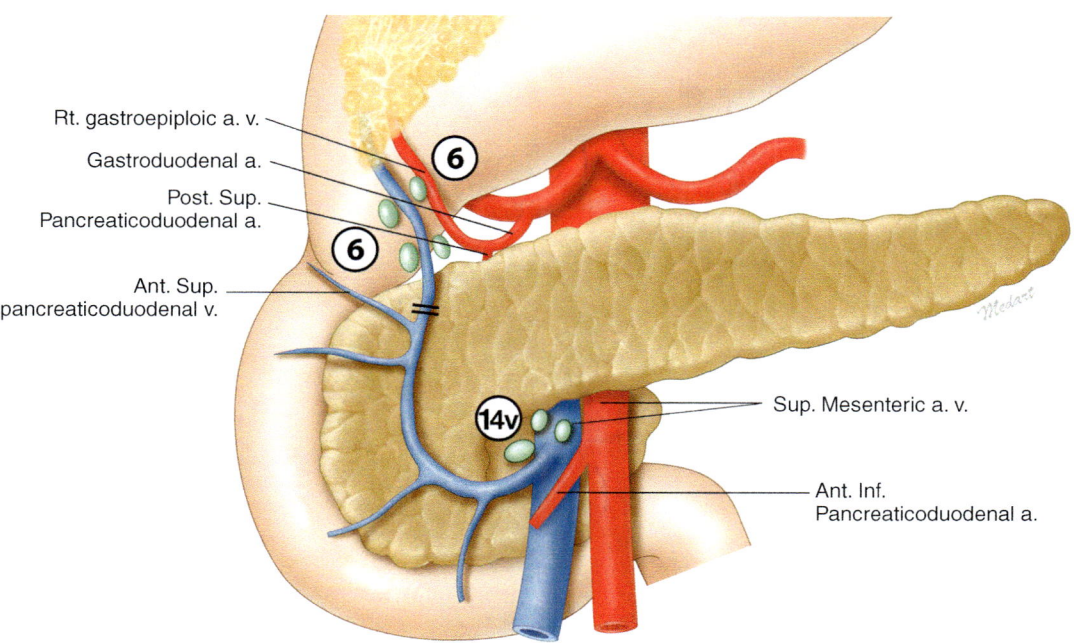

Rt. gastroepiploic a. v.
Gastroduodenal a.
Post. Sup.
Pancreaticoduodenal a.
Ant. Sup.
pancreaticoduodenal v.
Sup. Mesenteric a. v.
Ant. Inf.
Pancreaticoduodenal a.

Fig. 6.5 Anatomy around infra-pylorus of the stomach and the range for #6 lymph node dissection

Fig. 6.6 Anatomy and anatomical plane for dissecting left gastroepiploic vessels (#4sb)

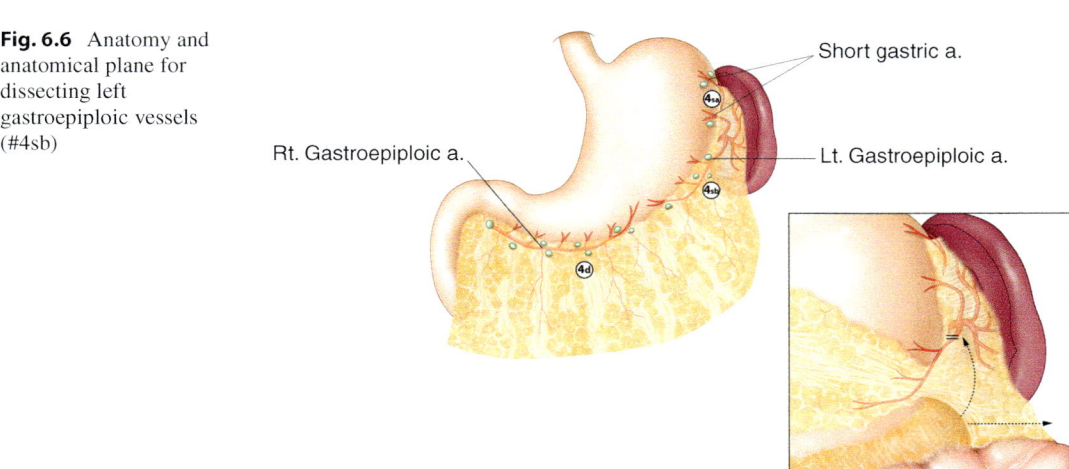

Short gastric a.
Rt. Gastroepiploic a.
Lt. Gastroepiploic a.

the proper hepatic artery and dissected from the right side to the left. At this point, the surgical tape that had been inserted in the superior border of the duodenum will be exposed, and the right gastric artery can be identified and ligated in the root. The small vessels around the pylorus should be cleared and the duodenum transected. The length of the duodenum to be transected should be determined according the planned type of reconstruction. If gastroduodenostomy with a circular staple is intended, a detachable anvil, 28–29 mm in diameter, should be inserted into the duodenal stump and a purse-string suture tied over the purse-string tying notch of the anvil. For other reconstruction, such as loop or Roux-en-Y gastrojejunostomy, the duodenum should be transected by a linear staple, and the staple line should be inverted by interrupted seromus-

Fig. 6.7 The procedures of no-touch technique for preventing the spillage of cancer cells during open surgery. The stomach is wrapped by surgical towel to prevent the surgeon from touching the tumor directly

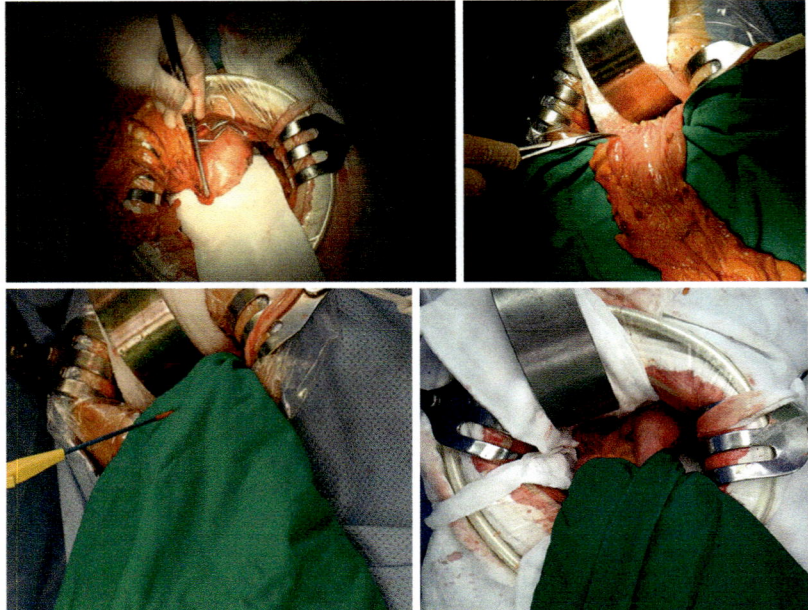

Fig. 6.8 Anatomy around supra-pylorus of the stomach and the range for #5 lymph node dissection

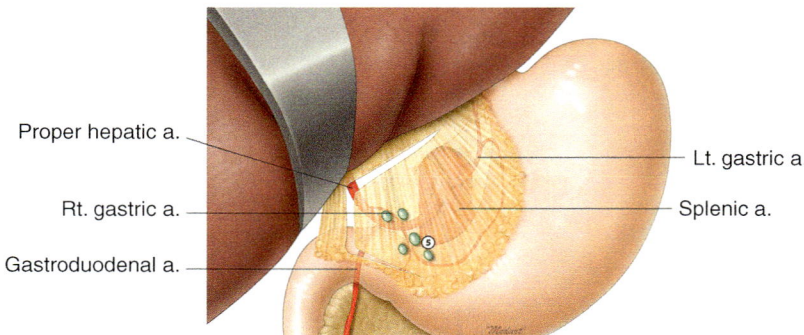

Proper hepatic a.

Rt. gastric a.

Gastroduodenal a.

Lt. gastric a.

Splenic a.

cular sutures. This will require putting the pyloric stump of the stomach into the surgical towel that was used earlier to wrap the stomach. The stomach should then be lifted up and retracted by the second assistant. The liver retraction should be maintained, and counter traction should be maintained by the first assistant, by gently pushing the pancreas toward the feet.

Suprapancreatic Lymph Node Dissection (#12a, #8a, #7, #11p, and #9)

Figure 6.9 depicts the anatomy of the suprapancreatic lymph nodes. After careful exposure of the proper hepatic artery and common hepatic artery, the soft tissues and lymph nodes around the left

side of the portal vein should be dissected (lymph node #12a). The lymph nodes of the pancreas upper portion should be dissected along the anterior portion of the common hepatic artery (lymph node #8a). Because the left gastric vein usually drains into the portal vein or the splenic vein, it can be identified and ligated during the dissection of these areas. Lymph nodes along the celiac axis should be dissected and the left gastric artery exposed and ligated at the root after isolation from the surrounding soft tissues, which includes lymph nodes (lymph node #7). It is recommended that the left gastric artery be ligated twice and its stump suture-ligated to ensure secure ligation. Next, lymph node dissection (lymph node #11p) should be performed

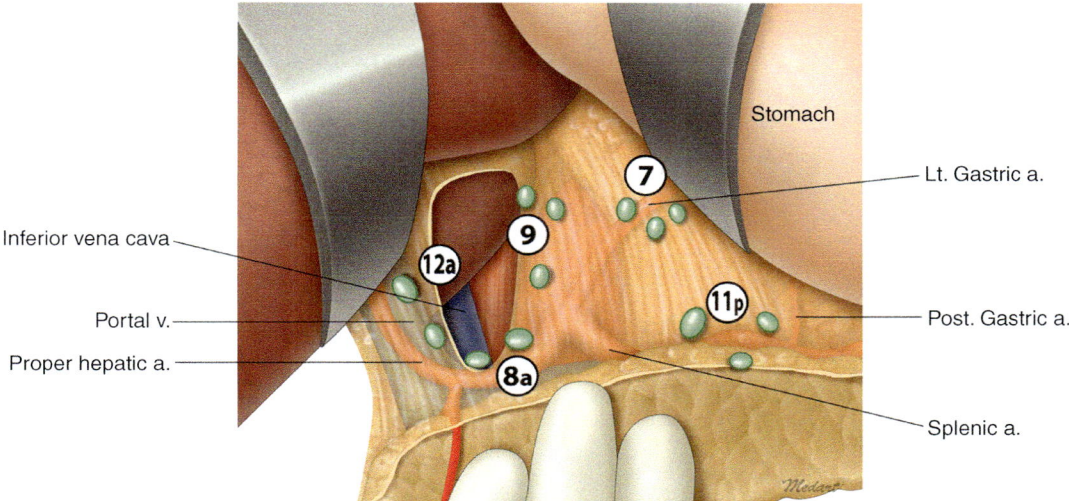

Fig. 6.9 Anatomy and the range of supra-pancreatic lymph nodes (#12a, #8a, #7, #9, #11p) for D2 lymph node dissection of subtotal gastrectomy

through the proximal splenic artery. One assistant should pull down the pancreas from the left of the ligated left gastric artery, exposing soft tissues on the superior border of the pancreas and along the splenic artery and permitting the #11p lymph node to be dissected. The left border of this node is usually posterior to the gastric artery, when it exists. The lymph node dissection (#9) should proceed cephalad to the esophagogastric junction from the ligated left gastric artery. After finalizing suprapancreatic lymph node dissection, a clean surgical tape should be placed above the area of the dissected lymph node #9 and behind the stomach.

Dissection of Lymph Nodes #1 and #3

A truncal vagotomy in esophagogastric junction area should be performed, and the lymph nodes along the lesser curvature of the stomach should be dissected (Fig. 6.10, video). The lymph nodes should be dissected to approximately 2–3 cm below the imaginary resection line of the lesser curvature of the stomach. The entire procedure is summarized in the video clip.

Gastric Resection to Achieve a Tumor-Free Proximal Margin

After dissection of all lymph nodes around the stomach, the resection line of the stomach should

be determined by confirming the distance from the tumor as approximately 60–70% of the stomach is transected. The proximal resection margin should be located 2–5 cm from the gastric cancer. In cases of non-palpable early gastric cancer, the clip applied during preoperative endoscopy is a useful indicator for determining the proximal resection line. When it is difficult to decide proximal margin that leaves tumor-free tissue, it should be confirmed by cryosection. If the tumor is identified in the frozen section, a total gastrectomy needs to be considered.

Checking the Status of Lymph Nodes According to Their Anatomical Location

The current pathological staging system (pN) from the American Joint Cancer Committee/ Union Internationale Contre le Cancer (AJCC/ UICC) is based only on the number of metastatic lymph nodes. Nonetheless, the anatomical extent of metastasis in the lymph nodes is still important for gastric cancer prognosis [18, 19]. Also, the location of metastatic lymph nodes relative to the location of the primary tumor in the stomach influences the probability and risk of lymph

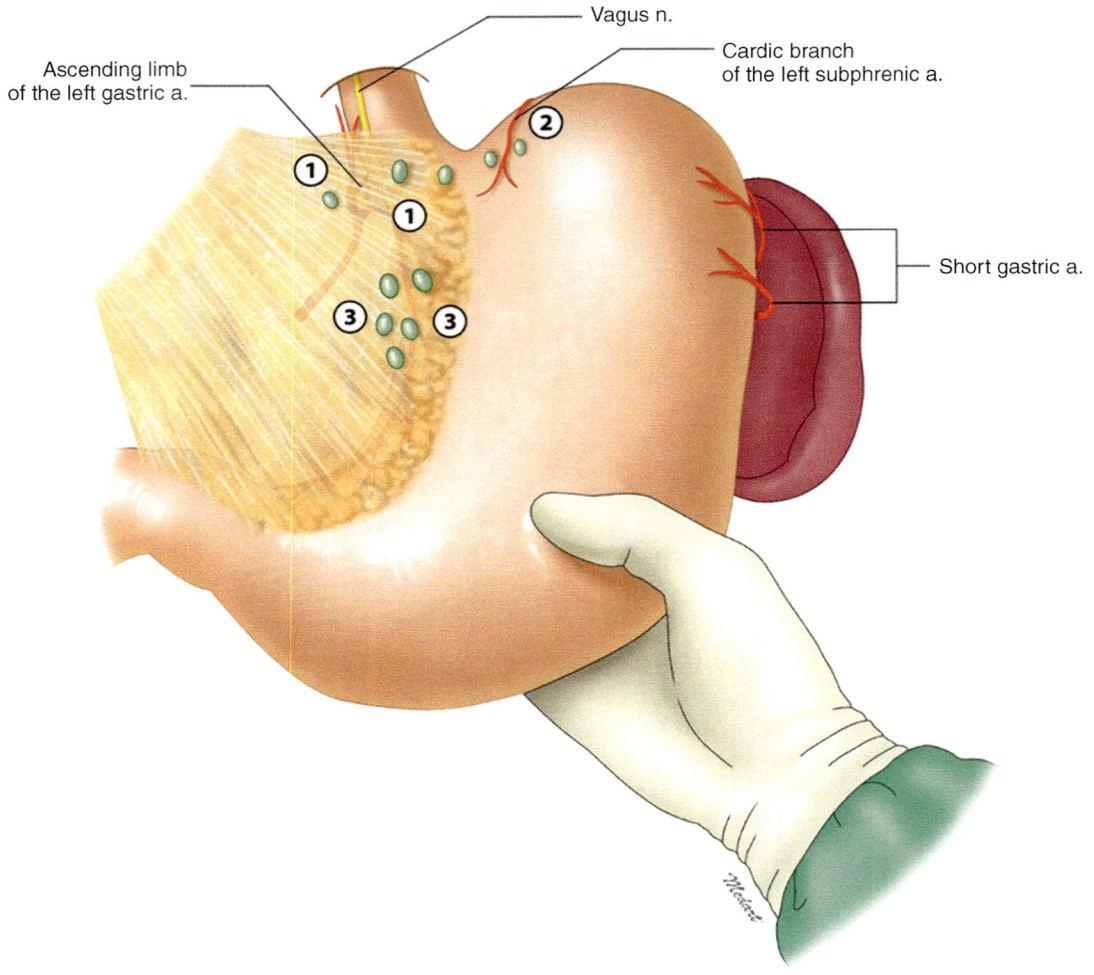

Fig. 6.10 Anatomy and the range for #1 and #3 lymph node dissection

node metastasis. This information will influence the decision on the surgical extent of lymph node dissection for gastric cancer.

Dividing lymph nodes according to their anatomical location in the specimen and recording their status is highly recommended. Figure 6.11 depicts the location of lymph nodes in the specimen.

Discussion

Good surgery for gastric cancer can be summarized in the mnemonic "**OPERATIONS**": Oncologic **P**rinciples, Good **E**xposure, Understanding

Anatomy, Comprehensive **T**otal Approach, Meticulous Lymph **N**ode Dissection, and Patients' **S**afety. Surgery is as much an art as a technique, and the surgeon's philosophy is an important component of practice. The surgeon should see the surgery, first and foremost, as for the patient's benefit and have the same concern and regard for the patient as for a family member. The patient with gastric cancer has only one chance to be cured by surgery. Often this requires innovation and the adaptation of new technology by the surgeon. However, innovations must always honor accepted oncologic principles and practices and be based on sound scientific rationale.

Fig. 6.11 The locations of each lymph node station in D2 level in the specimen after subtotal gastrectomy with D2 lymph node dissection

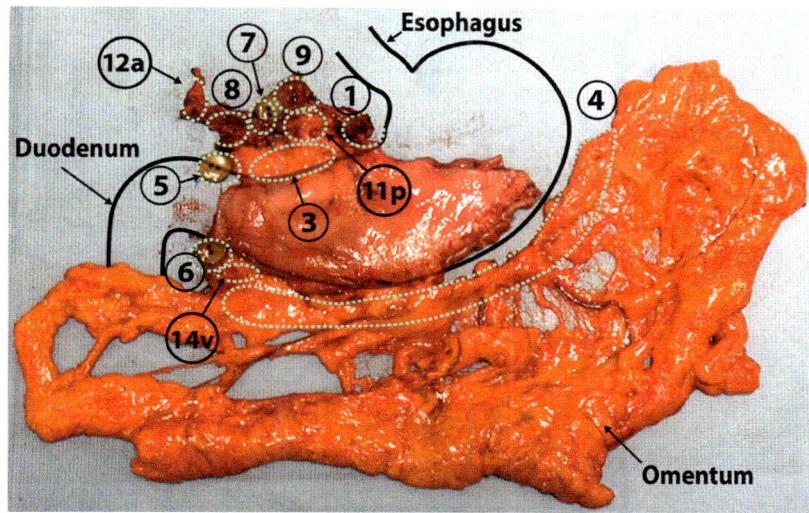

References

1. Torre LA, Bray F, Siegel RL, Ferlay J, Lortet-Tieulent J, Jemal A. Global cancer statistics, 2012. CA Cancer J Clin. 2015;65(2):87–108. https://doi.org/10.3322/caac.21262.
2. Japanese Gastric Cancer A. Japanese gastric cancer treatment guidelines 2010 (ver. 3). Gastric Cancer. 2011;14(2):113–23. https://doi.org/10.1007/s10120-011-0042-4.
3. Weinberg RA. The biology of cancer. 2nd ed. New York: Garland Science; 2014.
4. Kim HH, Han SU, Kim MC, Hyung WJ, Kim W, Lee HJ, et al. Long-term results of laparoscopic gastrectomy for gastric cancer: a large-scale case-control and case-matched Korean multicenter study. J Clin Oncol. 2014;32(7):627–33. https://doi.org/10.1200/JCO.2013.48.8551.
5. Cuschieri SA, Hanna GB. Meta-analysis of D1 versus D2 gastrectomy for gastric adenocarcinoma: let us move on to another era. Ann Surg. 2014;259(6):e90. https://doi.org/10.1097/SLA.0000000000000418.
6. Songun I, Putter H, Kranenbarg EM, Sasako M, van de Velde CJ. Surgical treatment of gastric cancer: 15-year follow-up results of the randomised nationwide Dutch D1D2 trial. Lancet Oncol. 2010;11(5):439–49. https://doi.org/10.1016/S1470-2045(10)70070-X.
7. Sasako M, Sano T, Yamamoto S, Kurokawa Y, Nashimoto A, Kurita A, et al. D2 lymphadenectomy alone or with Para-aortic nodal dissection for gastric cancer. N Engl J Med. 2008;359(5):453–62. https://doi.org/10.1056/NEJMoa0707035.
8. Wu CW, Hsiung CA, Lo SS, Hsieh MC, Chen JH, Li AF, et al. Nodal dissection for patients with gastric cancer: a randomised controlled trial. Lancet Oncol. 2006;7(4):309–15. https://doi.org/10.1016/S1470-2045(06)70623-4.
9. Ajani JA, Bentrem DJ, Besh S, D'Amico TA, Das P, Denlinger C, et al. Gastric cancer, version 2.2013: featured updates to the NCCN guidelines. J Natl Compr Cancer Netw. 2013;11(5):531–46.
10. Okines A, Verheij M, Allum W, Cunningham D, Cervantes A, Group EGW. Gastric cancer: ESMO clinical practice guidelines for diagnosis, treatment and follow-up. Ann Oncol. 2010;21(Suppl 5):v50–4. https://doi.org/10.1093/annonc/mdq164.
11. Japanese Gastric Cancer A. Japanese classification of gastric carcinoma – 2nd English edition. Gastric Cancer. 1998;1(1):10–24. https://doi.org/10.1007/s101209800016.
12. Liebermann-Meffert D. The greater omentum. Anatomy, embryology, and surgical applications. Surg Clin North Am. 2000;80(1):275–93, xii.
13. Hagiwara A, Takahashi T, Sawai K, Taniguchi H, Shimotsuma M, Okano S, et al. Milky spots as the implantation site for malignant cells in peritoneal dissemination in mice. Cancer Res. 1993;53(3):687–92.
14. Maruyama K, Okabayashi K, Kinoshita T. Progress in gastric cancer surgery in Japan and its limits of radicality. World J Surg. 1987;11(4):418–25.
15. Hagiwara A, Sawai K, Sakakura C, Shirasu M, Ohgaki M, Yamasaki J, et al. Complete omentectomy and extensive lymphadenectomy with gastrectomy improves the survival of gastric cancer patients with metastases in the adjacent peritoneum. Hepato-Gastroenterology. 1998;45(23):1922–9.
16. Hirao M, Kurokawa Y, Fujita J, Imamura H, Fujiwara Y, Kimura Y, et al. Long-term outcomes after prophylactic bursectomy in patients with resectable gastric cancer: final analysis of a multicenter randomized controlled trial. Surgery. 2015;157(6):1099–105. https://doi.org/10.1016/j.surg.2014.12.024.

17. Imamura H, Kurokawa Y, Kawada J, Tsujinaka T, Takiguchi S, Fujiwara Y, et al. Influence of bursectomy on operative morbidity and mortality after radical gastrectomy for gastric cancer: results of a randomized controlled trial. World J Surg. 2011;35(3):625–30. https://doi.org/10.1007/s00268-010-0914-5.

18. Son T, Hyung WJ, Kim JW, Kim HI, An JY, Cheong JH, et al. Anatomic extent of metastatic lymph nodes: still important for gastric cancer prognosis. Ann Surg Oncol. 2014;21(3):899–907. https://doi.org/10.1245/s10434-013-3403-x.

19. Choi YY, An JY, Katai H, Seto Y, Fukagawa T, Okumura Y, et al. A lymph node staging system for gastric cancer: a hybrid type based on topographic and numeric systems. PLoS One. 2016;11(3):e0149555. https://doi.org/10.1371/journal.pone.0149555. PubMed PMID: 26967161; PubMed Central PMCID: PMC4788413.

Open Surgery for Gastric Cancer: Total Gastrectomy with D2 Lymph Node Dissection

7

Yoon Young Choi and Sung Hoon Noh

Introduction

Total gastrectomy (TG), a total resection of the whole stomach including the cardia and pylorus, is a surgical procedure to treat gastric cancer which is located in proximal stomach and in a case that a satisfactory proximal resection safety margin cannot be guaranteed by distal gastrectomy. As like distal gastrectomy, the extent of lymph node (LN) dissection of TG for advanced gastric cancer is recommended in D2 level, and D2 level for TG additionally includes #2 (left paracardial LNs including those along the esophagocardiac branch of the left subphrenic artery), #4sa (left greater curvature LNs along the short gastric arteries), #10 (splenic hilar LNs including LNs in splenic artery distal to the

pancreatic tail, in the roots of the short gastric arteries, and along the left gastroepiploic artery proximal to its first gastric branch), and #11d (distal splenic artery LNs from halfway between its origin and the pancreatic tail end, usually from the beginning of posterior gastric artery from splenic artery, to the end of the pancreatic tail) LN groups along with those of distal gastrectomy. TG for gastric cancer is one of challenging surgical procedure because the extent of TG is wider than that of distal gastrectomy, LN dissection around spleen hilum is technically difficult, and surgical complications such as leak from esophagojejunostomy and pseudoaneurysm at splenic artery could be lethal. In addition, combined resection versus preservation of adjacent organs such as the pancreas and spleen for TG has long been in a debate. In this chapter, we will discuss about the historical changes of surgery for TG and technical aspects for TG with LN dissection. Detailed technique for reconstruction after open TG will be addressed in another chapter.

Electronic Supplementary Material The online version of this chapter (https://doi.org/10.1007/978-3-662-45583-8_7) contains supplementary material, which is available to authorized users.

Y. Y. Choi
Department of Surgery, Yonsei University Health System, Yonsei University College of Medicine, Seoul, Republic of Korea

S. H. Noh (✉)
Department of Surgery, Yonsei University Health System, Yonsei University College of Medicine, Seoul, Republic of Korea

Brain Korea 21 PLUS Project for Medical Science, Yonsei University Health System, Yonsei University College of Medicine, Seoul, Republic of Korea
e-mail: sunghoonn@yuhs.ac

Beginning of TG

The first total gastrectomy for cancer was performed by Carl B. Schlatter from the University of Zurich Switzerland who was a staff of Billroth in 1897 [1], and the first reconstruction type was loop esophagojeju-

© Springer-Verlag GmbH Germany, part of Springer Nature 2019
S. H. Noh, W. J. Hyung (eds.), *Surgery for Gastric Cancer*,
https://doi.org/10.1007/978-3-662-45583-8_7

nostomy without jejuno-jejunostomy. After the first case, the reconstruction type had developed, and Cesar Roux suggested "Roux-en-Y" anastomosis with end-to-end esophago-jejunostomy in 1907 [2]. The most popular type of reconstruction for TG now is modified Roux-en-Y, end-to-side esophagojejunostomy which was firstly reported by Thomas G. Orr in 1943 [3].

Extent of Lymph Node Dissection of TG for Gastric Cancer

In the initial efforts to identify lymphatic system around the stomach was performed based on the visible way by a kind of dye such as Prussian blue or India ink [4, 5]. Accumulated experience and knowledge about lymphatic system around the stomach were finally compiled, and the Japanese Research Society for Gastric Cancer reported Japanese manual that defined 16 regional LN stations based on their anatomical location in 1962 [6]. These regional LN stations were classified into N1, N2, N3, and N4 level, and the removal of LNs at N1 and N2 level was defined as D2 lymph node dissection. Propagation of D2 surgery in Japan led innovative improvement of prognosis of gastric cancer even in stage II and III [7], consequently D2 surgery has become a standard procedure for gastric cancer surgery. Once, there was a controversy in Western countries whether D2 surgery improves prognosis of patients with gastric cancer over D1 surgery or not, now D2 surgery is considered as an optimal extent of LN dissection for gastric cancer in the world [8–10].

D2 LN dissection for total gastrectomy includes all LN stations for distal gastrectomy with additional LNs around the pancreas tail and the hilum of the spleen [8]. The incidence of LN metastasis at the hilum of the spleen has been reported as 9–15% when cancer is located in upper third of the stomach [11–13]; consequently appropriate dissection in this region has been considered as one of the important procedures in total gastrectomy for gastric cancer.

Era of Combined Resection Moved to Organ Preservation for TG

During the 1900s, combined resection of adjacent organs was popular, and TG with distal pancreatectomy (including splenectomy) was a standard procedure for gastric cancer; consequently morbidity and mortality rate were high after TG. The reason of distal pancreatectomy was for removing LNs along the upper border of the pancreas and splenic hilum, and there was a clinical question that dissecting LNs around the pancreas without pancreatectomy could be feasible and reduce the complication after TG. Consequently a new procedure, pancreas-preserving TG, was proposed by Dr. Keiichi Maruyama in 1979 [14]. His operative outcomes were quite interesting; pancreas-preserving TG was related to a less postoperative mortality and morbidity (0.3% and 19.6% in pancreas-preserving group vs. 0.9% and 39.4% in pancreas resection group, respectively) and decreased newly developed diabetes mellitus (0% in pancreas preserving and 37% in pancreas resection group), with similar prognosis compared to TG with distal pancreatectomy; consequently pancreas-preserving TG had settled as a standard procedure for TG.

The next clinical question was the necessity of splenectomy for TG: how about removing LNs around the spleen hilum without splenectomy? Dr. Sung Hoon Noh presented the technical possibility and feasibility of spleen-preserving TG with splenic hilar lymph node dissection at the second International Gastric Cancer Congress in 1997 [15, 16]. He reported the outcomes of retrospective results, and spleen-preserving TG was related to less blood loss with morbidity, and the prognosis was similar that of TG with splenectomy [17, 18]. A following randomized controlled trial which compared splenectomy versus spleen-preserving TG for proximal gastric cancer showed similar outcomes: both group had similar number of retrieved LNs, postoperative morbidity, and prognosis [19]; however this trial did not calculate statistical power before the study; thus the outcome could be underpowered. A large-scale, multi-institutional randomized controlled trial was conducted in Japan, and the outcome was reported recently. The results showed that splenectomy was related to a higher morbidity (30.3% in splenectomy and 16.7% in spleen preservation group) and larger blood loss (390.5 vs. 315 mL, respectively), but the operation time, hospital mortality (0.4% vs. 0.8%, respectively), and prognosis were similar between two groups. Based on those results, the study concluded that splenectomy in TG for proximal gastric cancer should be avoided because it increases operative morbidity without prognostic benefit [20]. However, the real benefit from spleen preservation is still unanswered question because only 23% of spleen preservation group underwent #10 dissection or sampling in this study; consequently the benefit from spleen preservation could be attenuated by the harmful effect of LNs preservation at the spleen hilum.

On the contrary to a low mortality after TG regardless of splenectomy/pancreatectomy or not in Asian countries, results from United States showed TG for gastric cancer is still a challenging procedure because it is still related to high-mortality rate [21]. According to the results of American College of Surgeons National Surgical Quality Improvement Program database which were collected between 2005 and 2011, overall morbidity and mortality after TG were 36% and 4.7%, respectively. Also, splenectomy and pancreatectomy was risk factors of morbidity (odds ratio was 1.63 and 3.84, respectively), and pancreatectomy was related to a high mortality (odds ratio: 3.50). In conclusion, routine splenectomy should be avoided in a purpose of LN dissection for TG, and dissecting splenic hilar LNs is recommended if it is technically possible.

Surgical Procedure for Total Gastrectomy with D2 Lymph Node Dissection

The indication of TG is that cancer is located in proximal stomach. Sometimes huge tumor or Borrmann type IV gastric cancer can be indicated when appropriate safety margin cannot be achieved by distal gastrectomy. Other procedures including preoperative preparation, anesthesia,

position, incision, exposure, and preparation of main procedure are same to that of distal gastrectomy, and they will not be discussed in this chapter. Also, LN dissection for LNs that belong to D2 level of distal gastrectomy will be skipped, and readers would be directed to the chapter that dealing with these issues in this book. Readers can access to the detailed procedure for LN dissection of #11d and #10 by open surgery in the video clip.

Dissection of Lymph Nodes #11d

The borderline of #11p and #11d is posterior gastric vessels, and the area of #11d is from posterior gastric vessels to the spleen hilum through upper border of the pancreas. Through dissecting #11p, posterior gastric artery is identified and ligated to go through #11d. Operation surgeon grasps soft tissue on upper border of the pancreas, and assistant surgeon slightly presses the pancreas with stick sponge or hand with surgical tape (Fig. 7.1). When soft tissue of upper border of the pancreas is divided, splenic artery can be identified. Through the line of pancreas' upper border, from patients' right side to left side, LNs can be dissected from splenic artery. In the deeper portion of splenic artery, there is a splenic vein; thus LNs around them can be dissected with caution of thermal injury of adjacent vessels (Fig. 7.2).

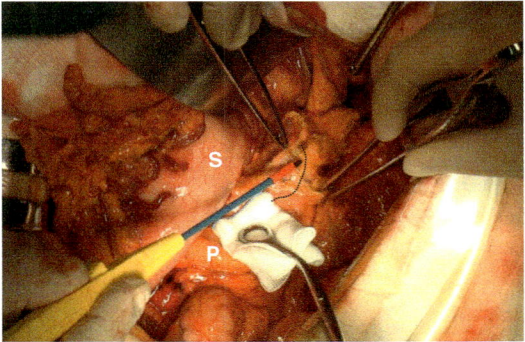

Fig. 7.1 Suprapancratic lymph node dissection between #11p and #11d. Dot line upper border of pancreas. S stomach, P pancreas

Dissection of Lymph Nodes #4sa, #10, and #2

To make good operative field to dissect #10 area, surgeon can insert surgical tapes behind the spleen for lifting up the spleen to anterior part that make surgeon able to access #10 area easily (Fig. 7.3). Because rough handling of the spleen can lead injury of posterior part of the spleen and sometimes it is difficult to handle the bleeding from spleen, surgeons should be careful not

to injure parenchyme of the spleen during this procedure. Surgeon's left hand slightly presses anterior portion of splenic hilum with surgical tape, and assistant surgeon makes countertraction with stick sponge (Fig. 7.4). Short gastric vessels (there are usually three to five vessels) are identified and ligated with dissecting LNs around them (#4sa) (Fig. 7.5). Behind the short gastric vessels, the main splenic artery and vein can be identified at splenic hilum. Surgeon grasps soft tissue around splenic vessels, and assistant surgeon makes countertraction with retracting splenic

Fig. 7.2 Exposed splenic vessels at the upper border of the pancreas. S stomach, P pancreas, SA splenic artery, SV splenic vein

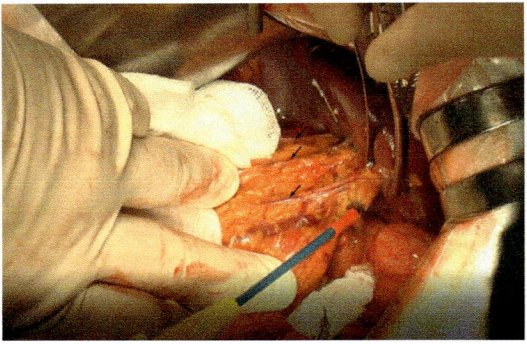

Fig. 7.4 Exposed short gastric vessels for #4sa lymph node dissection. Arrows: short gastric vessels

Fig. 7.3 The process of lifting the spleen up for achieving good operative field for splenic hilar (#10) lymph node dissection. The spleen is gently lifted up, and the rolled surgical tapes are inserted behind the spleen. S spleen

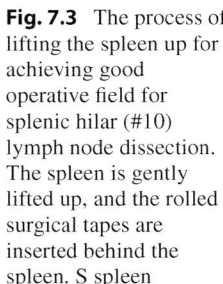

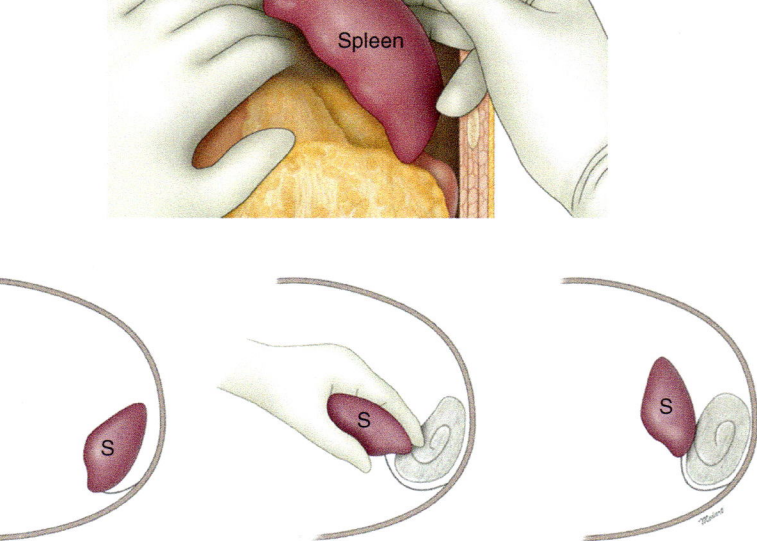

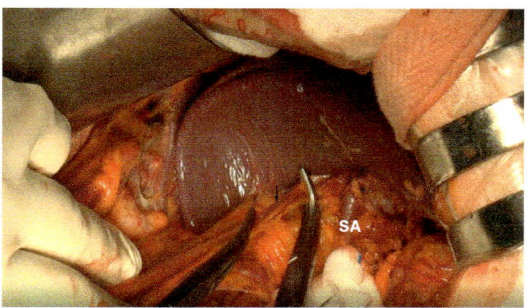

Fig. 7.5 Exposed short gastric vessel with ligation of it. Arrow: short gastric vessel

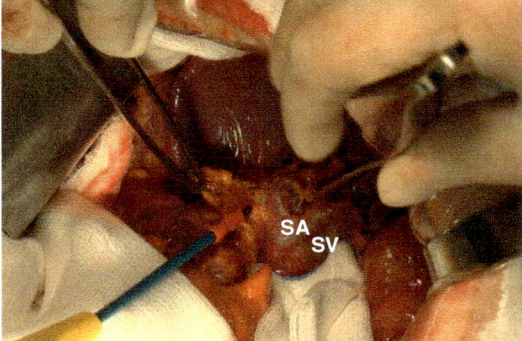

Fig. 7.6 Exposed splenic vessel at the hilum of the spleen for #10 lymph node dissection. SA splenic artery; SV splenic vein

artery and vein (Fig. 7.6). During dissecting this area (#10), surgeon should be careful not to make thermal injury around splenic artery because it sometimes can cause a critical complication, pseudoaneurysm. When dissecting soft tissue through splenic vessels to upper pole of spleen and esophagogastric junction, a branch from left inferior phrenic vessels can be identified at gastrophrenic ligament, and it should be ligated (#2).

References

1. Schlatter C. Vollstandiger Entfernung des Magens, Oesophagoenterostomie, beim Menschen. Beitr Klin Chir. 1897;19:757.
2. Roux C. L'esophago-jejune-gastrome. Nouvelle Operation Pour Retricissement Infranchissable de L'esophage. Semaine Med. 1907;27:37.
3. Orr TG. A modified technique for total gastrectomy. Arch Surg. 1947;54(3):279–86.
4. D. G. Zur Technik der Lymphagefass-injection, Eine neue Injectionsmasse fur Lymphagefasse. Polychrome Injection. Anat Anz. 1896;12:216–23.
5. T. K. Lymph node metastasis of gastric cancer. Jpn J Surg. 1944:15–6.
6. Cancer JRSfG. Japanese rules for gastric cancer study. 1st ed. (in Japanese). Tokyo/Osaka/Kyoto: Kanehara & Co LTD; 1962.
7. Cancer JRSfG. Annual report of nationwide registry of gastric cancer patients (in Japanese). Tokyo: National Cancer Center Press; 1972–1998. pp. 1–54.
8. Japanese Gastric Cancer Association. Japanese gastric cancer treatment guidelines 2014 (ver. 4). Gastric Cancer. 2017;20(1):1–19.
9. Ajani JA, Bentrem DJ, Besh S, D'Amico TA, Das P, Denlinger C, Fakih MG, Fuchs CS, Gerdes H, Glasgow RE, Hayman JA, Hofstetter WL, Ilson DH, Keswani RN, Kleinberg LR, Korn WM, Lockhart AC, Meredith K, Mulcahy MF, Orringer MB, Posey JA, Sasson AR, Scott WJ, Strong VE, Varghese TK Jr, Warren G, Washington MK, Willett C, Wright CD, McMillian NR, Sundar H, National Comprehensive Cancer Network. Gastric cancer, version 2.2013: featured updates to the NCCN guidelines. J Natl Compr Cancer Netw. 2013;11(5):531–46.
10. Waddell T, Verheij M, Allum W, Cunningham D, Cervantes A, Arnold D, European Society for Medical Oncology, European Society of Surgical Oncology, European Society of Radiotherapy and Oncology. Gastric cancer: ESMO-ESSO-ESTRO Clinical Practice Guidelines for diagnosis, treatment and follow-up. Ann Oncol. 2013;24(6):vi57–63.
11. Kosuga T, Ichikawa D, Okamoto K, Komatsu S, Shiozaki A, Fujiwara H, Otsuji E. Survival benefits from splenic hilar lymph node dissection by splenectomy in gastric cancer patients: relative comparison of the benefits in subgroups of patients. Gastric Cancer. 2011;14(2):172–7.
12. Sasada S, Ninomiya M, Nishizaki M, Harano M, Ojima Y, Matsukawa H, Aoki H, Shiozaki S, Ohno S, Takakura N. Frequency of lymph node metastasis to the splenic hilus and effect of splenectomy in proximal gastric cancer. Anticancer Res. 2009;29(8):3347–51.
13. Monig SP, Collet PH, Baldus SE, Schmackpfeffer K, Schroder W, Thiele J, Dienes HP, Holscher AH. Splenectomy in proximal gastric cancer: frequency of lymph node metastasis to the splenic hilum. J Surg Oncol. 2001;76(2):89–92.
14. Maruyama K, Sasako M, Kinoshita T, Sano T, Katai H, Okajima K. Pancreas-preserving total gastrectomy for proximal gastric cancer. World J Surg. 1995;19(4):532–6.
15. Choi YY, An JY, Kim HI, Cheong JH, Hyung WJ, Noh SH. Current practice of gastric cancer treatment. Chin Med J. 2014;127(3):547–53.

16. Choi YY, Noh SH, Cheong JH. Evolution of gastric cancer treatment: from the golden age of surgery to an era of precision medicine. Yonsei Med J. 2015;56(5):1177–85.

17. Oh SJ, Hyung WJ, Li C, Song J, Kang W, Rha SY, Chung HC, Choi SH, Noh SH. Yonsei gastric cancer C. the effect of spleen-preserving lymphadenectomy on surgical outcomes of locally advanced proximal gastric cancer. J Surg Oncol. 2009;99(5):275–80.

18. Lee KY, Noh SH, Hyung WJ, Lee JH, Lah KH, Choi SH, Min JS. Impact of splenectomy for lymph node dissection on long-term surgical outcome in gastric cancer. Ann Surg Oncol. 2001;8(5):402–6.

19. Yu W, Choi GS, Chung HY. Randomized clinical trial of splenectomy versus splenic preservation in patients with proximal gastric cancer. Br J Surg. 2006;93(5):559–63.

20. Sano T, Sasako M, Mizusawa J, Yamamoto S, Katai H, Yoshikawa T, Nashimoto A, Ito S, Kaji M, Imamura H, Fukushima N, Fujitani K, Stomach Cancer Study Group of the Japan Clinical Oncology Group. Randomized controlled trial to evaluate splenectomy in total gastrectomy for proximal gastric carcinoma. Ann Surg. 2017;265(2):277–83.

21. Bartlett EK, Roses RE, Kelz RR, Drebin JA, Fraker DL, Karakousis GC. Morbidity and mortality after total gastrectomy for gastric malignancy using the American College of Surgeons National Surgical Quality Improvement Program database. Surgery. 2014;156(2):298–304.

Gastrectomy with D3 Lymph Node Dissection

8

Mitsuru Sasako

Indication

Prophylactic Nodal Dissection

Japan Clinical Oncology Group (JCOG) carried out a phase III study on prophylactic nodal dissection of para-aortic lymph nodes (PAN) for potentially curable T3/T4 advanced gastric cancer [1]. This study, JCOG9501, is a multi-institutional prospective randomized control study carried out among 24 Japanese hospitals to evaluate superiority of D2 + PAN dissection (D) over D2 alone. Eligibility criteria are shown in Table 8.1. The primary end point was overall survival (OS), and the secondary were recurrent-free survival (RFS) and surgery-related complications and hospital death. The sample size was projected as 520 to detect 8% increase of 5-year survival rate for PAND with a one-sided alpha level of 0.05 and power of 80%. Between July 1995 and April 2001, 523 patients were randomly assigned to D2 alone (263) or D2 plus PAND (260) (Fig. 8.1). All except one underwent allocated nodal dissection and followed without any adjuvant treatment. In terms of patients' characteristics and prognostic factors, there was no difference between the two groups. Hospital death in both groups was as low as 0.8%. Incidence of

Table 8.1 Eligibility criteria

Inclusion criteria	Exclusion criteria
Pre-op	*Pre-op*
Adenocarcinoma 75 yrs or younger PaO2 > 70 mmHg, FEV1.0 > 50% CCr > 50 ml/min Written consent	Cancer in gastric stump Borrmann 4 (linitis) Other primary neoplasm History of MI or positive exercise ECG Liver cirrhosis or ICG15 > 10%
Intra-op	*Intra-op*
T2(SS), T3, T4 Curative resection (R0) Lavage cytology negative	Macroscopic N4 (frozen section not allowed)

major surgical complication such as anastomotic leak, intra-abdominal abscess, or pancreatic juice leak was the same between two groups, but that of total morbidity including minor complication was significantly higher after D2 + PAND than D2 [2]. Both OS and RFS curves were nearly completely overlapped, and HR was 1.03 (95% IC; 0.78–1.37; $p = 0.83$) (Fig. 8.2) and 1.08 (95% CI; 0.83–1.42; $p = 0.72$) (Fig. 8.3), respectively. Sites of initial recurrent did not show any difference between the two groups. In subgroup analysis, pathological tumor stage and lymph node stage (negative/positive) showed statistically significant interaction, but both of them cannot be known when performing surgery, and reasonable explanation could not be given. Although the interaction was not significant, hazard ratio for tumors of the upper third of the stomach was

M. Sasako (✉)
Department of Surgery,
Yodogawa Christian Hospital, Osaka, Japan
e-mail: msasako@hyo-med.ac.jp

© Springer-Verlag GmbH Germany, part of Springer Nature 2019
S. H. Noh, W. J. Hyung (eds.), *Surgery for Gastric Cancer*,
https://doi.org/10.1007/978-3-662-45583-8_8

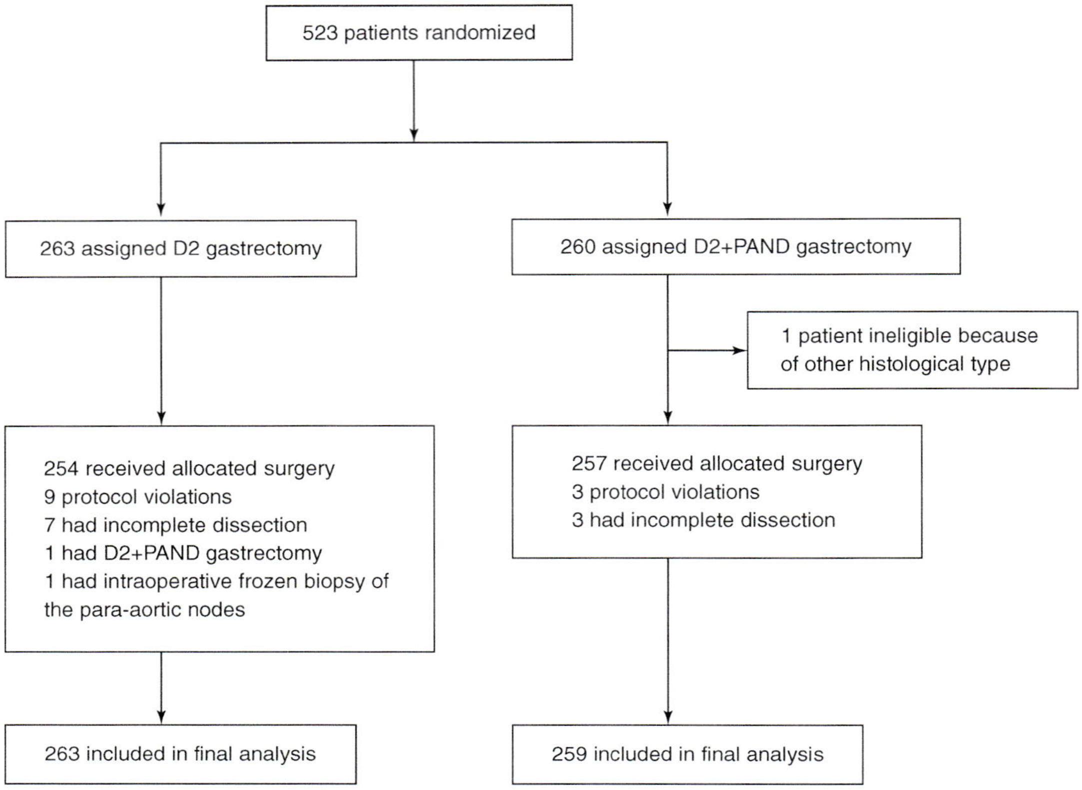

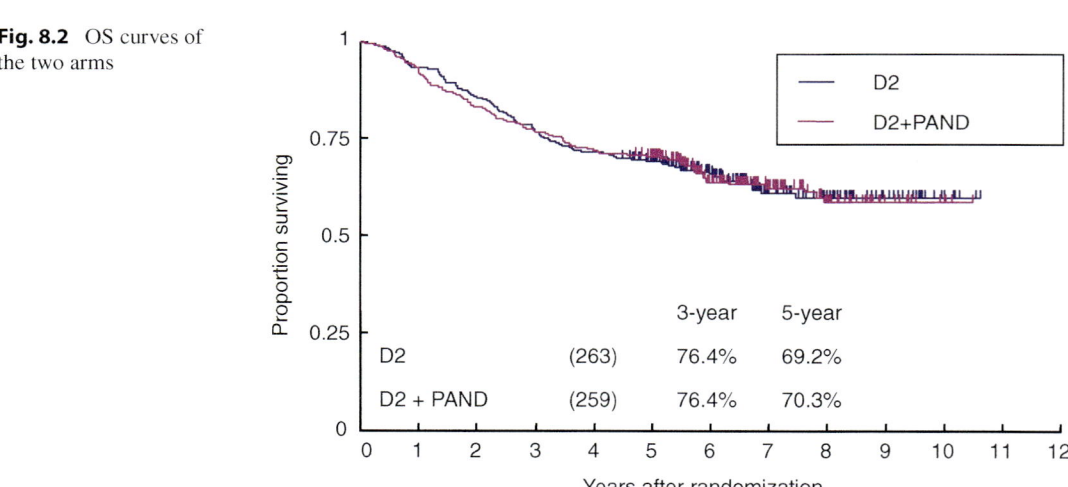

Fig. 8.1 Consort flow chart of the JCOG9501

Fig. 8.2 OS curves of the two arms

*: Survival analysis excluded ineligible patients (n=1).

Stratified log-rank test: P=0.57, HR=1.03 (0.77-1.37)

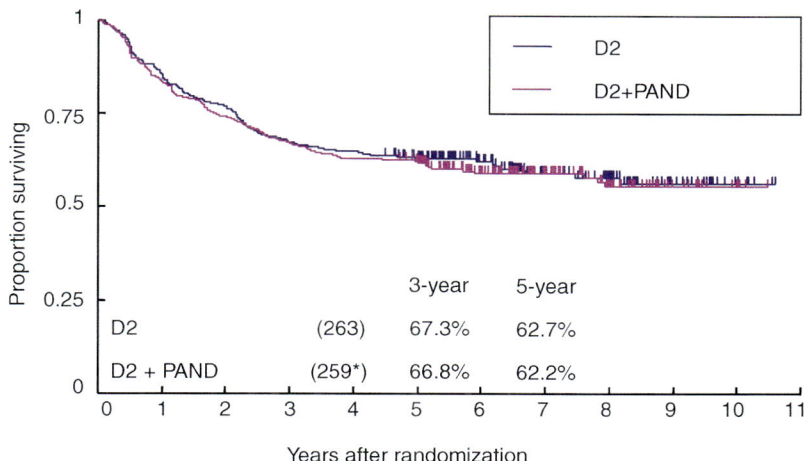

Fig. 8.3 RFS curves of the two arms

*: Survival analysis excluded ineligible patients (n=1).

Stratified log-rank test: 1 sided P=0.66, HR=1.06 (0.81-1.39)

0.58, while that of other locations was 1.10. Five-year OS of 22 out of 260 (8.5%) patients who had PAN metastasis was 18.2%, which was almost same as our expectation. In summary, PAND should be avoided in patients with potentially curable T3/4 tumors without any clinical evidence of PAN metastasis.

In JCOG9501 study, we excluded patients with tumors invading the cardia and esophagus, as we carried out at the same time another study JCOG9502 for these patients to test the superiority of left thoracoabdominal approach over transdiaphragmatic approach [3]. In the subgroup analysis of JCOG9501, tumors of the upper third of the stomach may have more benefit from PAND than tumors of other middle or lower third of the stomach [1]. In JCOG9502, the incidence of PAN metastasis was more than double of JCOG9501, 15.2%, and 5-year OS of these patients was 18.2%, showing much higher efficacy of PAND for these tumors [3]. Prophylactic PAND is not recommended, but partial PAND, area limited to the lateral to the aorta and above the left renal vein, might be considered for patients with Siewert type II or III tumors.

Therapeutic Dissection

It has long been known that some patients with PAN metastasis can be cured by dissection of all nodes including PA area, although the proportion of cured patients was as low as 10%. The Stomach Cancer Study Group (SCSG) of the JCOG has made several clinical studies on gastric cancer patients with extended lymph nodal disease, having either bulky metastatic nodes surrounding the celiac artery or its branches (conglomerate nodes of 3 cm or larger or two or more nodes of 1.5 cm or larger) or PAN larger than 10 mm. In the first study on this issue, neoadjuvant chemotherapy (NAC) by irinotecan plus cisplatin followed by D2 + PAND demonstrated 3-year OS of 27% (95% CI, 15–39%), while there were three treatment-related deaths [4]. In the second study, chemotherapy used for NAC was S-1 plus cisplatin. The 3- and 5-year OS of 51 eligible patients were 59% and 53%, respectively [5] (Fig. 8.4). The 5-year OS of those with clinical PAN metastasis without bulky N2 was 57 and that of those with both bulky N2 and PAN metastasis was 17%. In these two studies, histologically detected nodal metastasis of PAN among those without

Fig. 8.4 OS curve of
the patients enrolled in
the JCOG0405

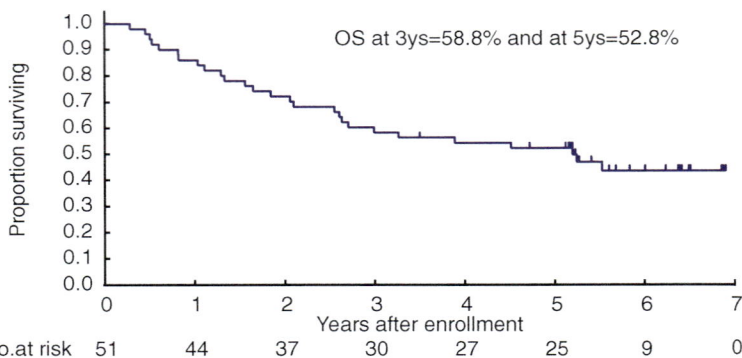

JCOG0405 OS curves of all eligible patients
including those who did not undergo surgery

OS at 3ys=58.8% and at 5ys=52.8%

No.at risk   51   44   37   30   27   25   9   0

clinical metastasis in PAN was seen in 30% and 20%, respectively. Thus even for bulky N2 without PAN metastasis, PAND should be carried out after prompt NAC.

Technique

1. *Extensive Kocher's maneuver (including mobilization of the hepatic flexure).*

    First step of PAND is extensive mobilization of the duodenum from the retroperitoneum. In this procedure, the hepatic flexure of the colon should be mobilized extensively to get a wide view of the PA area (Fig. 8.5). We should get in the layer immediately beneath the duodenum and the pancreas along the retro-pancreatic fascia covering the entire PAN area (Fig. 8.6). Dissection along this layer should be continued up to near the left kidney (Fig. 8.7). The inferior mesenteric vein can be seen from behind.

2. *Division of the membrane on the inferior vena cava (IVC).*

    The membrane covering the PA area, which also covers the vena cava, is divided longitudinally on the vena cava from about the position of the inferior mesenteric artery to the level of the left renal vein (Fig. 8.8). Following the exposed surface of the vena cava, the origin of the left renal vein can be easily found. Going caudally, the origin of the right gonadal vein is found, and the vein

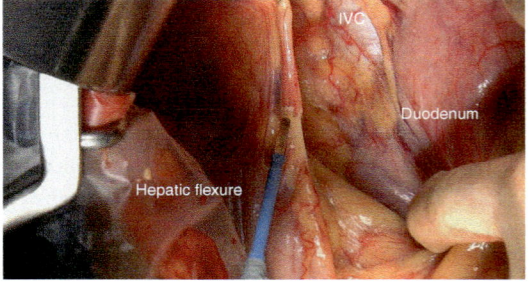

Fig. 8.5 Mobilization of the hepatic flexure

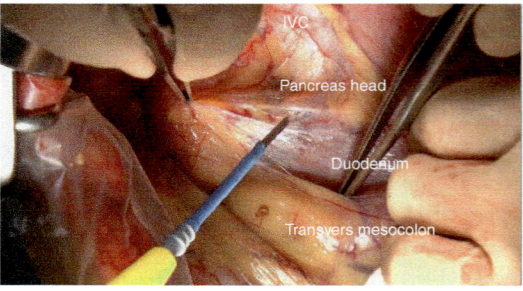

Fig. 8.6 Wide mobilization just beneath the retropancreatic fascia

should be cut at its origin (Fig. 8.9). The ventral surface of the left renal vein should be exposed till the origin of the left adrenal vein. As the whole PA area cannot be dissected en bloc in one piece, it should be divided at the level of the left renal vein. The tissue ventral to the left renal vein is ligated and divided (Fig. 8.10). As this tissue contains many large lymphatic vessels running

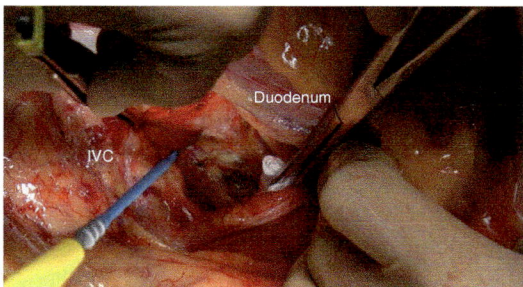

Fig. 8.7 Dissection along the retropancreatic fascia up to near the left kidney hilum

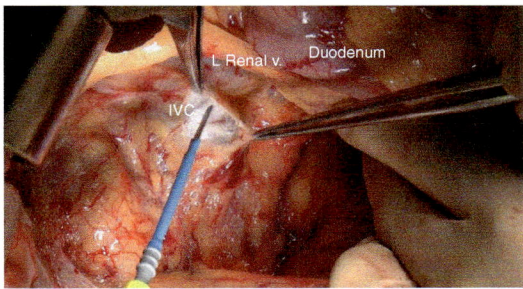

Fig. 8.8 Membrane covering the PA tissue is divided on the IVC to expose it

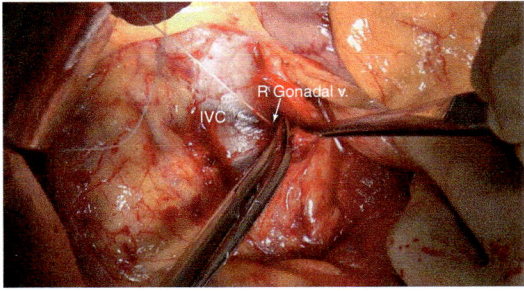

Fig. 8.9 Ligation and division of the right gonadal vein at its origin

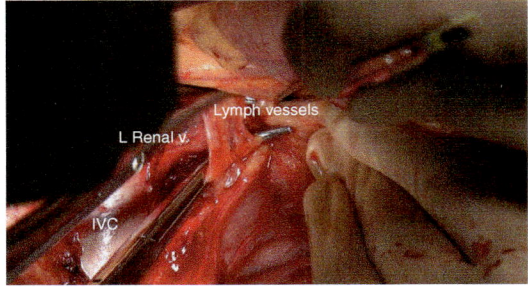

Fig. 8.10 PA tissue including large lymphatics should be ligated and divided upon the left renal vein

longitudinally, ligation is essential to avoid lymph ascites (chylo-ascites).

3. *Taping of the left renal vein (LRV) and exposing the surface of the aorta.*

    The left renal vein is taped around (Fig. 8.11) and pulled ventrally to expose the ventral surface of the aorta. The aorta is covered with thick adipose connective tissue, and it should be divided behind the left renal vein, as it is the thinnest at that level.

4. *Getting access to the bottom of the para-aortic tissue right to the aorta.*

    Dissecting the left lateral side of the IVC toward the back, we can expose the distal end of the right crus and the surface of the psoas muscle. Some autonomic nerve structures can be cut to access these structures. We can recognize the vein connecting with the azygos vein a few cm below the left renal vein, which can be divided at its root from the IVC (Fig. 8.12). The right renal artery can also be recognized.

5. *Dissection of the entire adipose connective tissue between the IVC and the aorta.*

    After reaching the bottom of the PA tissue, we start to dissect the tissue below the

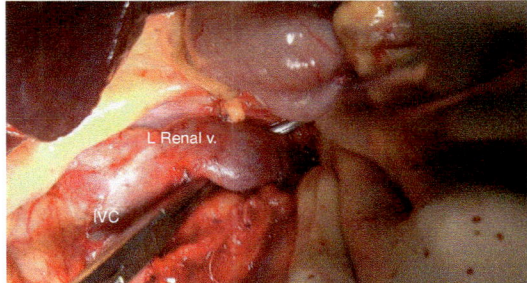

Fig. 8.11 The left renal vein is taped around

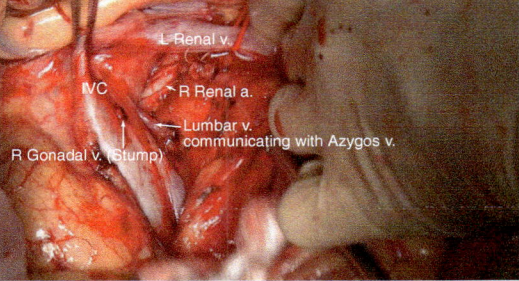

Fig. 8.12 Lumbar vein connecting with Azygous vein should be taken care

right renal artery and go along the surface of the psoas muscle caudally and from right to left toward the aorta (Fig. 8.12). The preaortic tissue is divided at the level of the left renal vein, and the origin of the left gonadal artery is exposed just a few cm below the left renal vein, and it should be divided at the origin (Fig. 8.13). In this process, the right lumbar arteries can be recognized, and the left lumbar veins cross over the psoas muscle and anterior vertebral ligament behind the aorta.

6. *Defining the caudal border of the dissection.*

   As we dissect the whole tissue between the IVC and the aorta caudally and right to left together with preaortic tissue, we can recognize the origin of the inferior mesenteric artery (IMA) after a while. It is the landmark of the inferior border of the dissection. Whole dissected tissue between the IVC and the aorta and that of pre-aorta should be ligated just below the level of the IMA (Fig. 8.14).

7. *Dissection along the left lateral side of the aorta to the posterior border.*

   Following the surface of the aorta toward left, the left gonadal artery is exposed, and it should be ligated and divided from the aorta (Fig. 8.15). Dissection is now continued along the left lateral wall of the aorta until the left lumbar veins and the anterior vertebral ligament are seen (Fig. 8.16). During this procedure, this layer is followed laterally on the fascia of the psoas muscle. Care should be taken not to injure the sympathetic nerve chain which is located on the psoas muscle.

8. *Separation of the PA tissue from the left Gerota's fascia.*

   The adipose tissue containing PAN is separated from that in the Gerota's fascia, which contains the ureter. Division from the left Gerota's fascia is performed along the left gonadal vein, which has only a couple of small branches draining from the PA area (Fig. 8.17). Separation from the left Gerota's fascia makes the lateral border of the PA tis-

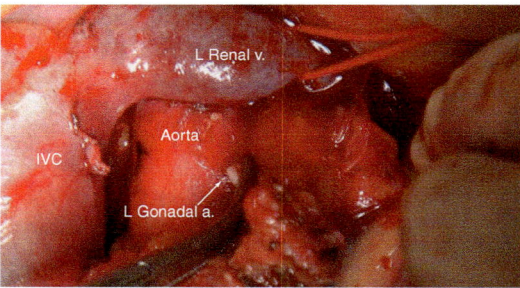

Fig. 8.13 Left gonadal artery should be divided at its origin

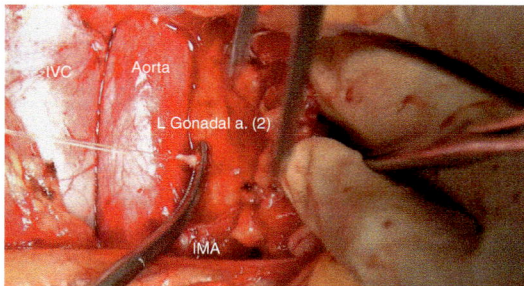

Fig. 8.15 Sometimes there are two left gonadal arteries

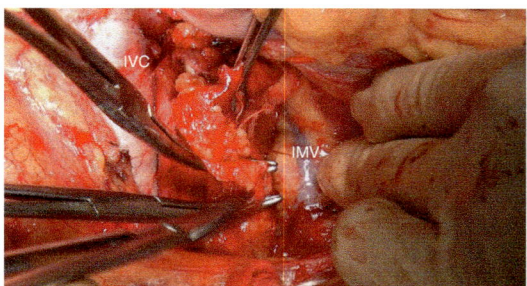

Fig. 8.14 Inferior border the the No.16 B1-int and -pre PA tissue. It should be divied just below the origin of the IMA level

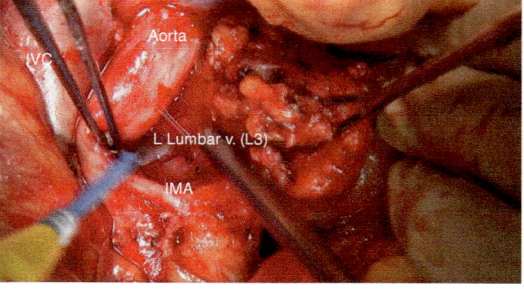

Fig. 8.16 Dissection along the left wall of the aorta is continued until the left lumbar vein and anterior vertebral ligamant are exposed

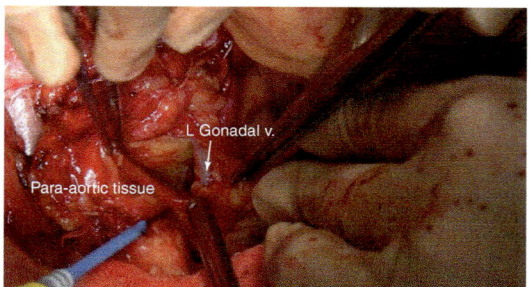

Fig. 8.17 Division along medial side of the left gonadal vein from the tissue encapsulated in the left Gerota's fascia

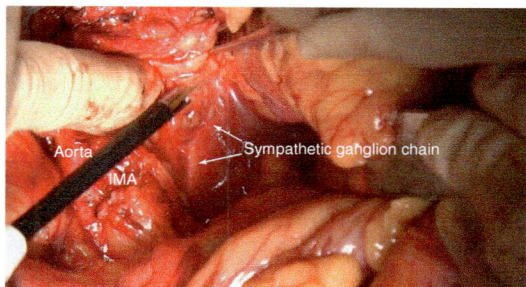

Fig. 8.19 Dissection should not go behind the left sympathetic ganglion chain, which should be preserved to avoid orthostatic hypotension after surgery

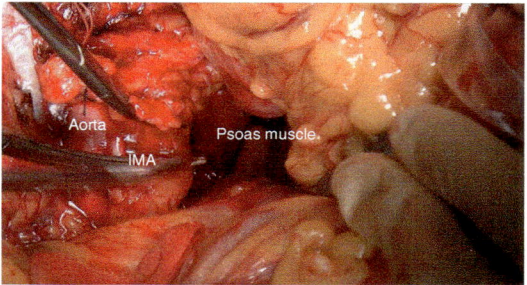

Fig. 8.18 PA tissue lateral to the aorta is divided just below the origin of the IMA

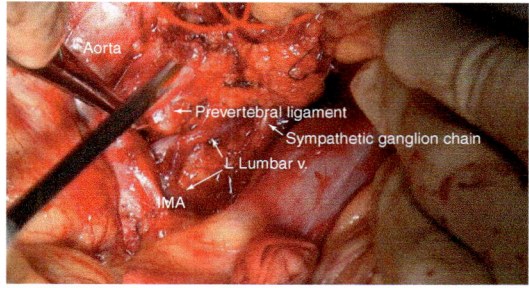

Fig. 8.20 View behind the aorta

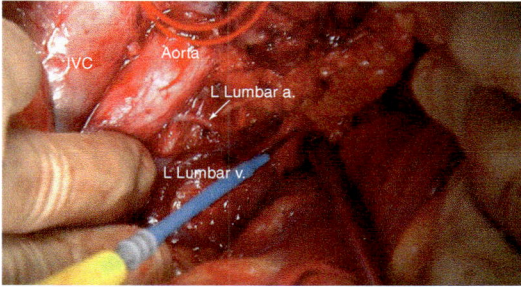

Fig. 8.21 View behind the aorta, slightly cranial to the Fig. 8.20

sue clear. Once the posterior Gerota's fascia is exposed, we can easily get into the space behind the posterior Gerota's fascia of the left kidney. To prepare the mobilization of the left kidney, quick and blunt dissection can separate the Gerota's fascia from the fascia of the psoas and quadratus lumborum muscles.

9. *Division of the PA tissue lateral to the aorta near the IMA.*

Just like the PA tissue between the IVC and the aorta, this part of PA tissue is ligated and divided at just below the level of the IMA (Fig. 8.18). Now the PA tissue is dissected from the posterior, inferior, and left lateral structures en bloc.

The left sympathetic ganglion chain can be recognized and preserved (Fig. 8.19). Median to the sympathetic ganglion chain and posterior to the aorta, left lumbar veins and artery can be seen and should be preserved (Figs. 8.20 and 8.21).

10. *Division of the PA tissue ventral to the renal left vein and exposure of the left renal artery.*

As the whole PA tissue cannot be dissected en bloc due to existence of the left renal vessels, the tissue lateral to the aorta is divided from the tissue cranial to the left renal vein. Firstly the tissue anterior to the left renal vein is divided. By this procedure, the left renal vein is clearly exposed, and the origin of the left adrenal vein can be recognized. Then the left renal artery, which exists in most cases a few centimeters cranial and behind the left renal vein, is exposed to avoid its injury (Fig. 8.22). Then the PA tissue

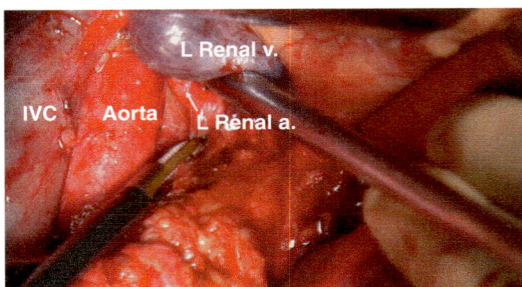

Fig. 8.22 Left renal arteries should be searched carefully along the left side of the aorta. Not commonly but occasionally there are a few of them

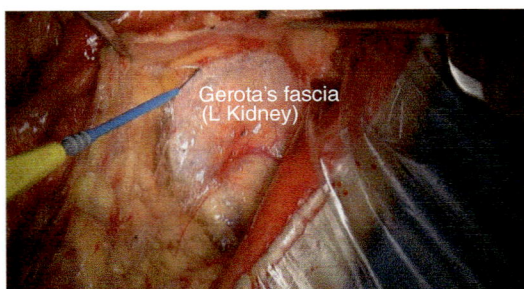

Fig. 8.24 The left colonic mesentery lying over the left Gerota's fascia is completely mobilized from it

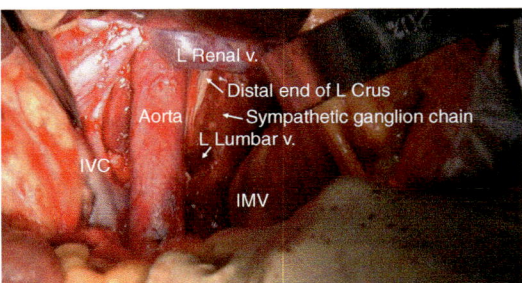

Fig. 8.23 View after dissection of No.16B1(-int, and -lat)

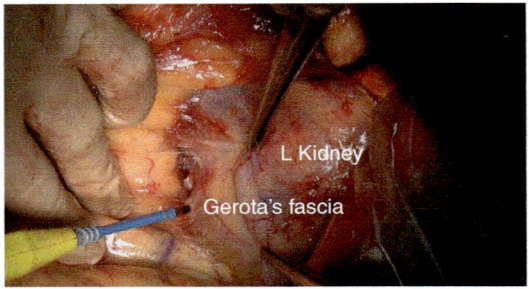

Fig. 8.25 Almost final point of the mobilization and dissection

below the left renal artery and dorsal to the left renal vein is divided from the cranial PA tissue. Figure 8.23 shows view after dissection of the 16B1 (para-aortic nodes between the left renal vein and the inferior mesenteric artery).

11. *Mobilization of the splenic flexure and exposure of the left Gerota's fascia.*

    After mobilizing the splenic flexure of the colon, the anterior Gerota's fascia is exposed widely until it is completely separated from the mesocolon (Figs. 8.24 and 8.25).

12. *Exposure of the left adrenal vein and the common trunk of hemiazygos and lumbar vein.*

    When the splenic flexure and the left half of the transverse colon are completely mobilized from the left retroperitoneum, the left kidney and the renal vein can be seen from anterior (Fig. 8.26). The origin of the left adrenal vein is also recognized. Near the origin of the left adrenal vein, the common trunk of lumbar vein and hemiazygos vein which goes caudally is ligated and divided from the left renal vein. The tissue

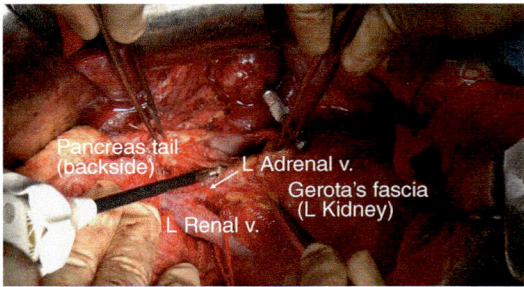

Fig. 8.26 When the left side colonic mesentery is mobilized widely together with the pancreas tail and the spleen, left renal vein and left adrenal vein are seen from anterior

containing lymph nodes along the left subphrenic vessels and median to the left adrenal gland is dissected. The dorsal border is the celiac ganglion.

13. *Mobilization of the left kidney and dissection of the tissue behind the renal vessels.*

    After putting the tapes on the left renal artery and vein, the left kidney is turned up, and tissue behind the left renal vessels is dissected carefully from these vessels (Figs. 8.27 and 8.28). The view after complete dissection of the PAN tissue is shown (Fig. 8.29).

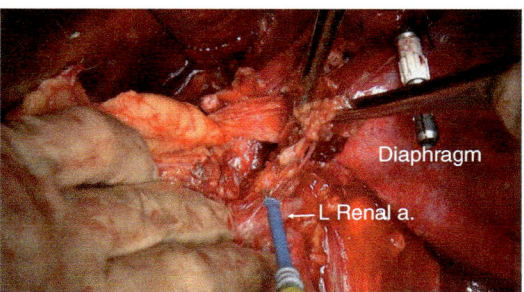

Fig. 8.27 Final step of the dissection of A2-lat: tissue surrounding the left renal vessels including that behind the vessels are completely dissected with the left kidney turned up

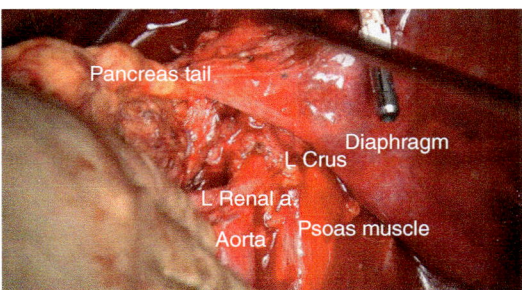

Fig. 8.28 View after complete dissection with the left kidney in operator's left hand

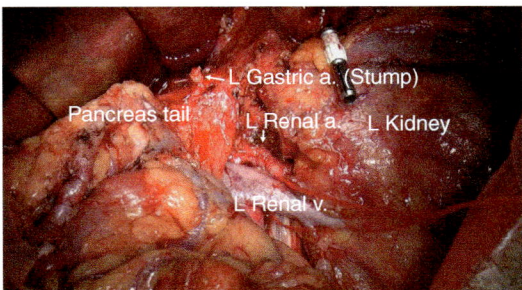

Fig. 8.29 Final view of the entire procedure

References

1. Sasako M, Sano T, Yamamoto S, et al. D2 lymphadenectomy alone or with para-aortic nodal dissection for gastric cancer. N Engl J Med. 2008;359:453–62.
2. Sano T, Sasako M, Yamamoto S, et al. Gastric cancer surgery: morbidity and mortality results from a prospective randomized controlled trial comparing D2 and extended para-aortic lymphadenectomy – Japan Clinical Oncology Group study 9501. J Clin Oncol. 2004;22:2767–73.
3. Sasako M, Sano T, Yamamoto S, et al. Left thoracoabdominal approach versus abdominal-transhiatal approach for gastric cancer of the cardia or subcardia: a randomised controlled trial. Lancet Oncol. 2006;7:644–51.
4. Yoshikawa T, Sasako M, Yamamoto S, et al. Phase II study of neoadjuvant chemotherapy and extended surgery for locally advanced gastric cancer. Br J Surg. 2009;96:1015–22.
5. Tsuburaya A, Mizusawa J, Tanaka Y, et al. Neoadjuvant chemotherapy with S-1 and cisplatin followed by D2 gastrectomy with para-aortic lymph node dissection for gastric cancer with extensive lymph node metastasis. Br J Surg. 2014;101:653–60.

Open Surgery for Gastric Cancer: Reconstruction

Joong Ho Lee and Woo Jin Hyung

Introduction

Restoring gastrointestinal continuity has remained an issue since the first successful gastrectomy. Although various reconstruction techniques are possible after gastrectomy, researchers and clinicians have yet to decide on an optimal or ideal reconstruction method. When choosing a reconstruction method, surgeons should seek to maintain, in addition to surgical and oncological stability, quality of life by ensuring nutritional intake after surgery.

Possible reconstruction methods after distal gastrectomy include gastroduodenostomy (also known as Billroth I reconstruction), gastrojejunostomy (also known as Billroth II reconstruction) with or without Braun anastomosis, and Roux-en-Y fashion gastrojejunostomy. After total gastrectomy, Roux-en-Y reconstruction is the most widely used procedure, although several modifications thereto have been devised.

J. H. Lee
Department of Surgery, National Health Insurance Service Ilsan Hospital, Goyang, Republic of Korea

W. J. Hyung (✉)
Department of Surgery, Yonsei University College of Medicine, Seoul, Republic of Korea
e-mail: wjhyung@yuhs.ac

Operative Technique

Reconstruction After Distal Gastrectomy

Gastroduodenostomy (Billroth I Reconstruction)

Gastroduodenostomy following distal subtotal gastrectomy is considered a preferred reconstruction method, especially in Asia [1]. Gastroduodenal anastomosis is performed end to end between the remnant stomach and the duodenum. Gastroduodenostomy has physiological advantages by affording duodenal passage preservation, and studies have described enhanced nutrient uptake and iron metabolism therewith, compared to other reconstruction methods, after distal gastrectomy [2, 3]. Anatomical advantages (e.g., single anastomosis) theoretically reduce the possibility of complications, such as anastomosis leakage, and allow for easier access to the biliary system.

Anastomosis can be performed manually or mechanically with a circular stapling device. Gastroduodenostomy with a circular stapler has been performed since the 1970s [4], and various modifications thereto have been reported. The use of a circular stapling device has been found to significantly shorten operation times, with similar incidences of complications, compared to other methods [5, 6].

© Springer-Verlag GmbH Germany, part of Springer Nature 2019
S. H. Noh, W. J. Hyung (eds.), *Surgery for Gastric Cancer*,
https://doi.org/10.1007/978-3-662-45583-8_9

Surgical Technique

To perform a gastroduodenostomy, a purse-string clamp is applied at the distal resection line of the duodenum. A straight clamp is applied just proximal to the purse-string clamp. The duodenum is then transected between two clamps (Fig. 9.1a). After a purse-string suture is made at the stump of the duodenum, a detachable anvil from a circular stapler with a diameter of 28–31 mm is gently inserted into the duodenal stump. Importantly, after the purse-string suture is tied over the anvil, the anvil should be grasped with the clamp to prevent its slippage down into the duodenal lumen (Fig. 9.1b).

A disposable automatic purse-string device can also be used. Performing a Kocher maneuver at the duodenum may reduce tension on the anastomosis site and readily allows the anvil to be inserted into the duodenum. Before transection of the duodenum, the Kocher maneuver can be more easily implemented.

After dividing the duodenum, anastomosis can be made before resection of the stomach, or gastrectomy can be performed first, followed by anastomosis. To perform the anastomosis before gastrectomy, a 3–4-cm gastrotomy in the distal part of the stomach is made to insert a circular stapler. The incision must avoid the area around the tumor and be opened along the greater curvature of the stomach, if possible (Fig. 9.2a). Through this gastrotomy, a lesion in the stomach can be grossly confirmed, and an adequate proximal resection margin can be determined.

After insertion of the anvil, the proximal cut edge of the gastrotomy is grasped, and the body of the circular stapler is inserted. The central rod of the circular stapler is then moved to penetrate through the posterior wall or the greater curvature of the stomach at the proper place of anastomosis (Fig. 9.2b). Afterward, the circular stapler is rotated toward the duodenum 180 degrees to lock the central rod and the anvil (Fig. 9.2c) to achieve side-to-end anastomosis of the gastroduodenostomy (Fig. 9.2d).

After anastomosis, any bleeding or disruption in the anastomosis is checked under direct vision through the opening of the gastrotomy. The donut ring in the anvil should be inspected carefully to ensure a complete ring is formed in the tissue. Following this procedure, the position of a nasogastric tube can be verified and gastric transection performed using linear staplers. The staple line is made about 1–2 cm from the anastomosis line of the gastroduodenostomy (Fig. 9.3a). Completed anastomosis of the stapled gastroduodenostomy is shown in Fig. 9.3b: the anastomosis was performed along the greater curvature of the remnant stomach, and note that the anastomosis did not cross the linear stapler lines of the gastric closure.

Anastomosis is easier to perform after retrieving the tumor specimen during resection of the stomach. After duodenal transection and completion of lymph node dissection, clamps are applied on the greater curvature of the stomach

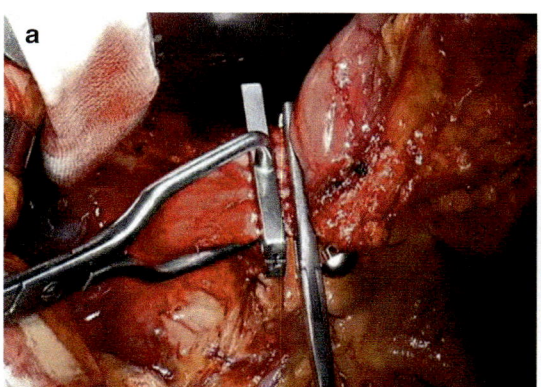
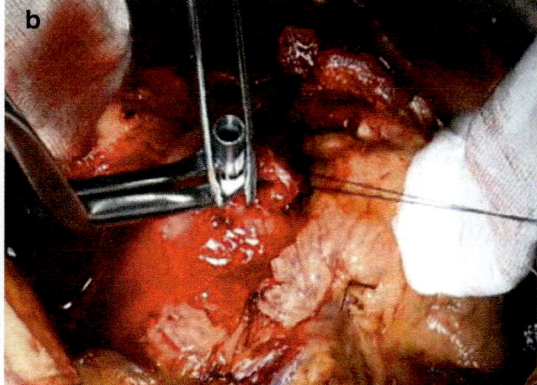

Fig. 9.1 Division of the duodenum for performing gastroduodenostomy. (**a**) A purse-string clamp is applied at the distal resection line of the duodenum. (**b**) The duodenum is transected, and the purse-string suture is tied over

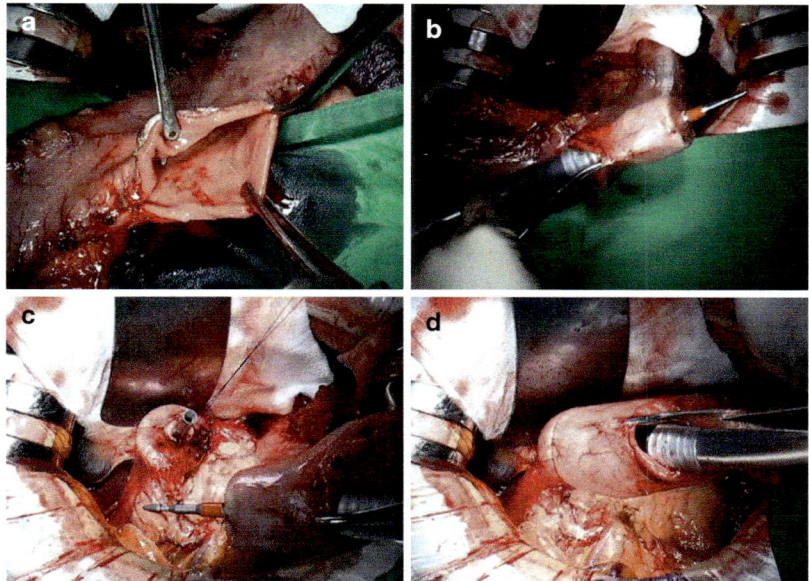

Fig. 9.2 Gastroduodenostomy with a circular stapler. (**a**) A gastrotomy in the distal part of the stomach is made. (**b**) Inserting a circular stapler through the gastrotomy, the central rod penetrates through the greater curvature of the stomach. (**c**) The stomach and stapler are rotated toward the duodenum. (**d**) The central rod and anvil are locked to perform side-to-end anastomosis

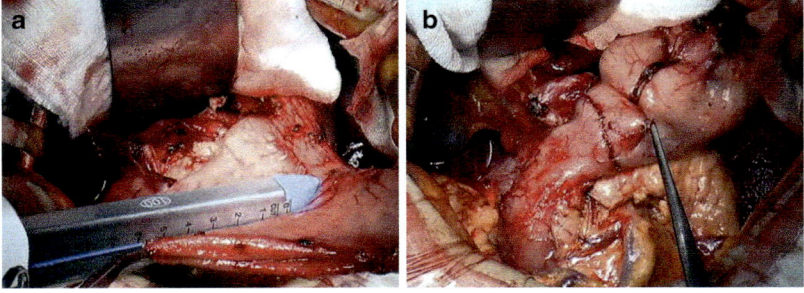

Fig. 9.3 Completed gastroduodenostomy with a circular stapler after distal subtotal gastrectomy. (**a**) The stomach is transected with linear staplers. (**b**) The staple line of the gastroduodenostomy does not cross the linear stapler lines of the gastric resection

along a determined proximal resection line, and then the greater curvature side of the stomach is divided between the clamps (Fig. 9.4a). Gastric resection is then carried out using a linear stapler, and the specimen is retrieved (Fig. 9.4b). For anastomosis, the body of a circular stapler is inserted at the entry hole in the remnant stomach upon removal of the applied clamp. The central rod of the stapler is advanced 1–2 cm away from the resection line to the posterior wall of the remnant stomach (Fig. 9.4c). After approximation of the central rod and the anvil, side-to-end anastomosis of the gastroduodenostomy is made by firing the stapler. Then, the entry hole of the remnant stomach is closed using a linear stapler (Fig. 9.4d). This method provides anastomosis on the posterior wall of the remnant stomach.

In both techniques, the circular and linear stapler lines do not cross one another, which is thought to lessen the risk of anastomotic leakage

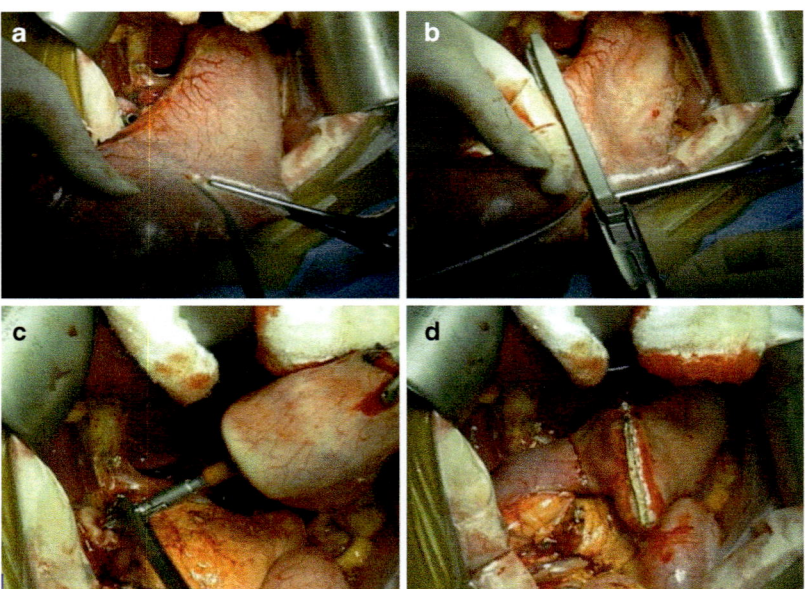

Fig. 9.4 Gastroduodenostomy after resection of the stomach. (**a**) A Payr's intestinal clamp is applied on the greater curvature side of the stomach. (**b**) The stomach is transected with linear staplers, and the tumor specimen is retrieved. (**c**) A circular stapler is inserted through the remnant stomach such that the central rod penetrates through the posterior wall of the stomach. (**d**) After finishing side-to-end gastroduodenostomy, the entry hole of the remnant stomach is closed using a linear stapler

[7]. To decrease tension during the gastroduodenostomy, incising the gastrophrenic ligament in the left edge of the fundus of the stomach is helpful, together with performing Kocher's maneuver [8].

Gastrojejunostomy (Billroth II Reconstruction)

Gastrojejunostomy provides anastomosis between the remnant stomach and the proximal loop of the jejunum after distal gastrectomy. A gastrojejunostomy is preferred over a gastroduodenostomy in cases in which only a small amount of remnant stomach is left because a larger portion of the stomach is removed due to a tumor located higher in the stomach. A gastrojejunostomy is also preferred when a tumor lesion is close to the pylorus ring of the stomach or when an ulcer is identified at the duodenal bulb. Unlike gastroduodenostomy reconstruction, gastrojejunostomy is always possible without unwarranted tension after anastomosis. The anastomosis can be performed manually or mechanically with a linear stapling device.

Gastrojejunostomy can be performed at the jejunal loop either behind the transverse colon (retrocolic) or in front of it (antecolic). While antecolic anastomosis is preferred because it is technically easier, both show similar long-term outcomes [9].

After resection of the stomach, gastrojejunostomy can be performed in a manner in which the remnant stomach is anastomosed to the antimesenteric side of the jejunum. Hand-sewn anastomoses are classically performed in an end-to-side fashion at the stump of the remnant stomach. On the other hand, mechanical anastomosis with a linear stapler is performed side to side in the greater curvature of the stomach. As end-to-side anastomosis allows for a greater range of stomach resection than side-to-end anastomosis, end-to-side hand-sewn anastomosis is preferred in cases of a tumor located higher in the stomach and of a small remnant stomach.

Surgical Technique

Here, the basic antecolic mechanical gastrojejunostomy is described. The side-to-side gastrojejunostomy can be performed using linear staplers. For mechanical anastomosis, the jejunal loop measuring approximately 10–15 cm from the ligament of Treitz is brought up to the stomach in an antecolic position after resection of the stomach. To create an isoperistaltic anastomosis, the afferent loop in the jejunum is fixed at the proximal part of remnant stomach, with the efferent loop at the stump. Thus, biliopancreatic secretions are emptied to efferent loop in direction because it is a dependent portion.

Anastomosis may be performed first after retrieval of the tumor specimen or before resection of the stomach. To begin, small holes are created at a proper site along the greater curvature of the stomach and the antimesenteric border of the jejunum. A linear stapler is then placed between the remnant stomach and jejunum, approximated, and then fired to achieve anastomosis (Fig. 9.5a). Following this procedure, gastric transection is performed using linear staplers (Fig. 9.5b). To finish, the common entry hole is closed with a single layer of running suture or using a linear stapler.

Roux-en-Y Gastrojejunostomy

Being increasingly performed, Roux-en-Y anastomosis after distal gastrectomy seeks to improve postoperative complications by preventing bile gastritis after vagotomy. Several studies have shown that this reconstruction method yields better long-term outcomes in terms of clinical symptoms and postoperative endoscopic findings [10, 11]. For these reasons, many surgeons prefer Roux-en-Y gastrojejunostomy for reconstruction after distal subtotal gastrectomy.

Surgical Technique

To begin the Roux-en-Y gastrojejunostomy, the jejunum, at a length 20–30 cm distal to the ligament of Treitz, is prepared as a Roux limb, transected using a linear stapler, and brought to the greater curvature of the remnant stomach via an antecolic route without any tension. A gastrostomy is then created at the distal edge of the greater curvature, and a small incision is made along the antimesenteric side of the jejunum, 6 cm from the stump, for side-to-side anastomosis. The linear stapler is inserted through enterotomies approximated along the edges of the stomach and jejunum, and the posterior wall of the stomach and the antimesenteric side of the jejunum are anastomosed by firing the stapler. The common enterotomy is closed in a single-layer fashion using a running suture or a linear stapler. Side-to-side or end-to-side jejunojejunostomy can then be performed at a length along the jejunum of approximately 25 cm from the gastrojejunostomy with a hand-sewn technique or stapled anastomosis (Fig. 9.6).

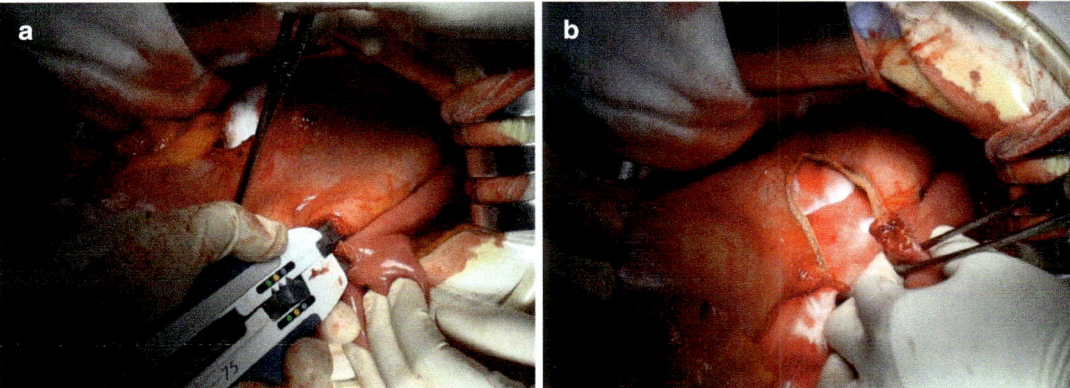

Fig. 9.5 Side-to-side gastrojejunostomy with a linear stapler. (**a**) A linear stapler is placed between the remnant stomach and jejunum then achieve anastomosis. (**b**) The stomach is transected with linear staplers, and the common entry hole is closed

Reconstruction After Total Gastrectomy

Roux-en-Y Esophagojejunostomy

Roux-en-Y reconstruction is a simple, well-codified method for achieving anastomosis after total gastrectomy. Recently, more complex constructions have been described, with the goals of preserving duodenal passage, creating a reservoir for ingested meals, and preventing reflux of biliopancreatic secretions [12]. In addition to restoring continuity

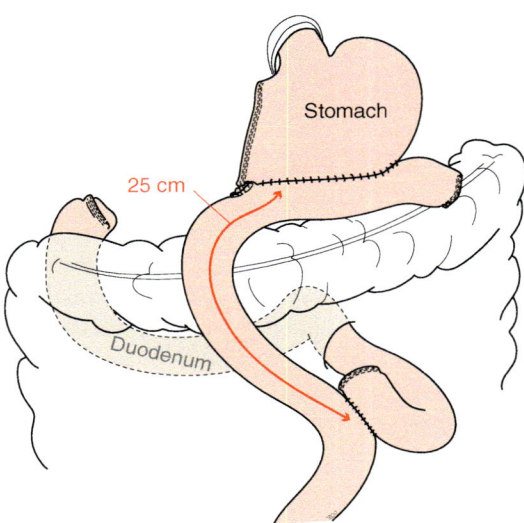

Fig. 9.6 Completed Roux-en-Y reconstruction after distal subtotal gastrectomy

of the digestive tract, these attempts seek to retain the nutritional status and to improve the quality of life of patients after gastrectomy. Notwithstanding, Roux-en-Y reconstruction is easy to perform and the most widely used procedure.

Surgical Technique

After the whole stomach is removed, a purse-string suture is applied at the stump of the esophagus as soon as possible to prevent shrinkage of the distal esophagus. An anvil with a diameter of 25–28 mm is carefully inserted into the esophagus. Following anvil placement at the distal esophagus, the purse-string suture is tied.

To prepare the jejunal loop, an appropriate area of the jejunum is transected distal to the ligament of Treitz while identifying the mesenteric vessel arcade. For esophagojejunostomy, the jejunal loop must be long, mobile, and well vascularized to reach the esophagus without tension.

In general, an esophagojejunostomy is created in an end-to-side fashion, bringing the jejunal loop in front of the transverse colon up to the esophagus. A circular stapler is inserted through the transected end of the jejunum, allowing the central rod to emerge in the antimesenteric wall at about 5 cm from the end of the jejunal loop (Fig. 9.7a). After attaching the anvil to the central rod, the stapler device is fired, and an end-to-side anastomosis is completed. The open end of the jejunal loop is then closed by a linear stapler (Fig. 9.7b).

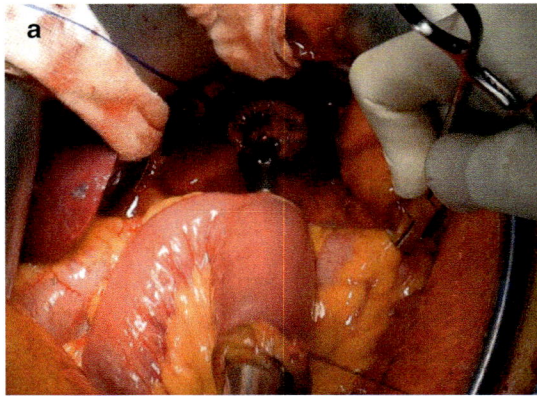
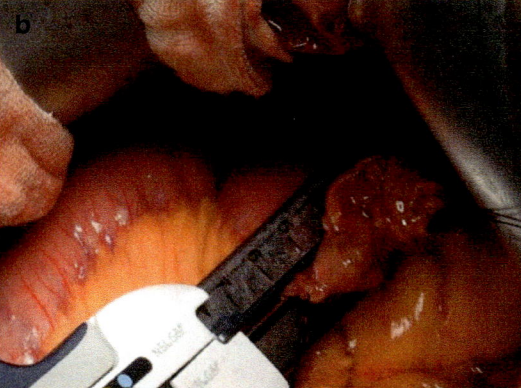

Fig. 9.7 Esophagojejunostomy with a circular stapler. (**a**) The circular stapler is inserted through the transected jejunal end such that the central rod penetrates the antimesenteric border of the jejunal loop. (**b**) The open end of the jejunal loop is closed by a linear stapler

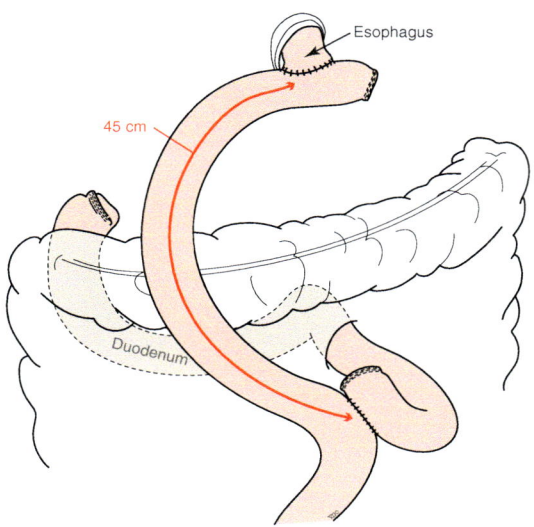

Fig. 9.8 Completed Roux-en-Y reconstruction after total gastrectomy

After the esophagojejunostomy, a jejunojejunostomy is performed to maintain biliopancreatic passage. Anastomosis between the proximal jejunum and the efferent limb is made in an end-to-side fashion at 15–20 cm distal to the ligament of Treitz. The length of the jejunal loop between the esophagojejunostomy and jejunojejunostomy should measure 45 cm to prevent regurgitation. A hand-sewn technique or a stapled anastomosis can be used (Fig. 9.8).

Summary

Gastrointestinal tract reconstruction after gastrectomy has evolved with the development of surgical techniques and stapling devices. A lot of effort has been exerted to make anastomosis safe, feasible, and functionally fit for patients after conventional open gastrectomy. Surgeons should consider surgical and oncological stability and quality of life by ensuring nutritional intake after surgery, although optimal or ideal reconstruction method is not clearly defined.

Disclosures This work was not supported by external or grant funding. None of the authors reports commercial associations or financial involvement that pose a conflict of interest in connection with the submitted article.

References

1. Information Committee of Korean Gastric Cancer A. Korean gastric cancer association nationwide survey on gastric cancer in 2014. J Gastric Cancer. 2016;16(3):131–40. https://doi.org/10.5230/jgc.2016.16.3.131.
2. Lee JH, Hyung WJ, Kim HI, Kim YM, Son T, Okumura N, Hu Y, Kim CB, Noh SH. Method of reconstruction governs iron metabolism after gastrectomy for patients with gastric cancer. Ann Surg. 2013;258(6):964–9. https://doi.org/10.1097/SLA.0b013e31827eebc1.
3. Kim BJ, O'Connell T. Gastroduodenostomy after gastric resection for cancer. Am Surg. 1999;65(10):905–7.
4. Nance FC. New techniques of gastrointestinal anastomoses with the EEA stapler. Ann Surg. 1979;189(5):587–600.
5. Hori S, Ochiai T, Gunji Y, Hayashi H, Suzuki T. A prospective randomized trial of hand-sutured versus mechanically stapled anastomoses for gastroduodenostomy after distal gastrectomy. Gastric Cancer. 2004;7(1):24–30. https://doi.org/10.1007/s10120-003-0263-2.
6. Takahashi T, Saikawa Y, Yoshida M, Otani Y, Kubota T, Kumai K, Kitajima M. Mechanical-stapled versus hand-sutured anastomoses in billroth-I reconstruction with distal gastrectomy. Surg Today. 2007;37(2):122–6. https://doi.org/10.1007/s00595-006-3361-z.
7. An JY, Yoon SH, Pak KH, Heo GU, Oh SJ, Hyung WJ, Noh SH. A novel modification of double stapling technique in Billroth I anastomosis. J Surg Oncol. 2009;100(6):518–9. https://doi.org/10.1002/jso.21368.
8. Kim YN, Aburahmah M, Hyung WJ, Noh SH. A simple method for tension-free Billroth I anastomosis after gastrectomy for gastric cancer. Transl Gastroenterol Hepatol. 2017;2:51. https://doi.org/10.21037/tgh.2017.05.08.
9. Umasankar A, Kate V, Ananthakrishnan N, Smile SR, Jagdish S, Srinivasan K. Anterior or posterior gastro-jejunostomy with truncal vagotomy for duodenal ulcer—are they functionally different? Trop Gastroenterol. 2003;24(4):202–4.
10. Kojima K, Yamada H, Inokuchi M, Kawano T, Sugihara K. A comparison of Roux-en-Y and Billroth-I reconstruction after laparoscopy-assisted distal gastrectomy. Ann Surg. 2008;247(6):962–7. https://doi.org/10.1097/SLA.0b013e31816d9526.
11. Inokuchi M, Kojima K, Yamada H, Kato K, Hayashi M, Motoyama K, Sugihara K. Long-term outcomes of Roux-en-Y and Billroth-I reconstruction after laparoscopic distal gastrectomy. Gastric Cancer. 2013;16(1):67–73. https://doi.org/10.1007/s10120-012-0154-5.
12. Chin AC, Espat NJ. Total gastrectomy: options for the restoration of gastrointestinal continuity. Lancet Oncol. 2003;4(5):271–6.

Laparoscopic Surgery for Gastric Cancer: Distal Subtotal Gastrectomy with D2 Lymph Node Dissection

10

Koichi Suda and Ichiro Uyama

Abbreviations

ASPDA	Anterior superior pancreaticoduodenal artery
ASPDV	Anterior superior pancreaticoduodenal vein
CHA	Common hepatic artery
GDA	Gastroduodenal artery
IPA	Infrapyloric artery
LGA	Left gastric artery
LGEA	Left gastroepiploic artery
PHA	Proper hepatic artery
PV	Portal vein
RGA	Right gastric artery
RGEA	Right gastroepiploic artery
RGEV	Right gastroepiploic vein
SPA	Splenic artery
SPV	Splenic vein

[2]. In terms of prognosis of gastric cancer, the 5-year relative survival was over 60% in Japan, whereas it was 25% in the Western countries [3]. There are two major factors which may cause such a great difference in long-term outcomes: the early detection of gastric cancer and the extended D2 lymph node dissection [1].

We introduced laparoscopic assistance into moderate to advanced gastrointestinal surgery in 1995 and developed techniques for laparoscopic distal and total gastrectomy with D2 dissection for advanced gastric cancer, which were published for the first time in the world [1, 4, 5]. Since then, we have performed more than 1500 laparoscopic gastrectomies. At present, the standard type of operation for curable gastric cancer is totally laparoscopic D2 gastrectomy [1].

We herein present the principles and methods of totally laparoscopic D2 distal gastrectomy.

Introduction

Gastric cancer remains a major public health problem in the world. Gastric cancer is the fourth most common cancer and the second leading cause of cancer-related death [1, 2]. The highest incidence of gastric cancer is found in East Asia

K. Suda · I. Uyama (✉)
Division of Upper GI, Department of Surgery, Fujita Health University, Toyoake, Aichi, Japan
e-mail: iuyama@fujita-hu.ac.jp

Setup

List of Instruments

The operating surgeon basically uses THUNDERBEAT (Olympus) and "Mancina" (Olympus) with his/her right and left hands, respectively. The assistant surgeon uses "Johann" (Olympus) and "Croce" (Olympus) with his/her cranial- and caudal-sided hands, respectively (Fig. 10.1). The 10 mm flexible high-definition

© Springer-Verlag GmbH Germany, part of Springer Nature 2019
S. H. Noh, W. J. Hyung (eds.), *Surgery for Gastric Cancer*,
https://doi.org/10.1007/978-3-662-45583-8_10

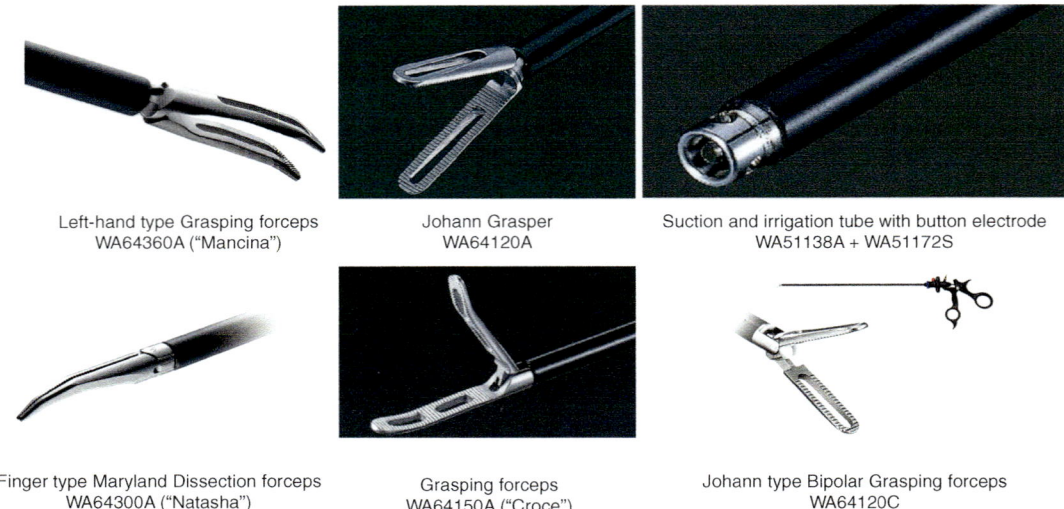

Left-hand type Grasping forceps
WA64360A ("Mancina")

Johann Grasper
WA64120A

Suction and irrigation tube with button electrode
WA51138A + WA51172S

Finger type Maryland Dissection forceps
WA64300A ("Natasha")

Grasping forceps
WA64150A ("Croce")

Johann type Bipolar Grasping forceps
WA64120C

Fig. 10.1 Forceps and hemostats specialized for advanced laparoscopic surgery

video laparoscope (LTF-S190-10, Olympus) is preferably used. All the details are shown in Table 10.1.

Patients

The stage of the cancer is classified according to the 14th edition of the Japanese Classification of Gastric Carcinoma [6]. Cancer staging is performed based on the findings of contrast-enhanced computed tomography, gastrography, endoscopic study, and endosonography before the beginning of any treatment and, when applicable, after the completion of chemotherapy. The patients with clinical T ≥ 2 cancer over 5 cm in size and/or a swollen locoregional lymph node over 1.5 cm in size undergo staging laparoscopy. Clinical stage ≤ IIIC is determined to be resectable. Neoadjuvant chemotherapy (S-1 80 mg/m2 day 1–21 + CDDP 60 mg/m2 day 8) is used for those with clinical T ≥ 2 as well as tumor ≥5.0 cm in size and/or a swollen locoregional lymph node ≥1.5 cm in size, unless the patients refuse it. Induction chemotherapy (S-1 80 mg/m2 day 1–14 + CDDP 35 mg/m2 day 8, or Docetaxel 30 mg/m2 day 1, 15 + CDDP 30 mg/m2 day 1, 15 + S-1 80 mg/m2 day 1–14)

is used for clinical stage IV disease, and radical gastrectomy is conducted when downstaging is achieved [7, 8].

Distal gastrectomy is used for the tumor localized to M and/or L area. D1+ lymphadenectomy is conducted for preoperative stage IA disease, whereas D2 is performed for preoperative stage IB, II, and III diseases in accordance with the fourth edition of the JGCA guidelines [9].

OR Setup

Basically, the operating surgeon stands on the patient's right side, except for #6 lymph node dissection (Fig. 10.2). When the operating surgeon stands on the patient's left side, the scrub nurse with the table should move from the caudal to the cranial side of the patient (Fig. 10.2) just to avoid the cables connecting between the forceps and generators from getting tangled.

Patient's Position

The patient is placed in a supine position with legs apart, left arm extended, and 15-degree head-up tilt.

Trocar Arrangement (Fig. 10.3)

- Camera port (CP): navel or midline below the navel
- Right upper port (RUP): one finger caudally from the right subcostal line, top of the right subphrenic "dome," affecting the comfortableness in grasping the adipose tissue including #11p

- Note: The distance between CP and RUP should be longer than eight fingers.
- Right lower port (RLP): caudally on the median line between CP and RUP
- Left upper port (LUP): eight fingers laterally to the bottom of the greater curvature of the stomach, affecting the comfortableness in #6 dissection

Table 10.1 List of instruments used for totally laparoscopic gastrectomy at Fujita Health University

Category	Description	Product name
Imaging	Monitor	OEV-261H
		NDS SC-WU26-A1511-1
	Video system	CV-190
	Light source	CLV-190
	Insufflations	UHI-4
	Scope	LTF-S190-10
		IMH20
		Video recorder
Energy	Ultrasonic(THUNDERBEAT)	USG400
		ESG400, WB50402W foot pedal
		TC-E400
		TD-TB400 (transducer)
		TD-TB400 (transducer)—spare
		TB-0545FC
		TB-0535FC
		MAJ-1871
		MAJ-1872
		MAJ-1873
		MAJ-1876
		MAJ-1870
		WB50403W (single foot pedal for bipolar)
		MAJ-814 (Pcode)
	Electrosurgical	FORCE TRIAD (Covidien)
HiQ	Dissector	WA64300A (with A60800A and A60201A) right-hand forceps
		WA64370A (with A60800A and A60201A) Fine Maryland
		WA64350A (with A60800A and A60201A) Maryland
		WA64150A Grasping forceps (Croce)
	Grasper	WA64360A (with A60800A and A60201A) left-hand forceps
		A64120A (with A60800A and A60201A) Johann grasper
	Bipolar	WA64120C (with WA60800C and WA60101C)
		*Bipolar cable: A60003C
	Others	WA51138A + **WA51172L**
		A60200A (ratchet hand)
		*Monopolar cable: A0358 (for FORCE TRIAD)
		Storz needle holder (Storz)
		WA64710A (Olympus Needle Holder)

(continued)

Table 10.1 (continued)

Category	Description	Product name
Consumables	First trocar	COR47 100 mm, balloon-type trocar (Applied Medical)
		12 mm × 75 mm (or 100 mm) trocar (Ethicon)
		5 mm ONB5STF(Covidien)
	Metzenbaum	A64810A (with A60800A + A60201A) or CB030
	Stapler	Tri-Staple, 45/60, Camel and Purple(distributed by Covidien)
		egia45avm
		egia60avm
		egia45amt
		egia60amt
	Clip	Covidien M clip
		Covidien M/L clip
	Suture	【3-0 Proline, 90 cm, SH-1 (Ethicon) 】 or 【3-0, Surgipro II, 90 cm, (Covidien, VP762X)】
		【3-0 Monocryl, 90 cm, SH-1 (Ethicon) 】 or 【3-0,75 cm, Caprosyn, (Covidien, UC-404)】 or 【3-0,75 cm, Biosyn (Covidien, GM324)】
		【PDS, SH (for open surgery) (Ethicon)】 or 【3-0, CR, Maxon (6229–43, Covidien)】
		【3-0 Vicryl CR SH-1(Ethicon) 】 or 【3-0 Polysorb (Covidien, GLJ-50M)】
		Polysorb, 2-0, 75 cm, 27 mm (Covidien, UL-878)
		Maxon, 1, CR, 48 mm (Covidien、GMMT540MG)
Others	Others	Surgical Octopus Retractor L, M, S (Nathanson Hook Liver Retractors® distributed by Yufu Itonaga Co.)
		Dr. Fog Endoscope Anti-Fog Solution, DF-3120 (distributed by AMCO)
		EndoClose 173022 (distributed by Covidien)
		Endo Universal Stapler 173052 (distributed by Covidien)
		Cherry Dissector BTD05 (distributed by Ethicon)
		PassSaver MD-49621 (Sumitomo)
		First option: Inzii 12/15 mm Retrieval System (Applied Medical) Second option: EndoCatch II 173049 (distributed by Covidien)
		Surgicel NU-KNIT 7.6 cm × 10.2 cm 15732 (Ethicon)
		Xylocaine Jelly (AstraZeneca)
		Pyoktanin Blue 25 g (KISHIDA)
		Storz Duomat (Storz)
		Tubes
		Y shape connector

These instruments were distributed by the Olympus unless otherwise noted

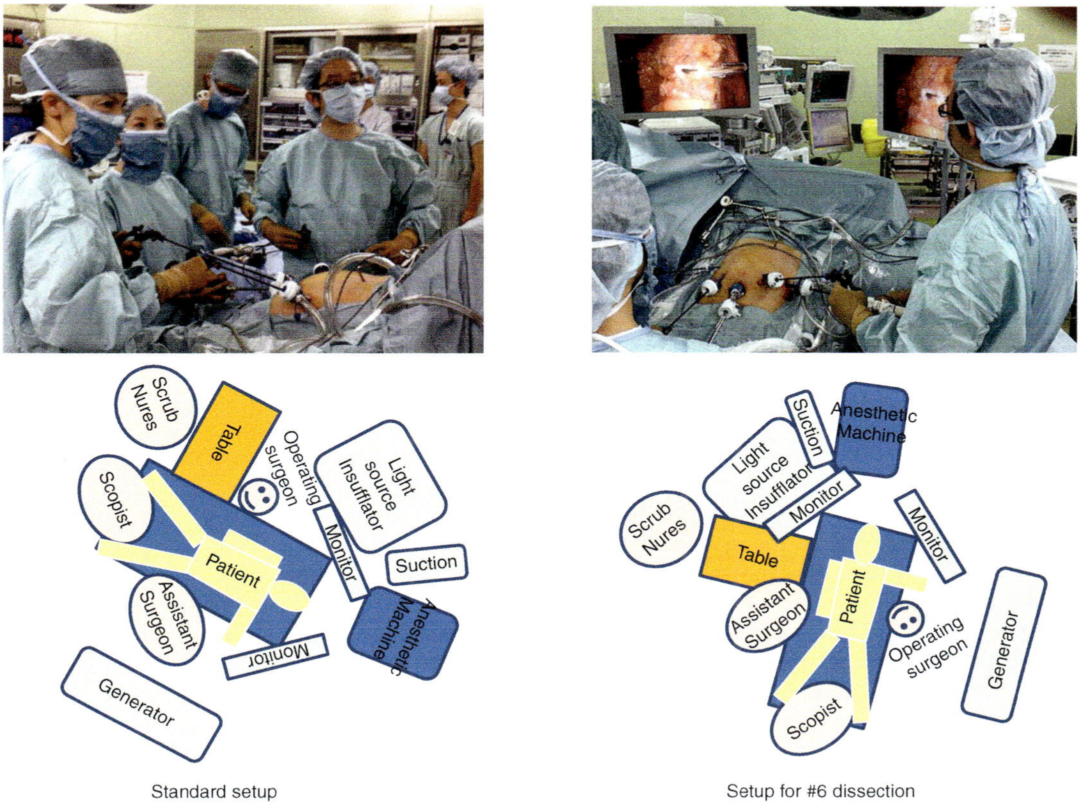

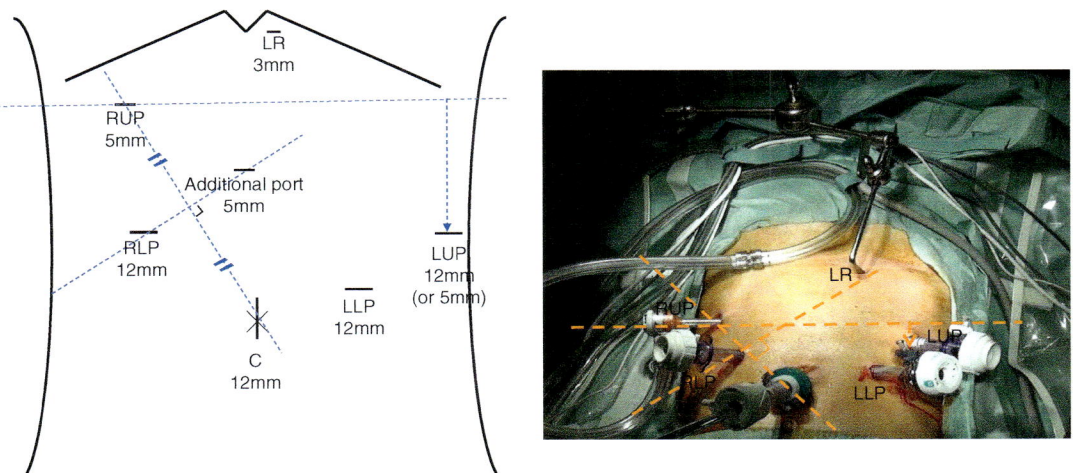

Fig. 10.2   OR setup

Fig. 10.3   Trocar arrangement in laparoscopic gastrectomy

- LLP: caudally on the median line between CP and LUP
- Additional port: cranially on the median line between CP and RUP, suitable for deeply dissecting suprapancreatic lymph nodes over the pancreas

D2 Lymph Node Dissection

Outermost Layer-Oriented Medial Approach

D2 dissection entails removal of the lymph nodes in the suprapancreatic area in distal gastrectomy [1]. Dissection of this area is technically demanding due to the serious risk of bleeding and/or pancreatic leakage derived from a major vessel or organ injury [1, 10, 12]. To improve the safety, efficacy, and reproducibility of suprapancreatic nodal dissection, we developed our original methodology called outermost layer-oriented medial approach [1, 10, 11]. In this approach, the layer between the autonomic nerve sheaths of the major arteries and the adipose tissue bearing the lymphatic tissue is dissected [1, 10, 11].

We termed this layer as the outermost layer of the autonomic nerve (Fig. 10.4) [1, 11]. To identify this layer throughout the dissection process, we developed an original surgical theory, "XYZ-axis" theory (Fig. 10.5), consisting of the following three steps—[1] cut the serosal membrane on the suprapancreatic border, [2] dissect suprapancreatic adipose tissue caudocranially toward the junction of the three arteries (zero point) to find the outermost layer, and [3] dissect the target adipose tissue mediolaterally along the layer spreading on the XZ and YZ axes.

Details of D2 Dissection in Distal Gastrectomy

#4d Dissection

The operating surgeon stands to the right of the patient. The assistant surgeon holds the greater curvature on the "watershed" dividing between the right and left gastroepiploic arteries (RGEA and LGEA) and raise it cranioventrally with his/her right hand. Subsequently, the assistant surgeon grasps the greater omentum near the transverse colon with his/her left hand. Then, the

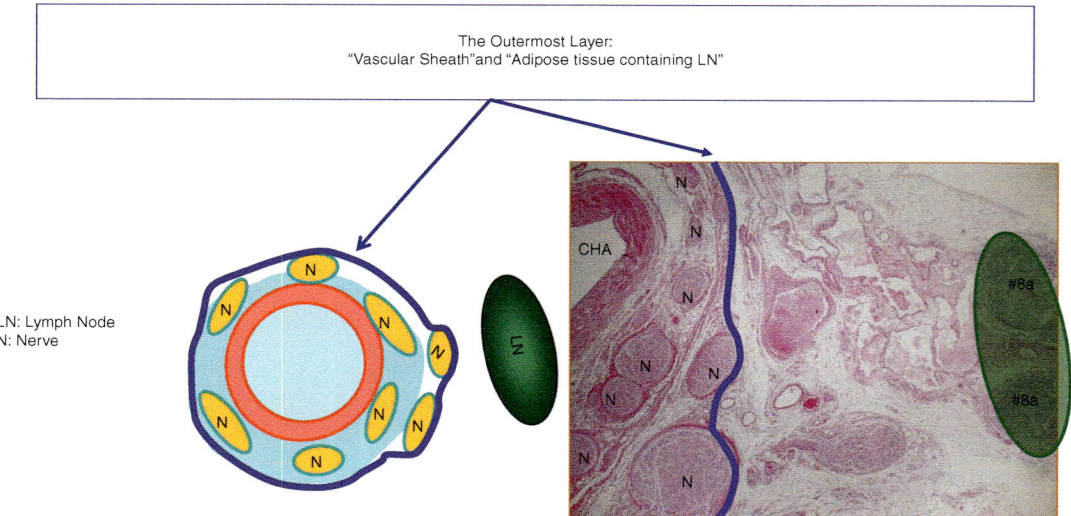

The Outermost Layer:
"Vascular Sheath" and "Adipose tissue containing LN"

LN: Lymph Node
N: Nerve

Appropriate tension generates thin space along the outermost layer
= Safe and adequate nodal dissection

Fig. 10.4 Outermost layer of the autonomic nerve

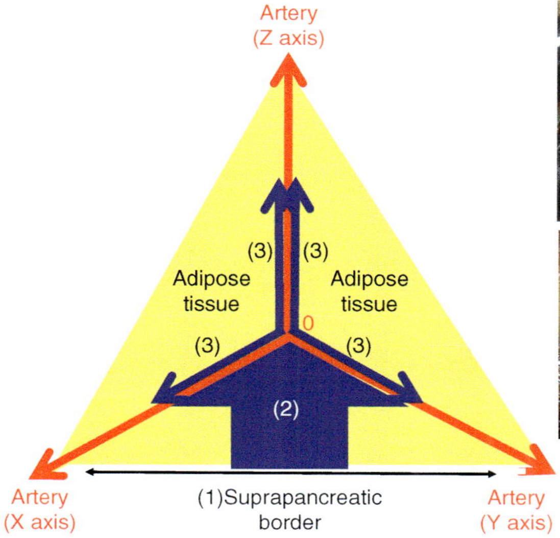

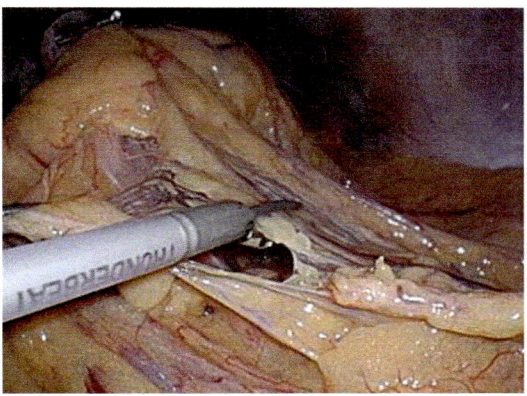

Fig. 10.5 XYZ-axis theory

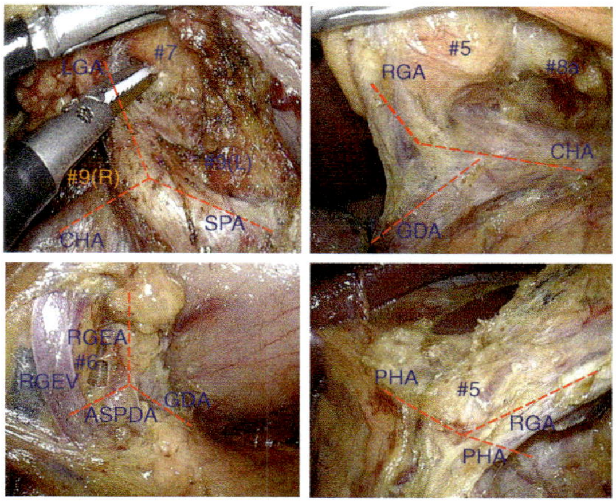

Fig. 10.6 #4d dissection

operating surgeon gently holds the pedicle of the right gastroepiploic artery and vein (RGEA and RGEV) to create a triangle. The operating surgeon starts opening the omental bursa at a thin part of the greater omentum (Fig. 10.6) and transects it along the border between the adipose tissue belonging to the stomach and that belonging to the transverse colon referring to the "line" generated by physiological adhesion (Fig. 10.7a). Adhesion between the posterior aspect of the stomach and the pancreatic body should also be detached as much as possible just to recover the original anatomy.

#4sb Dissection

The assistant surgeon holds the posterior aspect of the upper area of the stomach and determines the pedicle including the LGEA/LGEV originating from the pancreatic tail (Fig. 10.7a). By dividing the bursa along the physiological adhesion line mentioned above, the root of the gastric branch of LGEA is easily exposed preserving the omental branch (Fig. 10.7b). Then, the adipose tissue including #4sb is removed out of the greater curvature from the "watershed" up to the avascular area between LGEA and short gastric arteries (SGAs) (Fig. 10.7c).

#6 Dissection

The operating surgeon moves to the left of the patient. The transverse colon is mobilized by dissecting the fusion fascia, and the pancreatic head is widely exposed. The left aspect of the adipose tissue including #14v and 6 is dissected along the inferior border of the pancreas (Fig. 10.8a). Subsequently by dissecting on the edge of the pancreas continuously from the inferior to anterior aspects of the pancreatic neck, RGEA and the autonomic nerve on the right of RGEA are exposed (Fig. 10.8b). At this site, right gastroepiploic vein (RGEV) is running along the nerve, and the outermost layer of RGEA is widely

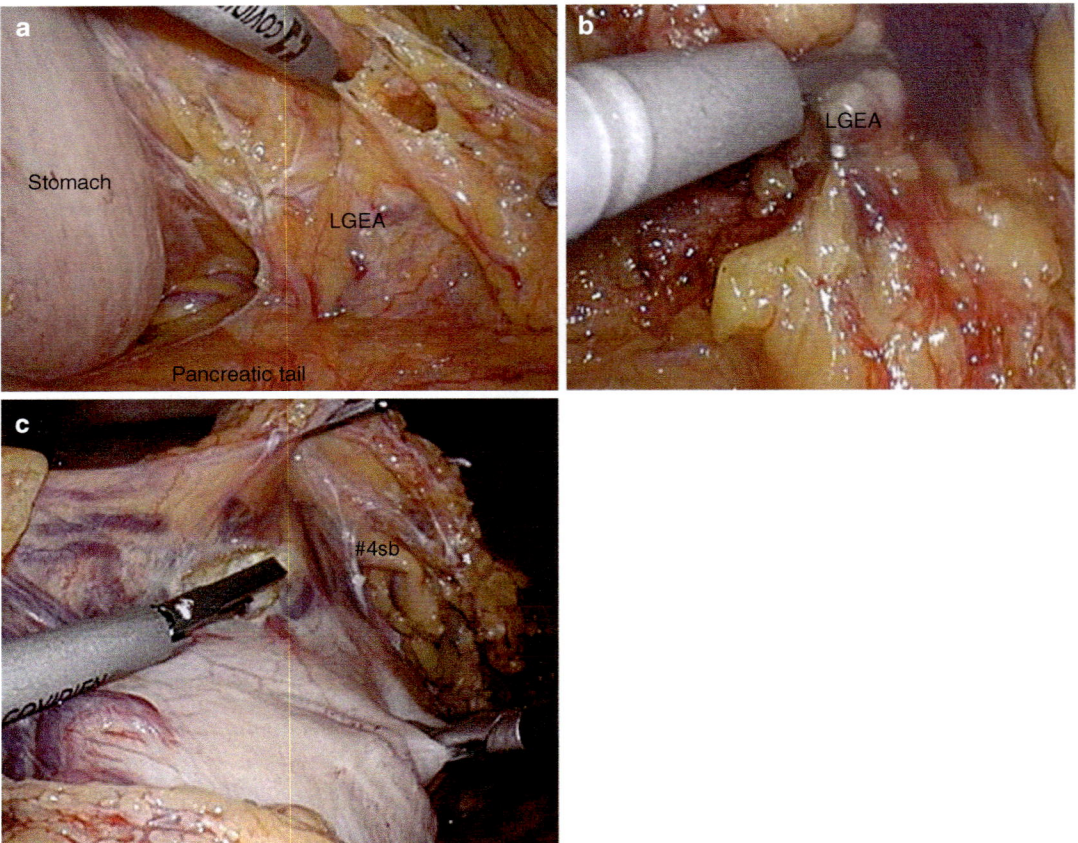

Fig. 10.7 #4sb dissection: (**a**) dissection of the physiological adhesion on the left field of the omental bursa, (**b**) transection of LGEA, (**c**) dissection of #4sb along the greater curvature of the stomach

exposed by dividing between the vein and nerve to facilitate #6v dissection (Fig. 10.8b). The prepancreatic fascia is dissected along the anterior superior pancreatoduodenal vein (ASPDV) (Fig. 10.8c). RGEV is transected right above ASPDV (Fig. 10.8d). Then, the adipose tissue bearing #6v is completely removed on the outermost layer of RGEA and anterior superior pancreatoduodenal artery (ASPDA) (Fig. 10.8e). During this process, infrapyloric veins are transected at their origins. As a next step, the cranial aspect of the fat tissue including station #6i and #6a is removed from the greater curvature side of the duodenum ("C-loop") (Fig. 10.9a). Finally, the RGEA and infrapyloric artery (IPA) are transected (Fig. 10.9b).

Transection of the Duodenum

The avascular area between the lesser curvature side of the duodenal bulb and the adipose tissue bearing #5 is opened from the posterior aspect of the stomach (Fig. 10.10a). Then, the duodenal bulb is transected in the posteroanterior direction (Fig. 10.10b).

Lesser Omentum, Top of #1

The operating surgeon moves back to the right of the patient. The lesser omentum is dissected along the most cranial hepatic branch of the vagal nerve ("reversed-L shape") (Fig. 10.11a). The anterior aspect of the subretroperitoneal fascia is exposed in front of the right diaphragmatic crus (Fig. 10.11b). The top of the #1 dissection

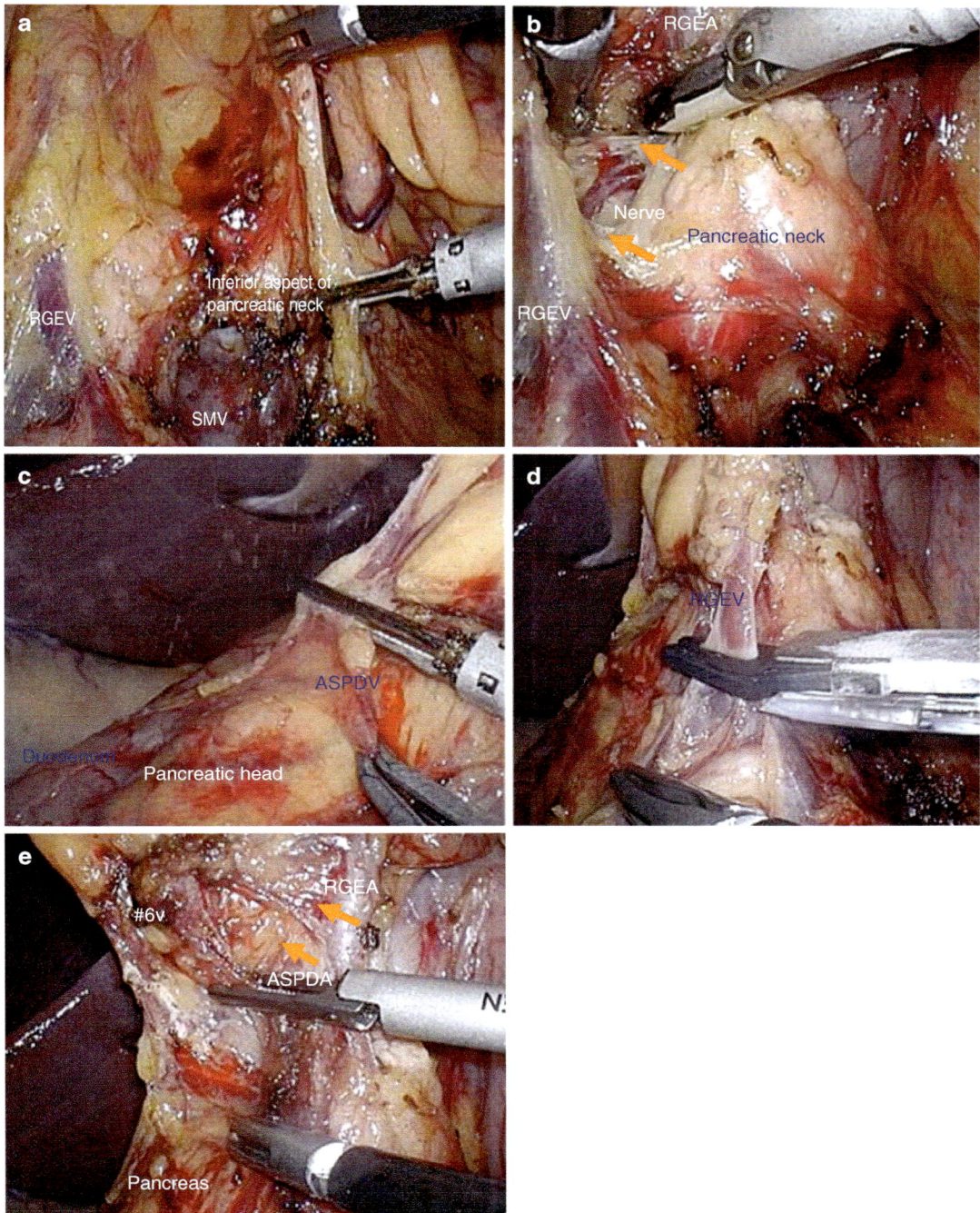

Fig. 10.8 #6v dissection: (**a**) exposure of the inferior aspect of the pancreatic neck; (**b**) continuous dissection on the edge of the pancreas from inferior to anterior aspects of the pancreatic neck, arrow: the outermost layer of RGEA; (**c**) dissection of the prepancreatic fascia along ASPDV; (**d**) transection of RGEV; (**e**) #6v dissection along the outermost layer (arrow) of RGEA and ASPDA

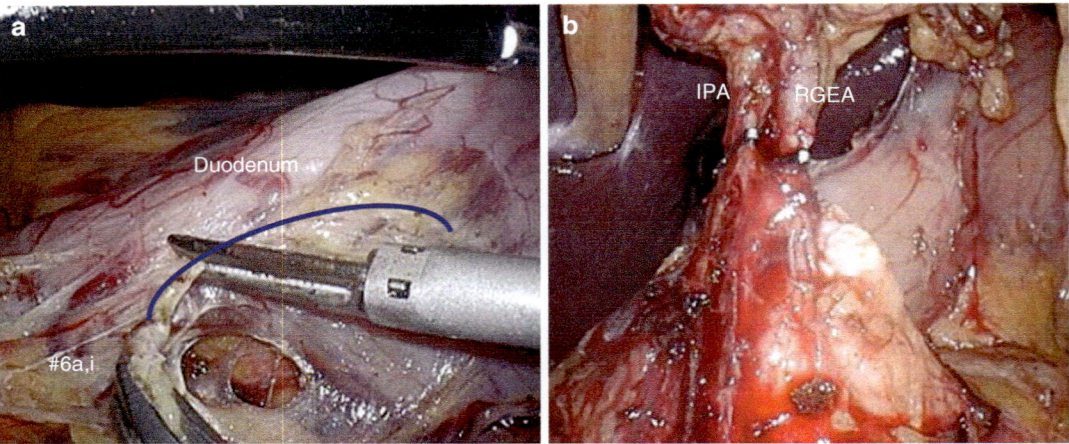

Fig. 10.9 #6a and i dissection: (**a**) dissection of the "C-loop," (**b**) transection of RGEA and IPA

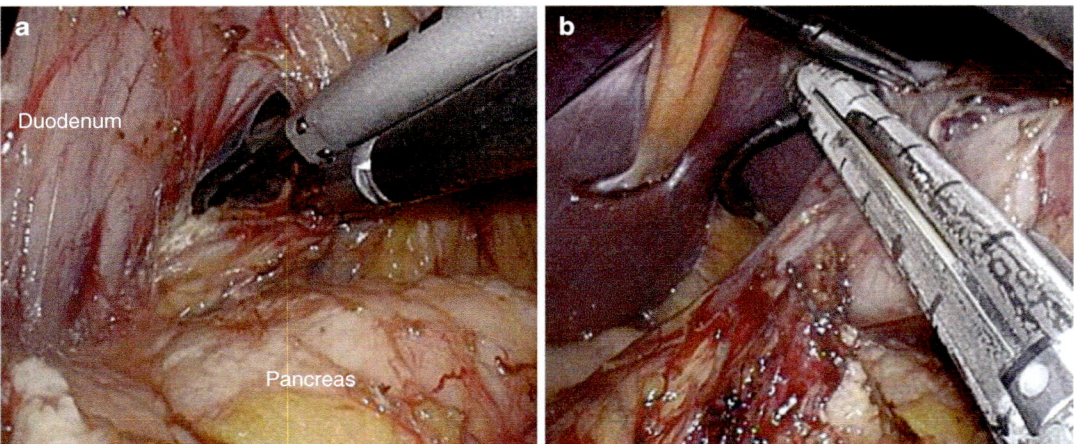

Fig. 10.10 Transection of the duodenum: (**a**) avascular area on the lesser curvature side of the duodenal bulb, (**b**) transection of the duodenal bulb

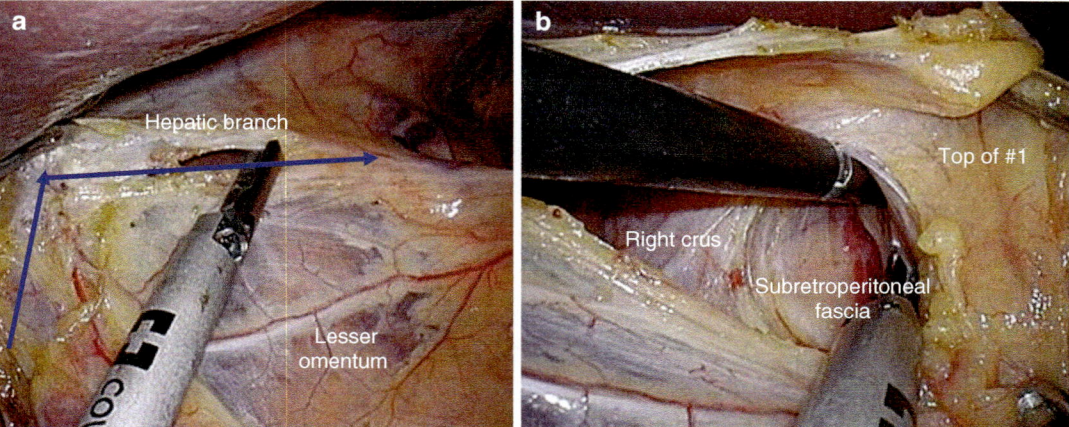

Fig. 10.11 Transection of the lesser omentum: (**a**) reversed L-shaped dissection of the lesser omentum, (**b**) the subretroperitoneal fascia on the right diaphragmatic crus

is determined confirming the final ascending branch of the left gastric artery (LGA).

Rolling Up the Stomach

To facilitate suprapancreatic lymph node dissection, the stomach is rolled up (Fig. 10.12).

Probing the Outermost Layer of CHA and SPA

The assistant surgeon retracts the caudal edge of the pancreatic body with his/her left hand (gauze-holding forceps) and stretches the gastropancreatic fold with his/her right hand. The operating surgeon stretches the adipose tissue containing #8a and #11p carefully and dissects it along the stably visualized outermost layer of the common hepatic artery (CHA) (Fig. 10.13a)

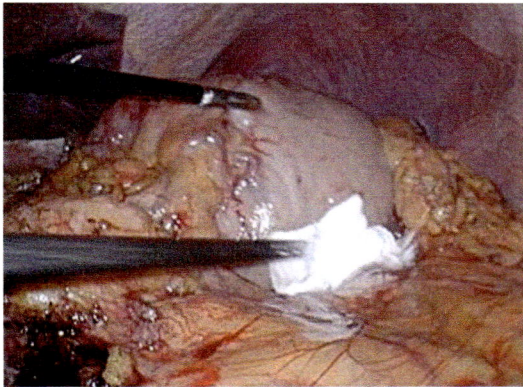

Fig. 10.12   Rolling up the stomach

and the proximal part of the splenic artery (SPA) (Fig. 10.13b). This dissection is continued along the outermost layer of the left lateral aspect of the proper hepatic artery (PHA) to the back of the right gastric artery (RGA).

#5 Dissection

The outermost layer along the cranial aspect of RGA and the distal part of PHA is exposed (Fig. 10.14a). The origin of RGA was divided by clips (Fig. 10.14b).

Medial Approach [1, 11]

The avascular space of the left gastric artery (LGA) is dissected bilaterally along the outermost layer (Fig. 10.15a, b).

#12a Dissection

The fat tissue containing #5, 8a, 9(R), and 12a is lifted ventrally. To create a good surgical field, the operating surgeon pulls the thick nerve fibers along the PHA laterodorsally, and the assistant surgeon pulls the nerve fibers on the cranial side of the CHA caudodorsally (Fig. 10.16a). Then, the portal vein (PV) is superficialized, and #12a lymph nodes are safely dissected along the PV (Fig. 10.16b).

#9(R) Dissection

The target fat tissue containing #8a, 9(R), and 12a is completely dissected along the outermost layer of the nerve plexus of the celiac artery, lead-

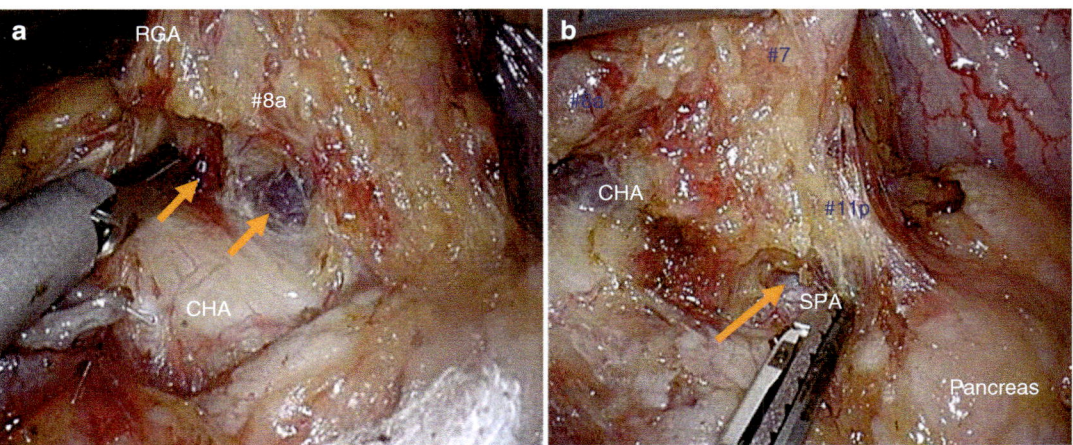

Fig. 10.13   Probing the outermost layer: (**a**) the outermost layer along CHA (arrow), (**b**) the outermost layer along SPA (arrow)

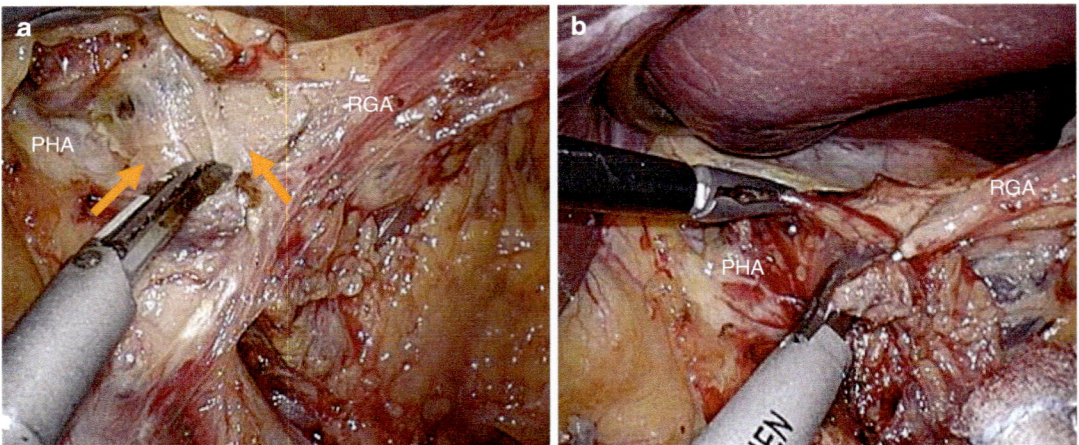

Fig. 10.14 #5 dissection: (**a**) the outermost layer along the cranial aspect of RGA, (**b**) transection of RGA

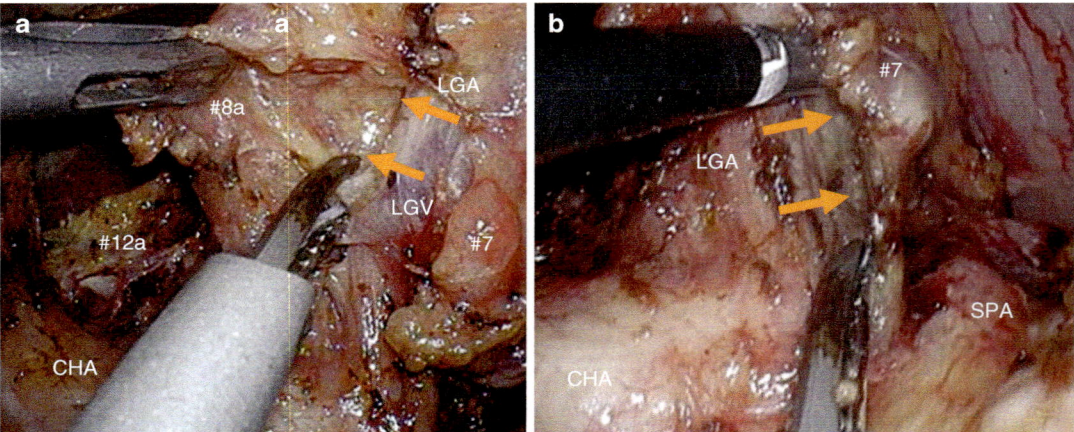

Fig. 10.15 Medial approach: (**a**) the outermost layer along the right aspect of LGA, (**b**) the outermost layer along the left aspect of LGA

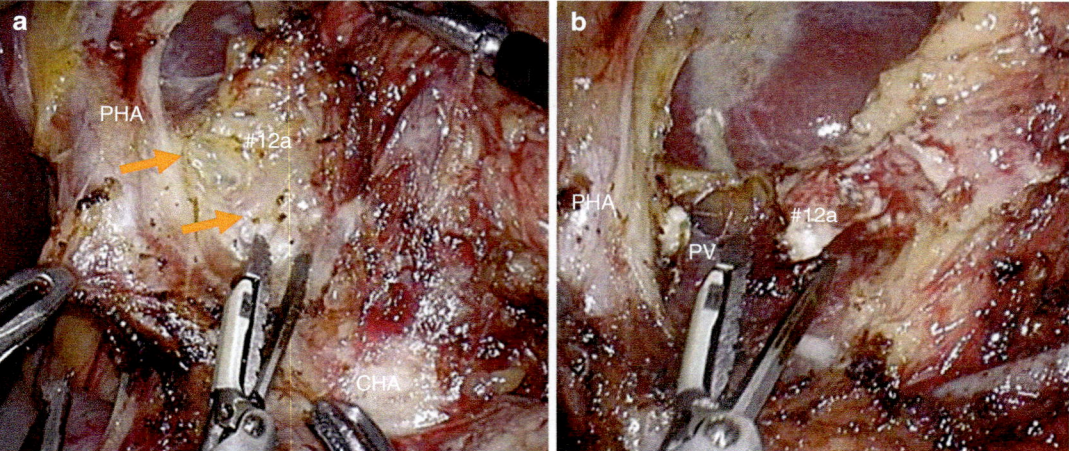

Fig. 10.16 #12a dissection: (**a**) creation of the good surgical field by pulling the nerves along PHA and CHA, arrow: outermost layer, (**b**) safe dissection on #12 along the superficialized PV

ing to sufficient mobilization of the target. Then, the lymphatic connection between the target fat tissue and #16a2-inter is divided and is dissected along the right diaphragmatic crus (Fig. 10.17). The left gastric vein (LGV) is transected on the way (Fig. 10.18a).

#7 Dissection
The origin of LGA is exposed and divided by clips (Fig. 10.18b).

#11p Dissection
The massive area of the target fat tissue bearing suprapancreatic lymph nodes is retracted laterally to the patient's left by the assistant surgeon. #11p lymph nodes are freed from the subretroperitoneal (Gerota's) fascia, delineating the dorsal

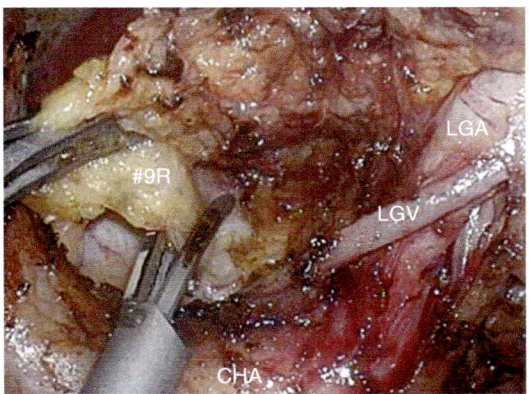

Fig. 10.17 #9(R) dissection: division of the lymphatic connection between #9(R) and #16a2-inter

aspect of #11p (Fig. 10.19a). The lateral aspect of the targeted fat tissue is dissected along the outermost layer of SPA (Fig. 10.19b). To obtain a good surgical view around the dorsal area of SPA, the assistant surgeon laterodorsally retracts the thick nerve fibers along the cranial aspect of SPA (Fig. 10.19b), and the operating surgeon pulls the target ventrally. Thus, SPV is superficialized and the bottom of #11p is dissected on the splenic vein (SPV) safely (Fig. 10.19c). #11p dissection is sometimes more easily conducted when it is done right after #4sb dissection.

#9(L) Dissection
The fat tissue containing #11p and 9(L) is lifted, and the lymphatic connection between #9(L) and 16a2-lat is divided (Fig. 10.20).

#1 and 3 Dissection
The adipose tissue bearing #1 and 3 is lifted by the assistant surgeon's right hand and the operating surgeon's left hand (Fig. 10.21a). The other hand of the assistant surgeon retracts the posterior aspect of the stomach dorsally (Fig. 10.21a). Using this surgical field, #1 and 3 are dissected in the caudocranial direction (Fig. 10.21b).

Transection of the Stomach
The stomach is transected from the greater to the lesser curvature on the line between the prefinal branch of LGEA and final ascending branch of LGA irrespective of the location of the tumor (Fig. 10.22).

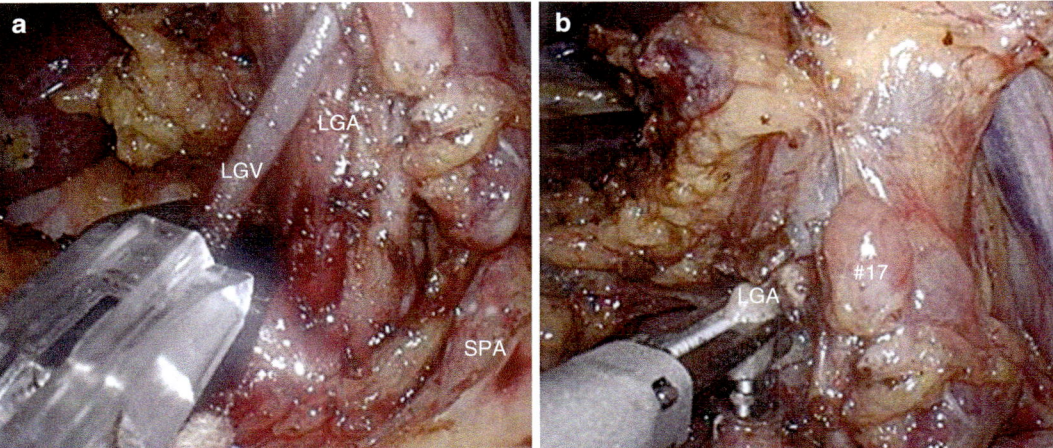

Fig. 10.18 #7 dissection: (**a**) transection of LGV, (**b**) transection of LGA

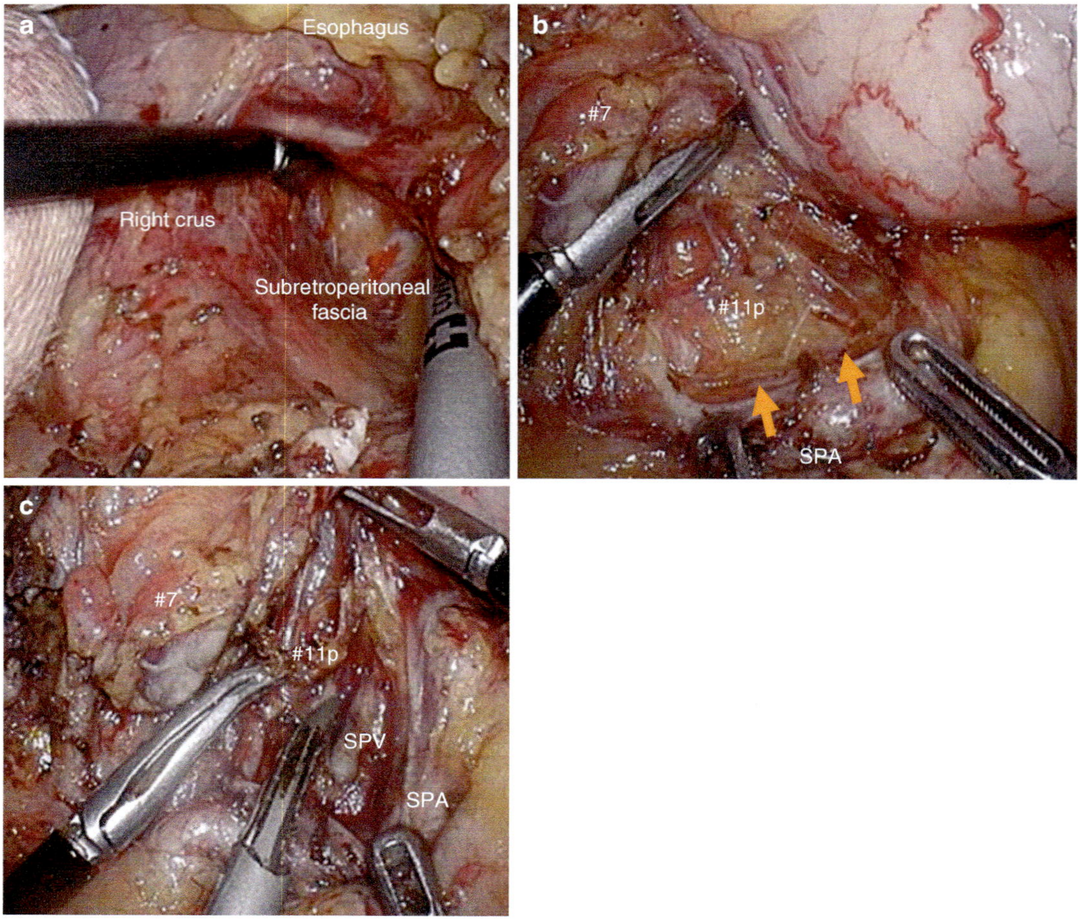

Fig. 10.19 #11p dissection: (**a**) mobilization of the dorsal aspect of #11p on the subretroperitoneal fascia, (**b**) dissection of the lateral aspect of #11p along the outermost layer of SPA, (**c**) dissection of the bottom of #11p on the superficialized SPV

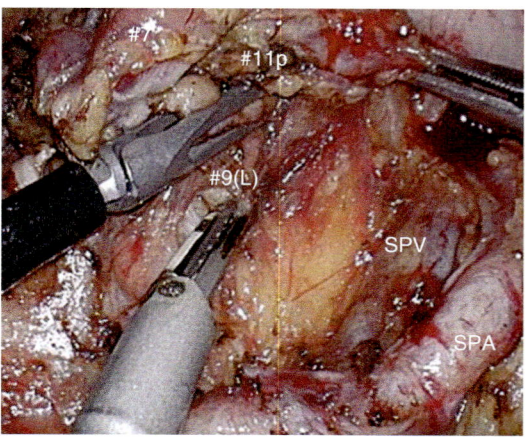

Fig. 10.20 #9(L) dissection

Results

According to our previous publication [8], operative time, blood loss, and the number of dissected lymph nodes were 354 (182–634) min, 34 (0–702) ml, and 40 (0–108), respectively. The morbidity and the incidence of pancreatic fistula were 6.7% and 2.5%, respectively. There has been no conversion to open procedure so far. The reoperation rate and mortality were both 0.6%. The duration of postoperative hospital stay was 14 (8–69) days.

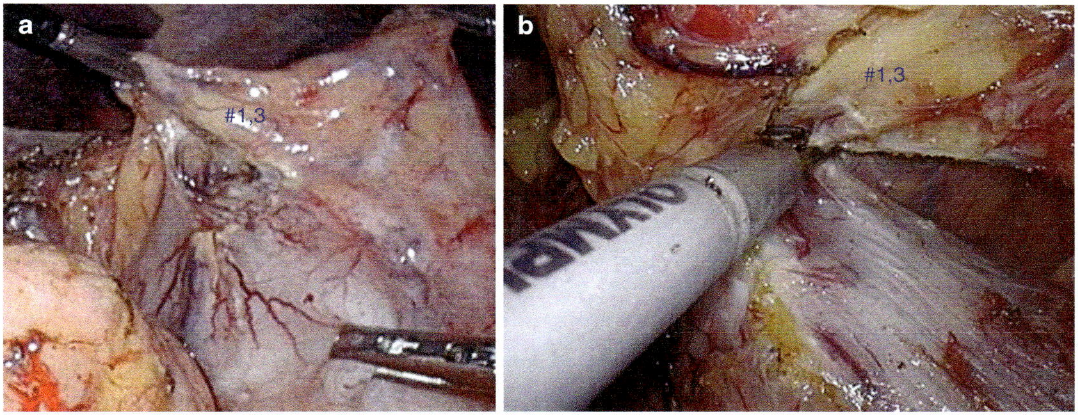

Fig. 10.21 #1 and 3 dissection: (**a**) surgical field for #1 and 3 dissection, (**b**) caudocranial dissection of #1 and 3 along the lesser curvature of the stomach

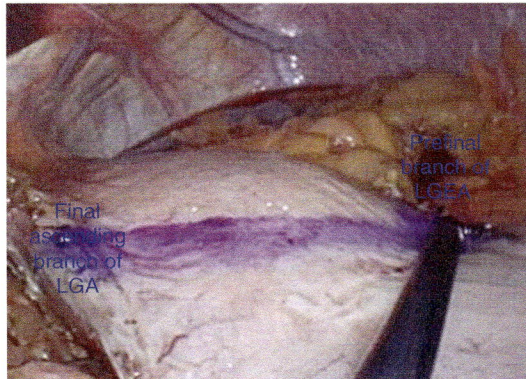

Fig. 10.22 Transection of the stomach

Discussion

Laparoscopic gastrectomy has been increasingly performed as a minimally invasive surgical approach that provides significant advantages for short-term outcomes as opposed to open surgical procedures for the early gastric cancer patients [13]. However, laparoscopic gastrectomy for advanced gastric cancer remains controversial because of its technical difficulties and lack of long-term results [1, 7–9, 13]. We have been demonstrated that use of laparoscopic approach, compared with open approach, not only for early but also for advanced gastric cancer, extended operative time, reduced blood loss and did not increase morbidity including pancreatic fistula

[7]. Moreover, no significant difference was observed in terms of long-term outcomes [7]. Thus, at our institute, laparoscopic D2 gastrectomy has been the standard type of operation for both early and advanced gastric cancer.

From the operating surgeon's point of view, to overcome the laparoscopic limited range of motion enjoying the high quality of laparoscopically magnified image, we believe mediolateral and/or caudocranial dissection must be the most important. Based on this philosophy, the XYZ-axis theory was established extending the outermost layer-oriented medial approach [10, 11]. Using this theory, the outermost layer could possibly be detected at any junction of three arteries, leading to smoother and more reproducible lymph node dissection.

There is no doubt that #11p and 12a dissection is the key to successful D2 distal gastrectomy. From the assistant surgeon's perspective, skillful laterodorsal retraction of the autonomic nerves along SPA, CHA, and PHA allows SPV and PV to come up closer to the suprapancreatic border, resulting in pancreas-protective safe D2 dissection.

Conclusions

It has been clearly shown that laparoscopic gastrectomy has considerable short-term benefits over open approach, even though further investigation would be required to demonstrate oncological safety of laparoscopic gastrectomy especially for advanced gastric cancer [1, 7, 13]. The principles and methods for totally laparoscopic gastrectomy based on our experience demonstrated in this article may help upper GI surgeons overcome technical difficulties in laparoscopic D2 gastrectomy.

Disclosures This work was not supported by any grants and fundings. No author has commercial association with or financial involvement that might pose a conflict of interest in connection with the submitted article.

References

1. Uyama I, Suda K, Satoh S. Laparoscopic surgery for advanced gastric cancer: current status and future perspectives. J Gastric Cancer. 2013;13:19–25.
2. Crew KD, Neugut AI. Epidemiology of gastric cancer. World J Gastroenterol. 2006;12:354–62.
3. Dikken JL, van de Velde CJ, Coit DG, Shah MA, Verheij M, Cats A. Treatment of resectable gastric cancer. Therap Adv Gastroenterol. 2012;5:49–69.
4. Uyama I, Sugioka A, Fujita J, Komori Y, Matsui H, Hasumi A. Laparoscopic total gastrectomy with distal pancreatosplenectomy and D2 lymphadenectomy for advanced gastric cancer. Gastric Cancer. 1999;2:230–4.
5. Uyama I, Sugioka A, Matsui H, Fujita J, Komori Y, Hasumi A. Laparoscopic D2 lymph node dissection for advanced gastric cancer located in the middle or lower third portion of the stomach. Gastric Cancer. 2000;3:50–5.
6. Japanese Gastric Cancer Association. Japanese classification of gastric carcinoma: 3rd English edition. Gastric Cancer. 2011;14:101–12.
7. Shinohara T, Satoh S, Kanaya S, Ishida Y, Taniguchi K, Isogaki J, Inaba K, Yanaga K, Uyama I. Laparoscopic versus open D2 gastrectomy for advanced gastric cancer: a retrospective cohort study. Surg Endosc. 2013;27:286–94.
8. Suda K, Man-I M, Ishida Y, Kawamura Y, Satoh S, Uyama I. Potential advantages of robotic radical gastrectomy for gastric adenocarcinoma in comparison with conventional laparoscopic approach: a single institutional retrospective comparative cohort study. Surg Endosc. 2015;29:673–85.
9. Japanese Gastric Cancer Association. JGCA gastric cancer treatment guidelines 2014 (ver. 4). Tokyo: Kanehara; 2014.
10. Kanaya S, Haruta S, Kawamura Y, Yoshimura F, Inaba K, Hiramatsu Y, Ishida Y, Taniguchi K, Isogaki J, Uyama I. Video: laparoscopy distinctive technique for suprapancreatic lymph node dissection: medial approach for laparoscopic gastric cancer surgery. Surg Endosc. 2011;25:3928–9.
11. Uyama I, Kanaya S, Ishida Y, Inaba K, Suda K, Satoh S. Novel integrated robotic approach for suprapancreatic D2 nodal dissection for treating gastric cancer: technique and initial experience. World J Surg. 2012;36:331–7.
12. Shinohara T, Kanaya S, Taniguchi K, Fujita T, Yanaga K, Uyama I. Laparoscopic total gastrectomy with D2 lymph node dissection for gastric cancer. Arch Surg. 2009;144:1138–42.
13. Nakauchi M, Suda K, Kadoya S, Inaba K, Ishida Y, Uyama I. Technical aspects and short- and long-term outcomes of totally laparoscopic total gastrectomy for advanced gastric cancer: a single-institution retrospective study. Surg Endosc. 2016;30(10): 4632–9. https://doi.org/10.1007/s00464-015-4726-4. Epub 2015 Dec 24.

Laparoscopic Surgery for Gastric Cancer, Total Gastrectomy with D2 Lymph Node Dissection

11

Yoo Min Kim and Woo Jin Hyung

Introduction

For advanced gastric cancer located in the upper body of the stomach, total gastrectomy with D2 lymph node dissection is recommended [1–4]. D2 lymph node dissection for proximal tumors requires the retrieval of the soft tissues around distal portions of the splenic vessels and splenic hilum, which contain lymph nodes at stations #10 and #11d [4, 5]. Two options – a total gastrectomy with splenectomy and a spleen-preserving total gastrectomy – exist for retrieval of lymph nodes at station #10. While splenectomy-related postoperative complications, such as subphrenic abscess and postsplenectomy syndrome, are well known, complete lymph node dissection of the splenic hilum during spleen-preserving total gastrectomy is a very complex procedure.

Currently, most surgeons only offer laparoscopic treatment of gastric cancer for early gastric cancer (cT1); splenectomy or spleen-preserving

hilar lymph node dissection is not recommended in laparoscopic gastric cancer surgery. Thus, spleen-preserving hilar lymph node dissection has not been mostly attempted in laparoscopic surgery procedures [6–8]. However, for the application of the laparoscopic gastrectomy for cT2 or more advanced lesions especially located greater curvature of the upper stomach, lymph node dissection of station 10 and station 11d should be performed during total gastrectomy for D2 lymph node dissection [9–12]. Laparoscopic total gastrectomy is considered technically more difficult than its distal gastrectomy counterpart and, therefore, less widely practiced [13–16].

Herein, we present the principles and detailed procedure of totally laparoscopic spleen-preserving total gastrectomy with D2 lymph node dissection.

Electronic Supplementary Material The online version of this chapter (https://doi.org/10.1007/978-3-662-45583-8_11) contains supplementary material, which is available to authorized users.

Y. M. Kim
Department of Surgery, CHA Bundang Medical Center, CHA University, Gyeonggi-do, Republic of Korea

W. J. Hyung (✉)
Department of Surgery, Yonsei University College of Medicine, Seoul, Republic of Korea
e-mail: wjhyung@yuhs.ac

Setup

Indications for Laparoscopic Total Gastrectomy with D2 Lymph Node Dissection

The preoperative diagnosis is made according to the findings of upper endoscopy with endoscopic ultrasound and abdominopelvic computed tomography. Unless patients have lesions suitable for endoscopic mucosal resection, patients with a preoperative diagnosis of T1 or T2 gastric cancers without evidence of lymph node metastasis in the extra-perigastric (N2) area by UICC and JGCA classification are candidates for laparoscopic surgery. The indication for the laparoscopic spleen-preserving splenic hilar lymph node dissection is gastric cancer in the upper body of the stomach with a high probability of deep submucosa (SM3) or proper muscle invasion without evidence of gross lymph node metastasis along splenic artery or splenic hilar area through preoperative evaluation.

OR Setup

The surgeon and scopist stand on the patient's right side, and an assistant surgeon and scrub nurse are on the patient's left side.

Alternatively, the scopist stands between the patient's legs if the patient lay on the table with legs apart.

Patient's Position

Basically, the patient is placed in a supine position, both arms extended, and 15-degree reverse Trendelenburg position, head-up tilt. The arms (right angle or alongside the body), legs (gathered or apart), and reverse Trendelenburg (10-degree ~ 30-degree tilt) positions are decided with surgeon's preference.

Port Placement

The camera is first inserted through the infraumbilical port, after which the other trocars are inserted under direct vision with laparoscope (Fig. 11.1).

- *Camera port*: 10–12 mm, midline below the umbilicus (Umbilicus or supraumbilicus is to the surgeon's preference.)
- *Right subcostal port*: 5 mm, one finger caudally from the right subcostal line, on top of the pylorus, adjusted to the surgeon's comfort for grasping and pulling over adipose tissue around celiac and splenic vessels

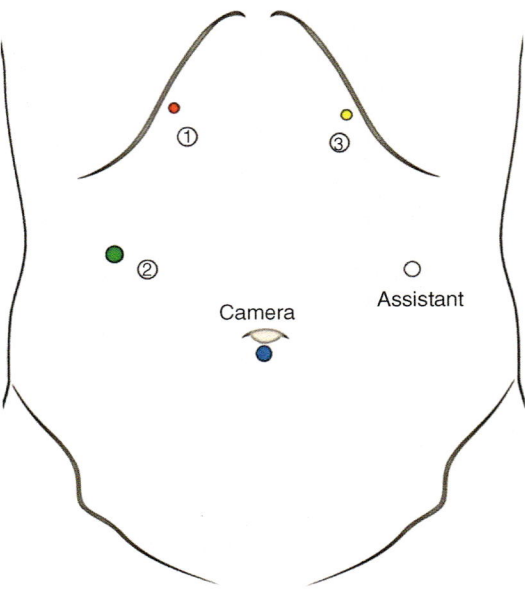

Fig. 11.1 Trocar arrangement in laparoscopic total gastrectomy. "1", red–Right subcostal port (5 mm); "2", green–Right lower port (main working, 5–12 mm); "3", yellow–Left subcostal port (5 mm); "assistant", white–Left lower port (assistant port, 6–12 mm); "camera", blue–camera port (10–12 mm)

- *Right lower port (main working)*: 5–12 mm, laterally from the right subcostal port, midline between the camera port and the right subcostal port, at the level of the head of the pancreas, to approach the splenic vessels superior to the pancreas with ultrasonic shears
- Note: This port can be inserted more medially in obese patient and laterally in patient with small abdominal cavity for a comfortable approach to the splenic hilum with laparoscopic instruments.
- *Left subcostal port*: 5 mm, one finger caudally from the left subcostal line, on top of the angle or midportion of the lesser curvature under laparoscope, inserted slightly caudally compared to the right subcostal port
- *Left lower port*: 5–12 mm, laterally from the left subcostal port, midline between the camera port and left subcostal port, at the level of greater curvature, to reach the greater curvature of the stomach for placing the endo-linear stapler

Liver Retraction

After trocar insertion is complete, the liver retraction is performed because it allows essential for clear visualization of the lesser curvature area and allows the assistant right hand to be free for dynamic use. For static retraction, we perform a liver suspension method, utilizing a suture and a gauze pad as a "sling" [17].

Details of D2 Dissection in Total Gastrectomy

Omentectomy

After establishment of pneumoperitoneum and trocar placement, the operation starts for omentectomy. A partial omentectomy divides and dissects the greater omentum at 4–5 cm from the greater curvature for the preservation of omentum. A total omentectomy divides the greater omentum from the transverse colon using ultrasonic shears from the mid-transverse colon toward the lower pole of the spleen. The assistant retracts the omentum toward the head with the right hand and pulls downward on the teniae coli of the transverse colon with atraumatic graspers in the left hand. It is important that no injury is made to the transverse colon when dissecting the attachment of the posterior greater omentum to the transverse colon (Fig. 11.2).

#4sb Dissection #4sa Dissection

The left gastroepiploic artery and left gastroepiploic vein are divided at the root for removal of splenic hilar lymph nodes. After division of the left gastroepiploic vessels at their roots, the gastrosplenic ligament is separated up to the left side of the esophageal hiatus by dividing the short gastric vessels from the surface of the spleen to dissect lymph nodes at #4sa around the short gastric vessels and to mobilize the upper part of the greater curvature of the stomach. For this procedure, the operating table is tilted left side up for better exposure of the gastrosplenic ligament and splenic hilar area using gravity. Because of the limitation in the number of instruments in laparoscopic surgery unlike open surgery, traction using gravity is important. To better expose the spleen and splenic hilar area during division of the gastrosplenic ligament, the posterior attachment of the spleen is not mobilized to keep it suspended within the splenic fossa against gravity as the dissection proceeds.

#11d and #10 Dissection

After fully exposing the splenic hilar area for the removal of the lymph nodes at #10 and #11d, the tail of the pancreas is retracted caudally with the left hand of the assistant, and the posterior wall of the upper stomach is pushed upward with the assistant's right hand. The splenic vessels are exposed at the junction between the stations #11p and #11d lymph nodes, and the dissection

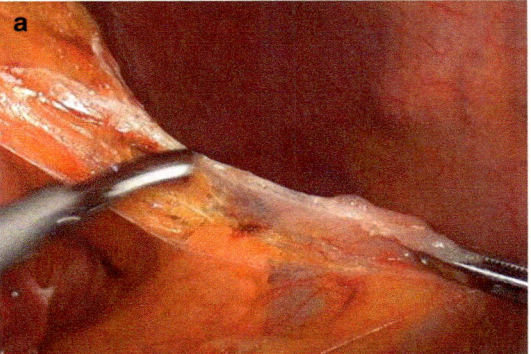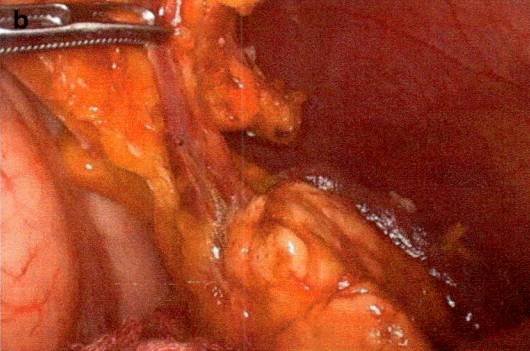

Fig. 11.2 Total omentectomy (**a**) and isolation of the left gastroepiploic vessels (**b**)

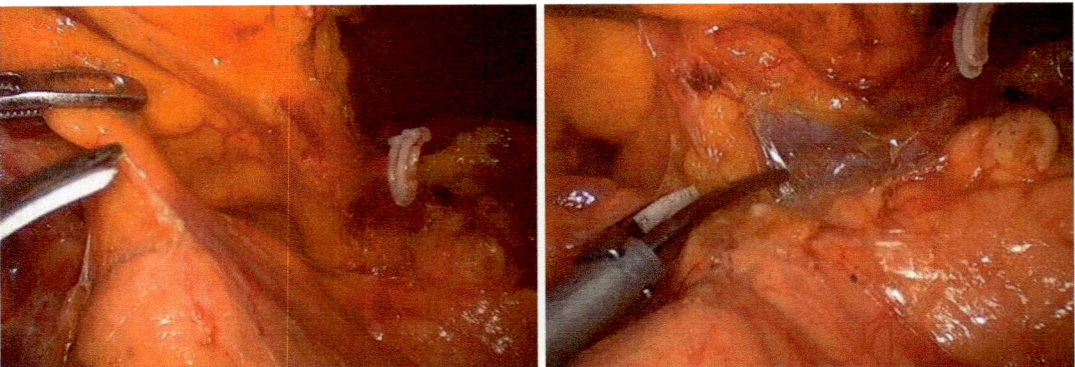

Fig. 11.3 Splenic vessel exposure at the junction between #11p and #11d

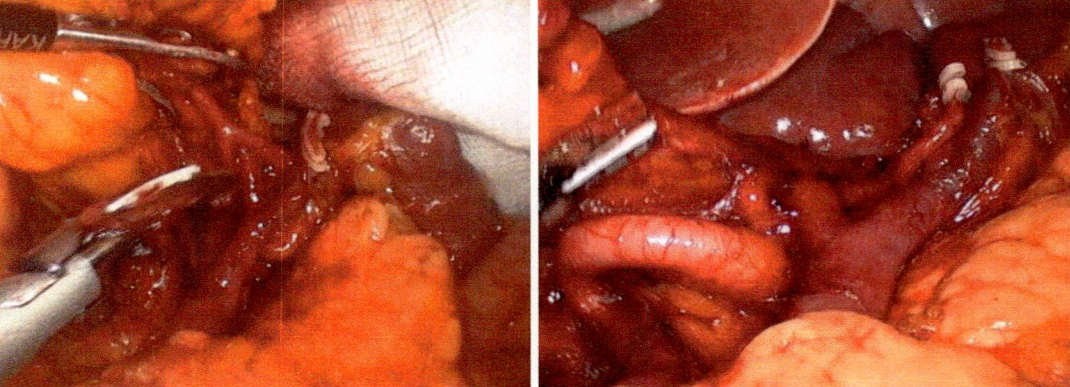

Fig. 11.4 Skeletonization of the splenic vessels from the distal of the posterior gastric vessels to the splenic hilar area

of station #11d lymph nodes starts there from the splenic vessels and then continues to the splenic hilum. By skeletonizing the splenic vessels from the posterior gastric vessels to the splenic hilar area, removal of the #11d and #10 lymph nodes bearing soft tissues is achieved, and all vessels in the splenic hilum are saved with preservation of the spleen. For a safe procedure, surgeon should take into account the splenic vascular anatomy preoperatively (Figs. 11.3, 11.4).

#2 Dissection

The retroperitoneal attachment of the posterior wall of the upper stomach is detached up to the diaphragmatic cruses, and the esophagocardiac branch of the left inferior phrenic artery is divided at its origin to enable dissection of the station 2 lymph nodes.

#4d and #6 Dissection and Duodenal Transection

After completing the operative procedure of the left side, the operating table is repositioned in neutral position. Then, the division of the greater omentum is continued distally toward the pylorus, and the right gastroepiploic vessels are divided at their roots. Soft tissues attached to the duodenum and head of the pancreas are dissected. The supra-duodenal vessels are ligated with ultrasonic shears, and the duodenum is transected 2 cm distal to the pylorus using an endoscopic linear stapler.

Suprapancreatic Dissection (#5, #12a, #8, #7, #9, #1, and #11p)

After duodenal transection, the right gastric artery is exposed and divided at its origin. After dissection along the gastroduodenal and proper hepatic artery and ligation of right gastric artery, soft tissues at the medial side of the portal vein are dissected. The pedicle of the left gastric artery and vein is carefully lifted with the assistant's right hand, and the pancreas is moved downward with gauze in the assistant's left hand. The gastropancreatic ligament is divided using ultrasonic shear, and the common hepatic artery is exposed. The soft tissues at the anterior part of the common hepatic artery and right side of the celiac artery are cleared, and the left gastric vein is exposed and divided at its draining point to the portal vein or splenic vein. The soft tissues above the upper edge of the pancreas are completely removed. The left gastric artery is then exposed and ligated at the root, while the lymph nodes are dissected around the celiac axis area. The stomach is freed from the retroperitoneal attachment up to the right diaphragmatic crus. The dissection is continued from the splenic vessels' origin toward the pancreatic tail to expose the proximal half of the splenic artery.

Distal Esophagus Transection

After the posterior surface of the upper stomach is separated from the retroperitoneum, the abdominal esophagus is mobilized by dividing the phrenoesophageal membrane and vagus nerves. The distal esophagus and the whole stomach are fully freed and transected with endolinear stapler.

Reconstruction and Specimen Retrieval

The stomach is packed within an endo-bag and placed in the right abdominal cavity. After laparoscopic total gastrectomy, bowel continuity is restored by Roux-en-Y esophagojejunostomy. There are several reconstruction methods: intracorporeally or extracorporeally, creating a side-to-side esophagojejunostomy with linear stapler or an end-to-side esophagojejunostomy with circular stapler. A jejunojenostomy is made at 45 cm distal to the esophagojejunostomy.

To determine the reconstruction method, the patient's condition, the location of tumor, the resection margins, and the surgeon's preference are considered. After reconstruction, the camera port site is extended to the lower abdominal wall about 2–3 cm, and the specimen is retrieved through the minilaparotomy site. The minilaparotomy is closed with interrupted 1-0 polydioxanone sutures. The trocar sites are closed with 2-0 polydioxanone sutures. The subcutis and cutis are restored with interrupted 3-0 polydioxanone sutures and skin staples.

Splenectomy for #10 Dissection

The complete clearance of splenic hilar lymph nodes by splenectomy should be considered for potentially curable T2–T4 tumors with invasion into the greater curvature of the upper stomach or into the spleen directly, even though splenectomy is not routinely performed during total gastrectomy for advanced gastric cancer on the upper stomach.

The gastrocolic ligament is first divided up to the spleen using ultrasonic shears or electrocautery. The splenocolic ligament is divided and lower pole of the spleen is mobilized. The splenophrenic and splenorenal ligament are divided up to the upper pole of the spleen to mobilize the spleen from the retroperitoneum. The splenectomy and dissection of the station #11d lymph nodes are performed after the mobilization of the lower stomach with lymph node dissection and esophageal transection. The upper body of the stomach is retracted downward and caudally after distal esophagus transection. The esophagocardiac branch of the left inferior phrenic artery is ligated at its origin for lymph node dissection at station 2. The #11d lymph node dissection is performed from the proximal part of splenic vessels to the splenic hilum. The splenic artery is skeletonized and ligated just distal to the bifurcation of the caudal pancreatic artery; the splenic vein is also skeletonized and ligated distal to the pancreatic tail to avoid pancreatic fistula. After skeletonization of splenic vessels, the splenic artery and vein are ligated with clips or vascular stapler.

Disclosures This work was not supported by external or grant funding. None of the authors have commercial associations or financial involvement that pose a conflict of interest in connection with the submitted article.

References

1. Degiuli M, Sasako M, Ponti A, et al. Randomized clinical trial comparing survival after D1 or D2 gastrectomy for gastric cancer. Br J Surg. 2014;101:23–31.
2. Songun I, Putter H, Kranenbarg EM, et al. Surgical treatment of gastric cancer: 15-year follow-up results of the randomised nationwide Dutch D1D2 trial. Lancet Oncol. 2010;11:439–49.
3. Sasako M, Sano T, Yamamoto S, et al. D2 lymphadenectomy alone or with para-aortic nodal dissection for gastric cancer. N Engl J Med. 2008;359:453–62.
4. Japanese Gastric Cancer Association. Japanese gastric cancer treatment guidelines 2014 (ver. 4). Gastric Cancer. 2017;20(1):1–19.
5. Japanese Gastric Cancer Association. Japanese classification of gastric carcinoma: 3rd English edition. Gastric Cancer. 2011;14:101–12.
6. Katai H, Yoshimura K, Fukagawa T, Sano T, Sasako M. Risk factors for pancreas-related abscess after total gastrectomy. Gastric Cancer. 2005;8(3):137–41.
7. Yoshino K, Yamada Y, Asanuma F, Aizawa K. Splenectomy in cancer gastrectomy: recommendation of spleen-preserving for early stages. Int Surg. 1997;82(2):150–4.
8. Maruyama K, Sasako M, Kinoshita T, Sano T, Katai H, Okajima K. Pancreas-preserving total gastrectomy for proximal gastric cancer. World J Surg. 1995;19(4):532–6.
9. Aikou T, Shimazu H, Takao T, et al. Significance of lymph nodal metastases in treatment of esophagogastric adenocarcinoma. Lymphology. 1992;25:31–6.
10. Maruyama K, Gunven P, Okabayashi K, et al. Lymph node metastases of gastric cancer. General pattern in 1931 patients. Ann Surg. 1989;210:596–602.
11. Mönig SP, Collet PH, Baldus SE, Schmackpfeffer K, Schröder W, Thiele J, Dienes HP, Hölscher AH. Splenectomy in proximal gastric cancer: frequency of lymph node metastasis to the splenic hilus. J Surg Oncol. 2001;76(2):89–92.
12. Ikeguchi M, Kaibara N. Lymph node metastasis at the splenic hilum in proximal gastric cancer. Am Surg. 2004;70(7):645–8.
13. Hyung WJ, Lim JS, Song J, Choi SH, Noh SH. Laparoscopic spleen-preserving splenic hilar lymph node dissection during total gastrectomy for gastric cancer. J Am Coll Surg. 2008;207(2):e6–11.
14. Shinohara T, Kanaya S, Taniguchi K, et al. Laparoscopic total gastrectomy with D2 lymph node dissection for gastric cancer. Arch Surg. 2009;144:1138–42.
15. Jia-Bin W, Chang-Ming H, Chao-Hui Z, Ping L, Jian-Wei X, Jian-Xian L. Laparoscopic spleen-preserving No. 10 lymph node dissection for advanced proximal gastric cancer in left approach: a new operation procedure. World J Surg Oncol. 2012;10:241.
16. Okabe H, Obama K, Kan T, Tanaka E, Itami A, Sakai Y. Medial approach for laparoscopic total gastrectomy with splenic lymph node dissection. J Am Coll Surg. 2010;211:e1–6.
17. Woo Y, Hyung WJ, Kim HI, Obama K, Son T, Noh SH. Minimizing hepatic trauma with a novel liver retraction method: a simple liver suspension using gauze suture. Surg Endosc. 2011;25(12):3939–45. https://doi.org/10.1007/s00464-011-1788-9.

Intracorporeal Reconstruction in Laparoscopic Gastrectomy

12

Hisahiro Hosogi, Yoshiharu Sakai, and Seiichiro Kanaya

Introduction

Since the introduction of laparoscopy-assisted distal gastrectomy (LADG) as a treatment for gastric cancer in the 1990s, the number of patients undergoing laparoscopic gastrectomy is rapidly increasing, particularly in eastern Asia [1, 2]. Initially, reconstruction was performed through a minilaparotomy after gastrectomy had been completed laparoscopically [3]. Laparoscopy-assisted gastrectomy provides several benefits including less blood loss, better cosmesis, and earlier recovery when compared with open gastrectomy [4]. However, the minilaparotomy required for an extracorporeal reconstruction decreases the advantages of the minimally invasive approach, especially in obese patients that need extension of the laparotomy to obtain a better view. To solve these problems, intracorporeal anastomosis techniques have been developed [5, 6], and a completely laparoscopic gastrectomy has become widespread not only in laparoscopic distal gastrectomy (LDG) but also in laparoscopic total gastrectomy (LTG) [7–10]. Recent studies of gastrectomy with intracorporeal anastomosis have reported acceptable surgical outcomes [7, 8, 11–13]. However, some technical pitfalls need to be understood, and adequate surgical skills should be acquired to ensure patient safety. In this chapter, common procedures of intracorporeal reconstruction in LDG and LTG with endoscopic linear staples are introduced, and reconstruction-related short-term results in our institution are reported.

Electronic Supplementary Material The online version of this chapter (https://doi.org/10.1007/978-3-662-45583-8_12) contains supplementary material, which is available to authorized users.

H. Hosogi (✉)
Department of Surgery, Graduate School of Medicine, Kyoto University, Kyoto, Japan

Department of Surgery, Osaka Red Cross Hospital, Osaka, Japan
e-mail: hisahoso@kuhp.kyoto-u.ac.jp

Y. Sakai
Department of Surgery, Graduate School of Medicine, Kyoto University, Kyoto, Japan
e-mail: ysakai@kuhp.kyoto-u.ac.jp

S. Kanaya
Department of Surgery, Osaka Red Cross Hospital, Osaka, Japan
e-mail: skanaya@osaka-med.jrc.or.jp

Materials and Methods

Patients

The records of 427 consecutive patients who underwent LDG or LTG for histologically proven adenocarcinoma of the stomach between April 2011 and March 2015 were retrieved from a prospective institutional database in the Osaka Red Cross Hospital. LDG was performed for 301 patients and LTG for

126 patients. Reconstruction-related short-term surgical outcomes were retrospectively investigated. Tumor stage was classified according to the seventh edition of TNM classification [14]. Postoperative complications, which occurred within 30 days after the operation, were classified according to the Clavien-Dindo classification system [15].

Operative Technique

The detailed procedure was described previously [6, 8, 16–18]. In all of the following reconstructive procedures, the surgeon stood on the right side of the patient. Endoscopic linear staplers were used in all the reconstructive procedures.

Reconstruction in LDG

For reconstruction in LDG, a delta-shaped anastomosis was the first choice when R0 resection was possible, with routine resection of two-thirds of the stomach [19]. The exception was patients with a hiatal hernia. Billroth II or Roux-en-Y reconstruction was performed when the extent of LDG resulted in a small remnant stomach due to the tumor location or when the duodenal bulb had to be resected due to tumor invasion. Billroth-II reconstruction was selected in elderly patients over 75 years of age, and the Roux-en-Y reconstruction was selected in younger patients or in those with a hiatal hernia.

(a) Delta-shaped anastomosis in Billroth-I reconstruction (Fig. 12.1 and Video 12.1).

After mobilization of the first portion of the duodenum, a linear stapler was introduced through the left lower trocar, and the duodenal bulb was transected in the ventro-dorsal (posterior-to-anterior) direction, not the usual craniocaudal (greater curvature to lesser curvature) direction (Fig. 12.1a). The blood supply to the anastomosis was thus preserved. After checking if an anastomosis was possible without undue tension, small enterotomies were created along the greater curvature of the remnant stomach and the posterior side of the duodenal stump. Supraduodenal arteries around the duodenal

stump were dissected, and a 2 cm length from the edge was devascularized in preparation for stapling. A 45-mm endoscopic linear stapler was applied through the left lower trocar, with one fork in each hole. The posterior wall of the stomach and that of the duodenum was apposed, and the stapler was fired (Fig. 12.1b). A V-shaped anastomosis was thus made along the posterior wall. After checking hemostasis of the staple line, the common enterotomy was closed temporarily with hernia staplers, and the anastomosis completed with one or two applications of a linear stapler (Fig. 12.1c).

(b) Gastrojejunostomy in Billroth-II reconstruction (Fig. 12.2 and Video 12.2).

The duodenal stump was reinforced with intracorporeal seromuscular suturing with extracorporeal Roeder's knots. Enterotomies were created on the greater curvature of the remnant stomach and the antimesenteric side of the jejunum located 25 cm distal to the ligament of Treitz. A 45-mm endoscopic linear stapler was applied through the right lower trocar. We routinely performed antecolic antiperistaltic gastrojejunostomy. The entry-hole closure with another stapler was not a painstaking task because the enterotomy for insertion of the stapler was made on the afferent loop, and the stoma size of the efferent loop was unaffected by the closure. Because a Braun anastomosis was not created, some sutures were added between the jejunal wall on the afferent loop and the staple line on the lesser curvature of the remnant stomach. This was done to help with food passage directly into the efferent loop.

(c) Gastrojejunostomy in Roux-en-Y reconstruction (Fig. 12.3 and Video 12.3).

Both antiperistaltic (functional end-to-end anastomosis) and isoperistaltic gastrojejunostomies have been reported [7, 9]. We prefer an antecolic, isoperistaltic gastrojejunostomy. Prior to the gastrojejunostomy, a jejunojejunostomy was made extracorporeally in the extended umbilical wound (Video 12.4). For intracorporeal gastrojejunostomy, a small enterotomy in the jejunal limb was

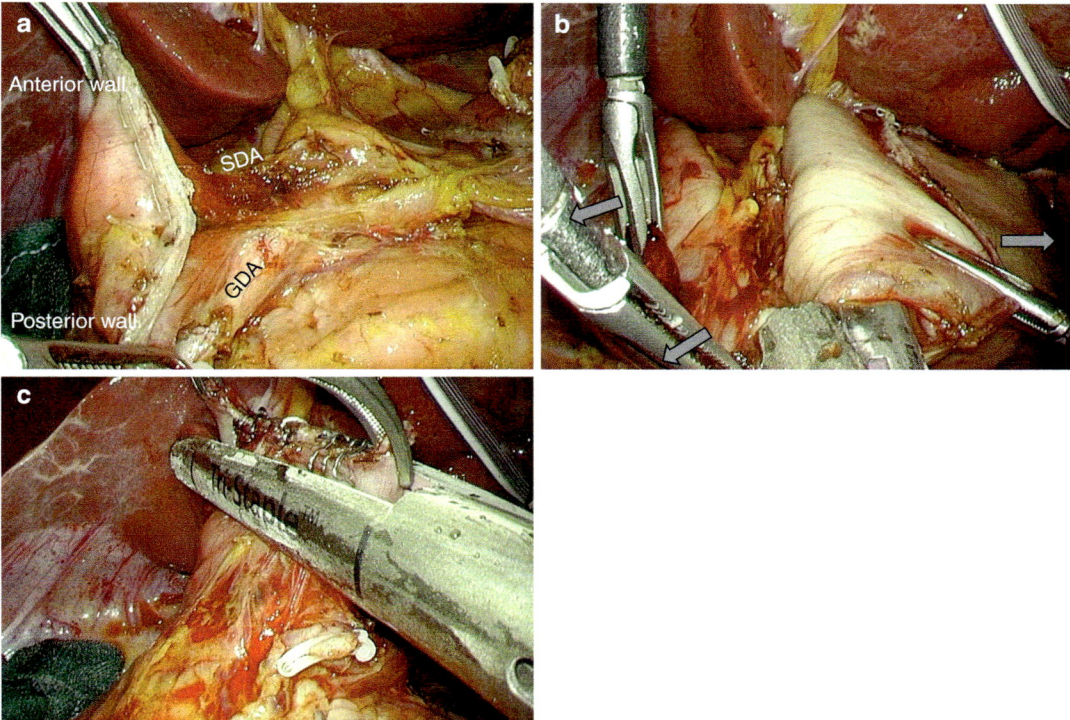

Fig. 12.1 Delta-shaped anastomosis in a Billroth-I reconstruction. (**a**) View after duodenal transection. Note that the duodenum was transected in the ventro-dorsal (posterior-to-anterior) direction, not the craniocaudal (greater curvature to lesser curvature) direction. The anterior and posterior walls are shown. SDA, supraduodenal artery; GDA, gastroduodenal artery. (**b**) First stapling in the delta-shaped anastomosis. A 45-mm stapler was applied through the left lower trocar. The posterior wall of the stomach and that of the duodenum were put together. Traction in the lateral direction by the surgeon and the assistant are important (boxed gray arrows). (**c**) Closing the common enterotomy with a stapler applied through the left lower trocar. The surgeon sets the transection line parallel to the axis of the stapler

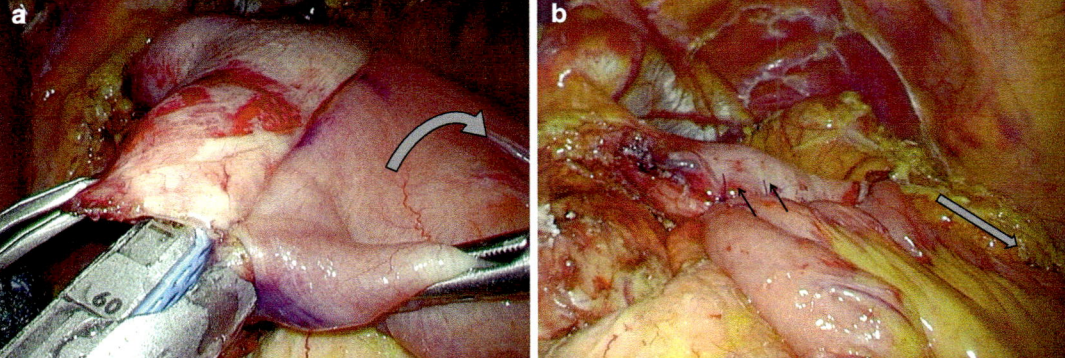

Fig. 12.2 Gastrojejunostomy in a Billroth-II reconstruction. (**a**) Antiperistaltic gastrojejunostomy. A 45-mm stapler was inserted through the right lower trocar. The efferent loop of the jejunum is shown by a boxed gray arrow. (**b**) Completion of a Billroth-II anastomosis. Sutures (dashed arrows) between the afferent loop of the jejunum and the remnant stomach make orientation into the efferent loop a straight line (boxed gray arrow)

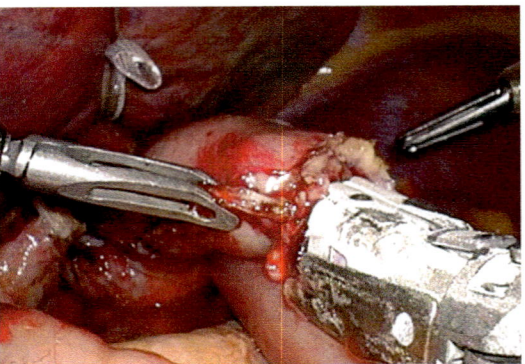

Fig. 12.3 Gastrojejunostomy in a Roux-en-Y reconstruction. First stapling in an isoperistaltic gastrojejunostomy. A 45-mm stapler was applied through the left lower trocar. Note that the anastomosis was made with the posterior wall of the remnant stomach

created on the antimesenteric side 45 mm from the edge, and the anastomosis was made on the posterior wall of the remnant stomach using a 45-mm stapler applied from the left lower trocar. This was done to prevent gastric stasis by avoiding a twist of the jejunal mesentery. During enterotomy closure with a linear stapler, care must be taken not to resect too much of the jejunal wall, which could potentially cause an anastomotic stricture. Petersen's defect was always closed with nonabsorbable sutures to prevent an internal hernia.

Reconstruction in LTG

The esophagus was transected in the right-to-left direction by a linear stapler inserted in the right lower trocar. Antecolic Roux-en-Y reconstruction was routinely selected. In some obese patients, reconstruction with a retrocolic route was selected. The esophagojejunostomy anastomosis was always made on the left side of the esophagus, as a redo anastomosis can be performed by widely opening the left diaphragm if necessary. Prior to esophagojejunostomy, a jejunojejunostomy was made extracorporeally in the extended umbilical wound (Video 12.4).

(a) Functional end-to-end anastomosis (FETE) in esophagojejunostomy (Fig. 12.4 and Video 12.5).

This procedure was the first choice as a reconstruction method in LTG when a sufficient length of the abdominal esophagus was preserved. After making small enterotomies on the left side of the esophageal stump and the antimesenteric side of the jejunal stump, a 45-mm stapler was applied through the left lower trocar. To avoid the insertion of the anvil fork into a submucosal "pseudolumen," a nasogastric tube was used as a guide (Fig. 12.4a). After confirming the fork insertion into the "true lumen" and absence of nasogastric tube involvement, the stapler was fired. A small stapling "gap" caused by slippage of the esophageal stump was managed by temporary laparoscopic continuous suture closure (Fig. 12.4b), and then another linear stapler for closure was applied from the right lower trocar. With this procedure, the jejunal mesentery runs in a straight fashion without any twist (Fig. 12.4c). Petersen's defect was always closed with nonabsorbable sutures.

(b) Isoperistaltic, side-to-side esophagojejunostomy (overlap method) (Fig. 12.5 and Video 12.6).

When sufficient length of the abdominal esophagus could not be preserved due to tumor invasion, and the anastomosis had to be made in the lower mediastinum, this procedure was selected. When the esophagus could not be transected with a linear stapler from the right lower trocar, opening the left diaphragm widely and using an intrathoracically inserted linear stapler through an additional intercostal trocar were helpful. Two forks of a linear stapler were inserted into the jejunum through a small enterotomy made 45-mm from the edge and another enterotomy on the esophageal stump. An isoperistaltic side-to-side anastomosis was constructed, and then the enterotomy was closed using hand-sewn

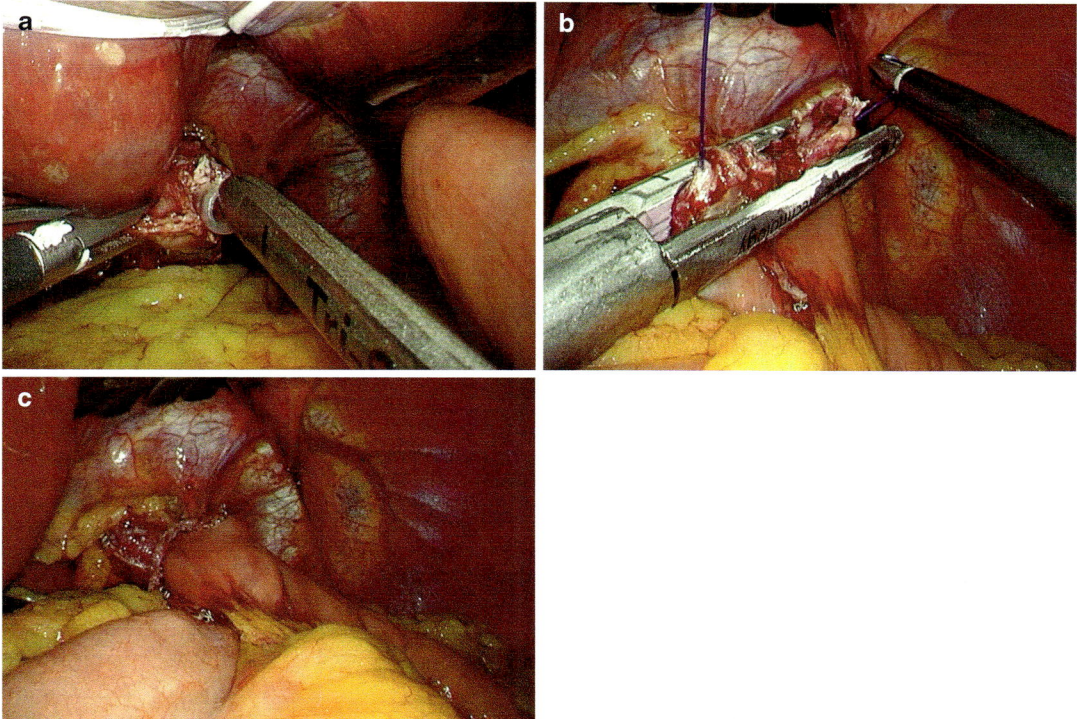

Fig. 12.4 Functional end-to-end anastomosis in esophagojejunostomy (FETE). (**a**) View during first stapling. A 45-mm stapler was applied through the left lower trocar. A nasogastric tube was used as a guide to confirm insertion of the anvil fork into the true lumen of the esophagus. (**b**) Closing the common enterotomy with a stapler from the right lower trocar. A small stapling "gap" caused by the slippage of the esophageal stump can be managed by temporary laparoscopic continuous suture. (**c**) Completion of the anastomosis. The jejunal mesentery runs straight without any twist. Petersen's defect was then closed with nonabsorbable sutures

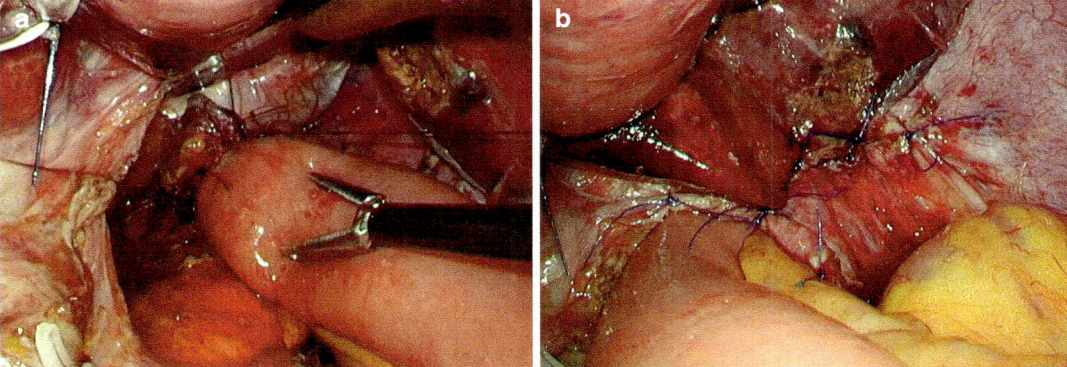

Fig. 12.5 Esophagojejunostomy with overlap method. (**a**) Completion of the anastomosis in the lower mediastinum. Stay sutures on the edges of the enterotomy were pulled out through the subcostal trocars while closing. (**b**) Closing the diaphragm with nonabsorbable sutures for prevention of hiatal hernia

interrupted sutures with extracorporeal Roeder's knots. Because the level of the anastomosis was in the mediastinum, stay sutures on the enterotomy were pulled out through the subcostal trocars so that the subsequent enterotomy closure was easier (Fig. 12.5a). After completing the anastomosis, the diaphragm was closed and sutures between the jejunal wall and the diaphragm were added to prevent a hiatal hernia (Fig. 12.5b). Nonabsorbable sutures were used for this procedure. Finally, the antimesenteric side of the jejunal limb was fixed to the duodenal stump to prevent the limb from falling into left dorsal subphrenic space and kinking off the esophagojejunal anastomosis.

Results

The clinicopathological characteristics of the 427 patients are summarized in Table 12.1. The reconstructive procedures and reconstruction-related short-term surgical outcomes are summarized in Table 12.2. Intraoperative problems during reconstruction were rare but were more often observed in LTG (4/126, 3%) than in LDG (1/301, 0.3%). There were no conversions to open surgery. The overall reconstruction-related morbidity rate was higher in LTG (8.0%) than in LDG (4.0%).

Table 12.1 Clinicopathological characteristics of the patients

Variables	LDG (n = 301)	LTG (n = 126)
Age, median (interquartile range)	70 (63–77)	70.5 (63–75)
Body mass index, median (interquartile range)	22.7 (20.8–24.8)	21.8 (20.1–24.0)
Sex, n, male/ female	207/94	84/42
Clinical stage, n		
IA/IB	168/43	40/18
IIA/IIB	25/20	13/19
IIIA/IIIB/IIIC	19/14/6	16/7/4
IV	6	9

Table 12.2 Reconstruction-related short-term surgical outcomes

Variables	LDG (n = 301)	LTG (n = 126)
Reconstructive procedures		
Billroth-I	211	
Billroth-II	62	
Roux-en-Y	28	126[a]
Functional end-to-end		88
Overlap		35
Trouble during reconstruction Conversion, n	1 0	4 0
Postoperative morbidity[b]		
Grade 2 or higher, in total, n, (%)	12 (4.0%)	10 (8.0%)
Grade 2, in total, n (%)	6 (2.0%)	5 (4.0%)
Anastomotic leakage	4 (1.3%)	3 (2.4%)
Ileus	2 (0.7%)	2 (1.6%)
Grade 3 or higher, in total, n (%)	6 (2.0%)	5 (4.0%)
Anastomotic leakage	4 (1.3%)	2 (1.6%)
Ileus	2 (0.7%)	1 (0.8%)
Anastomotic stenosis	0 (0.0%)	2 (1.6%)

[a]A circular stapler was used in one case, and intrathoracic overlap procedure was performed in two cases
[b]According to Clavien-Dindo classification

Discussion

Intracorporeal reconstruction in laparoscopic gastrectomy was first reported in 1992 in a Billroth-II gastrojejunostomy with a linear stapler [5]. Because of the technical difficulties of intracorporeal gastroduodenostomy, Billroth-II gastrojejunostomy was generally preferred over Billroth-I [20]. Gastroduodenostomy in laparoscopic gastrectomy was first introduced in 1994 [3], but it was performed extracorporeally with a circular stapler, in a similar fashion to open surgery. In 2002, we developed a technique for intracorporeal gastroduodenostomy with linear staplers [6], and short-term and long-term outcomes of 100 consecutive cases were validated [8]. There was no conversion to open surgery, and the mean time for the anastomosis was 13 minutes. Only one minor leak (1%) was observed as a postoperative anastomosis-related complication, and the incidence of dumping syndrome was as low as 5% according to the questionnaires administered at 6 months or more postoperatively. Although some technical pitfalls can occur, the delta-shaped anastomosis has become a widely used technique in Japan and Korea as a simple, quick, and safe method for intracorporeal gastroduodenostomy [7, 11–13].

With the increasing use of this procedure, the short-term outcomes of intracorporeal gastroduodenostomy with delta-shaped anastomosis were compared with those of extracorporeal gastroduodenostomy with a circular stapler [11–13, 21]. Some experienced surgeons reported satisfactory surgical outcomes of extracorporeal reconstruction [21], but intracorporeal gastroduodenostomy provided better results with less blood loss and faster recovery [11, 12], and further benefits were observed in obese patients [13], in whom extracorporeal anastomosis was difficult in a limited working space with a concern for excessive traction. Considering the limitation of the number of studies and selection biases, further evidence with prospective studies is required to confirm the advantage of intracorporeal reconstruction at this moment.

In gastrojejunostomy including both Billroth-II and Roux-en-Y reconstructions, linear staplers are preferred over circular staplers with advantages including easy access from a trocar, smooth insertion into the jejunum, anda better operative view [9] in the completely laparoscopic procedure. In gastrojejunostomy with a circular stapler, transoral placement of the anvil [22] or elimination of the purse-string suture [23] has been reported. While technically challenging, the rates of reconstruction-related complications, such as anastomotic stenosis, stricture, or Roux stasis, were low [7, 9, 22, 23].

The use of LTG remains limited because of the technically challenging esophagojejunostomy, but with the experience of intracorporeal reconstruction in LDG, techniques of intracorporeal esophagojejunostomy have been gradually established. In intracorporeal esophagojejunostomy with a circular stapler, insertion of the anvil head into the esophagus was the first obstacle, managed by hand-sewn purse-string sutures [24, 25], with the technique of attaching a thread or a tube with an anvil [26], or by transoral placement

of the anvil [27]. The handling of a circular stapler under a limited laparoscopic view is another obstacle, but it was managed by modifying the location of the camera port and the small incision in maintaining an adequate view [10].

Intracorporeal esophagojejunostomy with linear staplers is also a common procedure, with the advantages described above. Either the FETE or the isoperistaltic side-to-side anastomosis (overlap method) was selected. Laparoscopic FETE esophagojejunostomy following total gastrectomy was first reported by Uyama et al. in 1999 [28], with the principle of making the anastomosis with the first staple firing and closing the common enterotomy with the second stapler in an antiperistaltic manner. The anastomosis is temporarily closed with sutures or hernia staplers before applying the second staple firing. This is a simple and quick procedure that does not require hand-sewn suturing to complete the anastomosis, and the technique is similar to the delta-shaped anastomosis. The overlap method is another alternative, in cases with a tumor invading the esophagus. The first staple firing makes an isoperistaltic, side-to-side anastomosis, and the enterotomy is closed using a hand-sewn technique. Because the anastomosis is performed in the mediastinum, ensuring adequate working space with dissection into the mediastinum and adequate preparation of the esophagus is required for a safe anastomosis, without which the fork of the stapler cannot be inserted into the esophagus smoothly and may result in a long staple gap between the esophagus and jejunum. Advanced suturing and knotting skills are mandatory to close the enterotomy in this limited space.

Regarding anastomosis-related complications after LTG using either circular or linear staplers, the average leak rate was 3.9% with circular staplers and 2.8% with linear staplers. The frequency of stricture was 2.2% on average, which was not inferior to the reports on open total gastrectomy [10]. The apparent superiority of any particular method has not been confirmed. The optimal method should therefore be chosen based on the experience and technical proficiency of each surgical team.

Conclusions

With the development of laparoscopic technology and the accumulated experiences for 20 years, intracorporeal reconstruction has become the standard in laparoscopic gastrectomy. Several different techniques can be used and can achieve satisfactory outcomes. Understanding the concept and tips of each procedure is important to complete the reconstruction safely.

References

1. Jeong O, Park YK. Clinicopathological features and surgical treatment of gastric cancer in South Korea: the results of 2009 nationwide survey on surgically treated gastric cancer patients. J Gastric Cancer. 2011;11:69–77.
2. Kitano S, Shiraishi N. Current status of laparoscopic gastrectomy for cancer in Japan. Surg Endosc. 2004;18:182–5.
3. Kitano S, Iso Y, Moriyama M, et al. Laparoscopy-assisted Billroth I gastrectomy. Surg Laparosc Endosc. 1994;4:146–8.
4. Viñuela EF, Gonen M, Brennan MF, et al. Laparoscopic versus open distal gastrectomy for gastric cancer: a meta-analysis of randomized controlled trials and high-quality nonrandomized studies. Ann Surg. 2012;255:446–56.
5. Goh P, Tekant Y, Kum C, et al. Totally intra-abdominal laparoscopic Billroth II gastrectomy. Surg Endosc. 1992;6:160.
6. Kanaya S, Gomi T, Momoi H, et al. Delta-shaped anastomosis in totally laparoscopic Billroth I gastrectomy: new technique of intraabdominal gastroduodenostomy. J Am Coll Surg. 2002;195:284–7.
7. Okabe H, Obama K, Tsunoda S, et al. Advantage of completely laparoscopic gastrectomy with linear stapled reconstruction: a long-term follow-up study. Ann Surg. 2014;259:109–16.
8. Kanaya S, Kawamura Y, Kawada H, et al. The delta-shaped anastomosis in laparoscopic distal gastrectomy: analysis of the initial 100 consecutive procedures of intracorporeal gastroduodenostomy. Gastric Cancer. 2011;14:365–71.
9. Hosogi H, Kanaya S. Intracorporeal anastomosis in laparoscopic gastric cancer surgery. J Gastric Cancer. 2012;12:133–9.
10. Okabe H, Tsunoda S, Tanaka E, et al. Is laparoscopic total gastrectomy a safe operation? A review of various anastomotic techniques and their outcomes. Surg Today. 2015;45:549–58.
11. Kinoshita T, Shibasaki H, Oshiro T, et al. Comparison of laparoscopy-assisted and total laparoscopic Billroth-I gastrectomy for gastric cancer: a report of short-term outcomes. Surg Endosc. 2011;25:1395–401.
12. Kanaji S, Harada H, Nakayama S, et al. Surgical outcomes in the newly introduced phase of intracorporeal anastomosis following laparoscopic distal gastrectomy is safe and feasible compared with established procedures of extracorporeal anastomosis. Surg Endosc. 2014;28:1250–5.
13. Kim MG, Kawada H, Kim BS, et al. A totally laparoscopic distal gastrectomy with gastroduodenostomy (TLDG) for improvement of the early surgical outcomes in high BMI patients. Surg Endosc. 2011;25:1076–82.
14. UICC International Union Against Cancer. TNM classification of malignant tumours. 7th ed. New York: Wiley; 2009. p. 73–7.
15. Dindo D, Demartines N, Clavien PA. Classification of surgical complications: a new proposal with evaluation in a cohort of 6336 patients and results of a survey. Ann Surg. 2004;240:205–13.
16. Kanaya S, Haruta S, Kawamura Y, et al. Video: laparoscopy distinctive technique for suprapancreatic lymph node dissection: medial approach for laparoscopic gastric cancer surgery. Surg Endosc. 2011;25:3928–9.
17. Inaba K, Satoh S, Ishida Y, et al. Overlap method: novel intracorporeal esophagojejunostomy after laparoscopic total gastrectomy. J Am Coll Surg. 2010;211:e25–9.
18. Shinohara T, Kanaya S, Yoshimura F, et al. A protective technique for retraction of the liver during laparoscopic gastrectomy for gastric adenocarcinoma: using a Penrose drain. J Gastrointest Surg. 2011;15:1043–8.
19. Hosogi H, Kanaya S, Nomura H, et al. Setting the stomach transection line based on anatomical landmarks in laparoscopic distal gastrectomy. J Gastric Cancer. 2015;15:53–7.
20. Ballesta-Lopez C, Bastida-VilaX CM, et al. Laparoscopic Billroth II distal subtotal gastrectomy with gastric stump suspension for gastric malignancies. Am J Surg. 1996;171:289–92.
21. Kim DG, Choi YY, An JY, et al. Comparing the short-term outcomes of totally intracorporeal gastroduodenostomy with extracorporeal gastroduodenostomy after laparoscopic distal gastrectomy for gastric cancer: a single surgeon's experience and a rapid systematic review with meta-analysis. Surg Endosc. 2013;27:3153–61.
22. Ohashi M, Iwanaga T, Ohinata R, et al. A novel procedure for Roux-en-Y reconstruction following laparoscopy-assisted distal gastrectomy: transoral placement of anvil and intracorporeal gastrojejunostomy via umbilical mini-laparotomy. Gastric Cancer. 2011;14:188–93.
23. Omori T, Oyama T, Akamatsu H, et al. A simple and safe method for gastrojejunostomy in laparoscopic distal gastrectomy using the hemidouble-stapling technique: efficient purse-string stapling technique. Dig Surg. 2009;26:441–5.

24. Kinoshita T, Oshiro T, Ito K, et al. Intracorporeal circular-stapled esophagojejunostomy using hand-sewn purse-string suture after laparoscopic total gastrectomy. Surg Endosc. 2010;24:2908–12.
25. Kim HI, Cho I, Jang DS, et al. Intracorporeal esophagojejunostomy using a circular stapler with a new purse-string suture technique during laparoscopic total gastrectomy. J Am Coll Surg. 2013;216:e11–6.
26. Omori T, Oyama T, Mizutani S, et al. A simple and safe technique for esophagojejunostomy using the hemi-double stapling technique in laparoscopy-assisted total gastrectomy. Am J Surg. 2009;197:e13–7.
27. Jeong O, Park YK. Intracorporeal circular stapling esophagojejunostomy using the transorally inserted anvil (Orvil) after laparoscopic total gastrectomy. Surg Endosc. 2009;23:2624–30.
28. Uyama I, Sugioka A, Fujita J, et al. Laparoscopic total gastrectomy with distal pancreatosplenectomy and d2 lymphadenectomy for advanced gastric cancer. Gastric Cancer. 1999;2:230–4.

Part VII

Robotic Surgery for Gastric Cancer

Distal Subtotal Gastrectomy with D2 Lymph Node Dissection

13

Kun Yang and Woo Jin Hyung

Introduction

Since the first laparoscopic distal gastrectomy for gastric cancer was first reported in 1994 [1], the minimally invasive surgery has drawn much attention worldwide. As the accumulation of the data showed the favorable short-term outcomes and accelerated postoperative recovery without compromising the oncologic safety [2–4], laparoscopic distal gastrectomy has been widely accepted as an option of minimally invasive treatments for early cancer. However, the application of laparoscopic gastrectomy for advanced gastric cancer remains debatable, because of the technical difficulties of D2 lymphadenectomy and digestive tract reconstruction, as well as lack of long-term survival data of large-scale randomized controlled trials.

Meanwhile, new technology represented by robotic surgical systems has been proven useful in allowing surgeons to readily perform procedures regarded as difficult with conventional laparoscopic surgery, enabling complex procedures to be carried out with a minimally invasive approach [5–11]. To overcome the limitation associated with laparoscopic surgery, surgical robot was adopted as alternative minimally invasive surgery by experienced laparoscopic surgeons.

In this chapter, we demonstrated the current status, advantages, indication, and detailed procedures of robotic distal gastrectomy for gastric cancer.

K. Yang
Department of Gastrointestinal Surgery, West China Hospital, Sichuan University, Chengdu, Sichuan, China

Laboratory of Gastric Cancer, State Key Laboratory of Biotherapy, West China Hospital, Sichuan University, Chengdu, Sichuan, China

W. J. Hyung (✉)
Department of Surgery, Yonsei University College of Medicine, Seoul, Republic of Korea

Gastric Cancer Center, Yonsei Cancer Center, Yonsei University Health System, Seoul, Republic of Korea

Robot and Minimal Invasive Surgery Center, Severance Hospital, Yonsei University Health System, Seoul, Republic of Korea
e-mail: wjhyung@yuhs.ac

Advantages of Robotic Gastrectomy and Clinical Assessment of Its Application

Overview

The first case of robotic-assisted gastrectomy was reported in 2003 [5]. With the development of a decade, robotic gastrectomy has been proven to be safe and feasible in terms of mortality, morbidity, conversion rate, postoperative hospital stay, and oncological safety when compared with conventional laparoscopic gastrectomy.

© Springer-Verlag GmbH Germany, part of Springer Nature 2019
S. H. Noh, W. J. Hyung (eds.), *Surgery for Gastric Cancer*,
https://doi.org/10.1007/978-3-662-45583-8_13

Generally, compared with conventional laparoscopic surgery, robotic surgery may offer more precise lymphadenectomy around vessels by providing various technical advantages, such as three-dimensional image, motion scaling, tremor filtering, coaxial alignment, and articulated endoscopic wrist with seven degrees of freedom, which could minimize blood loss and invasiveness and improve the dexterity of surgeons [12]. Furthermore, ergonomic design of the robotic console could reduce the discomfort and fatigue of surgeons, especially for the operations with long durations. In addition, the camera arm and 30° endoscope could lift the abdominal wall, just like the gasless procedure in laparoscopic surgery, and expand the space for manipulation and provide excellent visions.

Specific Advantages in Robotic Gastrectomy with D2 Lymphadenectomy

With its mechanical superiority, robotic surgical systems provide 3-D views and ambidextrous tremor-filtered bidirectional dissection around complex vascular structures, contributing to constantly keeping the right surgical plane, such as the plane between lymph nodes bearing fatty tissues and major suprapancreatic vessels (or pancreatic parenchyma) in the process of suprapancreatic lymph node dissection, providing more thorough and precise dissection, and reducing the possibility of injuries to vessels or the pancreas [12]. Moreover, the equipment of wristed instruments via the robotic arms aids in the approach to and traction of the stomach and pancreas, as well as proper and stable exposure of the peripancreatic area, even to the dorsal side of the pancreas where it is difficult for current laparoscopic instrument and camera system to identify and reach. Stable retraction of tissues without tremor can reduce potential risk of injury to lymphatic tissues and bleeding from dissection plane. All of these features could make it somewhat easier for surgeons to perform D2 lymphadenectomy during gastrectomy. Additionally, the 3-D views and the scaled movements of robotic

instruments offer an optimal identification of vascular anomalies, such as an aberrant left hepatic artery originating from the left gastric artery, and allow the aberrant hepatic artery-preserving lymph node dissection. Furthermore, the robotic system facilitates intracorporeal hand-sewn sutures in all anastomosis even in deep and narrow spaces, which might promote the shift from extracorporeal to intracorporeal anastomosis in robotic surgery [13]. In addition, 3-D views and articulated instruments of robotic system could make the control of major bleeding due to vascular injury more easily [13]. Meanwhile, robotic distal gastrectomy exhibits a shorter learning curve than that for laparoscopic gastrectomy [14], which may enable a greater number of surgeons to perform D2 lymph node dissection during gastrectomy for gastric cancer. Shorter learning curves might also permit experienced surgeons to apply advanced or complicated procedures more easily for gastric cancer treatment.

Clinical Assessment of Robotic Gastrectomy

Although high-level evidence is still wanting since robotic gastrectomy for gastric cancer treatment is a relatively novel field, the feasibility, safety, and short-term outcomes of robotic gastrectomy have been reported to be comparable with conventional laparoscopic gastrectomy [15–17].

The morbidity and mortality rate, as well as conversion rate, did not differ significantly between laparoscopic gastrectomy and robotic gastrectomy [9, 15–17]. Some study even reported that the robotic gastrectomy could decrease the morbidity significantly, compared with laparoscopic gastrectomy [18]. Several studies have showed that robotic gastrectomy was associated with reduced intraoperative blood loss compared with laparoscopic gastrectomy, which can provide extra potential oncologic benefits through decreasing the intraperitoneal free cancer cell dissemination and immunosuppressing caused by perioperative transfusions, especially for locally advanced cancer [19].

The postoperative hospital stay after the robotic gastrectomy was much shorter than that of open gastrectomy [15, 16]. No significant differences were observed between robotic gastrectomy and laparoscopic gastrectomy in terms of time to ambulation, time to start food intake, and postoperative hospital stay [9, 20]. However, some studies showed shorter mean postoperative hospital stay in robotic gastrectomy group compared to laparoscopic gastrectomy group [18, 21]. Faster recovery allows patients to receive adjuvant chemotherapy timely.

Given the lack of long-term survival data of robotic gastrectomy, the numbers of harvested lymph nodes and the resection margin are often used to evaluate the oncological safety. Some meta-analysis which compared the robotic gastrectomy to laparoscopic gastrectomy showed that there was no significant difference in the number of retrieved lymph nodes [15–17]. Even some authors reported that robotic gastrectomy can yield more lymph nodes located in the extraperigastric area (2nd tier) in D2 lymphadenectomy [11, 22], compared with laparoscopic gastrectomy. For the resection margin, one study showed that no positive margins were observed in the robotic group, while some cases in the laparoscopic group had tumor involvement in the margin [23].

Regarding the comparisons of long-term survival between robotic gastrectomy with other approaches, retrospective studies revealed that long-term survival was similar between laparoscopic gastrectomy and robotic gastrectomy [11, 24]. However, because of the lack of randomized controlled trials demonstrating long-term outcomes, advantages of robotic gastrectomy from an oncologic view are still to be clarified.

Indication

Basically, the indications for robotic gastrectomy for gastric cancer are similar to those of the conventional laparoscopic gastrectomy. Candidates for robotic surgery include patients with a preoperative diagnosis of gastric cancer without serosa involvement and without evidence of lymph node metastasis to an extraperigastric area, except those with lesions suitable for endoscopic treatment. Distal gastrectomy is selected when a satisfactory proximal resection margin can be obtained. For early gastric cancer patients without lymph node involvement (cT1N0M0), limited lymphadenectomy (D1 or D1+) could be performed. The indications for D2 lymph node dissection comprise patients with a primary tumor of the deep submucosal layer or deeper invasion or patients with suspicious lymph node metastasis on preoperative diagnostic workup.

Patients with serosal involvement in locally advanced tumors, direct invasion to adjacent organs, or suspicion of extraperigastric lymph node metastasis are usually excluded from undergoing minimally invasive surgery. However, robotic gastrectomy for such cancers could be decided according to the surgeon's expertise and experience but should be performed within the context of clinical trials.

Operative Procedures [7, 25, 26]

Operating Room Setup

The patient cart is positioned at the head of the patient. The vision cart is located caudal to the patient. The surgeon's console is placed where the operator could see and check the patient cart and the patient. The assistant should have a position at the left side of the patient. And it is useful to have a second monitor on the right side of the table across from the assistant. Sterile back tables (instruments) are located at the patient's knee and at the foot of the bed. The scrub nurse locates at the lower right side of the table, opposing to the patient-side assistant. Operating room configuration is usually dependent on the room dimension as well as the preferences and experience of the surgeons. The operating room setup is shown in Fig. 13.1a.

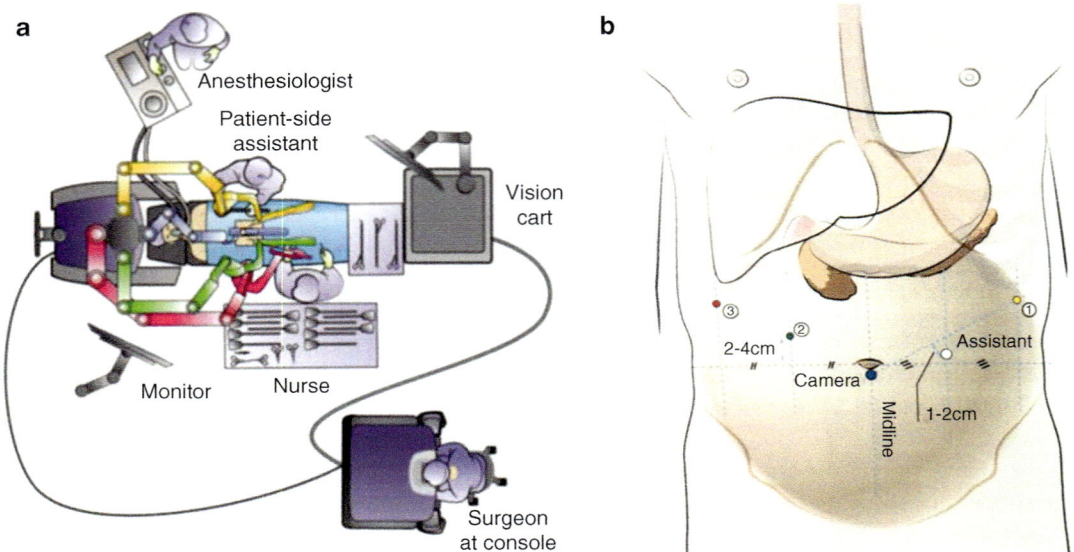

Fig. 13.1 Operating room setup and placements of trocars (cited from da Vinci Gastrectomy Procedure Guide [25]). (**a**) Operating room setup, (**b**) placements of trocars

Patient Positioning and Port Placement

Under general anesthesia, the patient's arms are placed alongside the body to prevent injury to the upper extremities by the robotic arms. In order to prevent the patients from translocation, the patients should be carefully secured and fixed by strap and gel pads across the thigh. After positioning, securing, and preparing the patient in the supine position, a 12-mm trocar is placed at the midline just below the umbilicus for inserting a dual lens laparoscope. After pneumoperitoneum of 12-mm Hg is achieved, the table is then placed in a reverse Trendelenburg position (15°). After laparoscopic exploration and checking for the optimal locations of the port sites, four additional ports could be inserted under camera visualization: one 12-mm and three 8-mm ports. Specifically, an 8-mm diameter port for the 1st arm of the robot is placed 1 cm below the costal angle, as far lateral as possible, on the patient's left side; the port should be at least 1 cm above the level of the bowel when viewed internally. Another 8-mm port for the 3rd arm should be inserted 1 cm below the costal angle, as far lateral as possible, on the patient's right side; it should

also be positioned 1 cm above the bowel. Another 8-mm port for the 2nd robotic arm should be inserted 2–4 cm above along an imaginary line that intersected the middle of the camera port and the right subcostal port; this step allows easier access to the pancreatic head and duodenum and achieves a proper angle with the non-wristed ultrasonic shears. The assistant port should be placed 1–2 cm below an imaginary line drawn from the insertion site of the 1st robotic arm to the umbilical camera port (Fig. 13.1b). Maximizing the distance between the ports (at least 8 mm, especially between 2nd arm and 3rd arm) for the robotic arms would help to prevent external collision of the robotic arms. If the patient is thin, the port for the 2nd arm must be placed more caudally; the ports for the 1st and 3rd arms can be positioned more medially for obese patients. During the operation, the camera port should be lifted as high as possible to make sufficient use of the space made by the pneumoperitoneum.

Docking

The position of the operating table should be reconfirmed before docking since it's impossible to adjust the operating table after docking. Adjust the camera arm setup joint toward the left side of the patient with only 1st arm and confirm sweet spot. The blue arrow should align within the blue marker on the second joint or assure an angle less than 90 degrees between the 1st and 3rd joints on the camera arm. The arm of the patient cart should be positioned high enough to provide space above the patient's head. Then, the patient cart is rolled up and positioned over the patient's head. The camera arm, camera arm setup joint, column, camera port, and target anatomy are aligned. Once the correct position is reached, the patient cart can be locked. Dock the camera arm firstly and then the other three robotic arms. The space between the 2nd and 3rd arms, as well as the space between the 1st arm and the camera arm, should be maximized by spreading these arms as far apart as possible. Remember to keep instruments in the center of their range of motion.

Instrumentations

The instrumentation and settings consist of a 30-degree down endoscope in the camera arm, Maryland bipolar forceps in the 1st arm, ultrasonic shears or the monopolar curved scissors in the 2nd arm, and Cadiere forceps in the 3rd arm, interchangeably. The 3rd arm is applied at the patient's right side because the 3rd arm should be at the opposite side of the 1st arm for better countertraction. Surgeons control the 1st arm by the right hand while 2nd and 3rd arms by the left hand through switching button. The assistant aids the surgeon to suck, irrigate, and apply stapler or other additional procedures through the assistant port.

Liver Retraction

Appropriate liver retraction to prepare for the sufficient operative field is very important, not only for maximizing the application of instruments by liberating the arm used for liver retraction but also for facilitating dissection, particularly for suprapancreatic lymph node dissection. Various methods of liver retraction such

as suspension using Penrose drains [27], the gauze suspension method [28], and retraction using liver retractor [29] have been described. Each of the aforementioned methods could be used provided that satisfied operative view is reached. To the authors' opinion, the gauze suspension method is simple and economic and almost harmless to the liver [28]. Briefly, two 4 × 4 inch gauze pads threaded by a 2-0 Prolene suture with 70-mm double straight needles are introduced into the intraperitoneal cavity via the assistant port. Next, the lesser omentum is divided up to the right side of the esophageal hiatus, and the Prolene suture is secured to the pars condensa with two Hemolocks. The straight needles are used to pierce the anterior abdominal wall directly on both sides of the xiphoid process and externally tied to suspend the liver toward the abdominal wall by the assistant.

Left-Side Dissection and Greater Curvature Mobilization (Lymph Node #4sb and #4d Dissection)

The greater omentum attaching to the greater curvature of the stomach is retracted cranially and ventrally by the 3rd arm, while the gravity of the transverse colon would act as countertraction. Left-side dissection and greater curvature mobilization begin by dividing the omentum and entering the lesser sac from the middle of the greater curvature, which comprises the fewest number of vessels, to the lower pole of the spleen using the ultrasonic shears. By continuing dissection, the left gastroepiploic artery and vein can be identified, ligated using clips via a robotic clip applier, and divided after giving the branch to the omentum (Fig. 13.2a). Division of adhesions between the lower pole of the spleen and greater omentum can prevent tearing of the splenic capsule. The short gastric vessels are usually preserved for a distal gastrectomy; however, if the tumor is in a high location, one or two short gastric arteries need to be divided for proper margins and create enough space for the resection and anastomosis. After ligating the left gastroepiploic vessels, all of the soft tissue along the greater curvature area

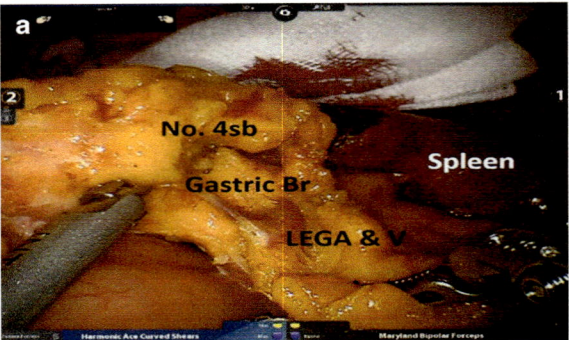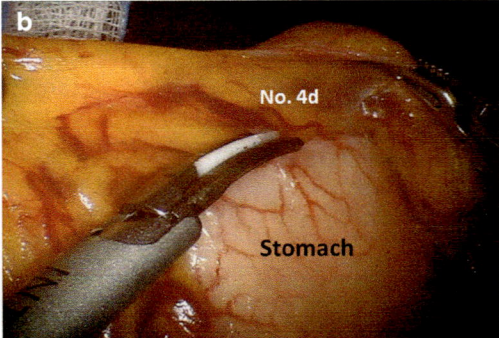

Fig. 13.2 Left-side dissection and greater curvature mobilization. (**a**) The left gastroepiploic artery and vein can be identified and divided after giving the branch to the omen-tum. (**b**) The greater curvature is skeletonized to remove No. 4sb and No. 4d lymph nodes. LEGA and V, left gastro-epiploic artery and vein; Br, branch

should be removed by skeletonizing along the greater curvature toward the pylorus to complete the No. 4sb and No. 4d lymph node dissection for a distal gastrectomy (Fig. 13.2b).

Right-Side Dissection and Infrapyloric Area Dissection (Lymph Node #6 and #14v Dissection)

Right-side dissection and infrapyloric dissection are performed by dissecting soft tissue from the middle colic vessels to the surface of the superior mesenteric vessels while exposing the head of the pancreas and removing lymph node-bearing tissues around the right gastroepiploic vessels.

Retract the gastroepiploic pedicle ventrally and appropriately by the 3rd arm. Before performing the infrapyloric dissection, the physiological adhesions between the posterior wall of the stomach and pancreas should be fully dissected, and the inferior pancreatic border is exposed, which is very helpful to seek and keep the correct dissected planes. Then, the transverse mesocolon should be detached from the gastroepiploic pedicle and the pancreatic head by identifying the middle colonic artery and following the pulsations to the inferior pancreatic border. The physiological adhesions between the transverse colon and the descending part of the duodenum should also be released at the same time. The right colonic vein and the Henle's trunk that drains into the superior mesenteric vein are used

as landmarks to identify the origin of right gastroepiploic vein. Soft tissues located on the right side and left side of the right gastroepiploic vein, as well as the soft tissues anterior to the anterior superior pancreaticoduodenal vein and Henle's trunk, should be dissected together using the Harmonic shears and the Maryland bipolar forceps until the pancreatic parenchyma is exposed. Next, the right gastroepiploic vein is clipped and divided distal to the confluence of the anterior superior pancreaticoduodenal vein (Fig. 13.3a). In case of No. 6 lymph node metastasis, the No. 14v lymph nodes should be also removed. Note that the venous drainage from the pancreatic head should be preserved when approaching the right side of the right gastroepiploic vein and the proper membrane of the pancreas which directly covers the pancreatic parenchyma should be kept intact to avoid the postoperative pancreatitis. If the middle colonic artery cannot be seen in some obese patients, dissect the opposite side first. Dissection to expose the right gastroepiploic artery is continued, and the artery is ligated and divided distal to the origin of anterior superior pancreaticoduodenal artery (Fig. 13.3b). Finally, the infrapyloric artery is identified and divided between clips. Thus, the right gastroepiploic vessels are dissected en bloc with lymphatic tissue (Fig. 13.3c). Sometimes, a ligule of pancreatic parenchyma is extended toward the duodenal bulb, or the pancreas is unexpectedly lifted up, which should be prevented from injuring. And there are many tiny branches around the root of

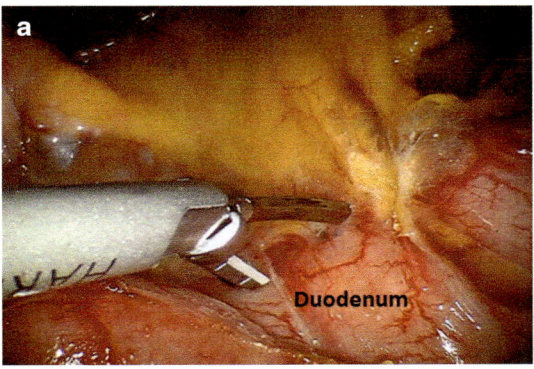

Fig. 13.3 Infrapyloric dissection. (**a**) The right gastroepiploic vein is clipped and divided distal to the confluence of the anterior superior pancreaticoduodenal vein. (**b**) The right gastroepiploic artery is ligated and divided distal to the origin of anterior superior pancreaticoduodenal artery. (**c**) View to show the dissection efficacy of No. 6 lymph node dissection. GCT, gastrocolic trunk; RGEV, right gastroepiploic vein; ASPDV, anterior superior pancreaticoduodenal vein; MCV, middle colonic vein; ARCV, accessory right colic vein; RGEA, right gastroepiploic artery; ASPDA, anterior superior pancreaticoduodenal artery; IPA, infrapyloric artery; GDA, gastroduodenal artery

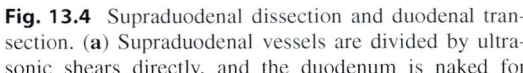

Fig. 13.4 Supraduodenal dissection and duodenal transection. (**a**) Supraduodenal vessels are divided by ultrasonic shears directly, and the duodenum is naked for transection. (**b**) The duodenum is stapled and divided about 2 cm distal to the pylorus using an endoscopic linear stapler through the assistant port

right gastroepiploic artery and infrapyloric artery; ultrasonic shears benefit to avoid bleeding and keep a clear surgical field.

Supraduodenal Dissection and Duodenal Transection

The duodenum is mobilized from the pancreas along the gastroduodenal artery to prepare for the duodenal transection, and the anterior side of the gastroduodenal artery is exposed. The dissection continues to the bifurcation of the proper hepatic artery and the gastroduodenal artery. Be sure to coagulate the small vessels from the head of the pancreas to the duodenum. After identification of the proper hepatic artery, a 4-inch by 4-inch gauze is inserted between the supraduodenal tissues and pancreas and acts like a "tent" to facilitate the dissection of the supraduodenal area and to avoid unexpected injuries to the pancreas and major vessels (such as the proper hepatic artery, gastroduodenal artery, or common hepatic artery). Supraduodenal vessels are divided by ultrasonic shears directly, and the duodenum is naked for transection (Fig. 13.4a). The duodenum is stapled and divided about 2 cm distal to the pylorus using an endoscopic linear stapler through the assistant port (Fig. 13.4b). The staple line of the duodenal stump could be reinforced by sutures if the Billroth-II or Roux-en-Y anastomosis is considered.

Suprapancreatic Area Dissection (Lymph Node #5, #7, #8a, #9, #11p, and #12a Dissection)

After transection of the duodenum, the stomach is retracted to the patient's left and ventral side to identify the right gastric vessels. In order to have an easier dissection of the anterior layer of the gastrohepatic ligament, the liver hilum is retracted by the Cadiere forceps of the 3rd robotic arm which is padded by a gauze. Dissection continues along the proper hepatic artery until the right gastric vessels are exposed. The anterolateral surface of proper hepatic artery is also exposed. Identify and skeletonize the root of the right gastric vessels for proper clip application. Divide the right gastric vessels at roots and dissect the No. 5 lymph node (Fig. 13.5a). When approaching the medial side of the proper hepatic artery, retraction of the liver hilum should be reduced. The tissues containing the vagus nerve around the proper hepatic artery are grasped by the Cadiere forceps and retracted to the right and caudal side, and the soft tissue located anterolateral to the proper hepatic artery which has been dissected before is countertracted to the left. Thus, a surgical plane could be created between the No. 12a lymph node-bearing tissue and the proper hepatic artery. Then all the tissues are removed en bloc along the surgical plane by Harmonic shears until the exposure of anterolateral wall of the portal vein (Fig. 13.5b). After finishing the No. 12a and No. 5 lymph node dissections, retract and tense the gastropancreatic fold using the Cadiere forceps ventrally. Lymph nodes bearing soft tissues at the surface of the common hepatic artery are gently pulled up by Maryland bipolar forceps, while the ultrasonic shears are used to skeletonize the common hepatic artery and dissect No. 8a lymph nodes from right to left. Avoid using active blade of Harmonic in direct contact with vessels; rotate the Harmonic shears away from vessels while skeletonizing. When dissecting the No. 8a lymph nodes cephalad to the common hepatic artery, retract the common hepatic artery dorsally and caudally by grasping the tissues around the artery, which is useful to expose easily and prevent injuries to major vessels. Complete the dissection of No. 8a and 12a lymph nodes around the proper and common hepatic artery and portal vein until the left gastric vein is identified. Clip and divide the left gastric vein at the root. Constantly dissect in the right plane between the nerve sheaths around the major arteries and lymph nodes bear-

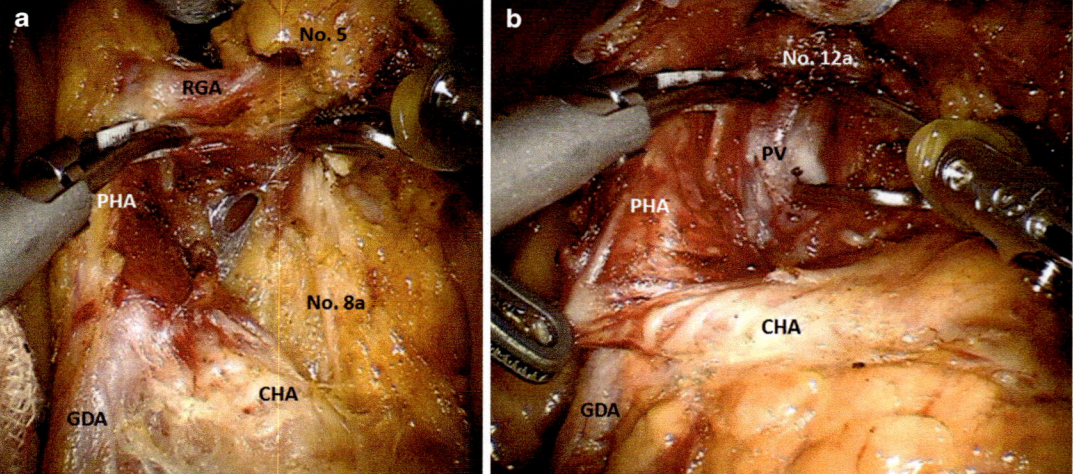

Fig. 13.5 Dissection of No. 5 and 12a lymph nodes. (**a**) Identify and skeletonize the root of the right gastric vessels for proper clip application, and divide the right gastric vessels at roots and dissect the No. 5 lymph nodes. (**b**) Dissection of No. 12a lymph nodes until the exposure of anterolateral wall of the portal vein. CHA, common hepatic artery; GDA, gastroduodenal artery; RGA, right gastric artery; PHA, proper hepatic artery; PV, portal vein

ing fatty tissues, and utilization of the articulation and grasping capabilities of the Cadiere and Maryland forceps to create the proper dissection angles for the non-wristed Harmonic shears during the process of suprapancreatic lymphadenectomy is necessary for a technically safe and radical lymphadenectomy.

Continue the dissection along the common hepatic artery toward the celiac trunk, and expose the origin of the splenic artery (Fig. 13.6a). Soft tissues around the celiac trunk are dissected and pulled up to the specimen side. The root of the left gastric artery is skeletonized, clipped, and divided (Fig. 13.6b). When skeletonizing the left gastric artery, rotating the camera can reveal the posterior side of the left gastric artery in the oblique view, making the following dissections easier. Also, division of the left gastric artery is important as it allows for greater exposure for the dissection of No. 11p lymph nodes. The nerve plexus around the celiac trunk could be preserved in the cases with prophylactic D2 lymph node dissection. If an aberrant left hepatic artery with thick diameter derived from the left gastric artery exists, or a normal left hepatic artery originating from the common hepatic artery is absent, the aberrant hepatic artery-preserving No. 7 lymph node dissection should be performed, which means to skeletonize the trunk of the left gastric artery without injuring and dividing and only divide the gastric branches at their origins.

With the 3rd arm padded with gauze to roll down the pancreas, compression and retraction provide the best possible exposure of the soft tissues containing No. 11p lymph nodes. Also, natural traction to the left side can be acquired with compression via the 3rd arm. If compression of the pancreas via the 3rd arm is insufficient, an assistant can help. Use the Maryland bipolar to create the proper angles and Harmonic shears to dissect the soft tissues along the superior border of the pancreas and the splenic artery until the origin of posterior gastric artery (if there is not an obvious posterior gastric artery, make sure to dissect at least 5 cm along the splenic artery) (Fig. 13.6c). If it is not possible to dissect the suprapancreatic area with traction via the Cadiere and Maryland forceps, the use of other endo-wristed devices (e.g., hook or monopolar scissors) may be helpful. For a complete No. 11p lymphadenectomy, the proximal part of the splenic vein should be exposed. Thereafter, the retroperitoneal attachment of the stomach was detached up to the diaphragmatic cruses, completing the removal of the perigastric lymph nodes. Utilization of the Cadiere forceps (3rd arm) to provide necessary countertraction and the articulated Maryland bipolar forceps to create proper angles is critical to the dissection of the soft tissues along the superior border of the pancreas and the proximal part of the splenic artery

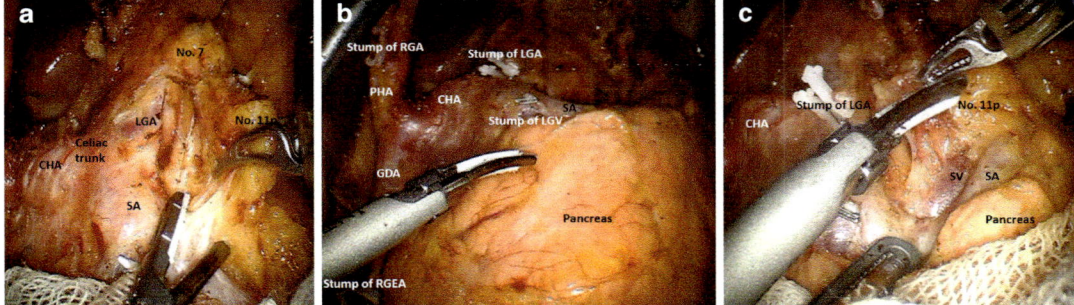

Fig. 13.6 Dissection of No. 7, 8a, 9, and 11p lymph nodes. (**a**) Continue the dissection along the common hepatic artery toward the celiac trunk, and expose the origin of the splenic artery. (**b**) Soft tissues around the celiac trunk are dissected, and the root of left gastric artery is skeletonized and divided. (**c**) Dissect the No. 11p lymph nodes along the superior border of the pancreas and the splenic artery until the origin of posterior gastric artery, and expose the proximal part of the splenic vein. CHA, common hepatic artery; LGA, left gastric artery; LGV, left gastric vein; SA, splenic artery; SV, splenic vein; GDA, gastroduodenal artery; RGA, right gastric artery; PHA, proper hepatic artery; RGEA, right gastroepiploic artery

(No. 11p lymph nodes), which facilitate surgeons to completely dissect the deep portion of No. 11p lymph nodes, one of the most technically complex procedures in conventional laparoscopic gastrectomy.

Lesser Curvature Dissection (Lymph Node #1 and #3 Dissection)

There are two ways to remove No. 1 and 3 lymph nodes. Posterior-side approach is known as dissection of soft tissues along the lesser curvature from the hiatus down to the transection line and from the posterior to the anterior side of the lesser curvature (Fig. 13.7), while anterior-side approach is characterized by keeping the dissection plane from anterior and from transection line up to the hiatus along the lesser curvature. The anterior and the posterior branches of vagal nerve should be divided.

Gastric Resection, Anastomosis, and Specimen Retrieval

After ensuring the proximal margin, the stomach is transected using endo-linear staplers via the assistant port for a distal gastrectomy. The specimen is bagged intracorporeally and placed aside for later removal. Various methods, such as Billroth-I, Billroth-II, or Roux-en-Y reconstruc-

tion, could be used to restore the digestive continuity [12, 24, 30, 31]. Both intracorporeal and extracorporeal anastomoses are acceptable. Either linear or circular staplers or hand-sewn sutures could be applied. Each method has its advantages and disadvantages. Surgeons could choose the optimal reconstruction method according to the tumor location, stage, life expectancy, and surgeon's preference, as well as their experience. If the robotic wristed linear stapler which could be applied by robotic arm can be introduced, the anastomoses would be more comfortable and stable.

Here, we describe our reconstruction procedures after distal gastrectomy as follows. After the resection of the stomach, gastroduodenostomy or gastrojejunostomy is performed intracorporeally, using an endo-linear stapler. Gastroduodenostomy is performed using linear staplers, similar to so-called delta-shaped anastomosis. The duodenum should be transected from the posterior to the anterior wall using an endoscopic linear stapler with blue cartilage inserted through the 12-mm assistant port. After the distal subtotal gastrectomy, small holes are created along the edge of the greater curvature of the remnant stomach and the medial edge of the duodenum. An endoscopic linear stapler is then placed between the remnant stomach and duodenum (cartridge in the stomach and anvil into the duodenum), and the posterior wall of the remnant stomach and the posterior wall of the duodenum

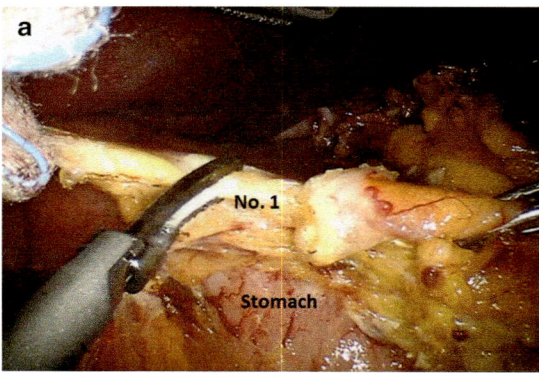
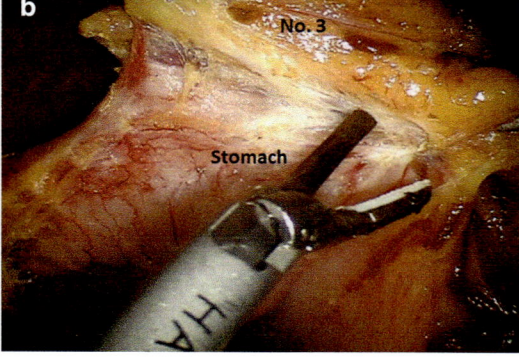

Fig. 13.7 Dissection of No. 1 and 3 lymph nodes. Dissection of soft tissues along the lesser curvature from the hiatus down to the transection line and from the poste-

rior to the anterior side of the lesser curvature. (**a**) Dissection of No. 1 lymph nodes. (**b**) Dissection of No. 3 lymph nodes

are approximated by the stapler. By firing the stapler, a common channel between the stomach and the duodenum is made. When closing the common entry hole, the previously stapled duodenal stump is also removed to secure the blood supply to the duodenum. For intracorporeal gastrojejunostomy, identification of the ligament of Treitz and creation of an enterotomy in the jejunum 15–20 cm from the ligament of Treitz using the ultrasonic shears are undertaken. After an enterotomy is created in the remnant stomach with ultrasonic shears, the endo-wristed grasping instrument is used to place endo-linear staplers first on the stomach and then on the jejunum. The stapler is fired after approximation, and the entry hole is closed with another stapler as well. Finally, a drain is placed below the left lobe of the liver. The specimen can then be retrieved through the extended infraumbilical trocar site.

Limitation and Future Perspectives

Higher cost and longer operative time seem to be the disadvantages of robotic surgery. Since robotic gastrectomy is considered to have little benefit compared with laparoscopic surgery, whether these disadvantages of robotic surgery can be justified by the advantages in radical lymphadenectomy still debatable. Although clinically negligible yet, the aforementioned benefits of robotic surgery undoubtedly make the minimally invasive gastrectomy easier, especially in the relatively complicated procedures such as aberrant hepatic artery-preserving lymph node dissection and function-preserving gastrectomy, compared with conventional laparoscopic surgery. Therefore, the surgeons are not reluctant to perform the robotic procedures [19].

The future developments of robotic gastrectomy are novel platforms, haptic feedback, improvement of flexible instruments, and application of diverse emerging technologies, such as fluorescent image-guided surgery or Tilepro™ function. The development of robotic system's advanced technology enables surgeons to challenge the new horizons of minimally invasive gastrectomy [32].

Conclusion

Robotic distal gastrectomy with radical lymphadenectomy is regarded as safe and feasible provided that the operations are performed by experienced surgeons, compared with conventional laparoscopy. Longer operation time, higher costs, and oncologic equivalency to its counterparts are still unresolved issues, which need further development and investigation. However, robotic distal gastrectomy for gastric cancer would be a promising approach by providing advantages in an accurate, complete, and delicate D2 lymphadenectomy.

References

1. Kitano S, Iso Y, Moriyama M, Sugimachi K. Laparoscopy-assisted Billroth I gastrectomy. Surg Laparosc Endosc. 1994;4(2):146–8.
2. Kim W, Kim HH, Han SU, et al. Korean Laparoendoscopic Gastrointestinal Surgery Study (KLASS) Group. Decreased morbidity of laparoscopic distal gastrectomy compared with open distal gastrectomy for stage I gastric cancer: short-term outcomes from a multicenter randomized controlled trial (KLASS-01). Ann Surg. 2016;263(1):28–35.
3. Inaki N, Etoh T, Ohyama T, et al. A multi-institutional, prospective, phase II feasibility study of laparoscopy-assisted distal gastrectomy with D2 lymph node dissection for locally advanced gastric cancer (JLSSG0901). World J Surg. 2015;39(11):2734–41.
4. Chen XZ, Hu JK, Yang K, Wang L, Lu QC. Short-term evaluation of laparoscopy-assisted distal gastrectomy for predictive early gastric cancer: a meta-analysis of randomized controlled trials. Surg Laparosc Endosc Percutan Tech. 2009;19(4):277–84.
5. Hashizume M, Sugimachi K. Robot-assisted gastric surgery. Surg Clin North Am. 2003;83(6):1429–44.
6. Uyama I, Kanaya S, Ishida Y, Inaba K, Suda K, Satoh S. Novel integrated robotic approach for suprapancreatic D2 nodal dissection for treating gastric cancer: technique and initial experience. World J Surg. 2012;36(2):331–7.
7. Kim YM, Son T, Kim HI, Noh SH, Hyung WJ. Robotic D2 lymph node dissection during distal subtotal gastrectomy for gastric cancer: toward procedural standardization. Ann Surg Oncol. 2016;23(8):2409–10.
8. Okumura N, Son T, Kim YM, et al. Robotic gastrectomy for elderly gastric cancer patients: comparisons with robotic gastrectomy in younger patients and laparoscopic gastrectomy in the elderly. Gastric Cancer. 2016;19(4):1125–34.

9. Kim HI, Han SU, Yang HK, et al. Multicenter prospective comparative study of robotic versus laparoscopic gastrectomy for gastric adenocarcinoma. Ann Surg. 2016;263(1):103–9.

10. Lee J, Kim YM, Woo Y, Obama K, Noh SH, Hyung WJ. Robotic distal subtotal gastrectomy with D2 lymphadenectomy for gastric cancer patients with high body mass index: comparison with conventional laparoscopic distal subtotal gastrectomy with D2 lymphadenectomy. Surg Endosc. 2015;29(11):3251–60.

11. Son T, Lee JH, Kim YM, Kim HI, Noh SH, Hyung WJ. Robotic spleen-preserving total gastrectomy for gastric cancer: comparison with conventional laparoscopic procedure. Surg Endosc. 2014;28(9):2606–15.

12. Song J, Oh SJ, Kang WH, Hyung WJ, Choi SH, Noh SH. Robot-assisted gastrectomy with lymph node dissection for gastric cancer: lessons learned from an initial 100 consecutive procedures. Ann Surg. 2009;249(6):927–32.

13. Coratti A, Annecchiarico M, Di Marino M, Gentile E, Coratti F, Giulianotti PC. Robot-assisted gastrectomy for gastric cancer: current status and technical considerations. World J Surg. 2013;37(12):2771–81.

14. Park SS, Kim MC, Park MS, Hyung WJ. Rapid adaptation of robotic gastrectomy for gastric cancer by experienced laparoscopic surgeons. Surg Endosc. 2012;26(1):60–7.

15. Marano A, Choi YY, Hyung WJ, Kim YM, Kim J, Noh SH. Robotic versus laparoscopic versus open gastrectomy: a meta-analysis. J Gastric Cancer. 2013;13(3):136–48.

16. Zong L, Seto Y, Aikou S, Takahashi T. Efficacy evaluation of subtotal and total gastrectomies in robotic surgery for gastric cancer compared with that in open and laparoscopic resections: a meta-analysis. PLoS One. 2014;9(7):e103312.

17. Xiong B, Ma L, Zhang C. Robotic versus laparoscopic gastrectomy for gastric cancer: a meta-analysis of short outcomes. Surg Oncol. 2012;21(4):274–80.

18. Suda K, Man-I M, Ishida Y, Kawamura Y, Satoh S, Uyama I. Potential advantages of robotic radical gastrectomy for gastric adenocarcinoma in comparison with conventional laparoscopic approach: a single institutional retrospective comparative cohort study. Surg Endosc. 2015;29(3):673–85.

19. Son T, Hyung WJ. Robotic gastrectomy for gastric cancer. J Surg Oncol. 2015;112(3):271–8.

20. Hyun MH, Lee CH, Kim HJ, Tong Y, Park SS. Systematic review and meta-analysis of robotic surgery compared with conventional laparoscopic and open resections for gastric carcinoma. Br J Surg. 2013;100(12):1566–78.

21. Noshiro H, Ikeda O, Urata M. Robotically-enhanced surgical anatomy enables surgeons to perform distal gastrectomy for gastric cancer using electric cautery devices alone. Surg Endosc. 2014;28(4):1180–7.

22. Junfeng Z, Yan S, Bo T, et al. Robotic gastrectomy versus laparoscopic gastrectomy for gastric cancer: comparison of surgical performance and short-term outcomes. Surg Endosc. 2014;28(6):1779–87.

23. Woo Y, Hyung WJ, Pak KH, et al. Robotic gastrectomy as an oncologically sound alternative to laparoscopic resections for the treatment of early-stage gastric cancers. Arch Surg. 2011;146(9):1086–92.

24. Pugliese R, Maggioni D, Sansonna F, et al. Subtotal gastrectomy with D2 dissection by minimally invasive surgery for distal adenocarcinoma of the stomach: results and 5-year survival. Surg Endosc. 2010;24(10):2594–602.

25. Hyung WJ. Da Vinci® Gastrectomy procedure guide PN 873058 Rev B 8/13. © 2014 Intuitive Surgical, Inc.

26. Obama K, Hyung WJ. Robotic gastrectomy for gastric Cancer. In: Watanabe G, editor. Robotic surgery. Tokyo: Springer; 2014. p. 49–62.

27. Shinohara T, Kanaya S, Yoshimura F, et al. A protective technique for retraction of the liver during laparoscopic gastrectomy for gastric adenocarcinoma: using a Penrose drain. J Gastrointest Surg. 2011;15(6):1043–8.

28. Woo Y, Hyung WJ, Kim HI, Obama K, Son T, Noh SH. Minimizing hepatic trauma with a novel liver retraction method: a simple liver suspension using gauze suture. Surg Endosc. 2011;25(12):3939–45.

29. Kinjo Y, Okabe H, Obama K, Tsunoda S, Tanaka E, Sakai Y. Elevation of liver function tests after laparoscopic gastrectomy using a Nathanson liver retractor. World J Surg. 2011;35(12):2730–8.

30. Kim MC, Heo GU, Jung GJ. Robotic gastrectomy for gastric cancer: surgical techniques and clinical merits. Surg Endosc. 2010;24(3):610–5.

31. Marano A, Hyung WJ. Robotic gastrectomy: the current state of the art. J Gastric Cancer. 2012;12(2):63–72.

32. Almadani ME, Abalajon DD, Yang K, Hyung WJ. Robotic gastrectomy: the future. Transl Gastrointest Cancer. 2015;4(6):448–52.

Total Gastrectomy with D2 Lymph Node Dissection

14

Hiroshi Okabe

Introduction

Robotic surgery is becoming a standard option for prostate cancer surgery, which requires fine anastomotic techniques in deep and physically limited surgical fields. Radical gastrectomy for gastric cancer also requires precise and complicated procedures; thus, robotic gastrectomy (RG) has been employed by some surgeons to provide better patient outcomes. Retrospective studies have shown that the advantages include fewer complications, less blood loss, shorter hospital stays, and retrieval of more lymph node. However, there are few studies showing definite evidence of the superiority of RG in randomized controlled trials [1, 2]. Levels of technical difficulty are different among several types of surgery for gastric cancer. RG would be expected to show more advantages in more complicated surgery. Total gastrectomy (TG) with D2 lymph node dissection is one of the most technically demanding surgeries. Therefore, advanced upper gastric cancer requiring a TG would be a good potential target of RG.

The previous Japanese gastric cancer treatment guidelines ver.3 stated that splenic hilar lymph nodes (lymph node station #10) should be removed in TG with D2 lymph node dissection [3]. The standard procedure for complete removal of the #10 lymph nodes has long been a combined splenectomy. However, the results of a randomized controlled trial comparing spleen-preserving surgery and splenectomy (JCOG 0110) recently revealed that splenectomy increases postoperative complications but does not improve the survival of patients, at least for tumors that do not invade the greater curvature of the stomach [4]. Therefore, spleen-preserving TG either with or without #10 lymphadenectomy is now considered to be a standard surgery for upper advanced gastric cancer, while splenectomy is still an important option for tumors on the greater curvature.

A comparative study of robotic and laparoscopic TG showed the feasibility of robotic TG and retrieved greater numbers of lymph nodes along the splenic artery and at the splenic hilum in the robotic surgery group [5]. However, studies evaluating robotic TG for advanced gastric cancer, especially with a #10 lymphadenectomy either with/without splenectomy, are still very limited [6]. Therefore, surgeons should be aware that robotic TG with D2 lymph node dissection is still in the developmental stage, and its feasibility and benefits need to be investigated by future clinical studies. This subchapter will focus on the technical aspects of robotic TG with D2 lymph node dissection and describe the setup of the robot, patient positioning, and surgical techniques

H. Okabe (✉)
Department of Gastroenterological Surgery,
New Tokyo Hospital, Matsudo, Japan
e-mail: h-okabe@shin-tokyohospital.or.jp

© Springer-Verlag GmbH Germany, part of Springer Nature 2019
S. H. Noh, W. J. Hyung (eds.), *Surgery for Gastric Cancer*,
https://doi.org/10.1007/978-3-662-45583-8_14

of TG, especially of the lymph node dissection around the splenic hilum and the supra-pancreatic area.

Indications for Robotic TG with D2 Lymph Node Dissection

TG with D2 lymph node dissection is generally indicated for patients with upper advanced gastric cancer. The current Japanese Society of Endoscopic Surgery (JSES) guidelines state that laparoscopic TG may be considered for clinical stage IA-IB gastric cancer [7]. However, the evidence supporting the feasibility of robotic TG is currently very weak. Therefore, robotic TG with D2 lymph node dissection for advanced cancer is recommended to be performed as prospective clinical studies. Experience in performing laparoscopic TG with D2 lymph node dissection is also strongly recommended for surgeons.

Robot Setup and Patient Positioning

A patient is placed in a modified lithotomy position with both legs fixed apart using the levitators. Upper arms are fixed alongside the body. The first port is inserted through the umbilicus using an open method. Pneumoperitoneum is established with 8–12 mmHg, and two 8-mm trocars for the robot and two 12-mm trocars are introduced using video imaging. 8-mm trocars are inserted at the lateral sides just below the costal margins. Twelve-mm trocars are placed 1–2 cm below the central points between the umbilicus and 8-mm trocars.

The patient cart is then placed above the patient's head, and the four robot arms are docked, while the patient is placed in a 15-degree reverse Trendelenburg position with the left side up for better exposure around the splenic hilar area. The camera arm is connected to the umbilical port. The first arm is connected to an 8-mm trocar that is inserted through the left lower 12-mm trocar for monopolar scissors. The second arm is used from the right lateral 8-mm tro-

car for fenestrated bipolar forceps. The third arm is used from the left lateral 8-mm trocar for Cadiere forceps. Nathanson's liver retractor is placed at the epigastric area (Fig. 14.1).

Surgical Technique

Splenic Hilar Dissection

The procedure starts with the division of the greater omentum. Serosal invasion of the tumor requires that the omentum be divided near the transverse colon to perform a total omentectomy. The omentum is freed from the left side of the transverse colon, followed by the division of the left gastroepiploic vessels. The left gastroepiploic artery (LGEA) should be divided at its origin in order to remove splenic hilar lymph nodes. Fat tissue associated with the LGEA is held by the Cadiere forceps and retracted to straighten the vessel. It is important to identify both the proximal and distal parts of the splenic lower polar artery to determine its origin, because the LGEA arises from it in the most common type of variations. Medial retraction of the LGEA helps to identify the distal portion of the lower polar artery, which is running into the lower pole of the spleen. Cranial retraction of the LGEA helps to identify the proximal portion of the lower polar artery (Fig. 14.2).

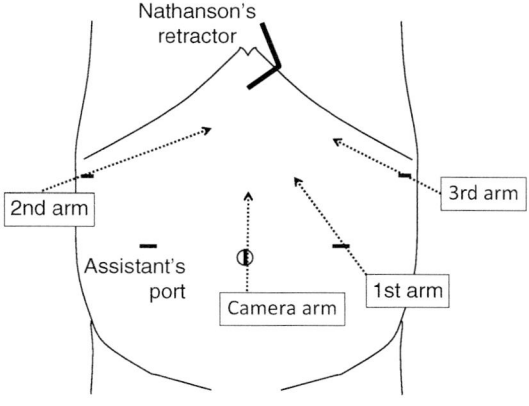

Fig. 14.1 Trocar placement for robotic total gastrectomy

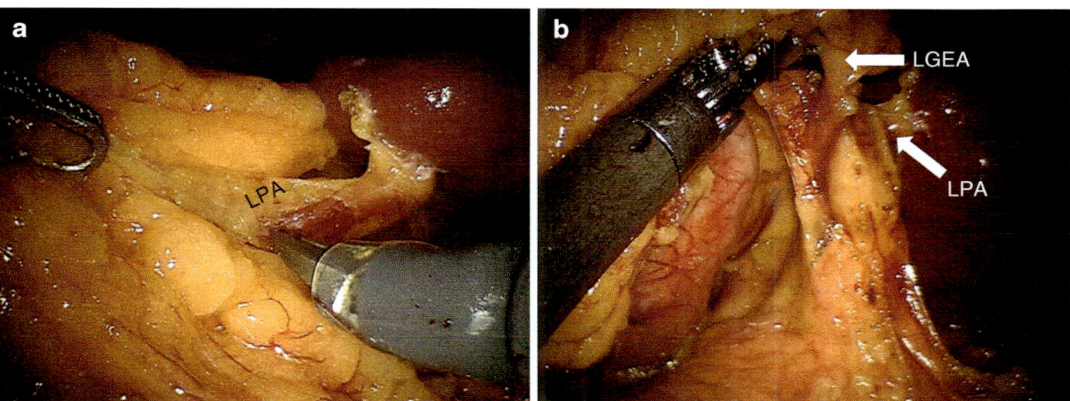

Fig. 14.2 (**a**) Dissection along the lower polar artery (LPA). (**b**) Isolation of the left gastroepiploic artery (LGEA) branching from the LPA

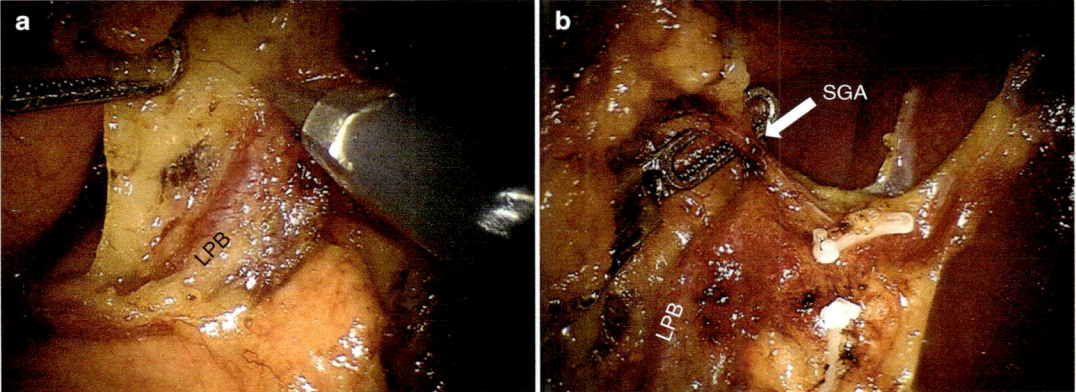

Fig. 14.3 (**a**) Dissection along the lower primary branch (LPB). (**b**) Isolation of the short gastric artery (SGA) branching from the LPB

The LGEA is divided at its root, and the omentum and the fat around the LGEA are lifted up over the stomach for better exposure of the splenic hilum. The gastrosplenic ligament involving the lowest short gastric artery is grasped by Cadiere forceps and retracted craniomedially. Stretching the gastrosplenic ligament with appropriate tension and dissection along the lower primary branch of the splenic artery help to identify the root of the short gastric artery (SGA; Fig. 14.3). Better visualization around the splenic hilum is obtained by further retraction of the gastrosplenic ligament with Cadiere forceps. Division of two or three SGAs allows identifying the bifurcation of the splenic artery (Fig. 14.4). It

is important to identify the bifurcation, because there are no short gastric branches in the area between the upper and lower primary branches of the splenic artery. However, it should be noted that three primary branches exist in 15–20% of cases.

Dissection along the distal splenic artery is done before dissecting the upper half of the splenic hilum. The perivascular nerve is preserved unless it is invaded by metastatic lymph nodes. The dissection progresses toward the distal side, and the remaining SGAs are identified. The origin of each SGA can be easily isolated by retracting the pedicle of the SGA with Cadiere forceps (Fig. 14.5). Division of SGAs allows further

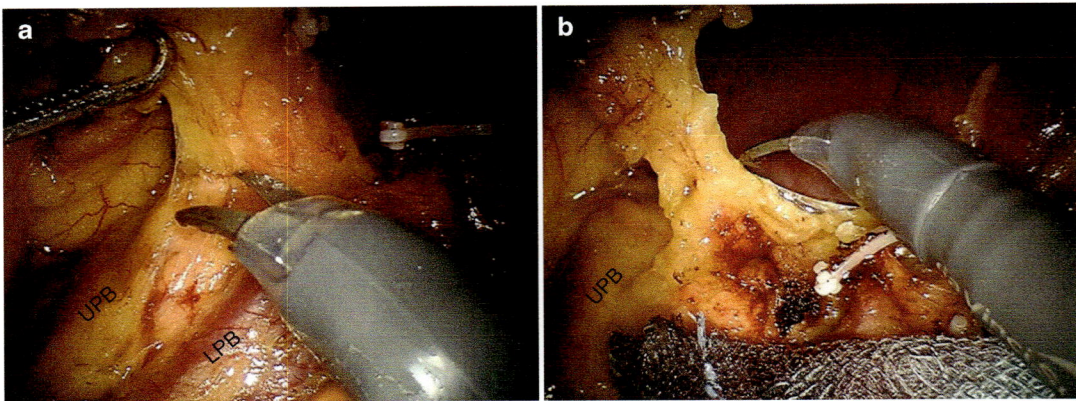

Fig. 14.4 (**a**) Bifurcation of the splenic artery. The pancreas is seen between the upper primary branch (UPB) and LPB. (**b**) Dissection of the area between the UPB and LPB

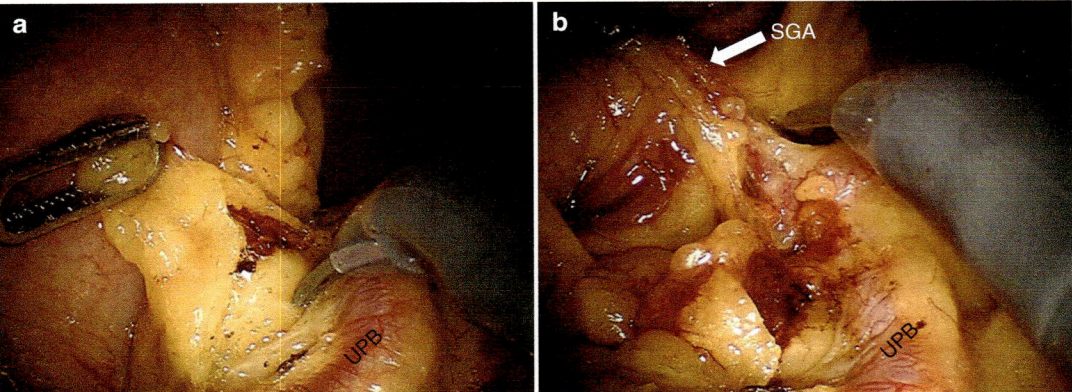

Fig. 14.5 (**a**) Dissection along the upper primary branch (UPB). The perivascular nerve is preserved. (**b**) Isolation of the short gastric artery (SGA). The pedicle is stretched to identify its origin

retraction of the gastropancreatic fold, and the fundic portion of the stomach is mobilized by dissection of Toldt's fusion fascia. The mobilized fundus is flipped over to obtain the better view around the splenic upper pole. The uppermost SGA is divided to finish the splenic hilar dissection (Fig. 14.6). It should be noted that the upper polar artery is found in about 40% of cases. The uppermost SGA usually branches from the distal end of the upper polar artery in those cases.

Dissection of the Left Side Gastropancreatic Fold

Division of all of the all SGAs is followed by cutting the gastrophrenic ligament to reach the left crus of the diaphragm. The gastropancreatic fold containing the splenic lymph nodes is cleanly dissected from the splenic vessels and the fusion fascia (Fig. 14.7). The dissection is continued in the medial direction, and the posterior gastric vessels are identified and divided at the roots. The splenic artery is then further dissected toward the proximal side to mobilize the #11p lymph nodes.

The gastropancreatic fold associated with the left gastric artery is retracted cranially with Cadiere forceps. Counter-traction is applied with the fenestrated forceps, allowing the common hepatic and splenic arteries to be dissected while the perivascular nerve is preserved. The coronary vein is divided, when it is drained to the splenic vein via the caudal side of the artery. Further

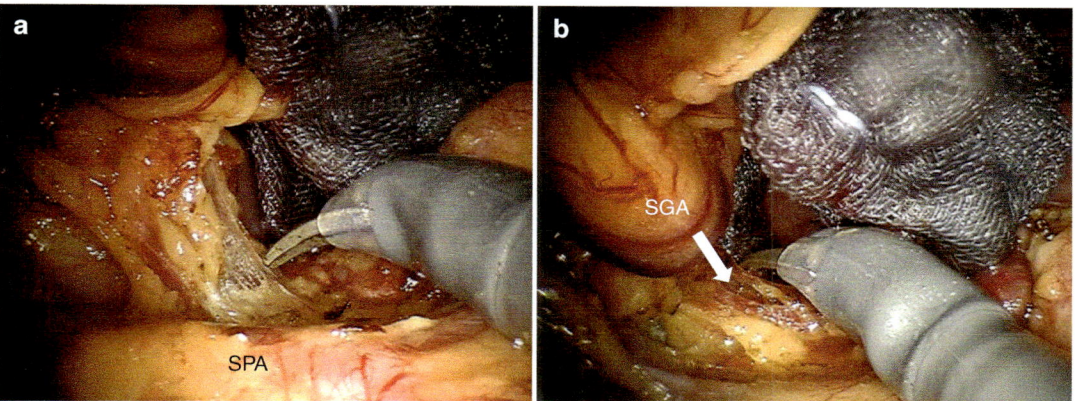

Fig. 14.6 (**a**) Mobilization of the fundus of the stomach by dissecting Toldt's fusion fascia. SPA, splenic artery. (**b**) The uppermost short gastric artery (SGA) at the splenic upper pole

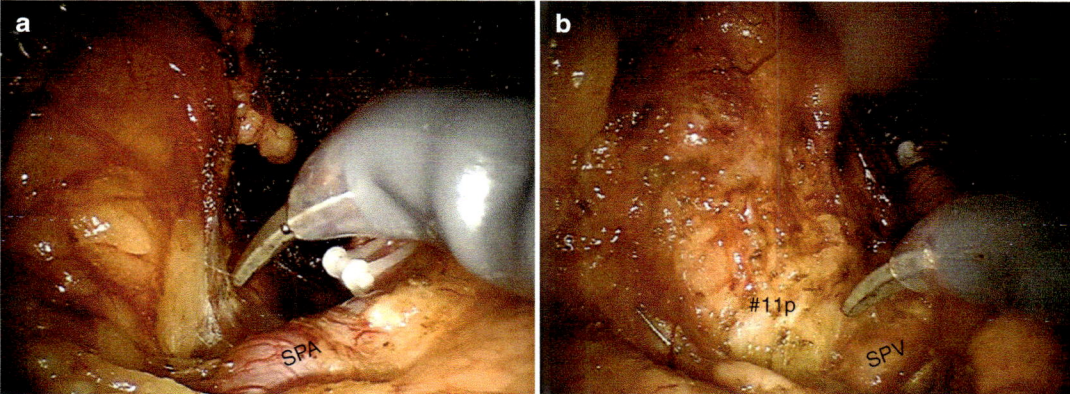

Fig. 14.7 (**a**) Dissection of the left side gastropancreatic fold. Dissection is done along the splenic artery (SPA) and Toldt's fusion fascia. (**b**) Dissection of the proximal splenic lymph nodes (#11p). The splenic vein (SPV) is seen at the bottom of the dissection

retraction of the gastropancreatic fold helps to identify the loose perivascular space alongside the left gastric artery. Dissecting the left space allows the #11p lymph nodes to be extracted from the retroperitoneum, with only the deep attachment to the pancreas remaining. Precise dissection is done to cut this attachment to completely remove the #11p lymph nodes. The splenic vein or the pancreas can be visualized at the bottom after the dissection (Fig. 14.7). The left gastropancreatic fold is dissected, exposing the left inferior phrenic artery. The fundic branch of the inferior phrenic artery is divided at its root to dissect the left paracardial lymph nodes, and the esophagus is isolated from the left crus. The

left crus of the diaphragm is exposed, and the left gastric artery is isolated and divided at its root (Fig. 14.8).

Dissection of the Right Side Gastropancreatic Fold

The right side omentum is next resected to expose the infrapyloric area. The robot may be undocked and the patient position reset to the simple head-up position in cases that underwent total omentectomy, in order to obtain better exposure of this area. The detailed technique of the dissection of the infrapyloric area is described in the previous

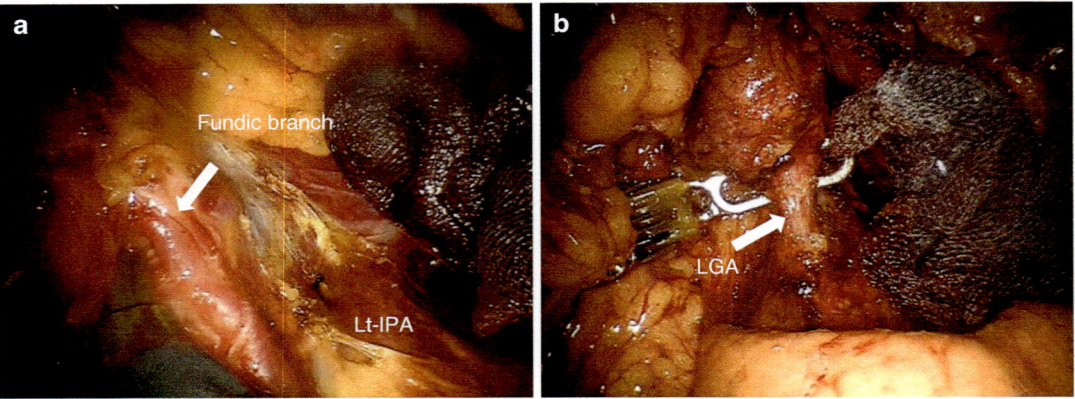

Fig. 14.8 (**a**) Isolation of the fundic branch of the left inferior phrenic artery (Lt-IPA). (**b**) Isolation of the left gastric artery (LGA)

subchapter. The dissection of the infrapyloric area is followed by transection of the duodenum with an endoscopic linear stapler, which is inserted through the left lower 12-mm port after removal of the da Vinci port for the first arm.

The pedicle of the right gastric artery is grasped with Cadiere forceps and retracted cranially. Applying the appropriate tension allows visualization of the loose dissection space between the #8a lymph nodes and the perivascular nerves of the common hepatic artery. The space is sharply dissected to mobilize the #8a lymph nodes. The direction of the retraction with Cadiere forceps is changed medially to approach the proper hepatic artery. A sharp dissection is done along the proper hepatic artery to isolate the right gastric artery. Division of the right gastric artery at its origin separates the right side gastropancreatic fold including the #8a, #12a, and #9 lymph nodes from the hepatic artery. Advancing the en bloc dissection of these lymph nodes requires the surgeon to control both the main traction by the Cadiere forceps and the counter-traction by the fenestrated forceps. The proper hepatic lymph nodes (#12a) are dissected by retracting the Cadiere forceps craniomedially, while the counter-traction is applied with the fenestrated forceps grasping the nerve fibers alongside the proper hepatic artery. The Cadiere forceps is retracted craniolaterally to dissect the right side celiac nodes (#9), and counter-traction is applied by the fenestrated forceps to dissect

along the perivascular nerves (Fig. 14.9). The #12a lymph nodes are dissected until the portal vein is exposed. The #9 lymph nodes are dissected until the celiac nerve plexus and the right crus of the diaphragm are exposed. The Hem-o-lok® is placed at the bottom of the lymph nodes to prevent the chyloleakage.

The dissection of the right side gastropancreatic fold along the right crus is continued to isolate the right side of the esophagus. The lesser omentum is divided toward the esophagogastric junction, and the anterior surface of the esophagus is released. The anterior and posterior vagal trunks are divided to completely isolate the esophagus (Fig. 14.10).

Reconstruction

The robot is undocked, and the transection of the esophagus and Roux-en Y reconstruction are performed laparoscopically. The esophagus is transected using an endoscopic linear stapler, which is inserted through the right lower 12-mm port. The umbilical trocar wound is extended, and the resected stomach is removed through it. Intracorporeal esophago-jejunal anastomosis is performed either with a functional end-to-end anastomosis or the overlap method. The detailed technique of the laparoscopic anastomosis is described in another chapter in this book or in a previous publication [8, 9]. A round-type suction

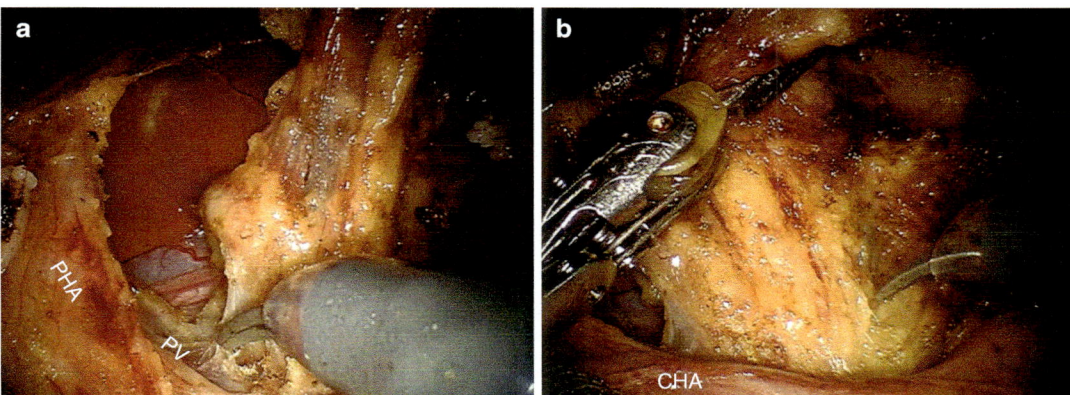

Fig. 14.9 (**a**) Dissection of the proper hepatic lymph nodes (#12a) along the portal vein (PV). PHA, proper hepatic artery. (**b**) Dissection of the right celiac lymph nodes (#9) along the celiac artery. Perivascular nerve is preserved. CHA, common hepatic artery

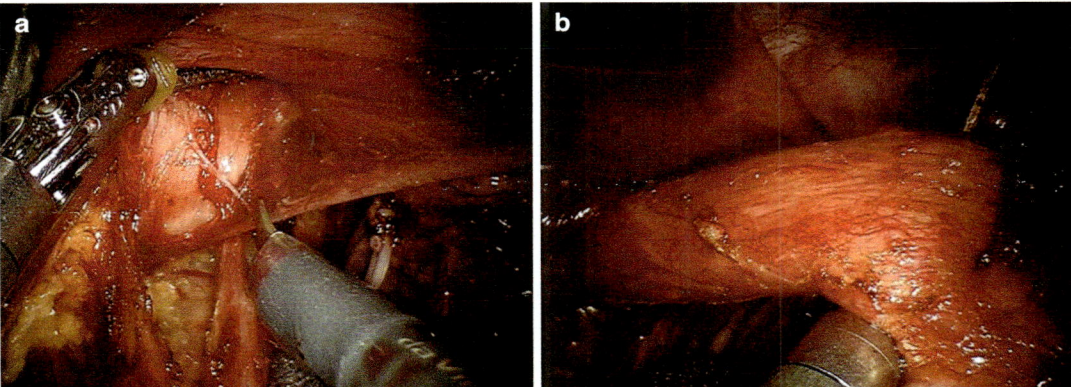

Fig. 14.10 (**a**) Division of the posterior vagal trunk. (**b**) Complete isolation of the esophagus

drain is inserted from the upper right port and placed behind the esophago-jejunal anastomosis. The operation is completed by closure of all trocar wounds.

Discussion

One potential advantage of robot is to make a technically difficult procedure, such as splenic hilar dissection and supra-pancreatic dissection, easier and safer by providing better dexterity. Pancreas-related complications, such as pancreatic fistula, peripancreatic abscess, or pancreatitis, are common complications following a D2 total gastrectomy. Heat injury and direct compression of the pancreas are potential causes of pancreas-related complications following laparoscopic surgery [10, 11]. Direct contact between the dissection device and the pancreas can be avoided in robotic surgery, thanks to its articulated shape, minimizing heat injury. In addition, the dissection around the pancreas can be done mostly without compression of the pancreas. Some retrospective studies suggest [5, 6] that major pancreas-related complications can be reduced by introduction of the robotic surgery.

On the other hand, there are still some technical issues to be resolved before robotic D2 TG can be accepted as a "technically feasible" option.

The first is the difficulty of the procedure in obese patients. It is very difficult to understand the vascular anatomy around the splenic hilum in obese patients during surgery. Careful dissection is necessary to identify each vessel, prolonging the length of the procedure. Preoperative evaluation of the branching pattern of the splenic vessels using CT imaging is strongly recommended in such cases. The second issue is how to obtain a good exposure of the splenic hilum in cases that require a total omentectomy or those with a large tumor. The exposure is usually obtained by lifting up the fundus with the omentum flipped over the stomach. However, the volume of the omentum can be so large that a portion of the organ obscures the view, especially in obese patients. Exposure of the upper part of the splenic hilum becomes more difficult in cases with a large tumor. One technique employed by some surgeons is suturing the stomach to the abdominal wall to prevent its falling down into the operative field. The third issue is the reconstruction. "Robotic" reconstruction generally uses endoscopic staplers that are operated by the assistant. The reconstruction method employed during laparoscopic surgery can be used in robotic surgery. However, this can be problematic when the assistant's stapler does not move where the surgeon intended it to be. A robotic stapler is under development, and further improvement in the future will yield the optimal technique.

References

1. Obama K, Sakai Y. Current status of robotic gastrectomy for gastric cancer. Surg Today. 2015;46: 528–34.

2. Kim HI, Han SU, Yang HK, Kim YW, Lee HJ, Ryu KW, Park JM, An JY, Kim MC, Park S, Song KY, Oh SJ, Kong SH, Suh BJ, Yang DH, Ha TK, Kim YN, Hyung WJ. Multicenter prospective comparative study of robotic versus laparoscopic gastrectomy for gastric adenocarcinoma. Ann Surg. 2016;263:103–9.

3. Japanese Gastric Cancer Association. Japanese gastric cancer treatment guidelines 2010 (ver. 3). Gastric Cancer. 2011;14:113–23.

4. Sano T, Sasako M, Mizusawa J, Katayama H, Katai H, Yoshikawa T. Randomized controlled trial to evaluate splenectomy in total gastrectomy for proximal gastric carcinoma (JCOG0110): final survival analysis. J Clin Oncol. 2015;33(abstr):103.

5. Son T, Lee JH, Kim YM, Kim HI, Noh SH, Hyung WJ. Robotic spleen-preserving total gastrectomy for gastric cancer: comparison with conventional laparoscopic procedure. Surg Endosc. 2014;28:2606–15.

6. Suda K, Man-I M, Ishida Y, Kawamura Y, Satoh S, Uyama I. Potential advantages of robotic radical gastrectomy for gastric adenocarcinoma in comparison with conventional laparoscopic approach: a single institutional retrospective comparative cohort study. Surg Endosc. 2015;29:673–85.

7. Uyama I, Okabe H, Kojima K, Satoh S, Shiraishi N, Suda K, Takiguchi S, Nagai E, Fukunaga T. Gastroenterological surgery: stomach. Asian J Endosc Surg. 2015;8:227–38.

8. Okabe H, Obama K, Tanaka E, Nomura A, Kawamura J, Nagayama S, Itami A, Watanabe G, Kanaya S, Sakai Y. Intracorporeal esophagojejunal anastomosis after laparoscopic total gastrectomy for patients with gastric cancer. Surg Endosc. 2009;23: 2167–71.

9. Inaba K, Satoh S, Ishida Y, Taniguchi K, Isogaki J, Kanaya S, Uyama I. Overlap method: novel intracorporeal esophagojejunostomy after laparoscopic total gastrectomy. J Am Coll Surg. 2010;211:e25–9.

10. Obama K, Okabe H, Hosogi H, Tanaka E, Itami A, Sakai Y. Feasibility of laparoscopic gastrectomy with radical lymph node dissection for gastric cancer: from a viewpoint of pancreas-related complications. Surgery. 2011;149:15–21.

11. Irino T, Hiki N, Ohashi M, Nunobe S, Sano T, Yamaguchi T. The hit and away technique: optimal usage of the ultrasonic scalpel in laparoscopic gastrectomy. Surg Endosc. 2015;30:245–50.

Reconstruction Methods After Robotic Distal or Total Gastrectomy

15

Sang-Yong Son and Sang-Uk Han

Introduction

Robotic technology has been introduced to gastric cancer surgery more recently than laparoscopic methods. Therefore, most robotic procedures, including radical lymphadenectomy and reconstructions, are based on those of laparoscopic surgery. Currently, various reconstruction techniques are used in laparoscopic gastrectomy, and these are currently reproduced by the robotic surgical systems, utilizing the improved dexterity resulting from the internal articulated endoscopic wrist [1–6].

Robotic systems provide surgeons with the possibility to perform precise sutures, even in deep and narrow spaces, and a few studies have reported on the feasibility of robot-sewn anastomoses. Hur et al. were amongst the first to report on the technical feasibility of robot-sewn anastomoses, applied in seven cases of robotic surgery for gastric cancer [1]. The median total operation time was 205 minutes and the median reconstruction time was 69 minutes, with the various reconstructions consisting of two Roux-en-Y esophagojejunostomies, two Roux-en-Y gastrojejunostomies, and three gastroduodenostomies. One patient was readmitted for stasis in the remnant stomach, but conservatively recovered.

Jiang et al. reported on the outcomes of robot-sewn esophagojejunostomy in 65 patients who underwent totally robotic total gastrectomy [2]. The mean times for total operation and esophagojejunostomy were 245 minutes and 45 minutes, respectively. One patient was readmitted for an intestinal obstruction and underwent reoperation; however, there were no strictures identified in any of the patients. Recently, a randomized clinical trial was conducted to evaluate the safety and efficacy of full robotic gastrectomy for gastric cancer with intracorporeal robot-sewn anastomosis [7]. A total of 364 patients with gastric cancer were recruited to this study, and 145 open gastrectomies and 151 robotic gastrectomies were finally analyzed. The operation time was significantly longer in the robotic gastrectomy group (242.7 vs. 192 min, $p = 0.002$), whereas blood loss was less (94 vs. 152 ml, $p < 0.001$), length of postoperative hospital stay was shorter (5.6 vs. 6.7 days, $p = 0.021$), and restoration of bowel function was earlier (2.6 vs. 3.1 days, $p = 0.028$). However, there was no significant difference in complication rate (10.3 vs. 9.3%, $p = 0.756$). The authors concluded that robotic gastrectomy with intracorporeal robot-sewn anastomosis is feasible and does not increase intraoperative or postoperative complication risk.

There is a recent trend for robotic gastrectomy reconstructions to move from extracorporeal procedures to intracorporeal procedures, referred to as "full or totally robotic gastrectomy," in which

S.-Y. Son · S.-U. Han (✉)
Department of Surgery, Ajou University School
of Medicine, Suwon, Republic of Korea
e-mail: hansu@ajou.ac.kr

© Springer-Verlag GmbH Germany, part of Springer Nature 2019
S. H. Noh, W. J. Hyung (eds.), *Surgery for Gastric Cancer*,
https://doi.org/10.1007/978-3-662-45583-8_15

all gastric resection and reconstruction are performed intracorporeally, under direct laparoscopic view, without a minilaparotomy. However, the advantages of the "totally robotic procedure" have not been firmly identified, even for laparoscopic surgery; its clinical benefits are assumed to be reduced postoperative pain, reduced surgical site complications, and enhanced postoperative recovery [8–11].

In this chapter, the technical details of intracorporeal reconstruction methods are discussed, including their advantages and disadvantages. A particular focus is paid to the Billroth I anastomosis after robotic subtotal gastrectomy and Roux-en-Y esophagojejunostomy after total gastrectomy.

Operative Setting and Preparation for Reconstructions

Patients are placed in the reverse Trendelenburg position to approximately 10–30°, which makes the stomach and colon retract downward due to gravity. This preoperative position setting is important for performing reconstruction after gastrectomy, as the ability to change the patient's position may be limited during the operation.

A five-port system is usually used for totally robotic gastrectomy. In distal gastrectomy, a symmetric port placement is recommended; two 12 mm trocars are placed on the infraumbilical area and the left lower abdomen because the first assistant usually stands or sits on the patient's left side. Three 8 mm trocars are placed on the right upper and lower abdomens and left upper abdomen (Fig. 15.1a). By contrast, an asymmetric port placement is recommended for total gastrectomy because the target organs such as the esophagus and spleen are located left of the midline. Especially of note is that the left-side trocars are placed more inferiorly than in distal gastrectomy, which allows the left-side robotic arm to have sufficient movement for splenic hilar dissection or esophagojejunostomy reconstruction (Fig. 15.1b).

After gastric resection with radical lymphadenectomy, the specimen is delivered via the extended umbilical incision. A pneumoperitoneum of 11–13 mmHg is then re-established, after temporary closure of the umbilical incision using towel clips or sutures. After the confirmation of free resection margins by frozen biopsy examination, intracorporeal anastomoses are performed, according to the extent of gastric resection and the surgeon's preference.

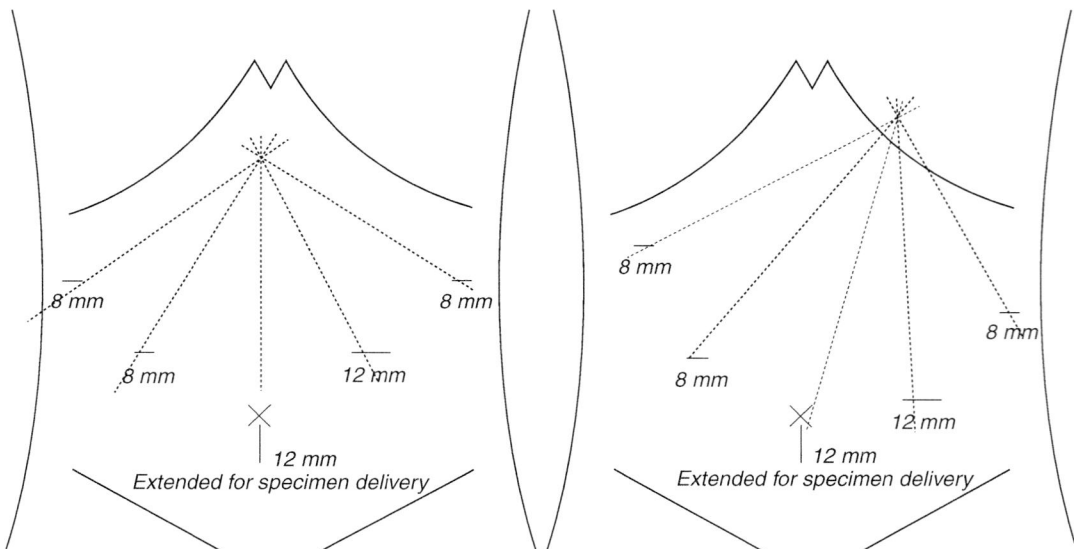

Fig. 15.1 Port placement for robotic gastrectomy. (**a**) The symmetric port placement for robotic distal gastrectomy. Two 12 mm trocars are placed on the infraumbilical area and the left lower abdomen. The left 12 cm trocar can be placed on the right side if the assistant stands or sits on

the patient's right side. (**b**) The asymmetric port placement for robotic total gastrectomy. The left-side trocars are placed more inferiorly than in distal gastrectomy because the target organs such as the esophagus and spleen are located left of the midline

Intracorporeal Billroth I Reconstruction after Robotic Distal Gastrectomy

The delta-shaped gastroduodenostomy was first introduced by Kanaya et al. for the intracorporeal Billroth I anastomosis [12]. The delta-shaped anastomosis is a functional end-to-end gastroduodenostomy technique performed using only linear staplers. Compared with extracorporeal Billroth I methods, it offers technical simplicity, wider lumen anastomosis, and a good surgical field (even in obese patients). There has been a general trend toward the use of delta-shaped gastroduodenostomy during the past decade; however, recent studies on delta-shaped anastomosis showed relatively high rates of anastomosis-related complications and bile reflux [11, 13–22]. Recently, an alternative method to delta-shaped anastomosis, so-called linear-shaped gastroduodenostomy, was introduced by Han et al. [23, 24]. At 6 months postoperation, endoscopic findings indicated that linear-shaped anastomoses showed significantly less food residue, gastritis, and bile reflux than delta-shaped anastomoses. However, there were no differences in endoscopic findings between the two groups at 12 months postoperation.

Surgical Techniques for Linear-Shaped Gastroduodenostomy

After infra- and supra-duodenal dissections, a 60 mm length of linear stapler is introduced through the left 12 mm port. The duodenum is transected in a cranio-caudal direction, without the 90° rotation that is crucial in the delta-shaped method (Fig. 15.2a). After completion of lymphadenectomy and gastric resection, an entry hole is created on the superior edge of the duodenal stump (Fig. 15.2b). Another entry hole is created on the greater curvature of the remnant stomach, about 60 mm away from the resection line (Fig. 15.2c). A 60 mm length of linear stapler is then introduced through the left 12 mm port, and the cartridge jaw is inserted into the stomach (Fig. 15.2d). The linear stapler is moved toward the duodenal stump, and the anvil jaw is inserted. The anastomosis is performed between the greater curvature side of the remnant stomach and the anterosuperior side

of the duodenum (Fig. 15.2e). After identifying the stapler line for bleeding, the common entry hole is closed by one or two 60 mm lengths of articulated linear staplers (Fig. 15.2f). In some cases, transient approximation of the entry hole using three stay sutures may be helpful for the tangential direction closure of the common entry hole.

Intracorporeal Roux-en-Y Esophagojejunostomy After Robotic Total Gastrectomy

Intracorporeal esophagojejunostomy remains the most critical and technically challenging step, even in laparoscopic surgery. Various methods for laparoscopic total gastrectomy have been introduced, but no standard protocol has been established. Intracorporeal reconstruction methods for Roux-en-Y esophagojejunostomy are categorized into the linear stapler and circular stapler methods, according to the type of stapler used for the esophagojejunostomy. Definitive evidence on the superiority of either method is still lacking. A recent review suggested that the circular stapler method is associated with a significantly higher risk of leakage and stenosis of the esophagojejunostomy: the rates of leakage for the circular and linear stapler methods were 4.7% and 1.1%, respectively ($p < 0.001$), while the rates of stenosis were 8.3% and 1.8%, respectively ($p < 0.001$). However, this study was not a systematic review but included 23 retrospective and 2 prospective studies [25].

The overlap method is one of the most favored linear stapler methods. It was first introduced by Inaba et al. in 2010 and has several advantages over conventional end-to-side anastomosis using a circular stapler [26]. Stapler handling is easier, even in a narrow space, and stapling can be performed regardless of the diameter of the esophagus [27, 28]. However, the overlap method that is currently being used has several technical shortcomings, namely, difficulties obtaining traction on the esophageal stump that necessitates the use of an additional stay suture, the risk of unintended stapling of the left crus, and the need for an additional stay suture when closing the common entry hole. Therefore, a modified technique that overcomes these shortcomings has been introduced, the so-called "modified overlap method using barbed sutures (MOBS)" [29].

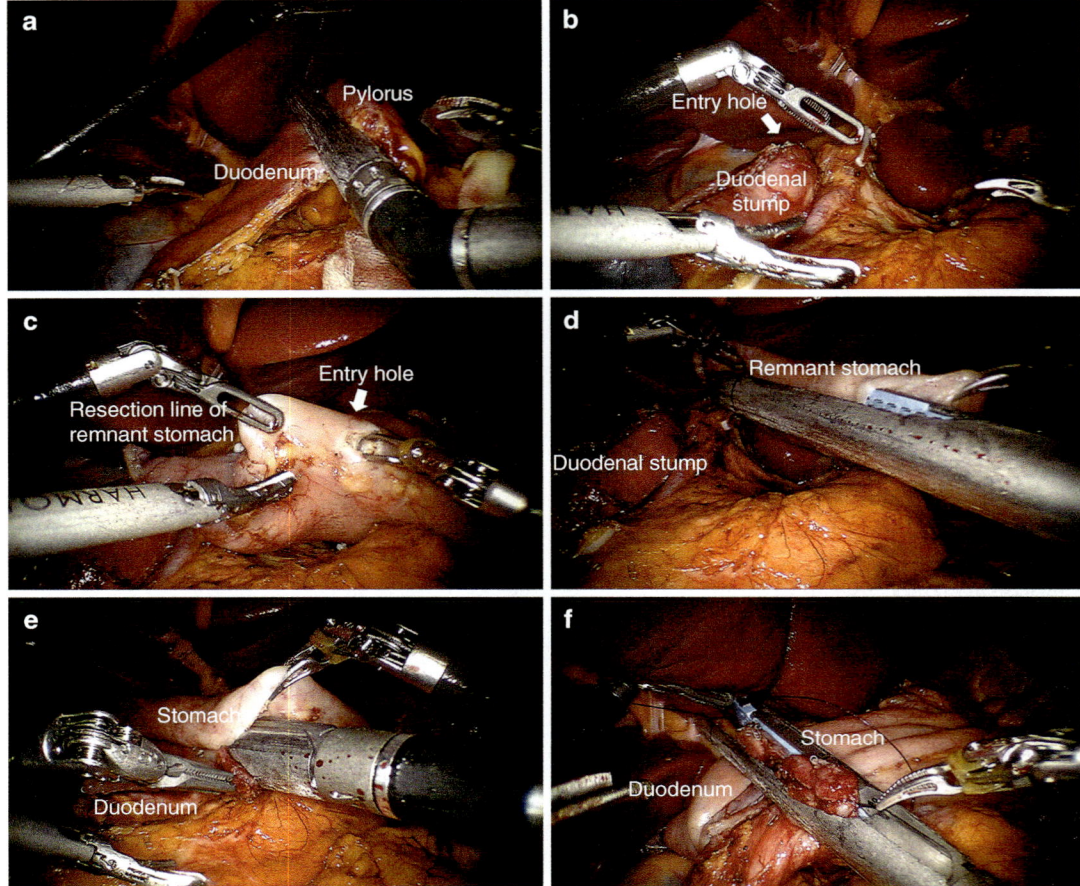

Fig. 15.2 Linear-shaped gastroduodenostomy (intracorporeal Billroth I method). (**a**) View of duodenal transection. Note that the duodenum is transected in a cranio-caudal direction. (**b**) Creating an entry hole on the superior edge of the duodenal stump. (**c**) Creating an entry hole on the remnant stomach. Note that this location is made on the greater curvature side, at least 6 cm away from the distal resection line. (**d**) Inserting the cartilage jaw of a 60 mm length linear stapler into the stomach. (**e**) First firing in the linear-shaped anastomosis. Note that the anastomosis is made between the greater curvature side of the remnant stomach and the anterosuperior side of the duodenum. (**f**) Closure of the common entry hole with an articulated linear stapler. Several stay sutures may be helpful for tangential direction closure of the common entry hole

Surgical Techniques for the Modified Overlap Method Using Barbed Sutures (MOBS)

After esophageal mobilization, a 60 mm length of stapler is introduced through the left 12 mm trocar, and the distal esophagus is transected transversely (Fig. 15.3a). After checking the free resection margins, two barbed threads are sutured on the stapled line of the esophageal stump (Fig. 15.3b). The distance between the two sutures is maintained at about 1 cm because their locations become lateral angles of the common entry hole after firing of the linear stapler. An entry hole is then made on the esophageal stump using ultrasonically activated shears (Fig. 15.3c). This technique is very useful for the surgeon to readily identify the intraluminal space with a sufficient opening because cutting the staple line means that the anterior and posterior walls are cut simultaneously. Another entry hole is made on the anti-mesenteric side of the jejunum, about 15–20 cm away from the Treitz ligament. The cartilage jaw of a 45 mm length of linear stapler is then introduced into the jejunum, and the jaws are closed, angled, and ascended toward the axis of the esophageal stump. Prior to esophagojejunostomy, the pre-sutured barbed threads are pulled downward to reduce the tension on the jejunal mesentery. The staple is then slightly opened, and the anvil jaw is introduced gently into the esophagus via the space between the right and left crura (Fig. 15.3d). After firing the stapler and checking the anastomosis, the com-

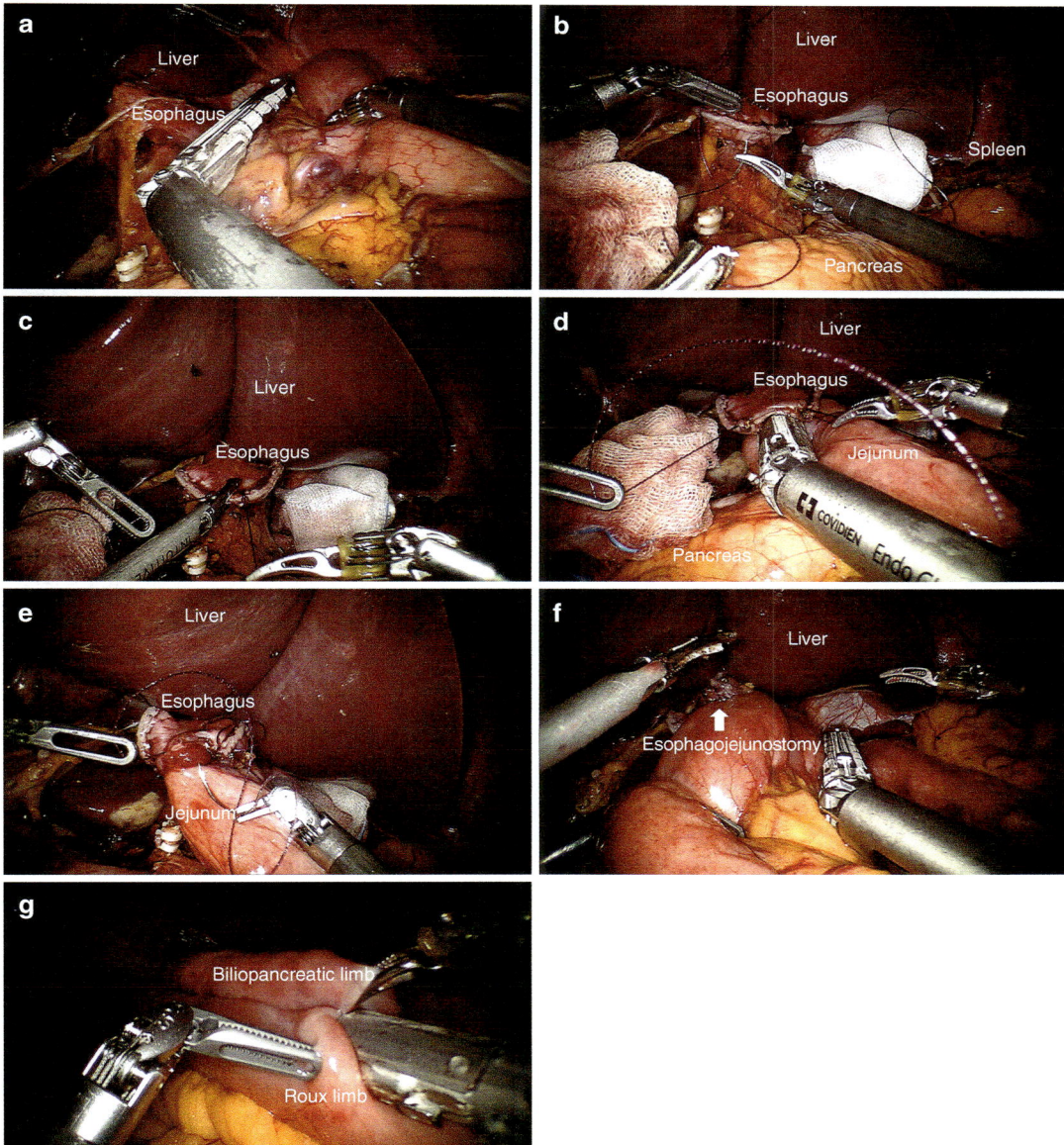

Fig. 15.3 Modified overlap method using knotless barbed sutures for intracorporeal Roux-en-Y esophagojejunostomy. (**a**) View of esophageal transection. Note that the esophagus is transected transversely. (**b**) Suture of two barbed threads on the stapled line of the esophageal stump. Note that the distance between them should be about 1 cm because their locations become lateral angles of the common entry hole after firing of the linear stapler. (**c**) Creating an entry hole on the esophageal stump using ultrasonically activated shears. (**d**) Firing a 45 mm length of linear stapler for esophagojejunostomy. Note that the pre-sutured barbed threads are pulled downward to reduce the tension on the jejunal mesentery during the anastomosis. (**e**) Closure of the common entry hole by the robot-sewn method using the pre-sutured barbed threads. (**f**) Division of the biliopancreatic limb and roux limb using a 60 mm length of linear stapler. (**g**) The making of a side-to-side jejunojejunostomy in a caudo-cranial direction

mon entry hole is closed bidirectionally by hand-sewing, using the pre-sutured barbed threads (Fig. 15.3e). Since the pre-sutured barbed threads are located at lateral angles to the common entry hole, they function both as a landmark and the stay sutures during the closure of the common entry hole. After completing the esophagojejunostomy, the roux limb and the biliopancreatic limb are separated by dividing the jejunum with a 60 mm length of linear staplers (Fig. 15.3f). A side-to-side jejunojejunostomy is made with two 60 mm lengths of staplers at the roux limb about 45–50 cm away from the esophagojejunostomy (Fig. 15.3g). At this moment, the stapler is introduced in a caudo-cranial direction. The mesenteric defect between the roux and biliopancreatic limbs should be repaired to prevent long-term complications such as internal hernia.

Conclusions

Recent advances in surgical instrumentation and techniques have allowed surgeons to perform intracorporeal reconstructions after robotic distal or total gastrectomy; these may reduce postoperative pain or complications and enhance postoperative recovery. Furthermore, the improved dexterity of robotic surgical systems may allow surgeons to perform precise sutures, even in deep and narrow spaces, such as in esophagojejunostomy. However, a meticulous and careful surgical technique with understanding of the concepts of each procedure is important for achieving optimal results and preventing anastomosis-related complications after robotic gastrectomy.

References

1. Hur H, Kim JY, Cho YK, Han SU. Technical feasibility of robot-sewn anastomosis in robotic surgery for gastric cancer. J Laparoendosc Adv Surg Tech A. 2010;20:693–7.

2. Jiang ZW, Liu J, Wang G, et al. Esophagojejunostomy reconstruction using a robot-sewing technique during totally robotic total gastrectomy for gastric cancer. Hepato-Gastroenterology. 2015;62:323–6.

3. Parisi A, Ricci F, Trastulli S, et al. Robotic total gastrectomy with intracorporeal Robot-Sewn anastomosis: a novel approach adopting the double-loop reconstruction method. Medicine. 2015;94:e1922.

4. Yang K, Bang HJ, Almadani ME, et al. Laparoscopic proximal gastrectomy with double-tract reconstruction by intracorporeal anastomosis with linear staplers. J Am Coll Surg. 2016;222:e39–45.

5. Quijano Y, Vicente E, Ielpo B, et al. Full robot-assisted gastrectomy: surgical technique and preliminary experience from a single center. J Robot Surg. 2016;10:297–306.

6. Kikuchi K, Suda K, Nakauchi M, et al. Delta-shaped anastomosis in totally robotic Billroth I gastrectomy: technical aspects and short-term outcomes. Asian J Endosc Surg. 2016;9:250–7.

7. Wang G, Jiang Z, Zhao J, et al. Assessing the safety and efficacy of full robotic gastrectomy with intracorporeal robot-sewn anastomosis for gastric cancer: a randomized clinical trial. J Surg Oncol. 2016;113:397–404.

8. Zhang YX, Wu YJ, Lu GW, et al. Systematic review and meta-analysis of totally laparoscopic versus laparoscopic assisted distal gastrectomy for gastric cancer. World J Surg Oncol. 2015;13:116.

9. Ikeda O, Sakaguchi Y, Aoki Y, et al. Advantages of totally laparoscopic distal gastrectomy over laparoscopically assisted distal gastrectomy for gastric cancer. Surg Endosc. 2009;23:2374–9.

10. Kim MG, Kim KC, Kim BS, et al. A totally laparoscopic distal gastrectomy can be an effective way of performing laparoscopic gastrectomy in obese patients (body mass index≥30). World J Surg. 2011;35:1327–32.

11. Kim MG, Kawada H, Kim BS, et al. A totally laparoscopic distal gastrectomy with gastroduodenostomy (TLDG) for improvement of the early surgical outcomes in high BMI patients. Surg Endosc. 2011;25:1076–82.

12. Kanaya S, Gomi T, Momoi H, et al. Delta-shaped anastomosis in totally laparoscopic Billroth I gastrectomy: new technique of intraabdominal gastroduodenostomy. J Am Coll Surg. 2002;195:284–7.

13. Kanaya S, Kawamura Y, Kawada H, et al. The delta-shaped anastomosis in laparoscopic distal gastrectomy: analysis of the initial 100 consecutive procedures of intracorporeal gastroduodenostomy. Gastric Cancer. 2011;14:365–71.

14. Kim DG, Choi YY, An JY, et al. Comparing the short-term outcomes of totally intracorporeal gastroduodenostomy with extracorporeal gastroduodenostomy

after laparoscopic distal gastrectomy for gastric cancer: a single surgeon's experience and a rapid systematic review with meta-analysis. Surg Endosc. 2013;27:3153–61.

15. Kitagami H, Morimoto M, Nozawa M, et al. Evaluation of the delta-shaped anastomosis in laparoscopic distal gastrectomy: midterm results of a comparison with Roux-en-Y anastomosis. Surg Endosc. 2014;28:2137–44.

16. Jeong O, Jung MR, Park YK, et al. Safety and feasibility during the initial learning process of intracorporeal Billroth I (delta-shaped) anastomosis for laparoscopic distal gastrectomy. Surg Endosc. 2015;29: 1522–9.

17. Lee HH, Song KY, Lee JS, et al. Delta-shaped anastomosis, a good substitute for conventional Billroth I technique with comparable long-term functional outcome in totally laparoscopic distal gastrectomy. Surg Endosc. 2015;29:2545–52.

18. Park KB, Kwon OK, Yu W, et al. Body composition changes after totally laparoscopic distal gastrectomy with delta-shaped anastomosis: a comparison with conventional Billroth I anastomosis. Surg Endosc. 2016;30:4286–93.

19. Lin M, Zheng CH, Huang CM, et al. Totally laparoscopic versus laparoscopy-assisted Billroth-I anastomosis for gastric cancer: a case-control and case-matched study. Surg Endosc. 2016;30:5245–54.

20. Lee SW, Tanigawa N, Nomura E, et al. Benefits of intracorporeal gastrointestinal anastomosis following laparoscopic distal gastrectomy. World J Surg Oncol. 2012;10:267.

21. Noshiro H, Iwasaki H, Miyasaka Y, et al. An additional suture secures against pitfalls in delta-shaped gastroduodenostomy after laparoscopic distal gastrectomy. Gastric Cancer. 2011;14:385–9.

22. Okabe H, Obama K, Tsunoda S, et al. Advantage of completely laparoscopic gastrectomy with linear stapled reconstruction: a long-term follow-up study. Ann Surg. 2014;259:109–16.

23. Byun C, Cui LH, Son SY, et al. Linear-shaped gastroduodenostomy (LSGD): safe and feasible technique of intracorporeal Billroth I anastomosis. Surg Endosc. 2016;30:4505–14.

24. Song HM, Lee SL, Hur H, et al. Linear-shaped gastroduodenostomy in totally laparoscopic distal gastrectomy. J Gastric Cancer. 2010;10:69–74.

25. Umemura A, Koeda K, Sasaki A, et al. Totally laparoscopic total gastrectomy for gastric cancer: literature review and comparison of the procedure of esophagojejunostomy. Asian J Surg. 2015;38:102–12.

26. Inaba K, Satoh S, Ishida Y, et al. Overlap method: novel intracorporeal esophagojejunostomy after laparoscopic total gastrectomy. J Am Coll Surg. 2010;211:e25–9.

27. Morimoto M, Kitagami H, Hayakawa T, et al. The overlap method is a safe and feasible for esophagojejunostomy after laparoscopic-assisted total gastrectomy. World J Surg Oncol. 2014;12:392.

28. Kitagami H, Morimoto M, Nakamura K, et al. Technique of Roux-en-Y reconstruction using overlap method after laparoscopic total gastrectomy for gastric cancer: 100 consecutively successful cases. Surg Endosc. 2016;30:4086–91.

29. Son SY, Cui LH, Shin HJ, et al. Modified overlap method using knotless barbed sutures (MOBS) for intracorporeal esophagojejeunostomy. Surg Endosc. 2017;31:2697–704.

Part VIII

Function-Preserving Surgery

Pylorous-Preserving Gastrectomy

16

Seung-Young Oh, Hyuk-Jun Lee,
and Han-Kwang Yang

Introduction

With the increasing proportion of early gastric cancer (EGC) and the excellent survival outcomes after treatment, surgeons are now paying attention to postoperative quality of life (QOL) to be as important as survival for these patients [1, 2]. Function-preserving surgery is a surgical approach which meets such trend. Pylorus-preserving gastrectomy (PPG) is a good example of function-preserving surgeries to reduce the surgical extent without compromising oncologic safety. PPG was firstly introduced by Maki et al. in 1967 for the treatment of peptic ulcers [3] and then was applied in gastric cancer in Japan and Korea. EGC located in the middle part of the stomach would be indicated, and with preserved pylorus, less postgastrectomy symptom or sequelae are expected.

Electronic Supplementary Material The online version of this chapter (https://doi.org/10.1007/978-3-662-45583-8_16) contains supplementary material, which is available to authorized users.

S.-Y. Oh · H.-J. Lee · H.-K. Yang (✉)
Seoul National University College of Medicine,
Seoul, Republic of Korea
e-mail: hkyang@snu.ac.kr

Indication

For PPG, to preserve pyloric branch of the vagus nerve, lymph node (LN) dissection around hepatic artery proper and right gastric artery is not done. Therefore, an important factor that should be considered before performing a PPG is the possibility of metastasis to LN station 5 around right gastric artery, and any case which can have LN metastasis in this area should not be indicated for PPG. In a study of the current status of PPG in Japan among 144 institutions, dissection of LN station 5 was not performed in 36.8% (53/144) and was partially performed in 56.2% (81/144) [4]. Our group had reported two important studies regarding the indication of PPG. Kong et al. analyzed the safety of lymph node station 5 and 6 in PPG using 1802 gastric cancer cohort [5]. In this study, if the tumor was located more than 5 cm from the pylorus, the metastasis rate of station 5 was 0% and 0.9% in T1a and in T1b, respectively. Similarly, the metastasis rate of station 6 was 0% and 1.8% in T1a and in T1b. Also, Yoo et al. reported the median and mean Maruyama index (MI, sum of the percentage of undissected lymph node station) of PPG as 0 and 0.8, respectively [6]. Both studies provided the background data of the oncologic safety of PPG and concluded PPG is safe for EGC located more than 5 cm from the pylorus.

Because the probability of LN metastasis increases as the depth of the lesion increases, the

© Springer-Verlag GmbH Germany, part of Springer Nature 2019
S. H. Noh, W. J. Hyung (eds.), *Surgery for Gastric Cancer*,
https://doi.org/10.1007/978-3-662-45583-8_16

depth of invasion should also be evaluated [5, 7]. For these reasons, PPG should only be considered only for patients with a cT1N0M0 gastric cancer. According to the Japanese gastric cancer treatment guidelines, PPG is indicated for the treatment of cT1N0M0 gastric cancers in the middle-third of the stomach, at least 4 cm away from the pylorus [8].

Surgical Techniques (Figs. 16.1, 16.2, 16.3, and 16.4 and Video)

The standard technique for PPG includes the preservation of the infra-pyloric vessels and the hepatic branch of the vagus nerve for the preservation of the pylorus functionally as well as structurally [4]. There are three types in accordance with the origin of the infra-pyloric artery, and the ligation points of the right gastroepiploic artery are different according to the anatomical type. According to a study by Haruta et al., the infra-pyloric artery originates from the anterior superior pancreaticoduodenal artery in 64.2% of cases (distal type), the right gastroepiploic artery in

23.1% of cases (caudal type), or the gastroduodenal artery in 12.7% of cases (proximal type) [9]. During LN dissection of station 6, the right gastroepiploic artery is ligated at its root in the distal or proximal types. In the caudal-type cases, the right gastroepiploic artery is ligated at a location distal to the origin of the infra-pyloric artery [4, 5, 10, 11]. The hepatic branch of the vagus nerve that innervates the pylorus usually follows the course of the supra-pyloric LNs (LN station 5) and should be preserved to maintain the motility of the pylorus. Most surgeons prefer to preserve the vagus nerve, rather than dissect supra-pyloric LN during PPG [7, 12–14], although surgeons commonly tried to completely dissect the supra-pyloric LNs in the early years of PPG [15].

Because an insufficient antral cuff length may lead to postoperative gastric stasis, a representative complication of PPG, the distance from the lesion to the pylorus needs to be carefully considered. When surgeons maintained an antral cuff length of 1.5 cm in the initial period of PPG, the incidence of postoperative delayed gastric emptying (DGE) was reported to range of 23–40% [12, 16, 17]. The relationship between the length of the antral seg-

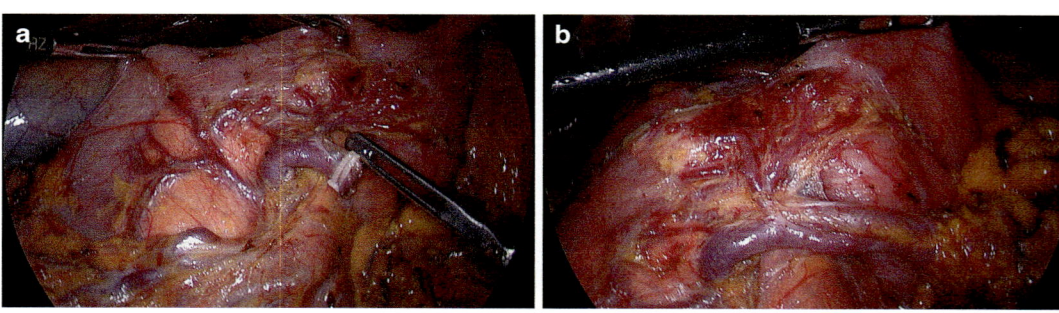

Fig. 16.1 (**a**, **b**) Preserving infra-pyloric vessels but lymph node around #6 station has been dissected

Fig. 16.2 Dissection of LN #8

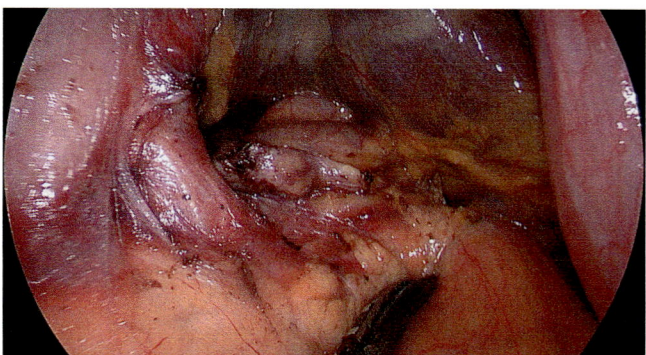

Fig. 16.3 Dissected LN #8, #7, #1, and #3. In this case, there was a replacing left hepatic artery from left gastric artery

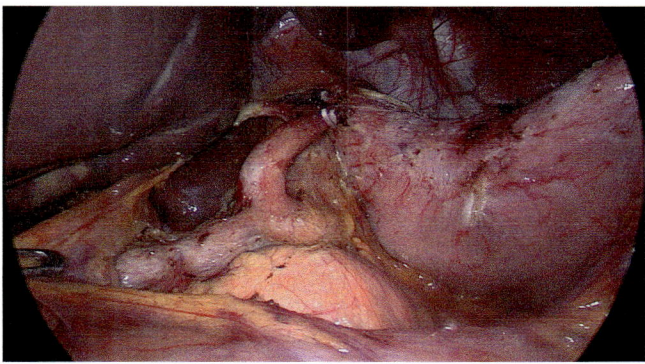

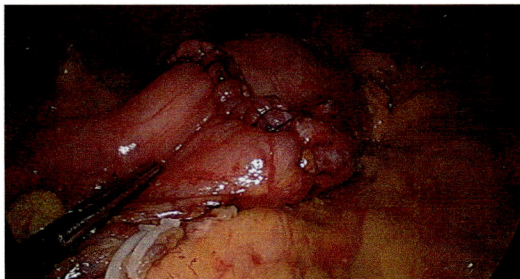

Fig. 16.4 Gastro-gastroanastomosis

ment and the incidence of DGE was investigated by Nakane et al. reporting an incidence rate of DGE of 35% (7/20) among patients with an antral cuff of 1.5 cm, compared to only 10% (1/10) among patients with an antral cuff of 2.5 cm, 1 year after PPG [18]. Nunobe et al. reported an incidence rate of DGE of 6–8% among 90 patients after PPG in whom vagus innervation and blood flow to the pylorus were preserved with 3 cm of antral cuff length [7]. As more studies on the PPG, the length of the antral cuff has tended to be longer. Considering a sufficient distal resection margin of >1 cm for EGC, current guidelines indicate that a minimum distance of 4.0 cm should be maintained between the side of the lesion to the pylorus. However, the optimal length for the antral cuff remains to be clarified.

Nowadays, pylorus-preserving gastrectomy (LAPPG) is commonly performed laparoscopically because patients who undergo PPG are diagnosed with EGC. Although the operation time is longer in LAPPG than in open PPG due to additional setting of laparoscopic surgery, LAPPG provides several benefits over PPG, such as reduced intraoperative blood loss and postoperative pain and a faster recovery [7, 15, 19].

For anastomosis, both extra- and intracorporeal methods can be performed for anastomosis in LAPPG. For the extracorporeal method, a hand-sewn anastomosis is usually applied. It generally requires an about 5 cm upper midline incision after laparoscopic dissection is finished (just before resection of the stomach). The distal part of the stomach is retracted through the incision and resected first. For the proximal side, after confirming the proximal margin by palpating a hemostatic clip applied preoperatively, lesser curvature side is resected by 10 cm linear stapler, and greater curvature side is anastomosed to antral cuff by continuous interlocking where hand-sewn gastro-gastrostomy is performed (or by interrupted Gambee suture). Intracorporeal anastomosis methods using linear staplers have recently been introduced. For the intracorporeal anastomosis, transection of the stomach in the sagittal direction (posterior to anterior direction), rather than in the *transverse* direction (greater curvature to lesser curvature direction), can facilitate the alignment of the linear staplers [20, 21]. After resection of the distal and proximal parts of the stomach, each arm of a 60 mm linear stapler is inserted into distal and proximal gastric remnants through the gastrostomy on the greater curvature side corner. The stapler has to be fired between the posterior walls on either side, and then the remaining gastrostomy can be closed using further staplers. [20, 21]

Robot-assisted pylorus-preserving gastrectomy (RAPPG) may provide another treatment option for EGC in the middle-third of the stomach considering benefits of robotic surgery including a three-dimensional and highly magnified imaging, a steady fixed camera, and an absence of a surgeon's tremors [22]. Han DS et al. reported that there was no significant difference in complication rates between the robot-assisted PPG and laparoscopic PPG groups. The mean number of examined lymph nodes (33.4 vs. 36.5; $P = 0.153$) and the mean number of lymph nodes at each station were not different between the two groups. RAPPG can be a safe treatment option for middle-third early gastric cancer in terms of surgical complications and oncologic outcomes. However, RAPPG has no benefit over LAPPG in this study [23]. In this study, the energy device was ultrasonic device in RAPPG group; future robotic device such as articulating energy device may improve the result. The benefits of RAPPG over LAPPG from patients' perspective remain controversial.

Oncologic Safety

Preservation of the vessel and nerves to maintain pyloric function may result in insufficient LN dissection at LN stations 5, 6, and 12a. An insufficient LN dissection would compromise the curative potential of radical gastrectomy in the treatment of gastric cancer. According to the Japanese gastric cancer treatment guidelines, D1+ lymphadenectomy should be performed in patients with a cT1N0 cancer [8]. LN dissection of station 6 with infra-pyloric artery preservation is a relatively easy technique, and LN station 12a is considered to be beyond the D1+ level in patients with cT1N0M0. However, LN station 5 is considered to be D1 level. In PPG, dissection of LN station 5 is not routinely performed in order to preserve function of the hepatic branch of the vagus nerve and, hence, of pyloric function. This could result in an incomplete D1 LN dissection, which is a concern regarding the oncologic safety of the procedure.

Sasako et al. used a new index (estimated by multiplying the incidence of metastasis and the 5-year survival rate of patients having metastasis to LN station 5) to evaluate the therapeutic value of LN dissection for gastric cancer, reporting a low index of 0.8 among patients with a cancer in the middle-third of the stomach [24]. The probability of metastasis to LN station 5 with an EGC localize to the middle-third of the stomach was also evaluated. Kodera et al. [25] reported the rate of metastasis rate to LN station 5 to be <5%, and Kone et al. [5] reported a rate of 4.2%. In both of

these studies, however, most patients with metastasis to LN station 5 were ultimately confirmed as having ≥T2 cancer after surgeries, whereas the metastasis rates to LN station 5 were very low among patients with T1 cancer. Furthermore, Hiki et al. [26] and Nunobe et al. [7] reported suprapyloric LN metastasis rates of 0.2% and 0.5%, respectively, among patients with T1 cancer located in the middle-third of the stomach.

In terms of long-term outcomes of PPG, Hiki et al. reported a 5-year survival rate of 98% among patients who underwent PPG for a cT1N0 gastric cancer without any case of recurrence [27]. Morita et al. reported a 5-year survival rate of 96.3%, with five cases of recurrence, among patients who underwent PPG for EGC [28]. Suh et al. reported a 3-year recurrence-free survival rate of 98.2% for LAPPG for EGC, which is comparable with the rate for LADG [14].

Advantages and Pitfalls

Compared to DG, PPG provides several benefits including a lower incidence of dumping syndrome, bile reflux, and gallstone formation, and better nutritional advantages, which is associated with a relatively small postoperative change in body weight [11, 14, 29–31]. Our group reported that PPG had fewer subjective postprandial symptoms, less bile reflux than distal gastrectomy [11]. Our group also reported that patients who underwent LAPPG had a better nutritional status, as compared with those who underwent LADG, including a smaller decrease in serum protein levels, serum albumin levels, and abdominal fat [14].

Gastric stasis is an annoying complication of PPG which makes surgeons to hesitate to perform PPG despite of many advantages. While the incidence of gastric stasis was as high as 40% during initial experiences with PPG [32], recent studies have reported the incidence of such complications after PPG of 6.2–10.3% [7, 14, 19, 28, 33, 34]. This value is still considered to be high, given that the rate of these complications after DG is about 1.0% [35]. Although the pathophysiologic mechanism of gastric stasis after PPG has not yet been fully defined, anastomotic edema and neurologic dysfunction, secondary to intraoperative damage, are known to be contributing factors [13, 32, 33].

Gastric stasis can be easily diagnosed based on a combination of symptoms, such as postprandial epigastric fullness or indigestion, with diagnosis confirmed by simple imaging, such as radiography or an upper gastrointestinal series [36]. Patients who developed gastric stasis after PPG may improve via conservative management and radiological interventions, such as balloon dilatation or stent insertion [23, 34, 36].

KLASS-04 Study: A Multicenter Prospective Randomized Controlled Trial

Currently, the comparison of the surgical, oncological, and patient-reported outcomes between LAPPG and LADG for the treatment of the middle-third of the stomach has only been evaluated in a few studies. Most of these studies were retrospective in nature, including data from a limited number of patients at a single center. To support the application of LAPPG in clinical practice, a comparative analysis of the short- and long-term outcomes of prospective randomized data is essential. In order to confirm whether the postoperative quality of life and nutritional status are better, and whether survival is comparable between LAPPG and LADG, the KLASS group has initiated a multicenter RCT (KLASS-04 study; NCT No.02595086) to compare LAPPG and LADG for the treatment of EGC located in the middle-third of the stomach.

A total of 256 patients, diagnosed with a cT1N0M0 primary gastric adenocarcinoma located in the middle-third of the stomach by EUS or CT, will be enrolled (128 patients in each group) (Table 16.1). The primary end point is the incidence of dumping syndrome, assessed using the Sigstad score (≥ 7 for dumping syndrome) at 1 year after surgery. The secondary end points are the 3-year relapse-free survival and overall survival; the 30-day operative morbidity and mortality; changes in body weight and fat volume on abdominal CT; postoperative changes in hemoglobin, protein, albumin, and prealbumin levels; symptoms and quality of life measurement using the JSGIS-Q, EORTC C30, and STO22; the incidence of gallstones; and the gross and microscopic findings on gastroscopy.

Table 16.1 Indications and contraindications for KLASS-04 study

Indications
$20 \leq$ age ≤ 80
Histologically proven gastric adenocarcinoma
Performance status of 0 or 1 on the eastern cooperative oncology group (ECOG) scale
$1 \leq$ American Society of Anesthesiologists class (ASA) ≤ 3
cT1N0M0 (by endoscopic ultrasonography or computed tomography scan)
Located at the middle-third of the stomach at least 5 cm away from the pylorus and resectable by distal gastrectomy
Written informed consent
Contraindications
Pyloric deformity due to ulcerative disease
History of gastric surgery (e.g., gastrojejunostomy or primary closure)
Synchronous early gastric cancer or adenoma in the antrum
Prior treatment with chemotherapy or radiotherapy against EGC diagnosed this time
Need for combined resection (e.g., cholecystectomy)
History of prior treatment (e.g., surgery, chemotherapy, or radiotherapy) against any other malignancies within the last 5 years (excluding cured basal cell carcinoma and in situ cervical cancer)
Lack of decision-making capacity
Pregnant or breast-feeding women
Currently involved or participated in another clinical trial within the last 6 months

References

1. Kim YW, Baik YH, Yun YH, Nam BH, Kim DH, Choi IJ, et al. Improved quality of life outcomes after laparoscopy-assisted distal gastrectomy for early gastric cancer: results of a prospective randomized clinical trial. Ann Surg. 2008;248:721–7.
2. Ahn HS, Lee HJ, Yoo MW, Jeong SH, Park DJ, Kim HH, et al. Changes in clinicopathological features and survival after gastrectomy for gastric cancer over a 20-year period. Br J Surg. 2011;98:255–60.
3. Maki T, Shiratori T, Hatafuku T, Sugawara K. Pylorus-preserving gastrectomy as an improved operation for gastric ulcer. Surgery. 1967;61:838–45.
4. Shibata C, Saijo F, Kakyo M, Kinouchi M, Tanaka N, Sasaki I, et al. Current status of pylorus-preserving gastrectomy for the treatment of gastric cancer: a questionnaire survey and review of literatures. World J Surg. 2012;36:858–63.
5. Kong SH, Kim JW, Lee HJ, Kim WH, Lee KU, Yang HK. The safety of the dissection of lymph node stations 5 and 6 in pylorus-preserving gastrectomy. Ann Surg Oncol. 2009;16:3252–8.
6. Yoo MW, Park do J, Ahn HS, Jeong SH, Lee HJ, Kim WH, et al. Evaluation of the adequacy of lymph node dissection in pylorus-preserving gastrectomy for early

gastric cancer using the maruyama index. World J Surg. 2010;34:291–5.

7. Nunobe S, Hiki N, Fukunaga T, Tokunaga M, Ohyama S, Seto Y, et al. Laparoscopy-assisted pylorus-preserving gastrectomy: preservation of vagus nerve and infrapyloric blood flow induces less stasis. World J Surg. 2007;31:2335–40.

8. Japanese Gastric Cancer Association. Japanese gastric cancer treatment guidelines 2010 (ver. 3). Gastric Cancer. 2011;14:113–23.

9. Haruta S, Shinohara H, Ueno M, Udagawa H, Sakai Y, Uyama I. Anatomical considerations of the infrapyloric artery and its associated lymph nodes during laparoscopic gastric cancer surgery. Gastric Cancer. 2015;18:876–80.

10. Sawai K, Takahashi T, Fujioka T, Minato H, Taniguchi H, Yamaguchi T. Pylorus-preserving gastrectomy with radical lymph node dissection based on anatomical variations of the infrapyloric artery. Am J Surg. 1995;170:285–8.

11. Park do J, Lee HJ, Jung HC, Kim WH, Lee KU, Yang HK. Clinical outcome of pylorus-preserving gastrectomy in gastric cancer in comparison with conventional distal gastrectomy with Billroth I anastomosis. World J Surg. 2008;32:1029–36.

12. Imada T, Rino Y, Takahashi M, Suzuki M, Tanaka J, Shiozawa M, et al. Postoperative functional evaluation of pylorus-preserving gastrectomy for early gastric cancer compared with conventional distal gastrectomy. Surgery. 1998;123:165–70.

13. Nishikawa K, Kawahara H, Yumiba T, Nishida T, Inoue Y, Ito T, et al. Functional characteristics of the pylorus in patients undergoing pylorus – preserving gastrectomy for early gastric cancer. Surgery. 2002;131:613–24.

14. Suh YS, Han DS, Kong SH, Kwon S, Shin CI, Kim WH, et al. Laparoscopy-assisted pylorus-preserving gastrectomy is better than laparoscopy-assisted distal gastrectomy for middle-third early gastric cancer. Ann Surg. 2014;259:485–93.

15. Hiki N, Shimoyama S, Yamaguchi H, Kubota K, Kaminishi M. Laparoscopy-assisted pylorus-preserving gastrectomy with quality controlled lymph node dissection in gastric cancer operation. J Am Coll Surg. 2006;203:162–9.

16. Kodama M, Koyama K, Chida T, Arakawa A, Tur G. Early postoperative evaluation of pylorus-preserving gastrectomy for gastric cancer. World J Surg. 1995;19:456–60; discussion 61.

17. Zhang D, Shimoyama S, Kaminishi M. Feasibility of pylorus-preserving gastrectomy with a wider scope of lymphadenectomy. Arch Surg. 1998;133:993–7.

18. Nakane Y, Michiura T, Inoue K, Sato M, Nakai K, Yamamichi K. Length of the antral segment in pylorus-preserving gastrectomy. Br J Surg. 2002;89:220–4.

19. Tanaka N, Katai H, Saka M, Morita S, Fukagawa T. Laparoscopy-assisted pylorus-preserving gastrectomy: a matched case-control study. Surg Endosc. 2011;25:114–8.

20. Lee SW, Bouras G, Nomura E, Yoshinaka R, Tokuhara T, Nitta T, et al. Intracorporeal stapled anastomosis following laparoscopic segmental gastrectomy for gastric cancer: technical report and surgical outcomes. Surg Endosc. 2010;24:1774–80.

21. Kumagai K, Hiki N, Nunobe S, Sekikawa S, Chiba T, Kiyokawa T, et al. Totally laparoscopic pylorus-

preserving gastrectomy for early gastric cancer in the middle stomach: technical report and surgical outcomes. Gastric Cancer. 2015;18:183–7.

22. Lee HJ, Yang HK. Laparoscopic gastrectomy for gastric cancer. Dig Surg. 2013;30:132–41.

23. Han DS, Suh YS, Ahn HS, Kong SH, Lee HJ, Kim WH, et al. Comparison of surgical outcomes of robot-assisted and laparoscopy-assisted pylorus-preserving gastrectomy for gastric cancer: a propensity score matching analysis. Ann Surg Oncol. 2015;22:2323–8.

24. Sasako M, McCulloch P, Kinoshita T, Maruyama K. New method to evaluate the therapeutic value of lymph node dissection for gastric cancer. Br J Surg. 1995;82:346–51.

25. Kodera Y, Yamamura Y, Kanemitsu Y, Shimizu Y, Hirai T, Yasui K, et al. Lymph node metastasis in cancer of the middle-third stomach: criteria for treatment with a pylorus-preserving gastrectomy. Surg Today. 2001;31:196–203.

26. Hiki N, Nunobe S, Kubota T, Jiang X. Function-preserving gastrectomy for early gastric cancer. Ann Surg Oncol. 2013;20:2683–92.

27. Hiki N, Sano T, Fukunaga T, Ohyama S, Tokunaga M, Yamaguchi T. Survival benefit of pylorus-preserving gastrectomy in early gastric cancer. J Am Coll Surg. 2009;209:297–301.

28. Morita S, Katai H, Saka M, Fukagawa T, Sano T, Sasako M. Outcome of pylorus-preserving gastrectomy for early gastric cancer. Br J Surg. 2008;95:1131–5.

29. Isozaki H, Okajima K, Momura E, Ichinona T, Fujii K, Izumi N, et al. Postoperative evaluation of pylorus-preserving gastrectomy for early gastric cancer. Br J Surg. 1996;83:266–9.

30. Song P, Lu M, Pu F, Zhang D, Wang B, Zhao Q. Meta-analysis of pylorus-preserving gastrectomy for middle-third early gastric cancer. J Laparoendosc Adv Surg Tech A. 2014;24:718–27.

31. Xiao XM, Gaol C, Yin W, Yu WH, Qi F, Liu T. Pylorus-preserving versus distal subtotal gastrectomy for surgical treatment of early gastric cancer: a meta-analysis. Hepato-Gastroenterology. 2014;61:870–9.

32. Tomita R, Fujisaki S, Tanjoh K. Pathophysiological studies on the relationship between postgastrectomy syndrome and gastric emptying function at 5 years after pylorus-preserving distal gastrectomy for early gastric cancer. World J Surg. 2003;27:725–33.

33. Fujita T. Outcome of pylorus-preserving gastrectomy for early gastric cancer. Br J Surg. 2008;95:1429; author reply −30.

34. Jiang X, Hiki N, Nunobe S, Fukunaga T, Kumagai K, Nohara K, et al. Postoperative outcomes and complications after laparoscopy-assisted pylorus-preserving gastrectomy for early gastric cancer. Ann Surg. 2011;253:928–33.

35. Kim W, Kim HH, Han SU, Kim MC, Hyung WJ, Ryu SW, et al. Decreased morbidity of laparoscopic distal gastrectomy compared with open distal gastrectomy for stage I gastric cancer: short-term outcomes from a multicenter randomized controlled trial (KLASS-01). Ann Surg. 2016;263:28–35.

36. Bae JS, Kim SH, Shin CI, Joo I, Yoon JH, Lee HJ, et al. Efficacy of gastric balloon dilatation and/or retrievable stent insertion for pyloric spasms after pylorus-preserving gastrectomy: retrospective analysis. PLoS One. 2015;10:e0144470.

Surgery for Gastric Cancer: Proximal Gastrectomy

Young Suk Park and Hyung-Ho Kim

Introduction

The incidence of gastric adenocarcinoma in the upper third of the stomach has steadily increased worldwide, and the incidence of early gastric cancer has increased sharply in East Asia. Because the long-term survival of patients with early-stage cancer is excellent, quality of life after surgery has become increasingly important. This has led to increases in function-preserving surgery, such as proximal gastrectomy and pylorus-preserving gastrectomy. However, conventional esophagogastrostomy after proximal gastrectomy has resulted in severe reflux esophagitis and anastomotic stenosis through acid regurgitation. Thus, many surgeons prefer to perform total gastrectomy rather than proximal gastrectomy for the upper-third gastric cancer.

According to the Japanese gastric cancer treatment guidelines [1], gastric resection can be modified for clinical T1 N0 tumors, and proximal gastrectomy can be utilized to treat proximal tumors. However, the proportion of patients undergoing proximal gastrectomy still remains low, and its oncologic safety and eligibility criteria remain unclear. New anastomotic methods after proximal gastrectomy may prevent reflux symptoms, as well as having nutritional benefits and improving quality of life.

Extent of Resection and Lymphadenectomy

Japanese gastric cancer treatment guidelines recommend proximal gastrectomy for early-stage proximal tumors, if more than half of the distal stomach can be preserved [1]. The extent of lymph node dissection in patients undergoing proximal gastrectomy is less than that in patients undergoing standard gastrectomy. D1 lymphadenectomy includes lymph node groups 1, 2, 3a, 4sa, 4sb, and 7, and D1+ lymphadenectomy adds groups 8a, 9, and 11p (Fig. 17.1). Lymph node groups 3b, 5, and 6, which are included in standard gastrectomy such as distal gastrectomy and total gastrectomy, are excluded in D1 lymphadenectomy of proximal gastrectomy to preserve the vascularity of the remnant distal stomach.

Lymph nodes in group 3a and 3b are anatomically defined as lesser curvature lymph nodes. Group 3a lies along the branches of the left gastric artery, whereas lymph nodes in group 3b are along the second branch and distal part of the right gastric artery (Fig. 17.2) [2]. By preserving

Y. S. Park
Department of Surgery, Seoul National University
Bundang Hospital, Seoul, Republic of Korea

H.-H. Kim (✉)
Department of Surgery, Seoul National University
Bundang Hospital, Seoul, Republic of Korea

Department of Surgery, Seoul National University
College of Medicine, Seoul, Republic of Korea
e-mail: hhkim@snubh.org

© Springer-Verlag GmbH Germany, part of Springer Nature 2019
S. H. Noh, W. J. Hyung (eds.), *Surgery for Gastric Cancer*,
https://doi.org/10.1007/978-3-662-45583-8_17

Fig. 17.1 The extent of
lymph node dissection
in proximal gastrectomy

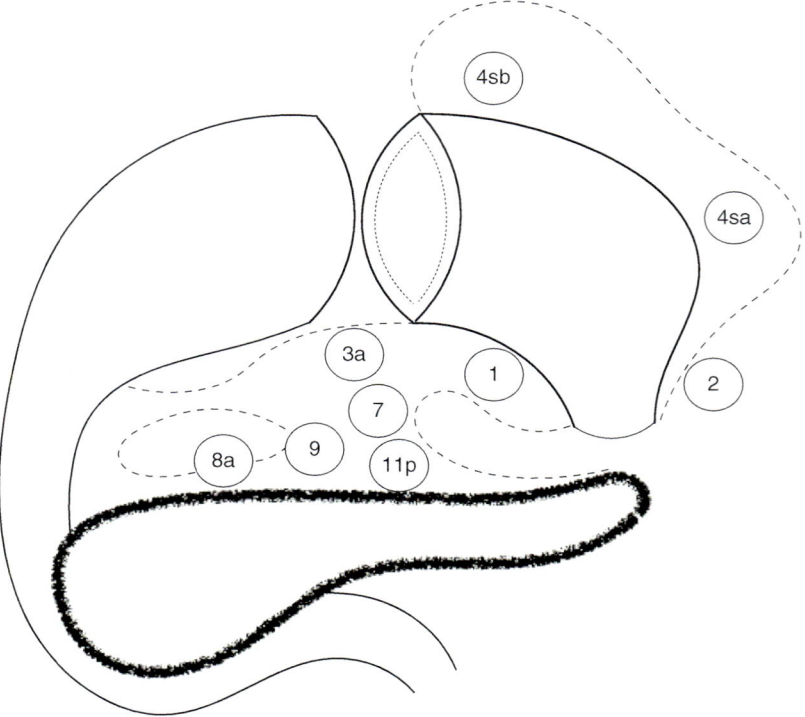

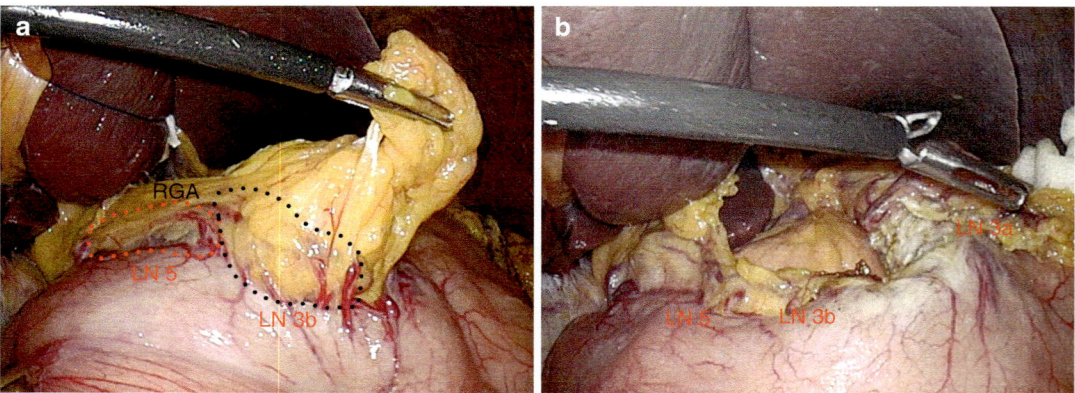

Fig. 17.2 Lymph node groups on the lesser curvature. (**a**) Lymph node group 3b and 5. (**b**) Lymph node group
3a, 3b, and 5

lymph nodes in area 3b and resecting the stomach
along the border between groups 3a and 3b, more
than half of the stomach can be preserved.
Therefore, the resection margin of the lesser curvature should be at or above the second branch of
the right gastric artery.

Reconstruction Methods and Complications

Esophagogastrostomy is a conventional reconstruction method widely used after proximal gastrectomy. Although esophagogastrostomy is a

simple, single-site anastomosis technique, it has been associated with high rates of long-term morbidities, such as reflux esophagitis and anastomosis stricture. These morbidities may be overcome by the addition of supplementary procedures, including (1) formation of a narrow (3–4 cm wide) gastric tube, with limited storage capacity, and esophagogastric tube anastomosis (Fig. 17.3) [3];

(2) preservation of the lower esophageal sphincter [4, 5]; (3) preservation of the hepatic and pyloric branches of the vagus nerve with or without pyloric drainage procedures, such as pyloromyotomy or pyloroplasty, to prevent delayed remnant gastric emptying which causes gastroesophageal reflux [3–5]; (4) creation of an acute angle at esophagogastrostomy, forming a new fundus (Fig. 17.4) [4, 6, 7]; (5) semicircular wrapping of the abdominal esophagus by the residual stomach, similar to a Toupet fundoplication (Fig. 17.5) [8]; and (6) a combination of the above procedures. These procedures were somewhat successful, reducing the rates of reflux esophagitis and stricture to 18–30% and 0–16%, respectively [3, 8–10]. Esophagogastrostomies with additional procedures are simple and easy compared to

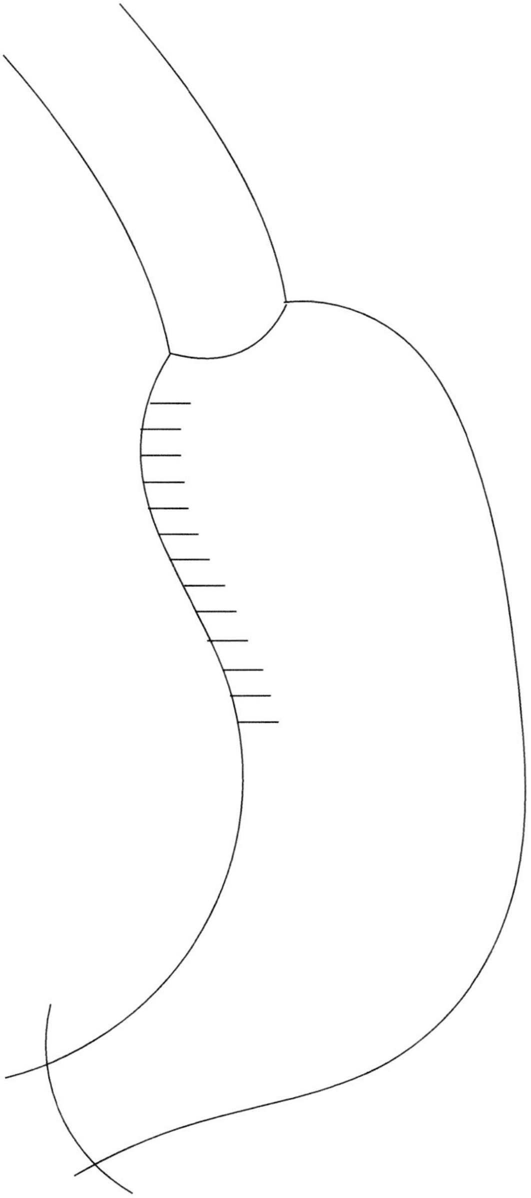

Fig. 17.3 Esophagogastric tube anastomosis

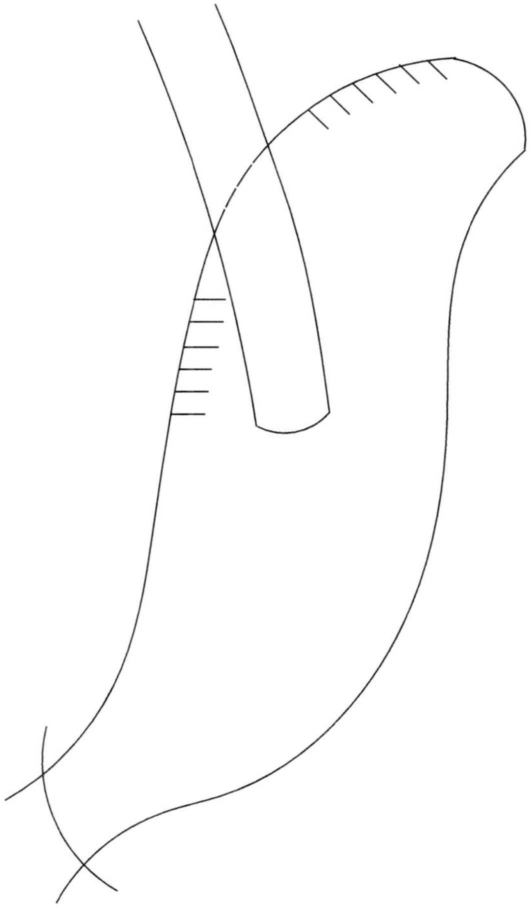

Fig. 17.4 Esophagogastrostomy with neo-fundus

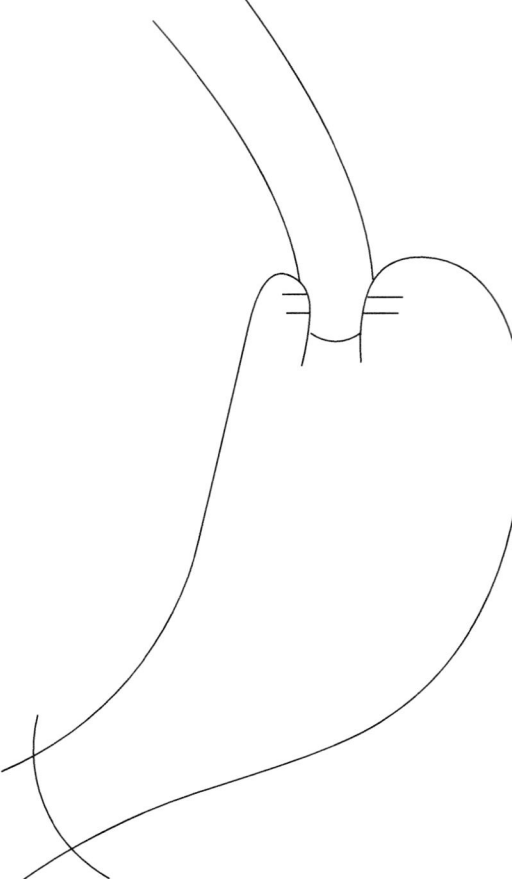

Fig. 17.5 Esophagogastrostomy with semicircular wrapping of the abdominal esophagus

the anterior wall of the gastric tube. After making a mucosal window at the bottom of the flap, 3–4 cm below the tip of the gastric tube, the esophageal and muco-submucosal layers of the stomach are sutured together. Finally, the completed esophagogastrostomy is wrapped with the seromuscular flaps. This double-flap technique can create a large pseudo-fornix, with the postoperative esophagogastrostomy shaped like the original cardia. Although this reconstruction is not simple, as well as being technically demanding, a laparoscopic double-flap method has been described recently [12].

The other alternative to esophagogastrostomy after proximal gastrectomy is esophagojejunostomy with additional anastomosis. Jejunal interposition consists of a short, 10–20 cm interposed jejunal limb and two anastomotic sites of esophagojejunostomy and gastrojejunostomy (Fig. 17.7). The rates of reflux esophagitis and esophagojejunal stricture after jejunal interposition have been reported to be 1.7–5.0% and 6.3%, respectively [13–15]. Although jejunal interposition is a powerful anti-reflux reconstruction method after proximal gastrectomy, the complexity of this procedure can induce internal herniation through the mesenteric window of the small intestine, which may result in the loss of a substantial proportion of the small intestine due to necrosis [6, 15].

Another method of esophagojejunostomy after proximal gastrectomy is double-tract reconstruction. This technique consists of three anastomoses: Roux-en Y esophagojejunostomy, gastrojejunostomy 15 cm below the esophagojejunostomy, and jejunojejunostomy 20 cm below the gastrojejunostomy (Fig. 17.8). Double-tract reconstruction therefore adds another anastomosis (gastrojejunostomy) to the conventional Roux-en Y esophagojejunostomy. Unlike jejunal interposition, this method maintains the continuity of the jejunum, making it easier to perform the procedure. Furthermore, it has a dual route for food passage, reducing the incidence of delayed remnant gastric emptying. The rates of reflux esophagitis and anastomosis stricture have been reported to be 0–25.0% and 4.7–10.0%, respectively [8, 17, 18]. To date, however, only a few

other anastomotic techniques after proximal gastrectomy. Therefore, these procedures are not difficult to apply to minimally invasive surgery such as laparoscopic or robotic proximal gastrectomy. This is another advantage of modified esophagogastrostomies.

In contrast to other modified esophagogastric reconstruction methods, the double-flap technique and valvuloplastic esophagogastrostomy are relatively time-consuming. Valvuloplastic esophagogastrostomy prevents gastroesophageal reflux by implanting the esophagus in a submuscular tunnel of the remnant stomach, which is expected to act as a one-way valve (Fig. 17.6) [11]. The first step in this reconstruction is to create double-door (H-shaped) seromuscular flaps in

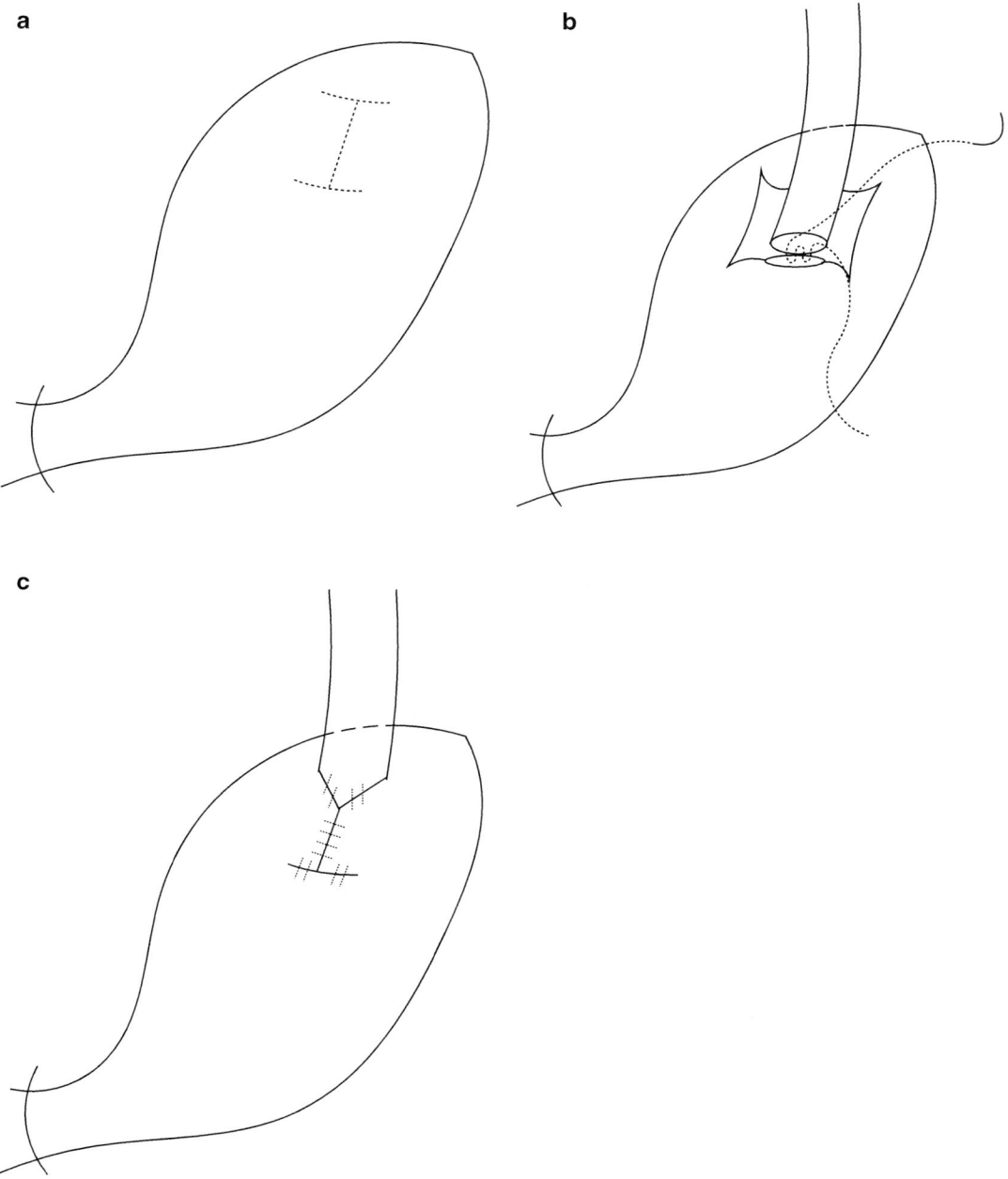

Fig. 17.6 Valvuloplastic esophagogastrostomy. (**a**) H-shaped seromuscular double flap. (**b**) Suturing of the esophagus and the gastric mucosal window. (**c**) Esophagogastrostomy covering with the double flap

studies have reported long-term functional benefits after double-tract reconstruction, indicating a need for additional studies to prove the functional superiority over other reconstruction methods.

Functional Benefits

The principal reason for choosing proximal rather than total gastrectomy is the preservation of a partial stomach. Patients are expected to eat suffi-

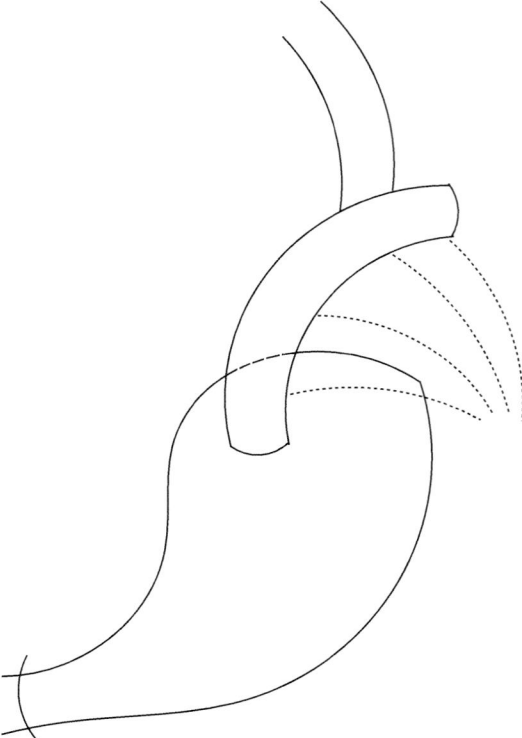

Fig. 17.7 Jejunal interposition

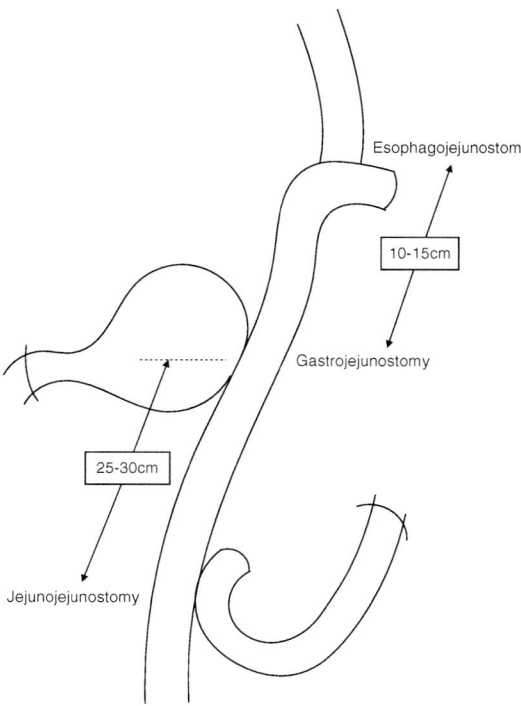

Esophagojejunostomy

10-15cm

Gastrojejunostomy

25-30cm

Jejunojejunostomy

Fig. 17.8 Double-tract reconstruction

cient food and maintain their preoperative body weight after gastrectomy. Maintenance of preoperative food intake is more frequent in patients who underwent proximal than total gastrectomy [19–21]. Ratios between postoperative 1 year and preoperative meal intake after proximal gastrectomy and total gastrectomy were found to be 68.3–71.0% and 63.6%, respectively [17, 22]. Consequently, in most studies, body weight maintenance was better in patients who underwent proximal than total gastrectomy [21, 23–25]. In contrast, one retrospective study reported similar body weight loss in both sets of patients, but the rates of long-term complications, such as stenosis (38.2%) and reflux (29.2%), were very high after gastric tube reconstruction in patients who underwent proximal gastrectomy [26]. These findings indicate that postoperative food intake and weight maintenance can be associated not only with the storage function of the remnant stomach but with late complications, including anastomosis strictures, reflux, and indigestion.

Several studies have used a standard questionnaire to evaluate gastrointestinal symptoms after proximal gastrectomy [3, 21]. Postgastrectomy symptoms, such as diarrhea, dumping syndrome, dysphagia, and reflux, are similar between proximal and total gastrectomy or less frequent following proximal gastrectomy [21]. A comparison of symptoms before and after proximal gastrectomy also showed no deterioration after surgery [3].

The rate of postoperative anemia was lower after proximal than after total gastrectomy [14, 20, 24, 25]. Anemia may be prevented after proximal gastrectomy due to the secretion of gastric intrinsic factor from residual gastric mucosa cells. Retrospective studies showed that serum vitamin B12 was significantly higher after proximal than after total gastrectomy [16, 25]. Moreover, iron may be better absorbed by the duodenum during food passage through the preserved natural gastrointestinal tract after proximal gastrectomy, but this should be clarified in future studies.

Oncologic Safety

Major concerns related to the oncologic safety of proximal gastrectomy for cancers in the upper third of the stomach include long-term survival;

metastasis of the supra- and infrapyloric lymph nodes, which may not be removed during proximal gastrectomy; and recurrent or metachronous cancer of the remnant stomach.

To date, no large-scale prospective randomized controlled trials have shown that proximal gastrectomy achieves oncologic outcomes equivalent to those of total gastrectomy. However, several prospective single-arm studies and meta-analyses [27, 28], as well as retrospective studies, suggest that long-term survival after proximal and total gastrectomy is comparable. Moreover, proximal gastrectomy in most East Asian countries is limited to patients with early-stage gastric cancer. Early gastric cancer of the upper third of the stomach seldom metastasizes to lymph nodes around the pylorus. Several retrospective studies [29, 30] have also reported that lymph node metastasis along the lower stomach (right-sided greater curvature nodes along the right gastroepiploic artery, and supra- and infrapyloric nodes, corresponding to lymph node groups 4d, 5, and 6, respectively, as defined by the Japanese Gastric Cancer Association [31]) was not observed in patients with proximal cancer confined to the muscularis propria. A retrospective analysis of a large cohort of Japanese patients with esophagogastric junctional adenocarcinoma found that the incidences of metastasis to nodal groups 5 and 6 were 1.7% and 0.8%, respectively, even when patients with advanced tumors were included [32]. This very low incidence of metastasis to lymph nodes along the lower stomach showed little impact on survival after proximal gastrectomy.

Although total gastrectomy eliminates the occurrence of cancer of the remnant stomach, it is not routinely performed in patients with lower-third gastric cancer to prevent remnant gastric cancer. Similarly, total gastrectomy should not be routinely performed in patients with upper-third gastric cancer solely to prevent cancer in the remnant stomach. However, the rate of remnant stomach cancer was reported higher after proximal (5.3–6.3%) than after distal gastrectomy [14, 15, 33]. Regular endoscopic screening of asymptomatic patients is therefore required for early detection of remnant gastric cancer after proximal as well as after distal gastrectomy. A retrospective

study revealed that endoscopic evaluation of the remnant stomach may be difficult after jejunal interposition or double-tract reconstruction if the distance between the esophagojejunostomy and gastrojejunostomy is longer than 10 cm [13]. However, shorter distance between them may lead to higher chance of gastroesophageal reflux. Therefore, surgeons have to carefully decide the distance between the two anastomosis sites when performing sphincter-substituting reconstructions, considering the postoperative endoscopic evaluation of the remnant stomach as well as reflux symptom.

Conclusion

Proximal gastrectomy may be a standard procedure for patients with early gastric cancer involving the upper third of the stomach because of its favorable outcomes. However, applicability of proximal gastrectomy to patients with advanced-stage cancer needs to be carefully debated.

Although the optimal reconstruction method after proximal gastrectomy remains unclear, current modified anastomotic techniques are sufficient to make proximal gastrectomy a useful function-preserving procedure. To confirm this conclusion, a large-scale randomized trial comparing the long-term survival and functional benefits of reconstruction techniques after proximal gastrectomy is required.

References

1. Japanese Gastric Cancer Association. Japanese gastric cancer treatment guidelines 2014 (ver. 4). Gastric Cancer. 2016;20(1):1–19.
2. Sano T, Aiko T. Japanese classifications and treatment guidelines for gastric cancer: revision concepts and major revised points. Gastric Cancer. 2011;14(2):97–100.
3. Ronellenfitsch U, Najmeh S, Andalib A, Perera RM, Rousseau MC, Mulder DS, et al. Functional outcomes and quality of life after proximal gastrectomy with esophagogastrostomy using a narrow gastric conduit. Ann Surg Oncol. 2015;22(3):772–9.
4. Tomita R. Surgical techniques to prevent reflux esophagitis in proximal gastrectomy reconstructed by esophagogastrostomy with preservation of the lower esophageal sphincter, pyloric and celiac branches of

the vagal nerve, and reconstruction of the new His angle for early proximal gastric cancer. Surg Today. 2015;46:827–34.

5. Huh YJ, Lee HJ, Oh SY, Lee KG, Yang JY, Ahn HS, et al. Clinical outcome of modified laparoscopy-assisted proximal gastrectomy compared to conventional proximal gastrectomy or total gastrectomy for upper-third early gastric cancer with special references to postoperative reflux esophagitis. J Gastric Cancer. 2015;15(3):191–200.

6. Yasuda A, Yasuda T, Imamoto H, Kato H, Nishiki K, Iwama M, et al. A newly modified esophagogastrostomy with a reliable angle of his by placing a gastric tube in the lower mediastinum in laparoscopy-assisted proximal gastrectomy. Gastric Cancer. 2015;18(4):850–8.

7. Ichikawa D, Komatsu S, Okamoto K, Shiozaki A, Fujiwara H, Otsuji E. Esophagogastrostomy using a circular stapler in laparoscopy-assisted proximal gastrectomy with an incision in the left abdomen. Langenbeck's archives of surgery. Deutsche Gesellschaft fur Chirurgie. 2012;397(1):57–62.

8. Sakuramoto S, Yamashita K, Kikuchi S, Futawatari N, Katada N, Moriya H, et al. Clinical experience of laparoscopy-assisted proximal gastrectomy with Toupet-like partial fundoplication in early gastric cancer for preventing reflux esophagitis. J Am Coll Surg. 2009;209(3):344–51.

9. Kosuga T, Ichikawa D, Komatsu S, Okamoto K, Konishi H, Shiozaki A, et al. Feasibility and nutritional benefits of laparoscopic proximal gastrectomy for early gastric cancer in the upper stomach. Ann Surg Oncol. 2015;22(Suppl 3):929–35.

10. Ichikawa D, Komatsu S, Okamoto K, Shiozaki A, Fujiwara H, Otsuji E. Evaluation of symptoms related to reflux esophagitis in patients with esophagogastrostomy after proximal gastrectomy. Langenbeck's archives of surgery. Deutsche Gesellschaft fur Chirurgie. 2013;398(5):697–701.

11. Kuroda S, Nishizaki M, Kikuchi S, Noma K, Tanabe S, Kagawa S, et al. Double-flap technique as an antireflux procedure in esophagogastrostomy after proximal gastrectomy. J Am Coll Surg. 2016;223(2):e7–e13.

12. Muraoka A, Kobayashi M, Kokudo Y. Laparoscopy-assisted proximal gastrectomy with the hinged double flap method. World J Surg. 2016;40:2419–24.

13. Tokunaga M, Ohyama S, Hiki N, Hoshino E, Nunobe S, Fukunaga T, et al. Endoscopic evaluation of reflux esophagitis after proximal gastrectomy: comparison between esophagogastric anastomosis and jejunal interposition. World J Surg. 2008;32(7):1473–7.

14. Nozaki I, Hato S, Kobatake T, Ohta K, Kubo Y, Kurita A. Long-term outcome after proximal gastrectomy with jejunal interposition for gastric cancer compared with total gastrectomy. World J Surg. 2013;37(3):558–64.

15. Katai H, Morita S, Saka M, Taniguchi H, Fukagawa T. Long-term outcome after proximal gastrectomy with jejunal interposition for suspected early cancer in the upper third of the stomach. Br J Surg. 2010;97(4):558–62.

16. Yoo CH, Sohn BH, Han WK, Pae WK. Proximal gastrectomy reconstructed by jejunal pouch interposition for upper third gastric cancer: prospective randomized study. World J Surg. 2005;29(12):1592–9.

17. Nomura E, Lee SW, Kawai M, Yamazaki M, Nabeshima K, Nakamura K, et al. Functional outcomes by reconstruction technique following laparoscopic proximal gastrectomy for gastric cancer: double tract versus jejunal interposition. World J Surg Oncol. 2014;12:20.

18. Ahn SH, do H J, Son SY, Lee CM, do J P, Kim HH. Laparoscopic double-tract proximal gastrectomy for proximal early gastric cancer. Gastric Cancer. 2014;17(3):562–70.

19. Ichikawa D, Ueshima Y, Shirono K, Kan K, Shioaki Y, Lee CJ, et al. Esophagogastrostomy reconstruction after limited proximal gastrectomy. Hepato-Gastroenterology. 2001;48(42):1797–801.

20. Zhao P, Xiao SM, Tang LC, Ding Z, Zhou X, Chen XD. Proximal gastrectomy with jejunal interposition and TGRY anastomosis for proximal gastric cancer. World J Gastroenterol. 2014;20(25):8268–73.

21. Takiguchi N, Takahashi M, Ikeda M, Inagawa S, Ueda S, Nobuoka T, et al. Long-term quality-of-life comparison of total gastrectomy and proximal gastrectomy by postgastrectomy syndrome assessment scale (PGSAS-45): a nationwide multi-institutional study. Gastric Cancer. 2015;18(2):407–16.

22. Namikawa T, Oki T, Kitagawa H, Okabayashi T, Kobayashi M, Hanazaki K. Impact of jejunal pouch interposition reconstruction after proximal gastrectomy for early gastric cancer on quality of life: short- and long-term consequences. Am J Surg. 2012;204(2):203–9.

23. Ohashi M, Morita S, Fukagawa T, Oda I, Kushima R, Katai H. Functional advantages of proximal gastrectomy with jejunal interposition over total gastrectomy with Roux-en-Y esophagojejunostomy for early gastric cancer. World J Surg. 2015;39(11):2726–33.

24. Ichikawa D, Komatsu S, Kubota T, Okamoto K, Shiozaki A, Fujiwara H, et al. Long-term outcomes of patients who underwent limited proximal gastrectomy. Gastric Cancer. 2014;17(1):141–5.

25. Son MW, Kim YJ, Jeong GA, Cho GS, Lee MS. Long-term outcomes of proximal gastrectomy versus total gastrectomy for upper-third gastric cancer. J Gastric Cancer. 2014;14(4):246–51.

26. An JY, Youn HG, Choi MG, Noh JH, Sohn TS, Kim S. The difficult choice between total and proximal gastrectomy in proximal early gastric cancer. Am J Surg. 2008;196(4):587–91.

27. Katai H, Sano T, Fukagawa T, Shinohara H, Sasako M. Prospective study of proximal gastrectomy for early gastric cancer in the upper third of the stomach. Br J Surg. 2003;90(7):850–3.

28. Wen L, Chen XZ, Wu B, Chen XL, Wang L, Yang K, et al. Total vs. proximal gastrectomy for proximal gastric cancer: a systematic review and meta-analysis. Hepato-Gastroenterology. 2012;59(114):633–40.

29. Kitamura K, Yamaguchi T, Nishida S, Yamamoto K, Ichikawa D, Okamoto K, et al. The operative indications for proximal gastrectomy in patients with gastric

cancer in the upper third of the stomach. Surg Today. 1997;27(11):993–8.

30. Kong SH, Kim JW, Lee HJ, Kim WH, Lee KU, Yang HK. Reverse double-stapling end-to-end esophagogastrostomy in proximal gastrectomy. Dig Surg. 2010;27(3):170–4.

31. Japanese Gastric Cancer Association. Japanese classification of gastric carcinoma: 3rd English edition. Gastric Cancer. 2011;14(2):101–12.

32. Yoshikawa T, Takeuchi H, Hasegawa S, Nozaki I, Kishi K, Ito S, et al. Theoretical therapeutic impact of lymph node dissection on adenocarcinoma and squamous cell carcinoma of the esophagogastric junction. Gastric Cancer. 2014;19(1):143–9.

33. Ohyama S, Tokunaga M, Hiki N, Fukunaga T, Fujisaki J, Seto Y, et al. A clinicopathological study of gastric stump carcinoma following proximal gastrectomy. Gastric Cancer. 2009;12(2):88–94.

Vagus-Preserving Gastrectomy

18

Masatoshi Nakagawa and Kazuyuki Kojima

Introduction

The radical surgical treatment of gastric cancer requires resection of a large portion of the stomach, as well as regional lymphadenectomy. It is well known that gastric resection and reconstruction of the gastrointestinal tract result in a variety of functional and physiological disorders such as dumping syndrome, malabsorption, diarrhea, and so on. These unpleasant alimentary and/or systemic symptoms are collectively referred to as postgastrectomy syndrome [1]. Vagus nerve preservation, which was first introduced in 1991, is one way to alleviate postgastrectomy syndrome [2]. In this chapter, we will describe the surgical anatomy, operational procedure, and postoperative outcomes of vagus-preserving gastrectomy (VPG).

Surgical Anatomy

There are three main parts of the vagus nerve in gastric surgery: (1) the hepatic branch from the anterior vagal trunk, (2) the celiac branch from the posterior vagal trunk, and (3) the hepatic nerve plexus (Fig. 18.1).

Hepatic Branch

The anterior vagal trunk bifurcates into the hepatic branch and the anterior gastric branch at the level of the right cardia. The hepatic branch consists of a few nerves traversing through the compact part of the lesser omentum caudal to the left lobe of the liver, and it joins the hepatic nerve plexus. The anterior gastric branch runs along the lesser curvature, innervating the anterior wall of the stomach from the cardia to the gastric body.

Celiac Branch

The posterior vagal trunk runs behind the abdominal esophagus through the gastropancreatic folds, bifurcating into the celiac branch and the posterior gastric branch. The celiac branch joins the right and left celiac ganglia. The celiac branch and the left gastric artery are often fused after they are joined together.

M. Nakagawa
Department of Gastric Surgery, Tokyo Medical and Dental University, Tokyo, Japan

K. Kojima (✉)
First Department of Surgery,
Dokkyo Medical University, Mibu-machi,
Shimotsuga-gun, Japan
e-mail: kojima-k@dokkyomed.ac.jp

© Springer-Verlag GmbH Germany, part of Springer Nature 2019
S. H. Noh, W. J. Hyung (eds.), *Surgery for Gastric Cancer*,
https://doi.org/10.1007/978-3-662-45583-8_18

Fig. 18.1 Schema of the vagus nerve around the stomach

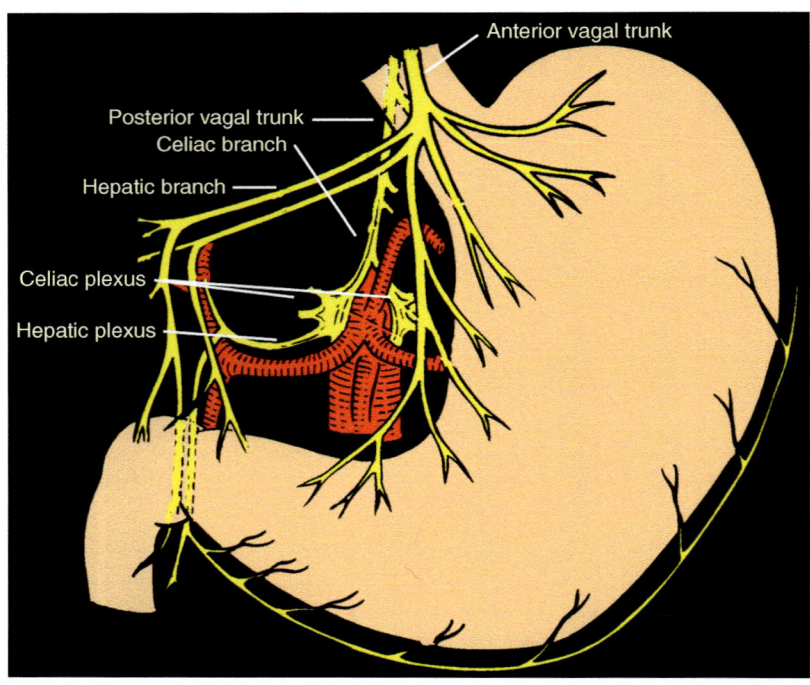

Hepatic Nerve Plexus

The hepatic nerve plexus arises from the celiac nerve plexus, which consists of the vagus nerve from the celiac ganglia and the sympathetic nerve from the greater splanchnic nerve. The nerve plexus surrounds the common and proper hepatic arteries, especially dorsal to their cranial circular location.

Operational Procedure

VPG was originally introduced in open surgery [2], but recently it has also been performed as a minimally invasive approach, and the magnified view of laparoscopic and robotic surgery facilitates identification of the vagus nerve, as well as a precise procedure. In this section, the laparoscopic procedure will be presented as described by Kojima et al. in their article [3].

The surgical procedure begins with port insertion and lymph node dissection around the greater omentum and infrapyloric area, followed by duodenal resection.

When the lesser omentum is resected, the hepatic branch from the anterior vagal trunk, which runs across the compact part of the lesser omentum near the liver, should be identified and preserved.

The posterior vagal trunk and celiac branches that run along the posterior wall of the abdominal esophagus and down to the celiac ganglion are identified. With exposure of the diaphragm's right crus and the anterolaterodorsal side of the abdominal esophagus, the posterior vagal trunk is isolated and retracted toward the right side with a vessel loop (Fig. 18.2).

After exposure of the common hepatic artery and gastropancreatic folds, the No. 8a lymph nodes, located along the common hepatic artery, are dissected. In this step, the hepatic nerve plexus that runs along the common hepatic artery must be preserved. Lymph nodes along the left gastric artery (No. 7) and celiac artery (No. 9) are dissected toward the position where the celiac branch of the posterior vagal trunk joins the left gastric artery (Fig. 18.3). The left gastric artery is divided with double clips after isolation of the celiac branches. The nerves of Latarjet are

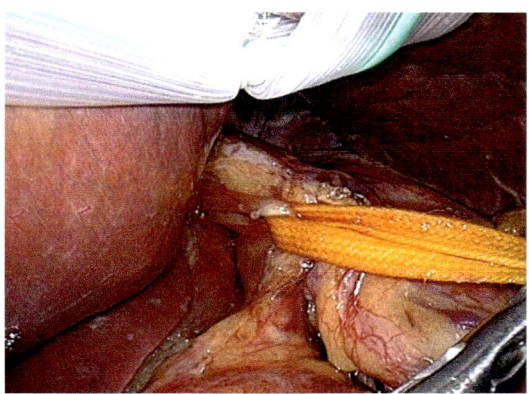

Fig. 18.2 Identification and isolation of the posterior vagal trunk. The posterior vagal trunk is isolated with a vessel loop

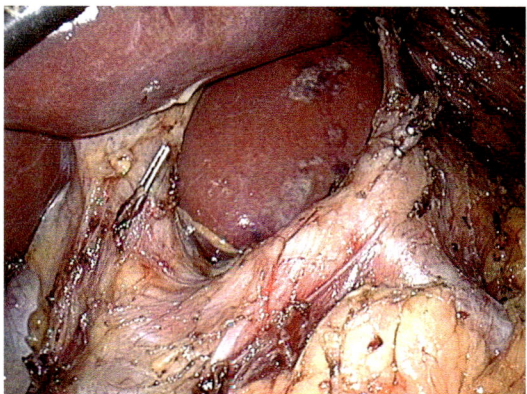

Fig. 18.4 Completion of vagus nerve-preserving lymph node dissection

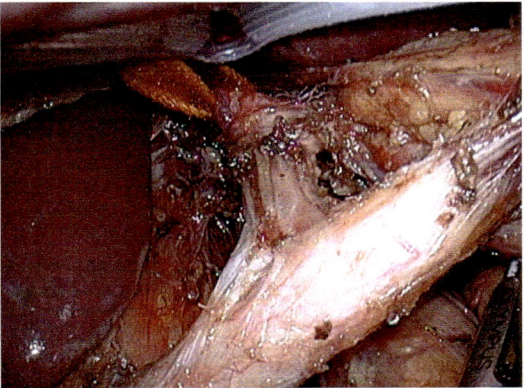

Fig. 18.3 Lymph node dissection around the left gastric artery and celiac axis with preservation of the celiac branch of the vagus nerve. The celiac branch and left gastric artery are joined together at the root of the left gastric artery

divided from the celiac branches, along with the perigastric lymph nodes. Retraction of the celiac branches toward the right side facilitates this procedure. The vagus nerve-sparing lymph node dissection is then completed (Fig. 18.4). After this procedure, resection of the stomach and reconstruction are performed.

Short-Term Results

As for the perioperative results, although only one article by Sakuramoto et al. reported that longer operative time and greater intraoperative bleeding were seen in the VPG group [4], two other articles showed comparable perioperative results, such as blood loss, operative time, morbidity, and postoperative hospital stay, between VPG and vagus nerve-resection gastrectomy (VRG) groups [3, 5]. The time to first flatus was also earlier in the VPG group than in the VRG group in some reports [5–7].

Two articles investigated the hormonal effects of vagus nerve preservation. Takiguchi et al. found that, on postoperative day 7, although plasma fasting ghrelin, which is a brain-gut peptide with GH-releasing and appetite-inducing properties, decreased significantly in both the VPG and VRG groups by about 50% of the baseline values, the postprandial reduction of ghrelin was maintained only in the VPG group [5]. Kim et al. reported that a lesser increase of peptide YY [8], acting as a satiety signal, was observed in the VPG group compared to the VRG group. They also concluded that less body weight loss was observed 1 month after surgery in the VPG group, which was related to less increase of peptide YY [9].

Long-Term Results

One article by Kim et al. showed less diarrhea 3 and 12 months after surgery and less appetite loss at 12 months in the VPG group. Yamada et al. reported that, at 1-year follow-up, the incidences of dumping syndrome and gallstone formation were significantly lower and significantly more residual food was seen on endoscopic examination in the VPG group than in the VRG group, although other clinical symptoms, endoscopic findings, and nutritional status were similar between the two groups. Uyama et al. also reported a lower incidence of diarrhea and gallstone formation in the VPG group with a median follow-up period of 23 months [10].

Two articles showed the data of VPG for up to 5 years. In the article by Inokuchi et al., the incidence of clinical symptoms such as gastroesophageal reflux, early dumping syndrome, and chronic diarrhea, endoscopic findings using the RGB score [11], and nutritional status were similar between the VPG and VRG groups, but gallstone formation was significantly less common in the VPG group 5 years after surgery [12]. Kim et al. compared the oncological outcomes between the two groups, concluding that there were no significant differences between the two groups in cancer recurrence and death over 5 years of follow-up [7].

Conclusion

Up to now, although there have been few reports of the feasibility and efficacy of VPG, and the results have varied article to article, based on the currently available evidence, it can be concluded that (1) it is a technically feasible and oncologically acceptable procedure as long as the appropriate inclusion criteria are applied; and (2) several positive postoperative outcomes, such as earlier first flatus after surgery, less diarrhea, less body weight loss, less appetite loss, less incidence of early dumping syndrome, and less gallstone formation, can be achieved by the procedure, which improves the patients' postoperative quality of life.

In order to further elucidate these issues, more research with larger sample sizes and diverse populations is needed, as well as research examining the molecular biological mechanisms that can explain the efficacy of vagus nerve preservation.

References

1. Carvajal SH, Mulvihill SJ. Postgastrectomy syndromes: dumping and diarrhea. Gastroenterol Clin N Am. 1994;23(2):261–79. Epub 1994/06/01.
2. Miwa K, Kinami S, Sato T, Fujimura T, Miyazaki I. Vagus-saving D2 procedure for early gastric carcinoma. Nihon Geka Gakkai Zasshi. 1996;97(4):286–90. Epub 1996/04/01.
3. Kojima K, Yamada H, Inokuchi M, Kawano T, Sugihara K. Functional evaluation after vagus-nerve-sparing laparoscopically assisted distal gastrectomy. Surg Endosc. 2008;22(9):2003–8. Epub 2008/07/03.
4. Sakuramoto S, Kikuchi S, Kuroyama S, Futawatari N, Katada N, Kobayashi N, et al. Laparoscopy-assisted distal gastrectomy for early gastric cancer: experience with 111 consecutive patients. Surg Endosc. 2006;20(1):55–60. Epub 2005/11/12.
5. Takiguchi S, Hiura Y, Takahashi T, Kurokawa Y, Yamasaki M, Nakajima K, et al. Preservation of the celiac branch of the vagus nerve during laparoscopy-assisted distal gastrectomy: impact on postprandial changes in ghrelin secretion. World J Surg. 2013;37(9):2172–9. Epub 2013/05/07.
6. Yamada H, Kojima K, Inokuchi M, Kawano T, Sugihara K. Efficacy of celiac branch preservation in Roux-en-y reconstruction after laparoscopy-assisted distal gastrectomy. Surgery. 2011;149(1):22–8. Epub 2010/04/27.
7. Kim SM, Cho J, Kang D, Oh SJ, Kim AR, Sohn TS, et al. A randomized controlled trial of vagus nerve-preserving distal gastrectomy versus conventional distal gastrectomy for postoperative quality of life in early stage gastric cancer patients. Ann Surg. 2016;263(6):1079–84. Epub 2016/01/05.
8. Halatchev IG, Ellacott KL, Fan W, Cone RD. Peptide YY3-36 inhibits food intake in mice through a melanocortin-4 receptor-independent mechanism. Endocrinology. 2004;145(6):2585–90. Epub 2004/03/16.
9. Kim HH, Park MI, Lee SH, Hwang HY, Kim SE, Park SJ, et al. Effects of vagus nerve preservation and vagotomy on peptide YY and body weight after subtotal gastrectomy. World J Gastroenterol. 2012;18(30):4044–50. Epub 2012/08/23.
10. Uyama I, Sakurai Y, Komori Y, Nakamura Y, Syoji M, Tonomura S, et al. Laparoscopic gastrectomy with preservation of the vagus nerve accompanied by lymph node dissection for early gastric carcinoma. J Am Coll Surg. 2005;200(1):140–5. Epub 2005/01/06.
11. Nagano H, Ohyama S, Sakamoto Y, Ohta K, Yamaguchi T, Muto T, et al. The endoscopic evaluation of gastritis, gastric remnant residue, and the incidence of secondary cancer after pylorus-preserving and transverse gastrectomies. Gastric Cancer. 2004;7(1):54–9. Epub 2004/03/31.
12. Inokuchi M, Sugita H, Otsuki S, Sato Y, Nakagawa M, Kojima K. Long-term effectiveness of preserved celiac branch of vagal nerve after Roux-en-Y reconstruction in laparoscopy-assisted distal gastrectomy. Dig Surg. 2014;31(4–5):341–6. Epub 2014/12/17.

Part IX

Sentinel Node Navigation Surgery

Hiroya Takeuchi and Yuko Kitagawa

Introduction

In Japan, early-stage gastric cancer (cT1) is found in many asymptomatic patients due to recent advances in endoscopic diagnosis, and the population with this condition currently reaches in excess of 50% in major institutions [1]. Endoscopic submucosal dissection (ESD) has already been accepted as the most minimally invasive procedure for the resection of early gastric cancer [1]. Laparoscopic gastrectomy represents an important intermediate option between ESD and open surgery for patients with gastric cancer [2]. The technique of laparoscopic gastrectomy has shifted from partial resection to more radical procedures such as laparoscopy-assisted distal gastrectomy (LADG) with D2 lymphadenectomy, which is comparable to conventional open distal gastrectomy and can be performed in clinical practices [3, 4].

Many patients with early gastric cancer are currently treated with advanced laparoscopic gastrectomy procedures, such as LADG and laparoscopy-assisted total gastrectomy (LATG) with standard lymph node dissection in Asian countries [1–4]. LADG and LATG contribute to both better esthetics and early postoperative

recovery [5]. However, patients' quality of life (QOL) is mainly affected by late-phase complications including dumping syndrome and body weight loss resulting from oral intake disturbance due to large extent of gastric resection. Therefore, both minimal invasiveness for early-phase recovery by laparoscopic surgery and additional late-phase function-preserving gastrectomy should be carefully considered in patients indicated for these procedures.

Function-preserving gastrectomy such as partial gastrectomy, segmental gastrectomy, and proximal gastrectomy with limited lymph node dissection is known to improve postoperative late-phase function. However, a certain incidence of skip metastasis in the 2nd or 3rd compartment of regional lymph nodes remains an obstacle to the wider application of these procedures. To overcome these issues, the concept of sentinel node (SN) mapping may become a novel diagnostic tool for the identification of clinically undetectable lymph node metastasis in early gastric cancer.

SNs are defined as the first draining lymph nodes from the primary tumor site [6, 7], and they are thought to be the first possible site of micrometastasis along the route of lymphatic drainage from the primary lesion (Fig. 19.1). The pathological status of SNs can theoretically predict the status of all regional lymph nodes. If SNs are recognizable and negative for cancer metastasis, unnecessary radical lymph node dissection

H. Takeuchi (✉) · Y. Kitagawa
Department of Surgery, Keio University School
of Medicine, Tokyo, Japan
e-mail: htakeuchi@a6.keio.jp; kitagawa@a3.keio.jp

© Springer-Verlag GmbH Germany, part of Springer Nature 2019
S. H. Noh, W. J. Hyung (eds.), *Surgery for Gastric Cancer*,
https://doi.org/10.1007/978-3-662-45583-8_19

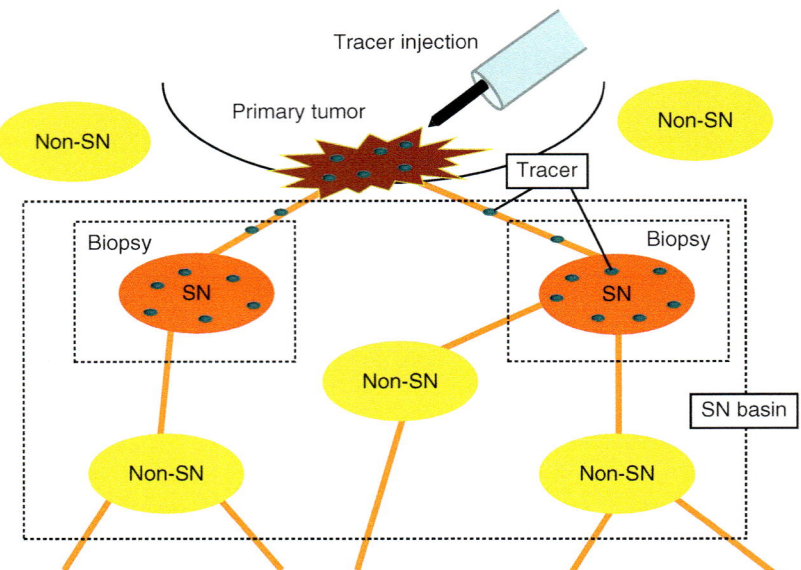

Fig. 19.1 Schema of gastric cancer and sentinel nodes (SN). The SN is defined as one or more lymph nodes that first receive lymphatic drainage from primary tumors. For intraoperative lymphatic mapping and SN biopsy, blue dye and/or radioisotope-labeled colloid is injected submu-cosally around primary tumor sites before surgery using endoscopy. Subsequently, the tracers pass through the afferent lymphatics, and blue-stained or radioactive nodes are regarded as the SN

could be avoided. SN navigation surgery is defined as a novel, minimally invasive surgery based on SN mapping and the SN-targeted diagnosis of nodal metastasis. SN navigation surgery can prevent unnecessary lymph node dissection, thus preventing the associated complications and improving the patient's QOL.

SN mapping and biopsy were firstly applied to melanoma and breast cancer patients and were subsequently extended to patients with many other solid tumors [7–9]. The clinical application of SN mapping for early gastric cancer has been controversial for years. However, single institutional results, including a recent multicenter trial of SN mapping for early gastric cancer, are considered acceptable in terms of the SN detection rate and accuracy of determination of lymph node status [10, 11]. On the basis of these results, we are developing a novel, minimally invasive function-preserving gastrectomy technique combined with SN mapping.

Laparoscopic SN Mapping Procedures for Gastric Cancer

A dual-tracer method that utilizes radioactive colloids and blue or green dyes is currently considered the most reliable method for the stable detection of SNs in patients with early gastric cancer [10, 11]. An accumulation of radioactive colloids facilitates the identification of SNs even in resected specimens by using a handheld gamma probe, and the blue dye is effective for intraoperative visualization of lymphatic flow, even during laparoscopic surgery. Technetium-99 m tin colloid, technetium-99 m sulfur colloid, and technetium-99 m antimony sulfur colloid are preferentially used as radioactive tracers. Isosulfan blue and indocyanine green (ICG) are the currently preferred choices as dye tracers.

In our institution, patients with clinical T1 tumors, primary lesions less than 4 cm in diameter, and clinical N0 gastric cancer undergo SN mapping and biopsy [10, 11]. In our procedures, 2.0 ml (150 MBq) of technetium-99 m tin colloid solution is injected the day before surgery into four quadrants of the submucosal layer of the primary tumor site using an endoscopic puncture needle. Endoscopic injections to the submucosal layer facilitate accurate tracer injection rather than laparoscopic injection from the seromuscular site of the gastric wall. Technetium-99 m tin colloid with relatively large particle size accumulates in the SNs after local administration.

The blue or green dyes are injected into four quadrants of the submucosal layer of the primary site using an endoscopic puncture needle at the beginning of surgery. Blue lymphatic vessels and blue-stained nodes can be identified by laparoscopy within 15 minutes after the injection of the blue or green dyes. Simultaneously, a handheld gamma probe is used to locate the radioactive SN. Intraoperative gamma probing is feasible in laparoscopic gastrectomy using a special gamma detector introducible from trocar ports [10, 11].

For intraoperative SN sampling, the pick-up method is well established for the detection of melanoma and breast cancer. However, it is recommended that the clinical application of intraoperative SN sampling for gastric cancer should include sentinel lymphatic basin dissection, which is a sort of focused lymph node dissection involving hot and blue nodes [10, 11]. The gastric lymphatic basins were considered to be divided in the following five directions along the main arteries: left gastric artery area, right gastric artery area, left gastroepiploic artery area, right gastroepiploic artery area, and posterior gastric artery area [12].

ICG is known to have excitation and fluorescence wavelengths in the near-infrared range [13]. Till date, some investigators have used infrared ray electronic endoscopy (IREE) to demonstrate the clinical utility of intraoperative ICG infrared imaging as a new tracer for laparoscopic SN mapping [13, 14]. IREE might be a useful tool to improve visualization of ICG-stained lymphatic vessels and SNs even in the fat tissues. More recently, ICG fluorescence imaging has been developed as another promising novel technique for SN mapping [15, 16]. SN could be clearly visualized by ICG fluorescence imaging compared to the naked eye. Further studies would be needed to evaluate the clinical efficacy of ICG infrared or fluorescence imaging and to compare those with radio-guided methods in prospective studies. However these new technologies might revolutionize the SN mapping procedures in early gastric cancer.

Results of SN Mapping in Gastric Cancer

To date, more than 100 single institutional studies have demonstrated acceptable outcomes of SN mapping for early gastric cancer in terms of the SN detection rate (90–100%) and accuracy (85–100%) of determination of lymph node status; these outcomes are comparable to those of SN mapping for melanoma and breast cancer [11]. A recent large-scale meta-analysis, which included 38 relevant SN mapping studies with 2128 gastric cancer patients, demonstrated that the SN detection rate and accuracy of prediction of lymph node metastasis based on SN status were 94% and 92%, respectively [17]. They concluded that the SN concept is technically feasible for gastric cancer, especially patients with early T stage (T1), with the use of combined tracers and submucosal injection methods during the SN biopsy procedures.

Our group in Japan had conducted a multicenter prospective trial (UMIN ID: 000000476) of SN mapping using a dual-tracer method with a radioactive colloid and blue dye [10]. In the trial, SN mapping was performed between 2004 and 2008 for 397 patients with early gastric cancer at 12 comprehensive hospitals, including our institution. Eligibility criteria were that patients had cT1N0M0 or cT2N0M0 single tumor with diameter of primary lesion less than 4 cm, without any previous treatments. As results, the SN detection rate was 98%, and the accuracy of determination of metastatic status was 99% [10]. The results of that clinical trial are expected to provide us with perspectives on the future of SN navigation surgery for early gastric cancer.

Clinical Application of Laparoscopic SN Navigation Surgery in Early Gastric Cancer

The distribution of sentinel lymphatic basins and the pathological status of SNs would be useful in deciding on the minimized extent of gastric resection and in avoiding the universal application of distal or total gastrectomy with D2 dissection. Appropriate indications for laparoscopic surgeries such as partial (wedge) resection, segmental gastrectomy, pylorus-preserving gastrectomy, and proximal gastrectomy (LAPG) for cT1N0 gastric cancer could be individually determined on the basis of SN status (Fig. 19.2) [18–20]. Earlier recovery after surgery and preservation of QOL in the late phase can be achieved by laparoscopic limited gastrectomy with SN navigation. Our study group in Japan has currently been conducting the multicenter prospective trial (UMIN ID: 000014401) which will evaluate the function-preserving gastrectomy with SN mapping in terms of long-term survival and patients' QOL as the next step. A Korean

group has also been conducting the multicenter prospective phase III trial to elucidate the oncologic safety including long-term survival of laparoscopic stomach-preserving surgery with sentinel lymphatic basin dissection compared to a standard laparoscopic gastrectomy [21].

A combination of laparoscopic SN biopsy and endoscopic mucosal resection (EMR)/endoscopic submucosal dissection (ESD) for early gastric cancer is another attractive option as a novel, whole stomach-preserved, minimally invasive approach. If all SNs are pathologically negative for cancer metastasis, theoretically, EMR/ESD instead of gastrectomy may be sufficient for the curative resection of cT1 gastric cancer beyond the ESD criteria [20, 22]. However, further studies are required to verify the safety and effectiveness of combined treatments involving laparoscopic SN biopsy and EMR/ESD.

Nowadays, LADG or LAPG is frequently applied to the patients with early gastric cancer according to the results of pathological assessment of primary tumor resected by EMR/ESD in clinical practices. To date, it has not been clarified whether the SN mapping is feasible even after EMR/ESD. One of the most important issues is whether lymphatic flow from the primary tumor to the original SNs might change after EMR/ESD. In our preliminary study,

Fig. 19.2 Individualized function-preserving approaches for cT1N0M0 gastric cancer based on sentinel node mapping. ESD, endoscopic submucosal dissection; EMR, endoscopic mucosal resection

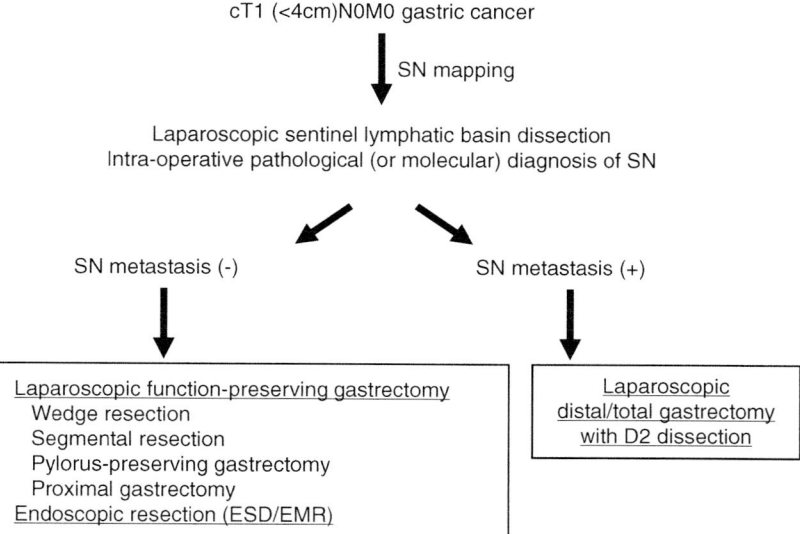

however, at least the sentinel lymphatic basin is not markedly affected by previous EMR/ESD [20, 22]. Modified gastrectomy according to SN distribution and metastatic status might be feasible even for the patients who underwent EMR/ESD prior to surgery.

Non-exposed Endoscopic Wall-Inversion Surgery Plus SN Mapping

In current function-preserving surgeries such as laparoscopic local resection or segmental gastrectomy, the approach of gastrectomy is only from the outside of the stomach, in which the demarcation line of the tumor cannot be visualized at the phase of resection. Therefore, the surgeons cannot avoid a wider resection of the stomach than is desired to prevent a positive surgical margin. The recent appearance of a new technique, referred to as non-exposed endoscopic wall-inversion surgery (NEWS), is a technique of full-thickness partial resection, which can minimize the extent of gastric resection using endoscopic and laparoscopic surgery without transluminal access mainly designed to treat gastric cancer. We have been accumulating cases of NEWS with SN biopsy for early gastric cancer

with the risk of lymph node metastasis in the clinical trial [23, 24].

In brief, after placing mucosal markings, ICG was injected endoscopically into the submucosa around the lesion to examine SNs (Fig. 19.3) [24]. The SN basin including hot or stained SNs was dissected, and an intraoperative pathological diagnosis confirmed that no metastasis had occurred. Subsequently, NEWS was performed for the primary lesion. Serosal markings were placed laparoscopically, submucosal injection was added endoscopically, and circumferential seromuscular incision and suturing were performed laparoscopically, with the lesion inverted toward the inside of the stomach. Finally, the circumferential mucosal incision was performed, and the lesion was retrieved perorally (Fig. 19.3).

The NEWS combined with the SN biopsy can minimize not only the area of lymphadenectomy but also the extent of gastric resection as partial gastrectomy for patients with SN-negative for metastasis [22]. Furthermore, NEWS does not need intentional perforation, which enables us to apply this technique to cancers without a risk of iatrogenic dissemination. The combination of NEWS with SN biopsy is expected to become a promising, ideal minimally invasive, function-preserving surgery to cure cases of cN0 early gastric cancer.

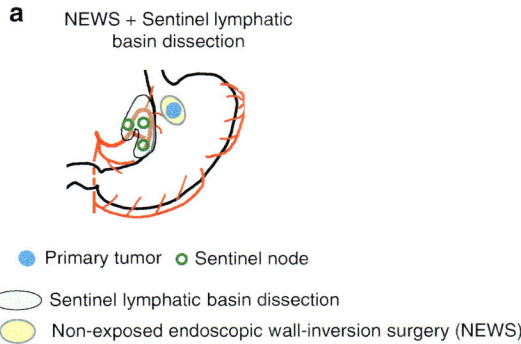

a   NEWS + Sentinel lymphatic
      basin dissection

● Primary tumor ○ Sentinel node

◯ Sentinel lymphatic basin dissection

◯ Non-exposed endoscopic wall-inversion surgery (NEWS)

Fig. 19.3 Non-exposed endoscopic wall-inversion surgery (NEWS) with SN biopsy and sentinel lymphatic basin dissection. (**a**) Schema of the NEWS with sentinel lymphatic basin dissection. (**b**) Marking was placed around the primary tumor. (**c**) Indocyanine green (ICG) was endoscopically injected to the gastric submucosal layer surrounding the primary tumor. (**d**) Laparoscopic observation of ICG with normal light. (**e**) Observation of ICG with infrared ray electronic endoscopy. Infrared ray electronic endoscopy can visualize SNs and lymphatics clearly. (**f**) Resection of sentinel lymphatic basin. (**g**) Laparoscopic circumferential seromuscular incision. (**h**) and (**i**) Laparoscopic seromuscular suturing and inversion of the primary lesion

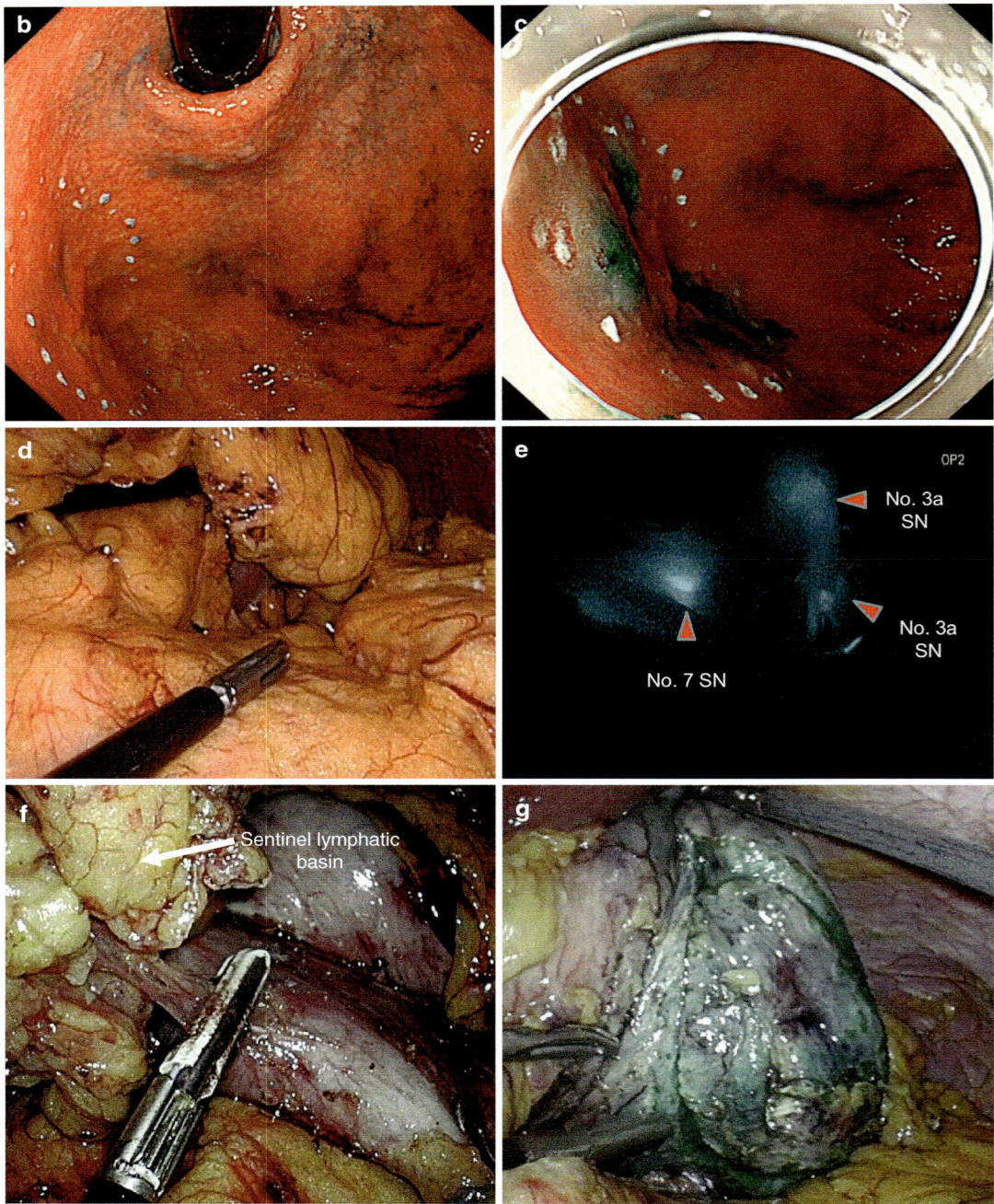

Fig. 19.3 (continued)

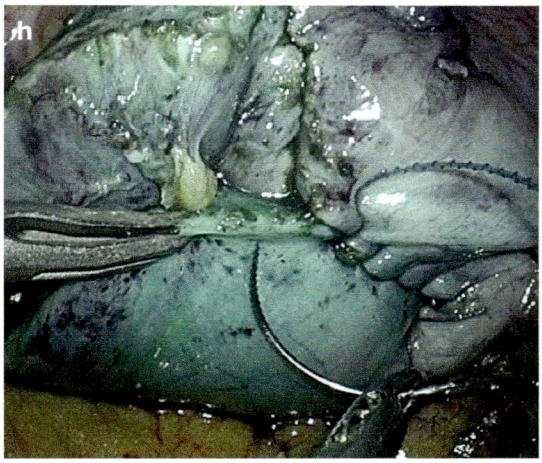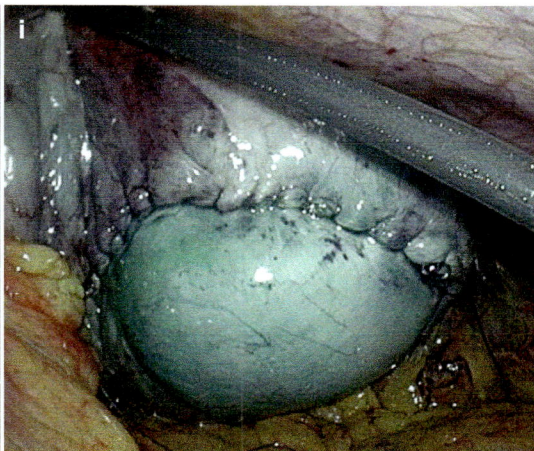

Fig. 19.3 (continued)

Conclusion

For early-stage gastric cancer, for which a better prognosis can be achieved through conventional surgical approaches, the establishment of individualized, minimally invasive treatments that may retain the patients' QOL should be the next surgical challenge. Although further studies are needed for careful validation, function-preserving gastrectomy based on SN navigation could be a promising strategy to achieve this goal.

References

1. Sano T, Hollowood K. Early gastric cancer: diagnosis and less invasive treatments. Scand J Surg. 2006;95:249–55.
2. Kitano S, Iso Y, Moriyama M, Sugimachi K. Laparoscopy-assisted Billroth I gastrectomy. Surg Laparosc Endosc. 1994;4:146–8.
3. Adachi Y, Shiraishi N, Shiromizu A, Shiromizu A, Bandoh T, Aramaki M, Kitano S. Laparoscopy-assisted Billroth I gastrectomy compared with conventional open gastrectomy. Arch Surg. 2000;135:806–10.
4. Shinohara T, Kanaya S, Taniguchi K, Fujita T, Yanaga K, Uyama I. Laparoscopic total gastrectomy with D2 lymph node dissection for gastric cancer. Arch Surg. 2009;144:1138–42.
5. Kim YW, Baik YH, Yun YH, Nam BH, Kim DH, Choi IJ, Bae JM. Improved quality of life outcomes after laparoscopy-assisted distal gastrectomy for early

gastric cancer: results of a prospective randomized clinical trial. Ann Surg. 2008;248:721–7.
6. Kitagawa Y, Fujii H, Mukai M, Kubota T, Ando N, et al. The role of the sentinel lymph node in gastrointestinal cancer. Surg Clin North Am. 2000;80:1799–809.
7. Morton DL, Wen DR, Wong JH, et al. Technical details of intraoperative lymphatic mapping for early stage melanoma. Arch Surg. 1992;127:392–9.
8. Giuliano AE, Kirgan DM, Guenther JM, Morton DL. Lymphatic mapping and sentinel lymphadenectomy for breast cancer. Ann Surg. 1994;220:391–401.
9. Bilchik AJ, Saha S, Wiese D, et al. Molecular staging of early colon cancer on the basis of sentinel node analysis: a multicenter phase II trial. J Clin Oncol. 2001;19:1128–36.
10. Kitagawa Y, Takeuchi H, Takagi Y, Natsugoe S, Terashima M, Murakami N, Fujimura T, Tsujimoto H, Hayashi H, Yoshimizu N, Takagane A, Mohri Y, Nabshima K, Uenosono Y, Kinami S, Sakamoto J, Morita S, Aikou T, Miwa K, Kitajima M. Sentinel node mapping for gastric cancer: a prospective multicenter trial in Japan. J Clin Oncol. 2013;31:3704–10.
11. Takeuchi H, Kitagawa Y. New sentinel node mapping technologies for early gastric cancer. Ann Surg Oncol. 2013;20:522–32.
12. Kinami S, Fujimura T, Ojima E, Fushida S, Ojima T, Funaki H, Fujita H, Takamura H, Ninomiya I, Nishimura G, Kayahara M, Ohta T, Yoh Z. PTD classification: proposal for a new classification of gastric cancer location based on physiological lymphatic flow. Int J Clin Oncol. 2008;13:320–9.
13. Tajima Y, Murakami M, Yamazaki K, Masuda Y, Kato M, Sato A, Goto S, Otsuka K, Kato T, Kusano M. Sentinel node mapping guided by indocyanine green fluorescence imaging during laparoscopic surgery in gastric cancer. Ann Surg Oncol. 2010;17:1787–93.

14. Ishikawa K, Yasuda K, Shiromizu T, Etoh T, Shiraishi N, Kitano S. Laparoscopic sentinel node navigation achieved by infrared ray electronic endoscopy system in patients with gastric cancer. Surg Endosc. 2007;21:1131–4.

15. Nimura H, Narimiya N, Mitsumori N, Yamazaki Y, Yanaga K, Urashima M. Infrared ray electronic endoscopy combined with indocyanine green injection for detection of sentinel nodes of patients with gastric cancer. Br J Surg. 2004;91:575–9.

16. Miyashiro I, Miyoshi N, Hiratsuka M, Kishi K, Yamada T, Ohue M, Ohigashi H, Yano M, Ishikawa O, Imaoka S. Detection of sentinel node in gastric cancer surgery by indocyanine green fluorescence imaging: comparison with infrared imaging. Ann Surg Oncol. 2008;15:1640–3.

17. Wang Z, Dong ZY, Chen JQ, Liu JL. Diagnostic value of sentinel lymph node biopsy in gastric cancer: a meta-analysis. Ann Surg Oncol. 2012;19:1541–50.

18. Takeuchi H, Saikawa Y, Kitagawa Y. Laparoscopic sentinel node navigation surgery for early gastric cancer. Asian J Endosc Surg. 2009;2:13–7.

19. Takeuchi H, Oyama T, Kamiya S, Nakamura R, Takahashi T, Wada N, Saikawa Y, Kitagawa Y. Laparoscopy-assisted proximal gastrectomy with sentinel node mapping for early gastric cancer. World J Surg. 2011;35:2463–71.

20. Takeuchi H, Kitagawa Y. Sentinel node navigation surgery in patients with early gastric cancer. Dig Surg. 2013;30:104–11.

21. Park JY, Kim YW, Ryu KW, Nam BH, Lee YJ, Jeong SH, Park JH, Hur H, Han SU, Min JS, An JY, Hyung WJ, Cho GS, Jeong GA, Jeong O, Park YK, Jung MR, Yoon HM, Eom BW. Assessment of laparoscopic stomach preserving surgery with sentinel basin dissection versus standard gastrectomy with lymphadenectomy in early gastric cancer-A multicenter randomized phase III clinical trial (SENORITA trial) protocol. BMC Cancer. 2016;16:340.

22. Mayanagi S, Takeuchi H, Kamiya S, Niihara M, Nakamura R, Takahashi T, Wada N, Kawakubo H, Saikawa Y, Omori T, Nakahara T, Mukai M, Kitagawa Y. Suitability of sentinel node mapping as an index of metastasis in early gastric cancer following endoscopic resection. Ann Surg Oncol. 2014;21:2987–93.

23. Goto O, Takeuchi H, Kawakubo H, Sasaki M, Matsuda T, Matsuda S, Kigasawa Y, Kadota Y, Fujimoto A, Ochiai Y, Horii J, Uraoka T, Kitagawa Y, Yahagi N. First case of non-exposed endoscopic wall-inversion surgery with sentinel node basin dissection for early gastric cancer. Gastric Cancer. 2015;18:440–5.

24. Takeuchi H, Kitagawa Y. Sentinel lymph node biopsy in gastric cancer. Cancer J. 2015;21:21–4.

Part X

Surgery for EG Junction Cancer

Yasuyuki Seto, Hiroharu Yamashita,
and Susumu Aikou

Gastric Cancer or Esophageal Cancer or Else?

Should esophagogastric junction (EGJ) cancer be classified or managed as gastric cancer or esophageal cancer or else? The debate focused on the issue has still remained [1], though EGJ cancer is increasing worldwide, in Asia [2–5] as well as western countries [6–8]. Squamous cell carcinoma developed in EGJ region is unanimously treated as esophageal cancer. For EGJ adenocarcinoma, Siewert classification has been widely applied: type I (adenocarcinoma of the distal esophagus), tumors with an epicenter located more than 1 cm above the EGJ; type II (true cardia cancer), tumors with an epicenter located within 1 cm oral and 2 cm aboral from the EGJ; and type III (subcardial cancer), tumors with an epicenter located below 2 cm from the EGJ [9, 10]. Among Siewert classifications, Siewert type I and III tumors are usually managed like esophageal and gastric cancers, respectively. However,

Electronic Supplementary Material The online version of this chapter (https://doi.org/10.1007/978-3-662-45583-8_20) contains supplementary material, which is available to authorized users.

Y. Seto (✉) · H. Yamashita · S. Aikou
Department of Gastrointestinal Surgery, Graduate School of Medicine, University of Tokyo,
Tokyo, Japan
e-mail: seto-tky@umin.ac.jp

in 7th AJCC TNM classification, both Siewert type II and III tumors had been classified as esophageal cancer. After some discussions [11–13], in 8th version, type III was changed to gastric cancer classification, while type II still stays in esophageal classification [14–15]. There have been many papers regarding the clinicopathologic features of Siewert type II tumors to identify the pathogenesis and appropriate treatment strategy. Some papers showed that the characteristics of Siewert type II were quite similar with gastric cancers [11, 12]. However, some papers reported that there were two distinct pathways of tumorigenesis of EGJ adenocarcinoma, related or unrelated to intestinal metaplasia, gastric atrophy, and gastric acid secretion [16–17]. The etiology as well as the treatment strategy has still remained controversy, especially for Siewert type II tumors.

In the EGJ region, the different tissues to be potentially cancerous lesion are known to exist: esophageal gland, Barrett epithelium, cardiac gland, fundic glands, etc. Therefore, some Siewert type II tumors might have different biological features from the esophageal and gastric cancers and, if so, should be regarded as the independent disease. Investigation by cancer genetics, etc. will be undoubtedly needed in the future.

Surgical Procedures

There have been various surgical approaches for EGJ cancers: Ivor Lewis (right thoracic and abdominal), left thoracoabdominal, transhiatal, and abdominal ones. Among them, Ivor Lewis or transhiatal approaches are mainly applied to Siewert type II tumor [18]. In the former, esophagectomy through right thoracotomy with reconstruction by gastric conduit and intrathoracic anastomosis is usually performed like esophageal cancer, while in the latter, extended total gastrectomy is done like gastric cancer. Why are those quite different procedures performed to Siewert type II EGJ cancer? Recent paper described that the choice of approach has been still based on surgeon's discretion [19]. A recent web-based worldwide questionnaire demonstrated that the majority of surgeons favor an extended gastrectomy for Siewert type II tumors (66% vs 27%) [20], while the big data based on 4996 NSQIP/SEER patients showed that esophagectomy was more frequently performed than gastrectomy (71% vs 29%) in the USA [21]. When the patients with Siewert type II tumor refer to thoracic surgeons, Ivor Lewis is likely to be indicated. Conversely, the abdominal surgeons prefer the transhiatal approach for Siewert type II tumors. The potential differences between the east and west in EGJ tumor biology were recently pointed out, and the optimal surgical approach in western countries was concluded to be Ivor Lewis [22]. That is why there have been two quite different approaches.

Several papers compared the short- and long-term outcomes between the esophagectomy and gastrectomy. No significant differences of postoperative morbidity and mortality were observed between those procedures [21, 23, 24]. As for the survival after surgery, two papers showed the better results in the esophagectomy than the gastrectomy groups [21, 23], while no difference between them was found in one report [24]. The comparison of long-term quality of life (QOL) between the two groups demonstrated the better QOL after the gastrectomy than the esophagectomy [25]. This should be considered at the decision of surgical procedures. Recently, a strong worldwide trend toward minimally invasive surgery is observed [20], and it is increasing gaining popularity over open surgery [19]. Intent to perform the minimally invasive surgery for EGJ cancers is, also, absolutely important. Laparoscopic resection of Siewert type II tumors was reported to be feasible and oncologically equivalent as compared to open procedures [26].

Lymphadenectomy

There have been many papers focusing the lymphadenectomy for EGJ cancers, to date. However, the strategy of lymphadenectomy, especially for Siewert type II tumors, has still remained controversial. The standard lymph node (LN) dissection for type II tumors has not been established, to date. However, most papers showed the significance of lymphadenectomy in the pericardial, lesser curvature and at the foot of the left gastric artery nodes (no.1, 2, 3, 7 LNs) [27–29]. Therefore, those LNs should be routinely dissected in all surgical cases with EGJ cancers, regardless of advanced or early stages. Optimal extent of lymph node dissection in the mediastinum for Siewert type II tumors has not been established. However, many papers showed the survival impact of lymphadenectomy in the lower mediastinum [27–30], while one paper described that mediastinal LN dissection was not essential in early Siewert type II tumors [31]. And, based on the analysis of recurrence pattern and lymph node metastasis, the complete mediastinal LN dissection was reported to be not mandatory for type II tumors arising within the stomach [32]. One paper showed that left renal vein nodal involvement (no.16a2; para-aortic LN) had a similar survival impact with the lower mediastinal and celiac axis LNs [29]. Now, multi-institutional prospective clinical trial to evaluate the significance of the lower mediastinal and no. 16a2 LN dissections for Siewert type II tumors is ongoing under the collaboration of the Japanese Gastric Cancer Association (JGCA) and the Japanese Esophageal Society (JES).

LNs along the distal portion of the stomach (no. 4, 5, 6) are located far from EGJ, though those LNs are simultaneously dissected when the total gastrectomy is performed. Many papers reported the poor prognosis and marginal therapeutic value of the Siewert type II cases with the nodal involvement in those LNs [27–29, 33]. The extended abdominal lymphadenectomy was suggested to improve survival because the poorer survival after D1 lymphadenectomy was shown in comparison with D1+/D2 lymphadenectomy [24]. Consistently, the nodal involvement around celiac axis (no. 9) was shown to impact the survival [29, 34].

To evaluate the optimal extent of LN dissection during EGJ cancer surgery, the JGCA and the JES conducted a nationwide survey to characterize the LN spread pattern of EGJ cancer in a large cohort. That was a questionnaire-based national retrospective study, in which clinical records of 3177 patients underwent R0 resection between 2001 and 2010 at the member hospitals of the JGCA and/or the JES were collected. And, the tumors of 40 mm or less in dimension were selected since large tumors were

apparently associated with poor macroscopic recognition of the anatomical EGJ. In Japan, EGJ cancers are defined as its epicenter within 2 cm proximal or distal to the EGJ according to the Japanese classification system (Nishi' classification), regardless of histological type. Among those 3177 patients, 2601 cases were proven to be histologically adenocarcinoma. The results were summarized in the previous paper [35]. The annual number of surgical cases was observed to increase steadily since 2001, especially for adenocarcinoma, in Japan. Figures 20.1, 20.2, 20.3, and 20.4 show the rates of the dissection (red bar) and LN metastasis (blue bar) according to each LN stations of all 2418 adenocarcinoma cases, 1430 early cases, 988 advanced cases, and 234 advanced cases with its epicenter within esophagus, respectively. The numbers of LN stationed are based on the Japanese classification. The cases with neoadjuvant therapy were excluded from the analysis. No. 100–112 and 107–109 LNs are located in the lower and middle mediastinum, respectively. All figures

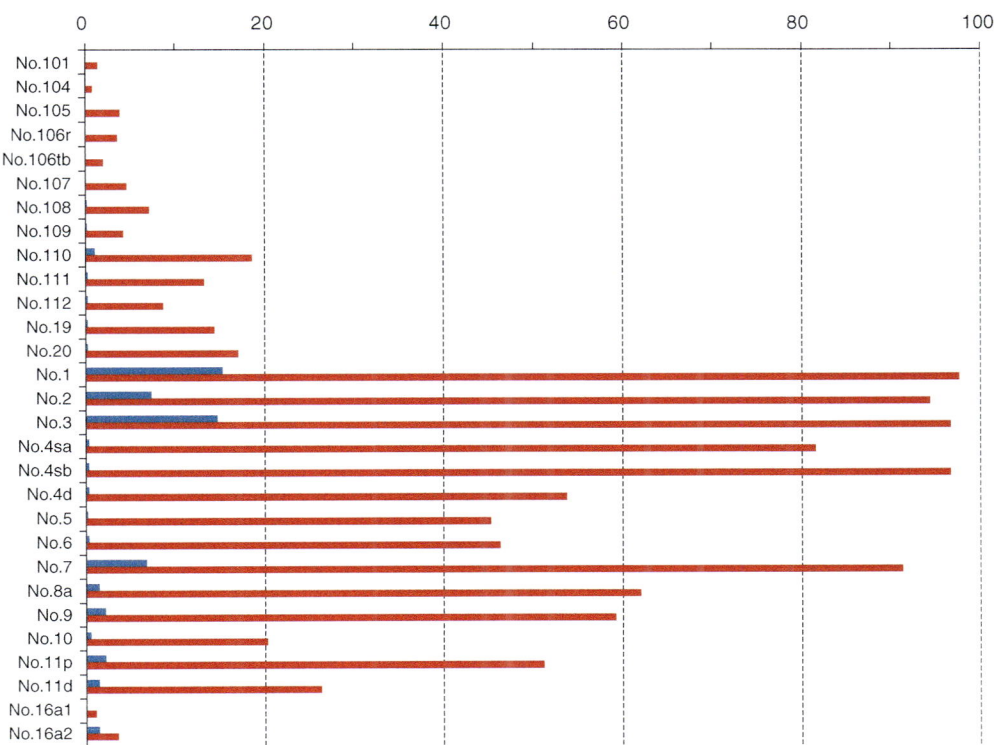

Fig. 20.1 Rate of dissection (red) and LN metastasis (blue) in all 2418 adenocarcinomas

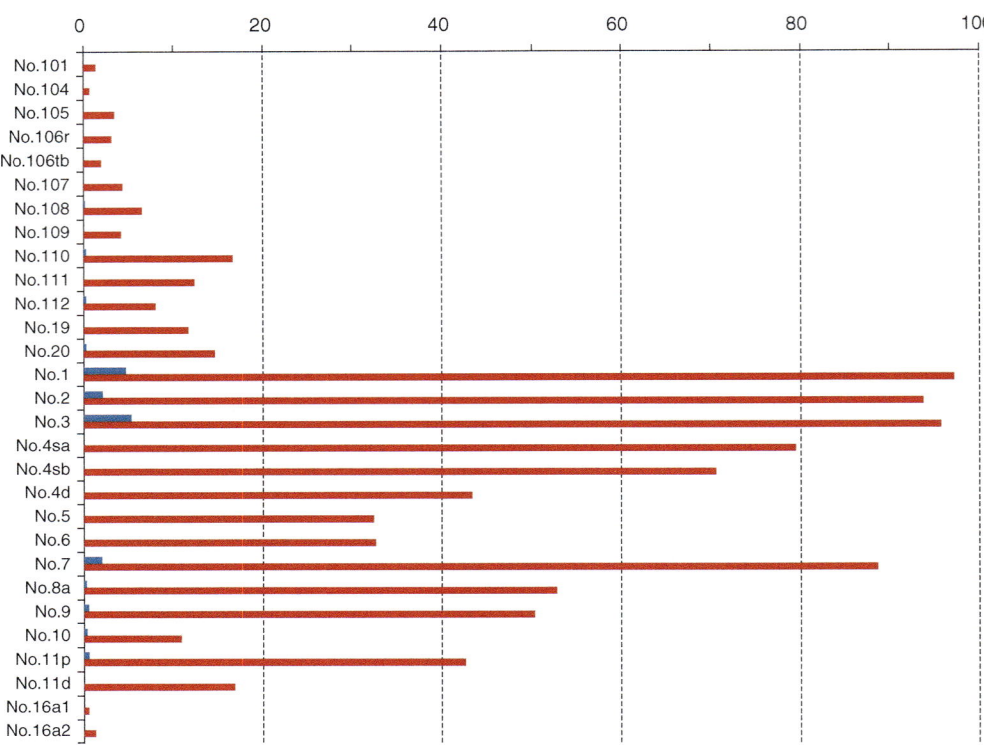

Fig. 20.2 Rate of dissection (red) and LN metastasis (blue) in 1430 early adenocarcinomas

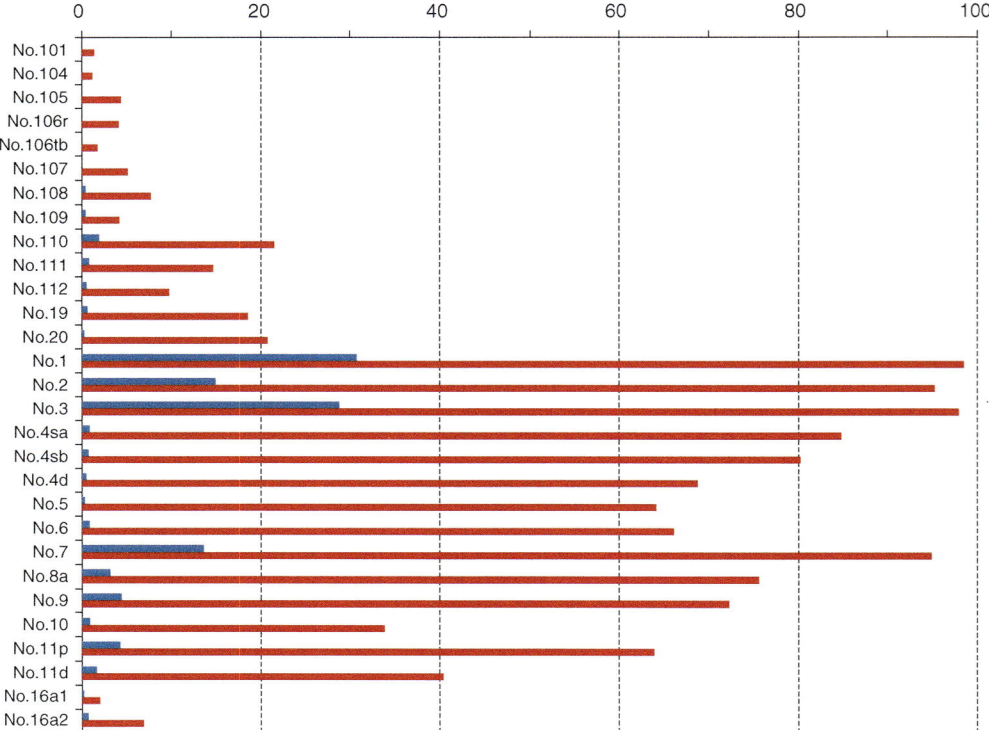

Fig. 20.3 Rate of dissection (red) and LN metastasis (blue) in 988 advanced adenocarcinomas

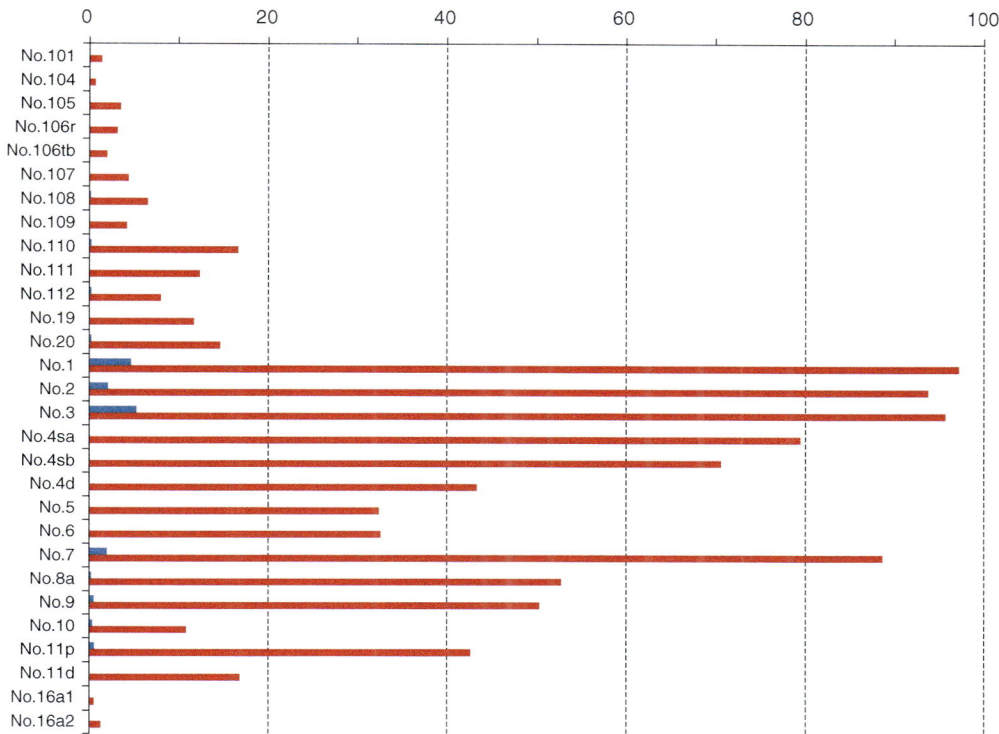

Fig. 20.4   Rate of dissection (red) and LN metastasis (blue) in 234 advanced cases with epicenter within esophagus

were shown in the final report of the abovementioned study (not published but delivered to the participating hospitals). The results were quite consistent with previous reports. Nodes along the distal portion of the stomach (no. 4, 5, 6) were much less often metastatic in any stages, though those were dissected in most cases. And, survival analysis failed to show the benefit of those dissections. Lower mediastinal LN dissection might contribute to improve survival for the EGJ cancer with esophagus-predominance or esophageal invasion.

Our Surgical Procedure

When more than half stomach can be preserved, the proximal gastrectomy (PG) is chosen, because the nutritional status after the PG were shown to be better than after the total gastrectomy (TG) by many studies [36–38], and no survival difference was observed between those procedures [39]. Furthermore, as the previous results showed, the dissections of no. 4, 5, and 6 LNs are not necessary for the radical resection of EGJ cancers. We

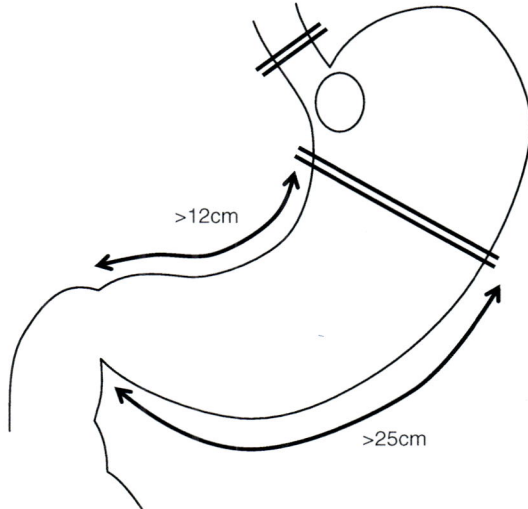

Fig. 20.5   Shema of remnant stomach

think that the TG should be avoided at the utmost. Usually, the stomach of 12 cm or more along the lesser curvature and 25 cm or more along the greater curvature from the pylorus ring is preserved (Fig. 20.5).

When the lower mediastinal LN dissection is considered to be beneficial, no. 110, 111, and 112 LNs are usually dissected (Video 20.1). Both side pleura are preserved, and the inferior pulmonary vein is a point of the upper margin of dissection. The reconstruction is usually done by jejunal interposition (JI) (Video 20.2). Frozen section analysis for the margin is usually submitted to confirm no cancer cells in the resection line. The jejuno-gastrostomy is created on the posterior wall of the remnant stomach by the circular stapler. That anastomotic site is at 5 cm distance from the resection line of the stomach (Fig. 20.6).

The length from the esophagojejunostomy to jejuno-gastrostomy is 8 cm. Some paper recommends the 15–25 cm distance between those anastomoses [40], but our data (Fig. 20.7, not published) showed that the frequency of reflux esophagitis was lower after the short than the long JIs. When the lower mediastinal LN dissection is thought to be unnecessary, laparoscopic proximal gastrectomy is done followed by esophagogastrostomy. That anastomotic site is at the anterior wall with 5 cm distance from the resection line of the stomach (Fig. 20.8). And, several stiches between the esophagus and stomach are added to

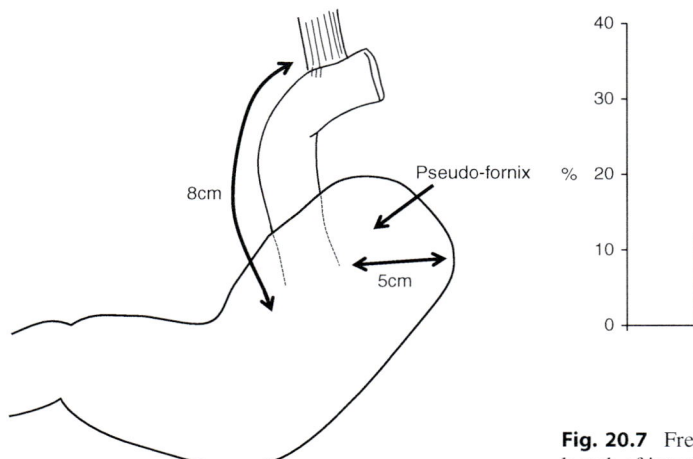

Fig. 20.6 Shema of reconstruction of jejunal interposition

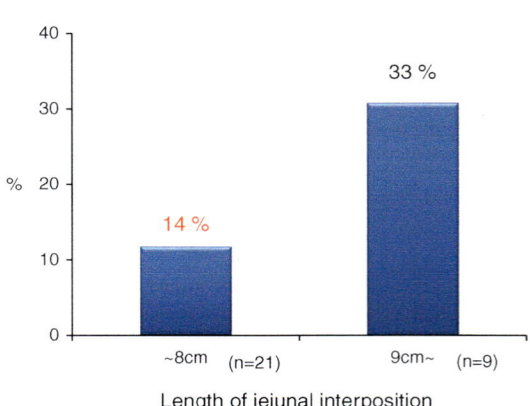

Fig. 20.7 Frequency of reflux esophagitis according to length of interposed jejunum

Fig. 20.8 Shema of esophagogastrostomy

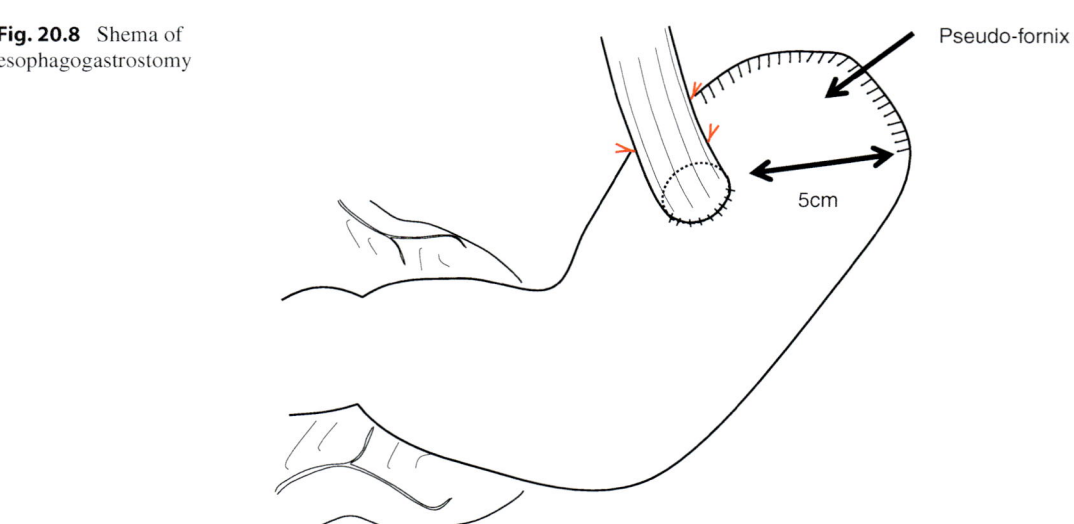

fix and prevent the reflux. Severe reflux esophagitis after PG has not been developed in our recent cases, though higher frequency of reflux esophagitis after PG was previously reported to be than TG [41].

References

1. Van Laethem JL, Carneiro F, Ducreux M, Messman H, Lordick F, Ilson DH, Allum WH, Haustermans K, Lepage C, Matysiak-Budnik T, Cats A, Schmiegel W, Cervantes A, Van Cutsem E, Rougier P, Seufferlein T. The multidisciplinary management of gastro-oesophageal junction tumours: European Society of Digestive Oncology (ESDO): expert discussion and report from the 16th ESMO World Congress on Gastrointestinal Cancer, Barcelona. Dig Liver Dis. 2016;48(11):1283–9. https://doi.org/10.1016/j.dld.2016.08.112. Epub 2016 Aug 20

2. Wang K, Yang CQ, Duan LP, Yang XS, Xia ZW, Cui RL, Jin Z, McNutt M. Changing pattern of adenocarcinoma of the esophagogastric junction in recent 10 years: experience at a large tertiary medical center in China. Tumori. 2012;98(5):568–74. https://doi.org/10.1700/1190.13196.

3. Liu K, Yang K, Zhang W, Chen X, Chen X, Zhang B, Chen Z, Chen J, Zhao Y, Zhou Z, Chen L, Hu J. Changes of esophagogastric junctional adenocarcinoma and gastroesophageal reflux disease among surgical patients during 1988–2012: a single-institution, high-volume experience in China. Ann Surg. 2016;263(1):88–95. https://doi.org/10.1097/SLA.0000000000001148.

4. Hatta W, Tong D, Lee YY, Ichihara S, Uedo N, Gotoda T. Different time trend and management of esophagogastric junction adenocarcinoma in three Asian countries. Dig Endosc. 2017;29(Suppl 2):18–25. https://doi.org/10.1111/den.12808.

5. Koizumi S, Motoyama S, Iijima K. Is the incidence of esophageal adenocarcinoma increasing in Japan? Trends from the data of a hospital-based registration system in Akita Prefecture, Japan. J Gastroenterol. 2017; https://doi.org/10.1007/s00535-017-1412-4. [Epub ahead of print]

6. Brown LM, Devesa SS, Chow WH. Incidence of adenocarcinoma of the esophagus among white Americans by sex, stage, and age. J Natl Cancer Inst. 2008;100(16):1184–7. https://doi.org/10.1093/jnci/djn211. Epub 2008 Aug 11

7. Pohl H, Sirovich B, Welch HG. Esophageal adenocarcinoma incidence: are we reaching the peak? Cancer Epidemiol Biomark Prev. 2010;19(6):1468–70. https://doi.org/10.1158/1055-9965.EPI-10-0012. Epub 2010 May 25

8. Buas MF, Vaughan TL. Epidemiology and risk factors for gastroesophageal junction tumors: understanding the rising incidence of this disease. Semin Radiat Oncol. 2013;23(1):3–9. https://doi.org/10.1016/j.semradonc.2012.09.008.

9. Siewert JR, Hölscher AH, Becker K, Gössner W. Cardia cancer: attempt at a therapeutically relevant classification. Chirurg. 1987;58(1):25–32. Chirurg 2003 Aug;74(8):703–8

10. Stein HJ, von Rahden BH, Höfler H, Siewert JR. Carcinoma of the oesophagogastric junction and Barrett's esophagus: an almost clear oncologic model? Chirurg. 2003;74(8):703–8.

11. Suh YS, Han DS, Kong SH, Lee HJ, Kim YT, Kim WH, Lee KU, Yang HK. Should adenocarcinoma of the esophagogastric junction be classified as esophageal cancer? A comparative analysis according to the seventh AJCC TNM classification. Ann Surg. 2012;255(5):908–15. https://doi.org/10.1097/SLA.0b013e31824beb95.

12. Mullen JT, Kwak EL, Hong TS. What's the best way to treat GE junction tumors? Approach like gastric cancer. Ann Surg Oncol. 2016;23(12):3780–5. Epub 2016 Jul 26

13. Adeshuko FA, Squires MH, Poultsides G, Pawlik TM, Weber SM, Schmidt C, Votanopoulos K, Fields RC, Maithel SK, Cardona K. A multi-institutional study comparing the use of the American joint committee on cancer 7th edition esophageal versus gastric staging system for gastroesophageal junction cancer in a Western population. Am Surg. 2017;83(1):82–9.

14. Rice TW, Patil DT, Blackstone EH. 8th edition AJCC/UICC staging of cancers of the esophagus and esophagogastric junction: application to clinical practice. Ann Cardiothorac Surg. 2017;6(2):119–30. https://doi.org/10.21037/acs.2017.03.14.

15. Rice TW, Gress DM, Patil DT, Hofstetter WL, Kelsen DP, Blackstone EH. Cancer of the esophagus and esophagogastric junction-major changes in the American joint committee on cancer eighth edition cancer staging manual. CA Cancer J Clin. 2017;67(4):304–17. https://doi.org/10.3322/caac.21399. Epub 2017 May 26

16. Nunobe S, Nakanishi Y, Taniguchi H, Sasako M, Sano T, Kato H, Yamagishi H, Sekine S, Shimoda T. Two distinct pathways of tumorigenesis of adenocarcinomas of the esophagogastric junction, related or unrelated to intestinal metaplasia. Pathol Int. 2007;57(6):315–21.

17. Horii T, Koike T, Abe Y, Kikuchi R, Unakami H, Iijima K, Imatani A, Ohara S, Shimosegawa T. Two distinct types of cancer of different origin may be mixed in gastroesophageal junction adenocarcinomas in Japan: evidence from direct evaluation of gastric acid secretion. Scand J Gastroenterol. 2011;46(6):710–9. https://doi.org/10.3109/00365521.2011.565069. Epub 2011 Mar 30

18. Mariette C, Piessen G, Briez N, Gronnier C, Triboulet JP. Oesophago-gastric junction adenocarcinoma: which therapeutic approach? Lancet Oncol. 2011;12(3):296–305. https://doi.org/10.1016/S1470-2045(10)70125-X. Epub 2010 Nov 23

19. Jezerskyte E, van Berge Henegouwen MI, Cuesta MA, Gisbertz SS. Gastro-esophageal junction cancers: what is the best minimally invasive approach? J Thorac Dis. 2017;9(Suppl 8):S751–S60. https://doi.org/10.21037/jtd.2017.06.56.

20. Haverkamp L, Seesing MF, Ruurda JP, Boone J, V Hillegersberg R. Worldwide trends in surgical techniques in the treatment of esophageal and gastroesophageal junction cancer. Dis Esophagus. 2017;30(1):1–7. https://doi.org/10.1111/dote.12480.

21. Martin JT, Mahan A, Zwischenberger JB, McGrath PC, Tzeng CW. Should gastric cardia cancers be treated with esophagectomy or total gastrectomy? A comprehensive analysis of 4,996 NSQIP/SEER patients. J Am Coll Surg. 2015;220(4):510–20. https://doi.org/10.1016/j.jamcollsurg.2014.12.024. Epub 2014 Dec 29

22. Giacopuzzi S, Bencivenga M, Weindelmayer J, Verlato G, de Manzoni G. Western strategy for EGJ carcinoma. Gastric Cancer. 2017;20(Suppl 1):60–8. https://doi.org/10.1007/s10120-016-0685-2. Epub 2016 Dec 30

23. Blank S, Schmidt T, Heger P, Strowitzki MJ, Sisic L, Heger U, Nienhueser H, Haag GM, Bruckner T, Mihaljevic AL, Ott K, Büchler MW, Ulrich A. Surgical strategies in true adenocarcinoma of the esophagogastric junction (AEG II): thoracoabdominal or abdominal approach? Gastric Cancer. 2018; https://doi.org/10.1007/s10120-017-0746-1. [Epub ahead of print].

24. Kneuertz PJ, Hofstetter WL, Chiang YJ, Das P, Blum M, Elimova E, Mansfield P, Ajani J, Badgwell B. Long-term survival in patients with gastroesophageal junction cancer treated with preoperative therapy: do thoracic and abdominal approaches differ? Ann Surg Oncol. 2016;23(2):626–32. https://doi.org/10.1245/s10434-015-4898-0. Epub 2015 Nov 12

25. Fuchs H, Hölscher AH, Leers J, Bludau M, Brinkmann S, Schröder W, Alakus H, Mönig S, Gutschow CA. Long-term quality of life after surgery for adenocarcinoma of the esophagogastric junction: extended gastrectomy or transthoracic esophagectomy? Gastric Cancer. 2016;19(1):312–7. https://doi.org/10.1007/s10120-015-0466-3. Epub 2015 Jan 28

26. Sugita S, Kinoshita T, Kaito A, Watanabe M, Sunagawa H. Short-term outcomes after laparoscopic versus open transhiatal resection of Siewert type II adenocarcinoma of the esophagogastric junction. Surg Endosc. 2018;32(1):383–90. https://doi.org/10.1007/s00464-017-5687-6. Epub 2017 Jun 27

27. Yamashita H, Katai H, Morita S, Saka M, Taniguchi H, Fukagawa T. Optimal extent of lymph node dissection for Siewert type II esophagogastric junction carcinoma. Ann Surg. 2011;254(2):274–80. https://doi.org/10.1097/SLA.0b013e3182263911.

28. Hasegawa S, Yoshikawa T, Rino Y, Oshima T, Aoyama T, Hayashi T, Sato T, Yukawa N, Kameda Y, Sasaki T, Ono H, Tsuchida K, Cho H, Kunisaki C, Masuda M, Tsuburaya A. Priority of lymph node dissection for Siewert type II/III adenocarcinoma of the esophago-

gastric junction. Ann Surg Oncol. 2013;20(13):4252–9. https://doi.org/10.1245/s10434-013-3036-0. Epub 2013 Aug 14

29. Mine S, Sano T, Hiki N, Yamada K, Nunobe S, Yamaguchi T. Lymphadenectomy around the left renal vein in Siewert type II adenocarcinoma of the oesophagogastric junction. Br J Surg. 2013;100(2):261–6. https://doi.org/10.1002/bjs.8967. Epub 2012 Nov 23

30. Nakamura M, Iwahashi M, Nakamori M, Naka T, Ojima T, Iida T, Katsuda M, Tsuji T, Hayata K, Mastumura S, Yamaue H. Lower mediastinal lymph node metastasis is an independent survival factor of Siewert type II and III adenocarcinomas in the gastroesophageal junction. Am Surg. 2012;78(5):567–73.

31. Lee IS, Ahn JY, Yook JH, Kim BS. Mediastinal lymph node dissection and distal esophagectomy is not essential in early esophagogastric junction adenocarcinoma. World J Surg Oncol. 2017;15(1):28. https://doi.org/10.1186/s12957-016-1088-x.

32. Suh YS, Lee KG, Oh SY, Kong SH, Lee HJ, Kim WH, Yang HK. Recurrence pattern and lymph node metastasis of adenocarcinoma at the esophagogastric junction. Ann Surg Oncol. 2017;24(12):3631–9. https://doi.org/10.1245/s10434-017-6011-3. Epub 2017 Aug 21

33. Wang JB, Lin MQ, Li P, Xie JW, Lin JX, Lu J, Chen QY, Cao LL, Lin M, Zheng CH, Huang CM. The prognostic relevance of parapyloric lymph node metastasis in Siewert type II/III adenocarcinoma of the esophagogastric junction. Eur J Surg Oncol. 2017;43(12):2333–40. https://doi.org/10.1016/j.ejso.2017.08.017. Epub 2017 Sep 8

34. Anderegg MC, Lagarde SM, Jagadesham VP, Gisbertz SS, Immanuel A, Meijer SL, Hulshof MC, Bergman JJ, van Laarhoven HW, Griffin SM, van Berge Henegouwen MI. Prognostic significance of the location of lymph node metastases in patients with adenocarcinoma of the distal esophagus or gastroesophageal junction. Ann Surg. 2016;264(5):847–53.

35. Yamashita H, Seto Y, Sano T, Makuuchi H, Ando N, Sasako M. Japanese gastric cancer association and the Japan esophageal society. Results of a nationwide retrospective study of lymphadenectomy for esopha-gogastric junction carcinoma. Gastric Cancer. 2017;20(Suppl1):69–83. https://doi.org/10.1007/s10120-016-0663-8. Epub 2016 Oct 28

36. Huh YJ, Lee HJ, Oh SY, Lee KG, Yang JY, Ahn HS, Suh YS, Kong SH, Lee KU, Yang HK. Clinical outcome of modified laparoscopy-assisted proximal gastrectomy compared to conventional proximal gastrectomy or total gastrectomy for upper-third early gastric cancer with special references to postoperative reflux esophagitis. J Gastric Cancer. 2015;15(3):191–200. https://doi.org/10.5230/jgc.2015.15.3.191. Epub 2015 Sep 30

37. Nishigori T, Okabe H, Tsunoda S, Shinohara H, Obama K, Hosogi H, Hisamori S, Miyazaki K, Nakayama T, Sakai Y. Superiority of laparoscopic proximal gastrectomy with hand-sewn esopha-gogastrostomy over total gastrectomy in improving postoperative

body weight loss and quality of life. Surg Endosc. 2017;31(9):3664–72. https://doi.org/10.1007/s00464-016-5403-y. Epub 2017 Jan 11

38. Jung DH, Lee Y, Kim DW, Park YS, Ahn SH, Park DJ, Kim HH. Laparoscopic proximal gastrectomy with double tract reconstruction is superior to laparoscopic total gastrectomy for proximal early gastric cancer. Surg Endosc. 2017;31(10):3961–9. https://doi.org/10.1007/s00464-017-5429-9. Epub 2017 Mar 24

39. Sugoor P, Shah S, Dusane R, Desouza A, Goel M, Shrikhande SV. Proximal gastrectomy versus total gastrectomy for proximal third gastric cancer: total

gastrectomy is not always necessary. Langenbeck's Arch Surg. 2016;401(5):687–97. https://doi.org/10.1007/s00423-016-1422-3. Epub 2016 May 4

40. Tao K, Dong JH. Phase I clinical research of jejunal interposition in adenocarcinoma of the esophagogastric junction II/III proximal gastrectomy. Gastroenterol Res Pract. 2016;2016:1639654. Epub 2016 Oct 19

41. Karanicolas PJ, Graham D, Gönen M, Strong VE, Brennan MF, Coit DG. Quality of life after gastrectomy for adenocarcinoma: a prospective cohort study. Ann Surg. 2013;257(6):1039–46. https://doi.org/10.1097/SLA.0b013e31828c4a19.

Surgery After Neoadjuvant Chemotherapy

21

Daniel Reim, Alexander Novotny, and Christoph Schuhmacher

Introduction

Neoadjuvant/perioperative chemotherapy (CT) for locally advanced gastric cancer has become a routine clinical procedure on the base of recent randomized controlled trials. This chapter describes the European prospective randomized controlled trials and focuses on their surgical results. Outcome-related measures are described from a surgical point of view. Numerous aspects are discussed, and the influence of surgical outcomes on oncologic results is critically reviewed.

Statement: This review fully has not been published or submitted before. All authors declare that they participated in the literature review and that they have seen and approved the final version. None of the authors have any conflicts of interest. No funds or grants or company gifts have been received, nor has the article been written by a third party.

D. Reim (✉) · A. Novotny · C. Schuhmacher (✉)
Klinik und Poliklinik für Chirurgie,
TUM School of Medicine,
Munich, Germany
e-mail: Daniel.reim@tum.de;
christoph.schuhmacher@ecrin.org

Clinical Trials for Neoadjuvant Chemotherapy and Their Surgical Outcomes

Neoadjuvant or perioperative CT is an accepted and recommended therapeutic approach of GC treatment in most European countries [1]. This goes back to the results of the British MAGIC [2] and the French FNLCC/FFCD trial [3], both of which included a rather large number of patients and were, thus, adequately powered. Both trials directly compared surgery with or without neoadjuvant or perioperative CT and showed a significant benefit for the multimodal approach.

Different theoretical advantages of neoadjuvant therapy over adjuvant therapy are discussed for potentially resectable GC [4]. One is the usually better general health condition of patients in the neoadjuvant setting. Another advantage is that downstaging of the tumor may lead to higher R0 resection rates. Several other benefits like effects on occult metastasis or single tumor cell dissemination (micrometastasis) at the earliest point in time are also discussed.

The MAGIC trial is the presently most recognized landmark study for perioperative CT [2]. Between 1994 and 2002 centers in the UK, Europe and Asia recruited patients with resectable GC and adenocarcinomas of the esophagogastric junction (EGJ). Patients were randomized to surgery with perioperative CT ($n = 250$) or surgery only ($n = 253$). CT consisted of three preoperative and three postoperative cycles of i.v. epirubicin, cisplatin, and continuous 5-FU. The fear that preoperative CT jeopardizes the perioperative outcome was not justified. Although remarkable and higher than common numbers presented by Asian authors, there was at least no significant difference in postoperative complications and 30-day mortality in both treatment arms (46% vs. 45% and 5.6% vs. 5.9%). For patients in the CT arm, a downstaging effect could be observed regarding the ypT and N-categories. OS as well as progression-free survival (PFS) of patients receiving perioperative CT was significantly increased compared to patients treated by surgery only ($p = 0.009$ and $p < 0.001$). The 5-year survival rate was 36% for patients receiving perioperative CT and 23% for patients treated by surgery only [2].

Critics of the perioperative treatment pointed out that many patients in the MAGIC trial did not receive the full number of postoperative CT cycles, because of poor performance status, complications, or compliance issues in the postoperative period. In fact, only about half (49.5%) of the patients who underwent preoperative treatment in the study also received the full courses of the planned postoperative CT.

Because the importance of the adjuvant component of the MAGIC regimen is uncertain, this issue was addressed by a retrospective study from the UK on a series of 66 patients undergoing perioperative CT according to the MAGIC protocol. The results of this study showed a considerable prognostic benefit in terms of disease-free survival (DFS) for patients receiving neoadjuvant as well as adjuvant treatment compared to patients who did not undergo postoperative CT, while OS was not significantly different between the two groups. So, administration of the adjuvant part of the regimen seemed to postpone tumor recurrence rather than preventing it [5].

The results of the French FNLCC ACCORD 07 FFCD 9703 trial confirmed data in favor of the establishment of perioperative CT for patients with resectable GC and esophageal adenocarcinoma [3]. The chemotherapeutic regimen consisted of two to three cycles of i.v. 5-FU and cisplatin. A postoperative CT was recommended in case of a response to the preoperative treatment or stable disease with positive lymph nodes. Two hundred twenty-four patients were randomized to receive either preoperative CT or primary surgery. The R0 resection rate among the patients receiving CT was significantly higher compared to the primary surgery arm (84% vs. 73%; $p = 0.04$). OS and DFS were significantly prolonged after CT ($p = 0.02$ and $p = 0.003$, respectively). The 5-year survival rates largely match those reported for the MAGIC trial (see above) with 38% in the CT and 24% in the surgery-only arm. [3]

The European Organization for Research and Treatment of Cancer (EORTC) 40954 Phase III trial investigated the same patient population as the MAGIC and the FNLCC ACCORD 07 FFCD 9703 trial, while adenocarcinomas of the distal esophagus (AEG I according to the Siewert's classification) were excluded [6]. Unfortunately the trial had to be closed early due to poor accrual after inclusion of 144 patients ($n = 72$ per treatment arm), while 360 patients were initially planned. The goal of the study was to achieve a surgical quality and higher grade of standardization. In contrast to the aforementioned, this trial solely relied on preoperative (neoadjuvant) CT with cisplatin, 5-FU, and folinic acid (PLF protocol). Resection was performed obeying strict surgical quality standards, including a D2 lymphadenectomy. The analysis of the patients included up to then showed a higher R0 resection rate among the patients treated with neoadjuvant CT compared to those undergoing primary surgery (81.9% vs. 66.7%; $p = 0.036$). A significant survival benefit could not be shown, but a downstaging and a tendency toward a prolonged OS and DFS for the neoadjuvant treatment arm were observed ($p = 0.113$ and $p = 0.065$). Postoperative complications and deaths were also more common among patients treated with neoadjuvant CT (27.1% vs. 16.2%; $p = 0.09$ and 4.3% vs. 1.5%), but did not differ significantly. With only 67 deaths occurring during the follow-up period, no survival benefit could be shown for the CT arm (median survival 64.6 mo. vs. 52.5 mo.;

$p = 0.466$) (in order to reach a power of 80%, 282 deaths would have been necessary). The fact that patient survival missed significance level in spite of higher R0 resection rates was attributed to the low patient number and the high surgical quality by the authors [6].

Ronellenfitsch et al. performed an interesting meta-analysis showing an absolute improvement in the survival of 9% at 5 years for patients undergoing perioperative CT [7]. This effect could be observed starting 18 months after surgery and was observable for 10 years. The odds of a R0 resection in patients treated with perioperative CT were 1.4 times higher than in untreated patients. Additionally no increase in postoperative morbidity and mortality as well as duration of hospitalization could be recognized. Also an interaction between age and treatment effect was considered. In contrast to a recently reported German series, no survival benefit from perioperative CT could be shown for elderly patients. Another remarkable point of a subgroup analysis was that there seemed to be a higher survival benefit for patients with tumors of the EGJ as compared to other sites [7], an observation which was basically confirmed in the patient population of a specialized German center [8].

There is also evidence in literature that patients with signet ring cell adenocarcinoma do not benefit from perioperative CT. Messager et al. investigated this issue in a multicenter comparative study including 3010 patients from 19 French centers including 1050 patients (34.9%) with signet cell histology [9]. In a patient cohort from the Klinikum rechts der Isar in Munich, Germany including 200 patients with diffuse-type histology having undergone neoadjuvant CT only, 14.5% showed a good histopathologic response (TRG1 according to Becker) [10]. In comparison 27.7% of patients with an intestinal type growth pattern ($n = 331$) showed a TRG1 in the histopathologic workup [unpublished data].

An ongoing British trial presently investigates the safety and efficacy of adding the monoclonal VEGF antibody bevacizumab to ECX CT administered perioperatively in patients with resectable gastric and EGJ adenocarcinomas [11]. This concept is based on the demonstrated beneficial effect of bevacizumab in the treatment of colorectal cancer and promising results in advanced GC (AVAGAST trial) [12].

Even though Asia is the traditional stronghold of adjuvant CT, neoadjuvant concepts recently gained interest for certain indications which are difficult to cure.

Currently the value of neoadjuvant CT in locally advanced, marginally resectable GC with poor prognosis, like tumors with paraaortal and/or bulky N2 and N3 nodal disease [13], large type 3 ($\geq$8 cm) or 4 (linitis plastica) tumors (JOCG0210 [14], JCOG0501 [15], JCOG1002 [16]), and T2–T3 N+ or T4 tumors (PRODIGY trial) [17], is investigated in Eastern Asia.

Despite promising results in the abovementioned trials, the outcomes appear to be difficult to evaluate due to the fact that the beneficial effects of perioperative chemotherapy are not directly attributed to either the neoadjuvant or the adjuvant part of the respective chemotherapeutic regimens. Therefore, careful consideration of the surgical outcomes within the trials is mandatory. One of the most debated issues regarding surgical technique and oncologic outcome is D2 lymphadenectomy. Recent data revealed the benefits even in the criticized Dutch gastric cancer trial [18]. The long-term results clearly demonstrated that adherence to D2 lymph node dissection resulted in reduced risk of death in gastric cancer patients. Therefore, it is important to review the abovementioned trials in the light of surgical procedures. Despite conceivable differences in ethnicity and biologic properties, survival outcomes between Eastern Asian and European patients appear to be enormous [19]. Whereas 5-year survival rates of around 60%–70% are reported in Japanese gastric cancer trials [20] in the surgery-only arms, a 20–30% 5-year survival rate is notable in the European trials for those patients undergoing surgery only for advanced gastric cancer [2, 3]. Therefore, surgical procedures appear to be relevant regarding the oncologic outcome also in patients having been treated by neoadjuvant or perioperative chemotherapy and have to be evaluated carefully in order to judge oncologic results.

MAGIC

The MAGIC trial was conducted in 104 centers in the UK, the Netherlands, Germany, Singapore, New Zealand, and Brazil between 1994 and 2002 [2]. Only 66–69% of the patients received curative resections, whereas 18–28% of all patients underwent palliative resection. The D2 dissection rates ranged from 40% to 43% of the patients, and 22–27% of the patients underwent esophago-gastrectomy for cardia cancer. Seventy-four percent of the patients suffered from stomach cancer, whereas all other patients had cancer of the lower esophagus or the cardia. The authors state that the extent of lymphadenectomy was left to the surgeons' discretion not making D2 dissection a prerequisite for the surgical procedure. The original paper does not report on preclinical stages but states that one of the inclusion criteria was at least stage II. The preoperative workup was not prescribed. Staging laparoscopy was not mandatory for the trial, and distant metastases were ruled out by CT scan. Additionally procedures involving the esophagus were not standardized regarding approach, luminal extent of resection, and lymphadenectomy.

ACCORD

The ACCORD trial was conducted in 28 French centers from 1995 to 2003 [3]. Seventy-five percent of the patients suffered from lower esophageal or gastric cardia cancer, whereas 25% of the patients had locally advanced gastric cancer. Forty-nine percent of the patients received esophagectomies, whereas gastrectomies were performed on 51% of the cases. D2 dissection was recommended for the study cohort, but the paper does not report on the success of D2 lymph node dissection. However, a median number of 19 dissected lymph nodes were reported. Preclinical stages were not reported in the original paper, and there is no data available if staging laparoscopy was performed in order to rule out peritoneal metastasis. Further surgical data is not available from the original publication.

EORTC

The EORTC trial was performed in ten experienced centers in Germany, Belgium, Portugal, the UK, and the Netherlands [6]. In contrast to the aforementioned trials, 96% of all patients had laparoscopic staging for pretherapeutic tumor classification. 51–54% of the patients revealed cancers of the GE junction or the proximal third of the stomach. All patients received gastrectomy (+/− transhiatal extension), and the D2 dissection rate was 93–96% with a median number of 31–33 dissected lymph nodes. Despite laparoscopic staging, 13–16% of the patients revealed metastatic disease in the final pathologic workup. The curative resection rate was 82% in those patients undergoing neoadjuvant chemotherapy compared to 67% for those patients undergoing surgery only. However, this effect did not translate into improved survival rates.

Implications of Surgical Outcomes After Neoadjuvant Chemotherapy

Regarding the heterogeneous (European) results derived from randomized controlled trials investigating the role of neoadjuvant/perioperative chemotherapy, it has to be stated that surgical quality reporting is underrepresented in the respective publications. Therefore, interpretation of the results, especially when it comes to comparisons with Eastern Asian data, has to be conducted carefully. First of all, reporting of preclinical data is insufficient. The landmark trials do not sufficiently report on the staging process. The EORTC trial may be considered an exemption, although only clinical T-stage is being reported. There is no information on the clinical N-stage, which may be related to the fact that not all centers perform endoscopic ultrasound. However, this factor could be negligible due to the fact that endoscopic N-staging did not demonstrate to be a reliable method, especially in cT2 cancers. Another point of criticism in the reported trials is that surgical procedures in the MAGIC and ACCORD trials did not adhere to

Eastern Asian standards, either D2 dissection rates are not reported or the number of dissected lymph nodes is too low in order to allow for sufficient surgical quality. The MAGIC trial reported that only 40% of the patients received D2 dissection and the ACCORD trial did not report on D2 dissection rates at all. However, adequate lymph node dissection was performed in the EORTC trial with a D2 dissection rate of 96% which is remarkable for European standards. Compared to results from Japanese trials, these results appear to be improvable in future trials. Here D2 dissection rates are 100%, and 5-year survival rate for the standard treatments for advanced gastric cancer accounts for over 60%. Nonetheless, D2 dissection cannot be considered as the only culprit for these survival differences. The Japanese trialists rigorously excluded patients from their trials when curative resections are not reached. In the S1 trials, for example, patients were even excluded when peritoneal washing cytology was not done. At least staging laparoscopy was performed in the EORTC trial to rule out occult peritoneal metastasis in contrast to the French and the British trial. Another issue could be the frequency of postoperative complications. In the MAGIC trial, a complication rate of over 40% was reported, whereas postoperative morbidity accounted for 20–30% in the ACCORD and EORTC trials. The postoperative complication rate in the S1 trial, for example, was below 20% [20]. Several groups reported that survival of postoperative complications leads to worsened long-term outcomes after oncologic surgery [21–23]. Toner et al. reported that survival of postoperative complications leads to worsened long-term outcomes after oncologic surgery [21]. The differences in postoperative complication rates could also be related to the various distributions of tumor location within the reported trials. At least half of the patients in all European trials had GE junction cancer. This stands in stark contrast to Eastern Asian patients where GE junction cancers rarely occur. This also leads to a higher amount of total gastrectomies or even esophagectomies leading to increased morbidity rates compared to Eastern Asian patients who usually undergo subtotal gastrectomy for cancer. Another issue could be the influence of obesity in the Western world. Another reason for higher complication rates in Western patient collectives could be the significantly higher BMI compared to Asians. Kodera et al. published that in Japanese patients higher BMIs were significantly related to postoperative complications after gastric cancer surgery [23].

Comparing the three European landmark studies, it appears remarkable that there could be a relation between surgical quality and the number of participating centers. The lower the number of trial sites became, the better the outcome in the surgery-only arm was. Surgery-related morbidity was highest in the MAGIC trial where over 100 centers took part, whereas the morbidity rate was lowest in the EORTC trial with only 10 participating trial centers. Several analyses in the past demonstrated a centralization effect for esophageal and gastric cancer surgery. One study reported specifically on gastric cancer which demonstrated that 30-day mortality could be reduced by over 7% per additional case in surgeons with an annual volume of at least 14 gastrectomies [24]. Another analysis from England reported that increasing hospital volume resulted in lower mortality, especially in the first 30 days after the surgical procedure [25]. Interestingly this effect was also detected in long-term outcomes leading to the intriguing suspicion that oncologic outcome could possibly be influenced just by hospital and individual surgeon's case volume. This also leads to the conclusion that the design of future trials should consider these facts and include only centers with the respective expertise in gastric cancer surgery.

Conclusions

In general, surgery after neoadjuvant chemotherapy should not be different from surgical procedures without multimodal treatments especially in advanced gastric cancer patients. The obvious advantages of D2 lymphadenectomy and radical surgery for complete tumor removal have been demonstrated in the past. Especially Eastern Asian surgical principles demonstrated their effectiveness before and should not be abandoned for Western patients undergoing treatment for locally advanced gastric cancers. The European trials on neoadjuvant/perioperative chemotherapy produced heterogeneous results regarding oncologic outcomes. Generally speaking, surgical aspects are underrepresented in these multicenter trials that led to the adoption of neoadjuvant chemotherapy in clinical routine for locally advanced gastric cancer. These trials are difficult to evaluate in their efficacy due to the heterogeneous surgical outcomes. This may be related to either an underreporting of surgical aspects or due to non-compliance with surgical (Eastern Asian) principles or to a non-efficient surgical quality control. The optimal staging modalities are still not defined yet and have to be consented on an international scale. From the author's point of view, EGD, endoscopic ultrasound, CT scans, and staging laparoscopy are considered to be mandatory for defining a clinical stage. Surgical quality controls of the respective trial participant should be mandatory before enrolling patients into clinical trials. This was demonstrated before by Korean trialists who claimed a surgical quality control study for the participating surgeons in order to demonstrate proficiency with the required techniques. A rigorous quality control by photo or video documentation or peer-reviewed trainings should be a prerequisite for future trials investigating on the outcome of neoadjuvant or perioperative chemotherapy for advanced gastric cancer. Centralization to trial sites with high surgical expertise should be held in mind to improve surgical outcomes. Therefore, interpretation of the respective trials in an international context and especially in comparisons with Eastern Asian trials will be difficult to perform. Nonetheless, Eastern Asian data from randomized controlled trials investigating the role of neoadjuvant/perioperative chemotherapy are not yet available and are desperately awaited to evaluate its value in a highly trained surgical community.

Most of the European landmark trials on perioperative CT were headed by medical oncologists. The lion's share of points of criticism on those trials could have been avoided by a closer involvement of surgeons when those trials were planned. These surgeons should not only be experienced in the performed procedures but also in the development of clinical trials. This is likewise a plea to all academic surgeons to involve themselves more in the conduct and initiation of clinical trials dealing with multimodal treatment strategies, not leaving this field solely to medical oncologists and/or radiooncologists.

References

1. Meyer HJ, Holscher AH, Lordick F, et al. Current S3 guidelines on surgical treatment of gastric carcinoma. Chirurg. 2012;83(1):31–7.
2. Cunningham D, Allum WH, Stenning SP, et al. Perioperative chemotherapy versus surgery alone for resectable gastroesophageal cancer. N Engl J Med. 2006;355(1):11–20.
3. Ychou M, Boige V, Pignon J-P, et al. Perioperative chemotherapy compared with surgery alone for resectable gastroesophageal adenocarcinoma: an FNCLCC and FFCD multicenter phase III trial. J Clin Oncol. 2011;29(13):1715–21.
4. Ott K, Lordick F, Blank S, et al. Gastric cancer: surgery in 2011. Langenbeck's Arch Surg. 2011;396(6):743–58.
5. Mirza A, Pritchard S, Welch I. The postoperative component of MAGIC chemotherapy is associated with improved prognosis following surgical resection in gastric and gastroesophageal junction adenocarcinomas. Int J Surg Oncol. 2013;2013:781742.
6. Schuhmacher C, Gretschel S, Lordick F, et al. Neoadjuvant chemotherapy compared with surgery alone for locally advanced cancer of the stomach and cardia: European Organisation for Research and Treatment of Cancer randomized trial 40954. J Clin Oncol. 2010;28(35):5210–8.
7. Ronellenfitsch U, Schwarzbach M, Hofheinz R, et al. Perioperative chemo(radio)therapy versus primary surgery for resectable adenocarcinoma of the stomach, gastroesophageal junction, and lower esophagus. Cochrane Database Syst Rev. 2013;5:CD008107.
8. Reim D, Gertler R, Novotny A, et al. Adenocarcinomas of the esophagogastric junction are more likely to respond to preoperative chemotherapy than distal gastric cancer. Ann Surg Oncol. 2012;19(7):2108–18.
9. Messager M, Lefevre JH, Pichot-Delahaye V, et al. The impact of perioperative chemotherapy on survival in patients with gastric signet ring cell adenocarcinoma: a multicenter comparative study. Ann Surg. 2011;254(5):684–93.
10. Becker K, Mueller JD, Schulmacher C, et al. Histomorphology and grading of regression in gastric

carcinoma treated with neoadjuvant chemotherapy. Cancer. 2003;98(7):1521–30.

11. Cunningham D, Stenning SP, Smyth EC, et al. Perioperative chemotherapy with or without bevacizumab in operable oesophagogastric adenocarcinoma (UK Medical Research Council ST03): primary analysis results of a multicentre, open-label, randomised phase 2-3 trial. Lancet Oncol. 2017;18(3):357–70.

12. Ohtsu A, Shah MA, Van Cutsem E, et al. Bevacizumab in combination with chemotherapy as first-line therapy in advanced gastric cancer: a randomized, double-blind, placebo-controlled phase III study. J Clin Oncol. 2011;29(30):3968–76.

13. Matsumoto T, Sasako M, Mizusawa J, et al. HER2 expression in locally advanced gastric cancer with extensive lymph node (bulky N2 or paraaortic) metastasis (JCOG1005-A trial). Gastric Cancer. 2015;18(3):467–75.

14. Iwasaki Y, Sasako M, Yamamoto S, et al. Phase II study of preoperative chemotherapy with S-1 and cisplatin followed by gastrectomy for clinically resectable type 4 and large type 3 gastric cancers (JCOG0210). J Surg Oncol. 2013;107(7):741–5.

15. Tanemura H, Oshita H, Yamada M, et al. Therapeutic outcome and prognosis in S-1+CDDP chemotherapy for advanced gastric cancer – postoperative histopathological assessment. Gan To Kagaku Ryoho. 2010;37(3):447–51.

16. Katayama H, Ito S, Sano T, et al. A phase II study of systemic chemotherapy with docetaxel, cisplatin, and S-1 (DCS) followed by surgery in gastric cancer patients with extensive lymph node metastasis: Japan Clinical Oncology Group study JCOG1002. Jpn J Clin Oncol. 2012;42(6):556–9.

17. Zang DY, Yang DH, Kim MJ, et al. Dose-finding study of docetaxel, oxaliplatin, and S-1 for patients with advanced gastric cancer. Cancer Chemother Pharmacol. 2009;64(5):877–83.

18. Songun I, Putter H, EM-K K, et al. Surgical treatment of gastric cancer: 15-year follow-up results of the randomised nationwide Dutch D1D2 trial. Lancet Oncol. 2010;11(5):439–49.

19. Merrett ND. Multimodality treatment of potentially curative gastric cancer: geographical variations and future prospects. World J Gastroenterol. 2014;20(36):12892–9.

20. Sasako M, Sakuramoto S, Katai H, et al. Five-year outcomes of a randomized phase III trial comparing adjuvant chemotherapy with S-1 versus surgery alone in stage II or III gastric cancer. J Clin Oncol. 2011;29(33):4387–93.

21. Toner A, Hamilton M. The long-term effects of postoperative complications. Curr Opin Crit Care. 2013;19(4):364–8.

22. Kodera Y, Ito S, Yamamura Y, et al. Obesity and outcome of distal gastrectomy with D2 lymphadenectomy for carcinoma. Hepato-Gastroenterology. 2004;51(58):1225–8.

23. Moriwaki Y, Kunisaki C, Kobayashi S, et al. Does body mass index (BMI) influence morbidity and long-term survival in gastric cancer patients after gastrectomy? Hepato-Gastroenterology. 2003;50(49):284–8.

24. Mamidanna R, Ni Z, Anderson O, et al. Surgeon volume and cancer esophagectomy, gastrectomy, and pancreatectomy: a population-based study in England. Ann Surg. 2016;263(4):727–32.

25. Coupland VH, Lagergren J, Luchtenborg M, et al. Hospital volume, proportion resected and mortality from oesophageal and gastric cancer: a population-based study in England, 2004–2008. Gut. 2013;62(7):961–6.

Part XII

Surgery for Remnant Gastric Cancer

Surgery for Remnant Gastric Cancer: Open Surgery

22

Yoon Young Choi and Sung Hoon Noh

Introduction

Remnant gastric cancer is a type of complicated gastric cancer. Although no consensus definition has been established to date, the most popular definition of remnant gastric cancer is a cancer in the remaining stomach at least 5 years after gastrectomy, regardless of the reason for the primary surgery (i.e., whether it was for benign or malignant disease). In the 1970s and 1980s, gastrectomy was frequently performed for complicated peptic ulcer disease, and most instances of remnant gastric cancer were located in the stomach remaining after surgery for this benign disorder. Nowadays, gastrectomy for benign disease has become less frequent because of the development

of effective medical treatment for peptic ulcer disease, which has led to a decrease in the frequency of remnant gastric cancer after surgery for benign disease. By contrast, nationwide mass screening for gastric cancer has increased the proportion of early gastric cancers detected in Korea and Japan, and treatment strategies for gastric cancer have improved, leading to longer survival of patients with gastric cancer. Unlike gastric cancers in Western countries, which generally occur in the upper third of the stomach, 60–70% of gastric cancers in Korea and Japan occur in the distal stomach and are usually treated by distal gastrectomy. Consequently, the incidence of remnant gastric cancer is expected to increase, especially in East Asia.

Despite the clinical importance of remnant gastric cancer, the molecular carcinogenesis and clinical features of this cancer have not been well characterized; consequently, optimal treatment strategies for remnant gastric cancer have not been established. Reasons for the lack of clinical knowledge about this disease may include its low incidence (follow-up after gastrectomy has demonstrated remnant gastric cancer incidence rates of 1–3% [1–3]) and the use of variable definitions of remnant gastric cancer in the available studies (which is especially apparent as we are now in a transition period, with the incidence after surgery for benign disease decreasing and the incidence after surgery for cancer increasing).

Electronic Supplementary Material The online version of this chapter (https://doi.org/10.1007/978-3-662-45583-8_22) contains supplementary material, which is available to authorized users.

Y. Y. Choi
Department of Surgery, Yonsei University Health System, Yonsei University College of Medicine, Seoul, Republic of Korea

S. H. Noh (✉)
Department of Surgery, Yonsei University Health System, Yonsei University College of Medicine, Seoul, Republic of Korea

Brain Korea 21 PLUS Project for Medical Science, Yonsei University Health System, Yonsei University College of Medicine, Seoul, Republic of Korea
e-mail: sunghoonn@yuhs.ac

Because of the paucity of information regarding treatment options for remnant gastric cancer per se, clinical practice has generally been based on knowledge about primary gastric cancer, especially in terms of staging of the disease [4], extent of surgical resection, and chemotherapy regimens. The available knowledge about remnant gastric cancer, derived from retrospective studies at large-volume hospitals and multiple centers, suggests that the prognosis of this cancer is comparable to that of primary gastric cancer. However, this does not mean that the treatment of remnant gastric cancer does not need to be distinguished from that of primary gastric cancer because the lymphatic structure and molecular carcinogenesis of the two types of cancer could differ [5].

Detailed discussions of the molecular mechanisms of, and perioperative chemotherapy and radiotherapy for, remnant gastric cancer are beyond the scope of the current section. In this chapter, we introduce the clinicopathologic characteristics of remnant gastric cancer and the expected patterns of lymphatic metastases according to the type of previous reconstruction. In addition, we briefly introduce the possibility of endoscopic treatment and minimally invasive surgery (laparoscopic or robotic surgery) for remnant gastric cancer. Finally, the issues surrounding, and the detailed procedures of, gastrectomy and lymph node dissection for remnant gastrectomy will be addressed and related to treatment outcomes of remnant gastric cancer.

Clinicopathologic Characteristics of Remnant Gastric Cancer

Remnant gastric cancer has an incidence of 1–3% and is much more common in males than females (the male/female ratio is 3–5:1). The time interval between primary gastrectomy and the diagnosis of remnant gastric cancer depends on the reason for the initial surgery: the interval is generally shorter after surgery for malignant disease (approximately 10 years) than after gastrectomy for benign disease (approximately 30 years). In addition, remnant gastric cancer is more frequent after

gastrojejunostomy than after gastroduodenostomy. Chronic inflammation due to bile reflux is one of the putative mechanisms responsible for the development of remnant gastric cancer, whereas the etiology of other remnant gastric cancers may be similar to that of primary gastric cancer.

Lymph Node Metastases in Remnant Gastric Cancer

Lymphatic flow around the remnant stomach is changed because of the altered anatomy caused by the previous surgery; lymphatic drainage of the remnant stomach after gastroduodenostomy is different from that after gastrojejunostomy. In addition, lymphatic drainage is also affected by the reason for the initial surgery because a more extended lymph node dissection would have been performed for malignant disease, whereas a more limited or no lymph node dissection would have been performed for benign disease. Therefore, the surgical approach should be distinguished according to the type of reconstruction and reason for the initial surgery.

After gastroduodenostomy, cancer in the remnant stomach can spread to the hepatoduodenal ligament, superior mesenteric vein, splenic vessels, and short gastric vessels (Fig. 22.1). After gastrojejunostomy, the lymphatic flow is similar to that observed gastroduodenostomy, so the cancer can spread through the splenic and short gastric vessels. However, lymphatic flow differs after gastrojejunostomy in that metastases can also spread to the mesentery of the jejunum through the anastomosis site (Fig. 22.2). Of course, when the right gastroepiploic, right gastric, and left gastric vessels are retained after the previous surgery (mainly after surgery for benign disease), cancer in the remnant stomach can spread through the lymphatics around these remaining vessels as well. Thus, although there is no definition of D2 for remnant stomach cancer, all D2 lymph nodes for primary gastric cancer should be removed. Furthermore, because lymphatics around the splenic vessels are the main lymphatic flow of the remnant stomach, lymph node dissection in this area should be performed meticulously. Routine

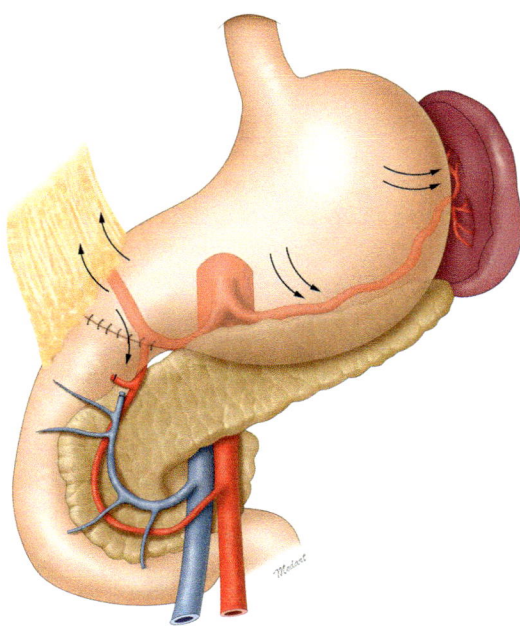

Fig. 22.1 The lymphatic flows of remnant stomach after gastroduodenostomy. The cancer can spread to hepatoduodenal ligament, superior mesenteric vessels, splenic vessels, and short gastric vessels

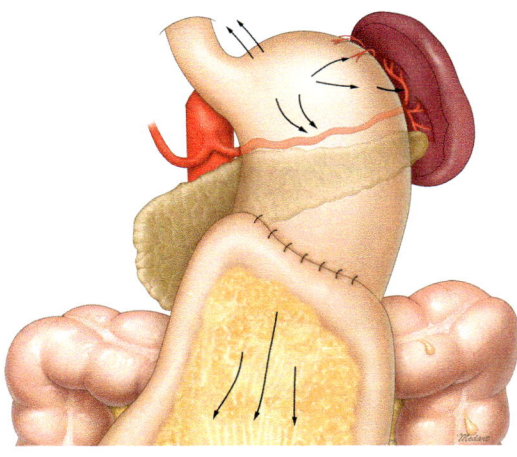

Fig. 22.2 The lymphatic flows of remnant stomach after gastrojejunostomy. The cancer can spread not only through vessels around stomach but also through the mesentery of the jejunum

splenectomy for lymph node dissection around the splenic vessels is not recommended, which is similar to the situation for primary gastric cancer in the upper third of the stomach; however, com-

plete removal of lymph nodes is a prerequisite for spleen-preserving completion total gastrectomy for remnant gastric cancer.

Minimally Invasive Treatment for Remnant Gastric Cancer

Endoscopic Treatment

Endoscopic resection of gastric cancer, such as by endoscopic mucosal resection and endoscopic submucosal dissection, has become widely used to treat primary gastric cancer in the very early stages. The absence of lymph node metastases is a prerequisite for endoscopic resection of gastric cancer because the procedure only involves removal of the primary cancer, without any lymph node dissection. Selection of which patients can be candidates for this treatment was based on a large-scale review of pathologic results from surgical specimens. Gotoda et al. reviewed the pathologic results of 5265 patients who underwent gastrectomy with lymph node dissection for early gastric cancer and developed a stratification system regarding the risk of lymph node metastasis [6]. Based on these results, patients with a very low risk of lymph node metastases have been treated with endoscopic resection. It is not yet clear whether endoscopic resection is feasible or efficacious for remnant gastric cancer, however, because of the limited number of cases of this type of tumor. In addition, endoscopic resection would be technically challenging because of the narrow space and fibrotic changes around the stapled anastomosis site. Despite these difficulties, recent studies have shown that endoscopic resection for remnant gastric cancer is feasible [7–12], and it has been suggested that the same indications for endoscopic resection of primary gastric cancer might be applied to remnant gastric cancer as well [13]. Considering the high degree of difficulty performing completion total gastrectomy for remnant gastric cancer because of fibrosis, adhesions, and changed anatomy, endoscopic resection could be a reasonable treatment option for remnant gastric cancer with a very low risk of lymph node metastases, especially in patients with severe comorbidities.

Laparoscopic and Robotic Surgery

Surgery for remnant gastric cancer is technically challenging because of fibrosis, adhesions, and altered anatomy caused by previous surgery. Thus, minimally invasive surgery (such as laparoscopic or robotic surgery) for remnant gastric cancer is difficult to perform, and substantial surgical skills and experience, as well as a comprehensive understanding of the anatomy, are required to perform this procedure. Some surgeons with advanced laparoscopic skills have attempted this seemingly impossible surgery and reported it to be feasible and possible to perform safely, with morbidity and mortality rates comparable to those of open surgery [14–18]. When surgeons try to perform completion total gastrectomy by laparoscopic or robotic methods, there should be no hesitation to convert to open surgery if a problem arises. Detailed results and surgical techniques for minimally invasive surgery of remnant gastric cancer are addressed in another chapter.

Open Surgery for Remnant Gastric Cancer

Difficulties with performing completion total gastrectomy for remnant gastric cancer arise from two distinct characteristics of remnant gastric cancer: (1) the presence of adhesions and fibrosis caused by the previous surgery and (2) changes in the lymphatic drainage. It is generally agreed that there will be more adhesions and fibrosis when the previous surgery was for cancer rather than for benign disease. There will be adhesions around the remnant stomach extending to the wound, other peritoneal surfaces, small bowel, colon, and liver, but the most critical region for completion total gastrectomy will be the supra-pancreatic area. Especially when the

reason for previous surgery was cancer, lymph nodes around the celiac axis would have been dissected, which in turn produces more adhesions and fibrosis in the supra-pancreatic area. Consequently, surgeons should be very careful to avoid injuring major vessels, such as the common hepatic artery, portal vein, splenic artery and vein, and even the aorta and inferior vena cava. Dissecting the lymph nodes from the patient's left to right side rather than right to left side may help identify the appropriate anatomical plane because the anatomy of the left side (around the splenic hilum) may not be affected by the previous surgery. The right gastroepiploic and right gastric vessels would usually have been ligated during the prior surgery, but the left gastroepiploic and left gastric vessels would rarely have been ligated when the reason for previous gastrectomy was benign disease. Although the right gastroepiploic and right gastric vessels would have already been ligated by the previous surgery, careful lymph node dissection around #5 and #6 would be required if the previous surgery was for benign disease. Lymph nodes around the superior mesenteric vein (#14v) are not included in the current D2 lymph node dissection for primary gastric cancer, but if this node remains and the tumor in the remnant stomach is located near the gastroduodenostomy site, dissecting #14v would be helpful for accurate staging and prognosis determination.

After careful dissection between the abdominal wall and intestines, the anatomy around remnant stomach should be identified through adhesiolysis. When the greater omentum remains, total omentectomy is performed in the same manner as during primary gastric cancer surgery. Usually adhesions exist between the liver and the ventral side of the stomach, and gentle dissection of the plane between the liver surface and gastric wall is required. When the tumor is located on the anterior side of the stomach, the surgeon should be careful not to injure the gastric wall during the dissection.

When the previous surgery involved a gastroduodenostomy, the duodenum is transected by stapling, after fully identifying the borders of the duodenum, stomach, and pancreas. Sometimes the gastroduodenostomy was performed by stapling during the previous surgery and is close to the head of the pancreas; if so, resecting the duodenum by stapling will be difficult. In this situation, the duodenum can be transected by a scalpel and the opening repaired by hand suturing (recently, delta anastomosis for laparoscopic gastroduodenostomy has become popular [19], and it would be difficult to secure enough space for duodenectomy with stapling after this type of anastomosis because the previous staple line may extend into the deep part of the duodenum).

Previous gastrojejunostomy would have been performed via an antecolic or retrocolic route. When the previous anastomosis was anterior to the transverse colon, if the cancer does not invade the transverse colon, adhesions between the stomach, jejunum, and transverse colon should be carefully dissected, and both the afferent and efferent jejunum should be divided and transected. Because remnant gastric cancer can spread through the mesentery of the jejunum (Fig. 22.2), the lymph nodes around this mesentery should be removed as appropriate. When the previous gastrojejunostomy was performed by the retrocolic route, the mesocolon should be carefully divided without damaging the vessels supplying the transverse colon. If the cancer invades the transverse colon or vessels of the transverse colon, segmental resection of the transverse colon should be considered.

After resection of the duodenum following gastroduodenostomy or resection of both the afferent and efferent jejunum (and sometimes the transverse colon as well) following gastrojejunostomy, the remnant stomach is lifted upward and retracted by a second assistant. There will be fibrotic adhesions in the supra-pancreatic area if the reason for previous surgery was cancer. Adhesions in the supra-pancreatic area are divided, and any lymph nodes at #12a, #8a, #7, #11p, or #9 remaining from the previous surgery are dissected in the same manner as for primary gastric cancer.

Splenic hilar lymph node dissection is one of the most important parts of surgery for remnant gastric cancer, but relatively fewer adhesions are located here because this area will not have been affected by the previous gastrectomy, regardless of the reason for the surgery. When the left gastroepiploic vessels were not previously dissected, dissecting #4Sb and ligating the short gastric vessels (#4Sa) can expose the hilum of the spleen. If it is technically difficult to dissect the lymph nodes at the splenic hilum, splenectomy must be considered. However, routine splenectomy for completion total gastrectomy is not recommended, which is similar to the situation with total gastrectomy for primary gastric cancer. Note that spleen-preserving completion total gastrectomy is not the same as lymph nodes-around-the-splenic-hilum-preserving gastrectomy.

Figures 22.3 and 22.4 depict the extent of resection of the remnant stomach for remnant gastric cancer according to the type of previous anastomosis. The attached video clip summarizes the procedure of open completion total gastrectomy for remnant gastric cancer. This 71-year-old female patient underwent gastrectomy with gastrojejunostomy (loop, antecolic) for peptic ulcer disease 35 years previously. The order of dissection can be changed according to the surgeon's preferences.

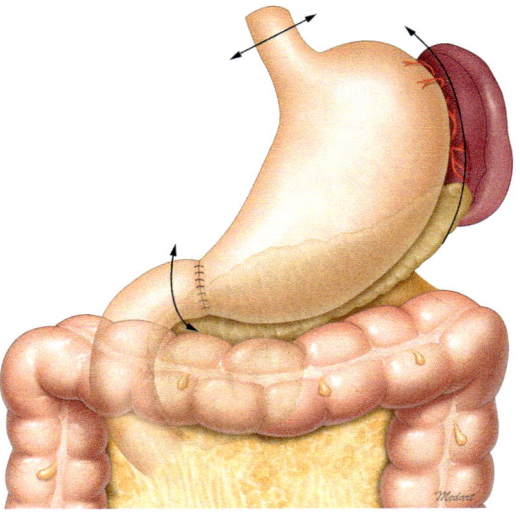

Fig. 22.3 The extent of resection of remnant stomach after gastroduodenostomy for remnant gastric cancer

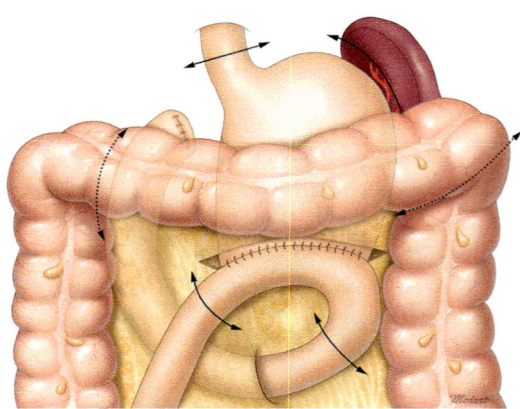

Fig. 22.4 The extent of resection of remnant stomach after gastrojejunostomy for remnant gastric cancer

Treatment Outcomes of Remnant Gastric Cancer

Short-term outcomes of completion total gastrectomy for remnant gastric cancer have been reported by several studies. Postoperative morbidity rates have varied from 20% to 40%, and postoperative mortality rates have ranged from 0% to 12.5% [20–24]. Of note, most of these studies were conducted in East Asia, including Korea, Japan, and China. The mortality was relatively high in a study from the West [24]; however, this report was too old (published in 1986) to allow one to conclude that there is difference in mortality after completion total gastrectomy between the East and West. Overall, the morbidity and mortality rates after completion total gastrectomy for remnant gastric cancer seem to be generally similar to those reported after gastrectomy for primary gastric cancer. Few studies have directly compared short-term outcomes after remnant gastric cancer surgery to those after primary gastric cancer surgery; in these reports, outcomes were similar after both types of surgery [21, 25].

Whether the prognosis of remnant gastric cancer is poorer than that of primary gastric cancer in the upper third of the stomach is controversial [3, 26–34]. A recent systematic review that conducted pooled analyses examining this issue found that the outcomes among previous studies were significantly heterogeneous [5]. In subgroup analyses, the prognosis of remnant gastric cancer was similar in the early stages (stage I/II according to the current TNM staging system for primary gastric cancer) but poorer in the advanced stages (stage III/IV), compared to the prognosis after primary gastric cancer in the upper third of the stomach. These findings cannot be considered conclusive, and the reason for these results is not yet clear. However, they emphasize the importance of early detection of remnant gastric cancer.

Discussion

Remnant gastric cancers that we encounter clinically are mixtures of cancers that are similar to primary gastric cancers, tumors caused by chronic inflammation secondary to bile reflux, and other cancers caused by mechanisms that are not yet well understood. These varying etiologies of remnant gastric cancer lead to heterogeneous clinical responses to standard treatments, which are generally based on our current knowledge regarding primary gastric cancer. In addition, remnant gastric cancer in recent years primarily involves cancer in the remnant stomach after distal gastrectomy. Recently, function-preserving gastrectomy (e.g., proximal gastrectomy) has become popular to improve the quality of life of patients with early-stage gastric cancer, and survivors who have undergone this type of surgery are becoming more common. If we consider that two-thirds of gastric cancers in Korea and Japan occur in the lower third of the stomach, remnant gastric cancer after proximal gastrectomy for gastric cancer will likely increase in frequency, as the lower third of the stomach remains after this surgery; consequently, the landscape of remnant gastric cancer will change again. However, whether this type of remnant gastric cancer would or would not be similar to primary gastric cancer is another unclear issue.

Even amidst the aforementioned complexity, it is clear that radical surgery for remnant gastric cancer is the only treatment strategy available to provide a true cure. Nevertheless, radical surgery for remnant gastric cancer is technically difficult and challenging because of adhesions and fibrosis due to the previous surgery and because of alterations in the anatomy, including changes in the lymphatic drainage. Therefore, surgeons should refine their surgical skills and experience to conquer the present and upcoming complex disease, remnant gastric cancer. In addition, it cannot be overemphasized that following oncologic principles for cancer surgery is important for all operations involving remnant gastric cancer.

References

1. Kodera Y, Yamamura Y, Torii A, Uesaka K, Hirai T, Yasui K, et al. Incidence, diagnosis and significance of multiple gastric cancer. Br J Surg. 1995;82(11):1540–3.. Epub 1995/11/01. PubMed PMID: 8535813
2. Viste A, Bjornestad E, Opheim P, Skarstein A, Thunold J, Hartveit F, et al. Risk of carcinoma following gastric operations for benign disease. A historical cohort study of 3470 patients. Lancet. 1986;2(8505):502–5. PubMed PMID: 2875248
3. Kaneko K, Kondo H, Saito D, Shirao K, Yamaguchi H, Yokota T, et al. Early gastric stump cancer following distal gastrectomy. Gut. 1998;43(3):342–4. PubMed PMID: 9863478; PubMed Central PMCID: PMC1727245
4. Nakagawa M, Choi YY, An JY, Hong JH, Kim JW, Kim HI, et al. Staging for remnant gastric cancer: the metastatic lymph node ratio vs. the UICC 7th edition system. Ann Surg Oncol. 2016; https://doi.org/10.1245/s10434-016-5390-1. PubMed PMID: 27370654
5. Shimada H, Fukagawa T, Haga Y, Oba K. Does remnant gastric cancer really differ from primary gastric cancer? A systematic review of the literature by the Task Force of Japanese Gastric Cancer Association. Gastric Cancer. 2015; https://doi.org/10.1007/s10120-015-0582-0. Epub 2015/12/17. PubMed PMID: 26667370
6. Gotoda T, Yanagisawa A, Sasako M, Ono H, Nakanishi Y, Shimoda T, et al. Incidence of lymph node metastasis from early gastric cancer: estimation with a large number of cases at two large centers. Gastric Cancer. 2000;3(4):219–25. PubMed PMID: 11984739
7. Ojima T, Takifuji K, Nakamura M, Nakamori M, Katsuda M, Iida T, et al. Endoscopic submucosal dissection for gastric tumors in various types of remnant stomach. Endoscopy. 2014;46(8):645–9. https://doi.org/10.1055/s-0034-1365454. PubMed PMID: 24777426
8. Takenaka R, Kawahara Y, Okada H, Tsuzuki T, Yagi S, Kato J, et al. Endoscopic submucosal dissection for cancers of the remnant stomach after distal gastrectomy. Gastrointest Endosc. 2008;67(2):359–63. https://doi.org/10.1016/j.gie.2007.10.021. Epub 2008/01/30. PubMed PMID: 18226704
9. Hirasaki S, Kanzaki H, Matsubara M, Fujita K, Matsumura S, Suzuki S. Treatment of gastric remnant cancer post distal gastrectomy by endoscopic submucosal dissection using an insulation-tipped diathermic knife. World J Gastroenterol. 2008;14(16):2550–5. Epub 2008/04/30. PubMed PMID: 18442204; PubMed Central PMCID: PMCPMC2708368
10. Nonaka S, Oda I, Makazu M, Haruyama S, Abe S, Suzuki H, et al. Endoscopic submucosal dissection for early gastric cancer in the remnant stomach after gastrectomy. Gastrointest Endosc. 2013;78(1):63–72. https://doi.org/10.1016/j.gie.2013.02.006. Epub 2013/04/10PubMed PMID: 23566640
11. Tanaka S, Toyonaga T, Morita Y, Fujita T, Yoshizaki T, Kawara F, et al. Endoscopic submucosal dissection for early gastric cancer in anastomosis site after distal gastrectomy. Gastric Cancer. 2014;17(2):371–6. https://doi.org/10.1007/s10120-013-0283-5. Epub 2013/07/23. PubMed PMID: 23868403
12. Lee JY, Choi IJ, Cho SJ, Kim CG, Kook MC, Lee JH, et al. Endoscopic submucosal dissection for metachronous tumor in the remnant stomach after distal gastrectomy. Surg Endosc. 2010;24(6):1360–6. https://doi.org/10.1007/s00464-009-0779-6.. PubMed PMID: 19997930
13. Choi YY, Kwon IG, Lee SK, Kim HK, An JY, Kim HI, et al. Can we apply the same indication of endoscopic submucosal dissection for primary gastric cancer to remnant gastric cancer? Gastric Cancer. 2014;17(2):310–5. https://doi.org/10.1007/s10120-013-0265-7.. Epub 2013/05/23. PubMed PMID: 23695167
14. Kwon IG, Cho I, Guner A, Choi YY, Shin HB, Kim HI, et al. Minimally invasive surgery for remnant gastric cancer: a comparison with open surgery. Surg Endosc. 2014;28(8):2452–8. https://doi.org/10.1007/s00464-014-3496-8. Epub 2014/03/14. PubMed PMID: 24622766
15. Tsunoda S, Okabe H, Tanaka E, Hisamori S, Harigai M, Murakami K, et al. Laparoscopic gastrectomy for remnant gastric cancer: a comprehensive review and case series. Gastric Cancer. 2016;19(1):287–92. https://doi.org/10.1007/s10120-014-0451-2. Epub 2014/12/17. PubMed PMID: 25503677
16. Nagai E, Nakata K, Ohuchida K, Miyasaka Y, Shimizu S, Tanaka M. Laparoscopic total gastrectomy for remnant gastric cancer: feasibility study. Surg Endosc. 2014;28(1):289–96. https://doi.org/10.1007/s00464-013-3186-y. Epub 2013/09/10. PubMed PMID: 24013469
17. Son SY, Lee CM, Jung DH, Lee JH, Ahn SH. Park do J, et al. laparoscopic completion total gastrectomy for remnant gastric cancer: a single-institution experience. Gastric Cancer. 2015;18(1):177–82. https://doi.org/10.1007/s10120-014-0339-1. Epub 2014/01/31. PubMed PMID: 24477417

18. Kim HS, Kim BS, Lee IS, Lee S, Yook JH, Kim BS. Laparoscopic gastrectomy in patients with previous gastrectomy for gastric cancer: a report of 17 cases. Surg Laparosc Endosc Percutan Tech. 2014;24(2):177–82. https://doi.org/10.1097/SLE.0b013e31828f6bfb. Epub 2014/04/02. PubMed PMID: 24686356

19. Kanaya S, Kawamura Y, Kawada H, Iwasaki H, Gomi T, Satoh S, et al. The delta-shaped anastomosis in laparoscopic distal gastrectomy: analysis of the initial 100 consecutive procedures of intracorporeal gastro-duodenostomy. Gastric Cancer. 2011;14(4):365–71. https://doi.org/10.1007/s10120-011-0054-0. Epub 2011/05/17. PubMed PMID: 21573920

20. Kodera Y, Yamamura Y, Torii A, Uesaka K, Hirai T, Yasui K, et al. Gastric stump carcinoma after partial gastrectomy for benign gastric lesion: what is feasible as standard surgical treatment? J Surg Oncol. 1996;63(2):119–24. https://doi.org/10.1002/(SICI)1096-9098(199610)63:2<119::AID-JSO9>3.0.CO;2-H. PubMed PMID: 8888805

21. Imada T, Rino Y, Takahashi M, Shiozawa M, Hatori S, Noguchi Y, et al. Clinicopathologic differences between gastric remnant cancer and primary cancer in the upper third of the stomach. Anticancer Res. 1998;18(1A):231–5. Epub 1998/05/06. PubMed PMID: 9568082

22. Wang Y, Huang CM, Wang JB, Zheng CH, Li P, Xie JW, et al. Survival and surgical outcomes of cardiac cancer of the remnant stomach in comparison with primary cardiac cancer. World J Surg Oncol. 2014;12:21. https://doi.org/10.1186/1477-7819-12-21. PubMed PMID: 24468299; PubMed Central PMCID: PMC3906884

23. Kwon IG, Cho I, Choi YY, Hyung WJ, Kim CB, Noh SH. Risk factors for complications during surgical treatment of remnant gastric cancer. Gastric Cancer. 2015;18(2):390–6. https://doi.org/10.1007/s10120-014-0369-8. Epub 2014/04/08. PubMed PMID: 24705942

24. Viste A, Eide GE, Glattre E, Soreide O. Cancer of the gastric stump: analyses of 819 patients and comparison with other stomach cancer patients. World J Surg. 1986;10(3):454–61. PubMed PMID: 3727608

25. Thorban S, Bottcher K, Etter M, Roder JD, Busch R, Siewert JR. Prognostic factors in gastric stump carcinoma. Ann Surg. 2000;231(2):188–94.. PubMed PMID: 10674609; PubMed Central PMCID: PMC1420985

26. Sasako M, Maruyama K, Kinoshita T, Okabayashi K. Surgical treatment of carcinoma of the gastric stump. Br J Surg. 1991;78(7):822–4. PubMed PMID: 1873711

27. Pointner R, Wetscher GJ, Gadenstatter M, Bodner E, Hinder RA. Gastric remnant cancer has a better prognosis than primary gastric cancer. Arch Surg. 1994;129(6):615–9.. Epub 1994/06/01. PubMed PMID: 8204036

28. Newman E, Brennan MF, Hochwald SN, Harrison LE, Karpeh MS Jr. Gastric remnant carcinoma: just another proximal gastric cancer or a unique entity? Am J Surg. 1997;173(4):292–7. https://doi.org/10.1016/s0002-9610(96)00403-5. Epub 1997/04/01. PubMed PMID: 9136783

29. Bruno L, Nesi G, Montinaro F, Carassale G, Lassig R, Boddi V, et al. Clinicopathologic findings and results of surgical treatment in cardiac adenocarcinoma. J Surg Oncol. 2000;74(1):33–5. PubMed PMID: 10861606

30. An JY, Choi MG, Noh JH, Sohn TS, Kim S. The outcome of patients with remnant primary gastric cancer compared with those having upper one-third gastric cancer. Am J Surg. 2007;194(2):143–7. https://doi.org/10.1016/j.amjsurg.2006.10.034. Epub 2007/07/10. PubMed PMID: 17618792

31. Schaefer N, Sinning C, Standop J, Overhaus M, Hirner A, Wolff M. Treatment and prognosis of gastric stump carcinoma in comparison with primary proximal gastric cancer. Am J Surg. 2007;194(1):63–7. https://doi.org/10.1016/j.amjsurg.2006.12.037. PubMed PMID: 17560911

32. Mezhir JJ, Gonen M, Ammori JB, Strong VE, Brennan MF, Coit DG. Treatment and outcome of patients with gastric remnant cancer after resection for peptic ulcer disease. Ann Surg Oncol. 2011;18(3):670–6. https://doi.org/10.1245/s10434-010-1425-1. Epub 2010/11/11. PubMed PMID: 21063791

33. Li F, Zhang R, Liang H, Zhao J, Liu H, Quan J, et al. A retrospective clinicopathologic study of remnant gastric cancer after distal gastrectomy. Am J Clin Oncol. 2013;36(3):244–9. https://doi.org/10.1097/COC.0b013e3182467ebd. Epub 2012/04/13. PubMed PMID: 22495457

34. Tokunaga M, Sano T, Ohyama S, Hiki N, Fukunaga T, Yamada K, et al. Clinicopathological characteristics and survival difference between gastric stump carcinoma and primary upper third gastric cancer. J Gastrointest Surg. 2013;17(2):313–8. https://doi.org/10.1007/s11605-012-2114-0. PubMed PMID: 23233273

Laparoscopic Surgery

23

Eishi Nagai and Masafumi Nakamura

Introduction

Recently, a declining incidence and mortality rate of gastric cancer has been observed in western countries, as well as Asian countries [1]. However, gastric cancer is still considered as the third most common cause of cancer death worldwide [2]. Despite the development of chemotherapy, surgical resection still remains the only potentially curative treatment. Among the surgical procedures for gastric cancer (e.g., total gastrectomy, distal gastrectomy, and proximal gastrectomy), distal gastrectomy is the most common procedure, which risks the occurrence of a synchronous and/or metachronous gastric lesion. The clinical entity of remnant gastric cancer (RGC) was initially reported in 1922 [3]. According to the 2011 Japanese classification of gastric cancer [4], RGC is defined as all carcinomas arising in the remnant stomach following a gastrectomy, irrespective of the histology of the primary lesion. The incidence of RGC has been reported as 2–3% in patients who have undergone an initial gastrectomy [5–7] and was reported to account for 1.8% of all gastric cancers in a large series [8].

Laparoscopic gastrectomy is now a widely accepted treatment of primary early gastric cancer, because of its less invasive nature and shorter recovery time [9, 10]. And laparoscopic gastrectomy has gradually gained acceptance for the treatment of advanced gastric cancer [11]. On the other hand, laparoscopic total gastrectomy (LTG) for remnant gastric cancer is still not a standard surgical treatment, because of the presence of severe adhesions of adjacent organs and displacement of anatomical structures due to initial surgery. There are very few reports indicating the feasibility of laparoscopic surgery for remnant gastric cancer, and the number of cases reported was very small. The benefit of laparoscopic surgery for RGC is still controversial; thus the indication for laparoscopic surgery should be based on surgeon or institutional experience.

Indications

LTG is our procedure of choice for all cases of resectable remnant gastric cancer. We do not hesitate to convert to an open procedure when we cannot achieve good operative exposure due to large tumor size or when we encounter unexpected complications such as injury to major blood vessels or adjacent organs.

E. Nagai (✉) · M. Nakamura
Department of Surgery and Oncology, Graduate School of Medical Sciences, Kyushu University, Fukuoka, Japan
e-mail: eishi@surg1.med.kyushu-u.ac.jp

© Springer-Verlag GmbH Germany, part of Springer Nature 2019
S. H. Noh, W. J. Hyung (eds.), *Surgery for Gastric Cancer*,
https://doi.org/10.1007/978-3-662-45583-8_23

Preoperative Evaluation

Preoperative clinical factors, including clinical classification of tumor depth (cT), nodal involvement (cN), and distant metastasis (cM), are evaluated by upper gastrointestinal contrast studies, esophagogastroduodenoscopy, endoscopic ultrasonography, abdominal ultrasonography, and computed tomography (CT), consistent with the TNM staging system. Three-dimensional CT is especially useful to check for the presence of vascular anatomical variations in patients with RGC (Fig. 23.1a–c).

Operating Room Setup and Patient Position

Our preference is to use a high-definition video system with two monitors for use by the primary and assistant surgeon. Under general anesthe-

sia, five trocars are inserted into the abdomen with the patient in supine position with legs slightly apart. The patient is then placed in reverse Trendelenburg position as the operation commences. The primary surgeon stands on the patient's right, the assistant on the patient's left, and the camera operator stands between the patient's legs.

Trocar Placement

First, a 12-mm trocar is inserted at the umbilical area using the open technique. If severe adhesions are expected, the left lateral abdomen would be another option for entry of the first 12-mm trocar in order to avoid injury. A 5-mm trocar is then inserted at the left hypochondriac region, and/ or a 12-mm trocar is inserted at the right lateral abdominal in an area without adhesions. These

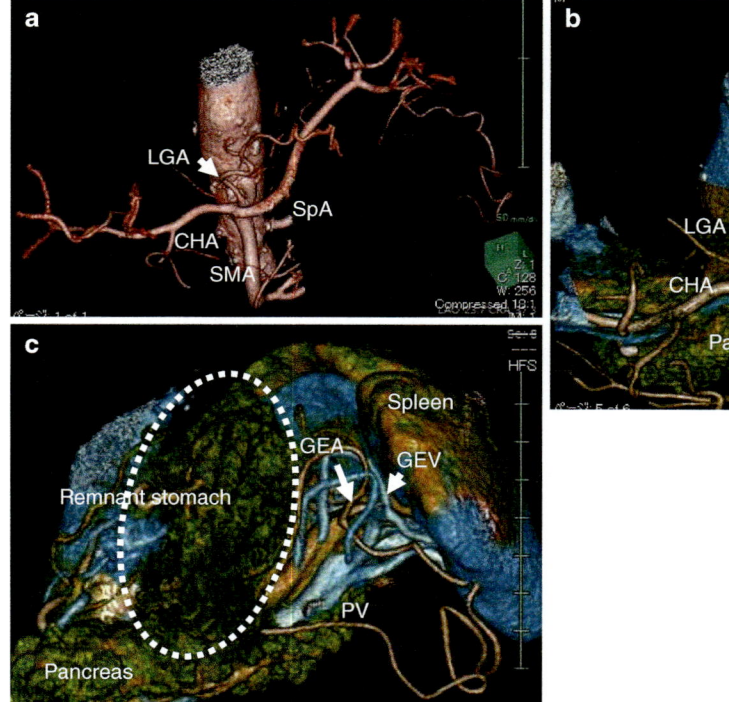
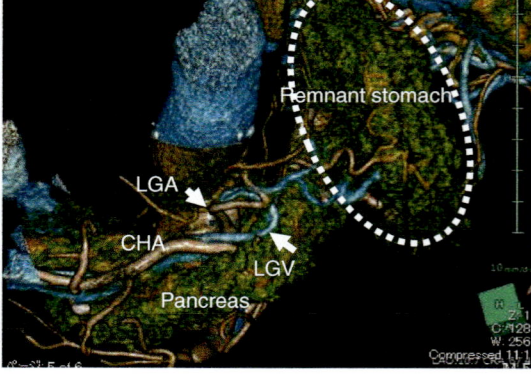
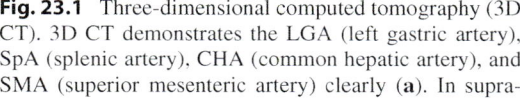

Fig. 23.1 Three-dimensional computed tomography (3D CT). 3D CT demonstrates the LGA (left gastric artery), SpA (splenic artery), CHA (common hepatic artery), and SMA (superior mesenteric artery) clearly (**a**). In supra-pancreatic area (**b**) and splenic hilum (**c**), the relation between artery and vein is also clearly seen (**b**). (LGV, left gastric vein; GEA, gastroepiploic artery; GEV, gastroepiploic vein)

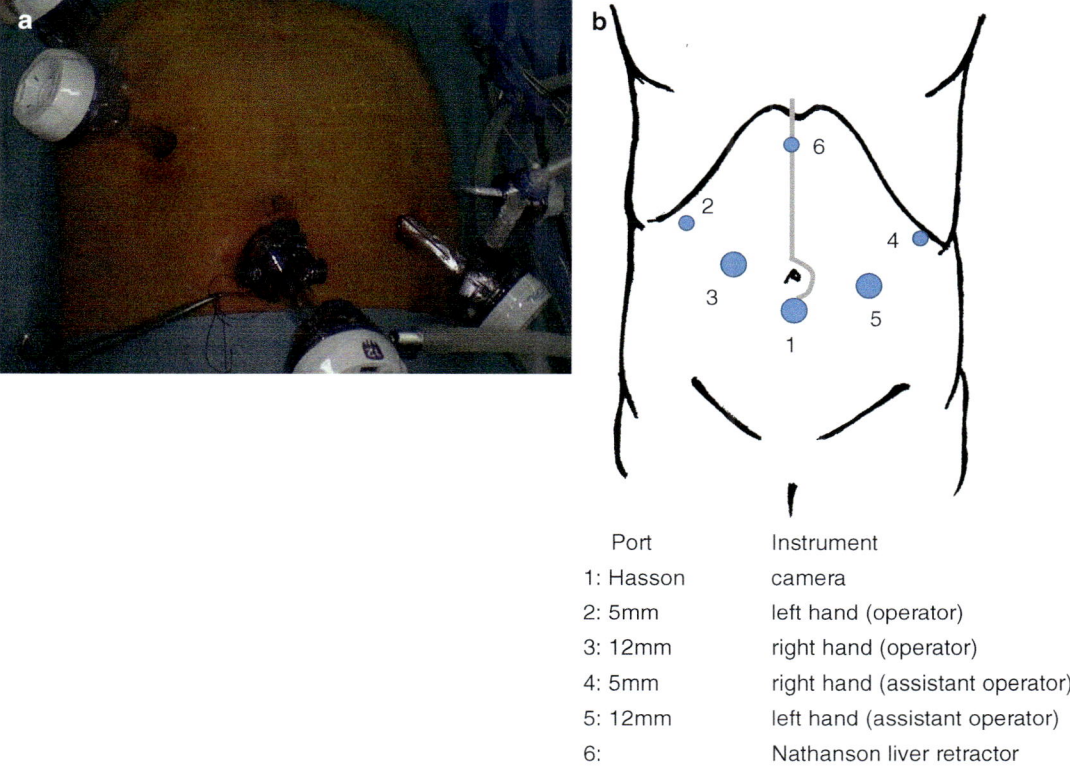

Port	Instrument
1: Hasson	camera
2: 5mm	left hand (operator)
3: 12mm	right hand (operator)
4: 5mm	right hand (assistant operator)
5: 12mm	left hand (assistant operator)
6:	Nathanson liver retractor

Fig. 23.2 Trocar positions in LTG for RGC (**a**) and schematic diagram of the trocar positions (**b**)

two or three trocars are then used for adhesiolysis due to initial surgery. Subsequent trocars are then inserted until there are five trocars in total sequentially (Fig. 23.2), as shown in the figure. Liver retractor is inserted at the epigastric region (Fig. 23.2a, b).

Surgical Procedures

The choice of surgical procedure is influenced by the type of reconstruction (Billroth I vs. Billroth II) as well as disease entity (malignant vs. benign) of the initial surgery. The lymphatic pathway along the left gastric artery and left gastroepiploic artery is preserved in patients with initial surgery for benign disease. Lymph node dissection at the supra-pancreatic area and along the left gastroepiploic artery is necessary for these patients. On the other hand, severe adhesions at the supra-pancreatic area are expected in the

patients with initial surgery for gastric cancer. In our series, Billroth I reconstruction is associated with malignant initial disease. Here, we present two types of surgical technique of laparoscopic gastrectomy for RGC: Billroth I reconstruction with malignant initial disease and Billroth II with benign initial disease.

Patients Who Previously Underwent Billroth I Reconstruction

After doing adhesiolysis between the abdominal wall and the intestines (Fig. 23.3), the greater omentum is dissected along the gastrocolic ligament, avoiding injury of transverse colon and mesocolon (Fig. 23.4a). The root of the first short gastric artery is then exposed, clipped, and cut (Fig. 23.4b). Short gastric arteries are subsequently cut at their roots. Adhesions between the posterior wall of the stomach and the pancreas

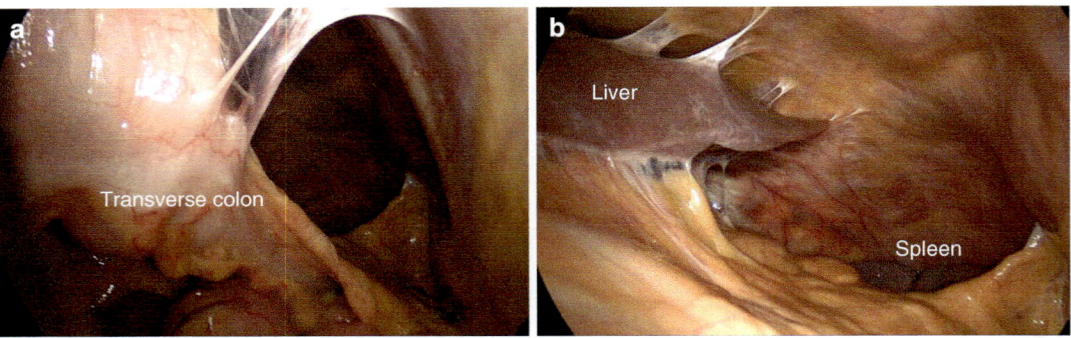

Fig. 23.3 The transverse colon (**a**) is adherent to the previous surgical scar and the upper abdominal wall. Omentum (**b**) is adherent to the dorsal surface of the liver

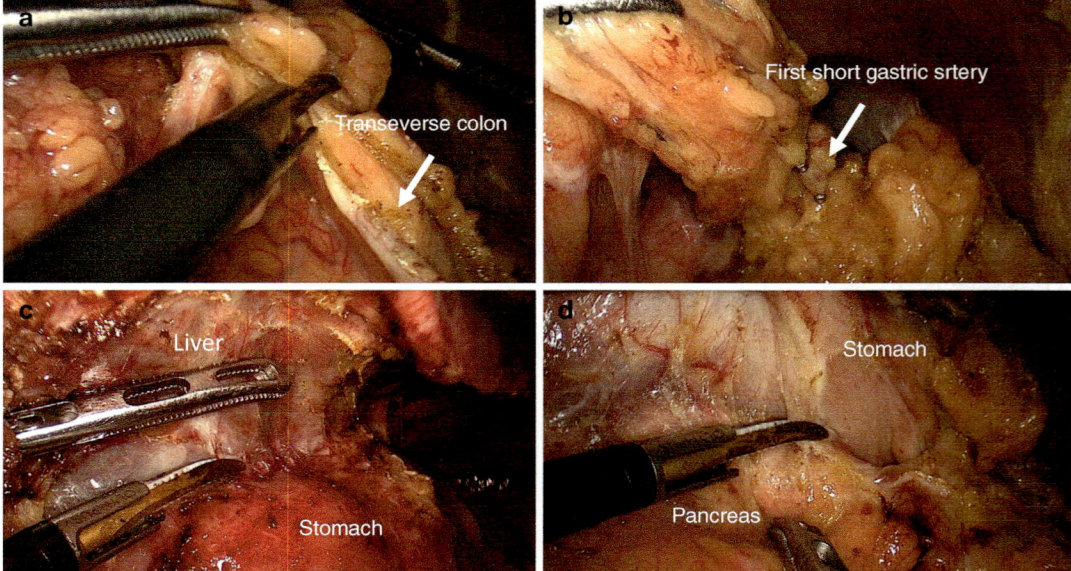

Fig. 23.4 The greater omentum is dissected along the transverse colon (**a**). The first short gastric artery is identified (**b**). Adhesiolysis is performed around the gastric wall (**c, d**)

are then dissected (Fig. 23.4c, d). Because of the presence of severe adhesions between the inferior surface of the left lateral segment of the liver and the ventral surface of the remnant stomach, this area is dissected carefully to avoid gastric wall injury. After separating the gastric wall and duodenal wall from the pancreatic parenchyma, the gastroduodenal anastomosis is completely exposed (Fig. 23.5a). The duodenum is then divided at just the aboral side of the anastomosis with the use of a linear stapler (Fig. 23.5b).

The gastric remnant is retracted upwards to obtain adequate operative view for gastric mobilization and lymphadenectomy (Fig. 23.5c). When the adhesions between the inferior surface of the left lateral segment of the liver and the remnant stomach are very severe, the hepatic capsule is removed to avoid injury to the gastric wall (Fig. 23.5d). The connective tissues along the common hepatic artery, celiac trunk, and splenic artery are then dissected, avoiding injury of these vessels. If the root of the left gastric vessel was left intact during the initial surgery, meticulous dissection is necessary to avoid inadvertent injury (Fig. 23.6a, b). After lymph node dissection along the surface of the diaphragmatic crus, the esophagus is exposed (Fig. 23.6c) and is divided at a sufficient

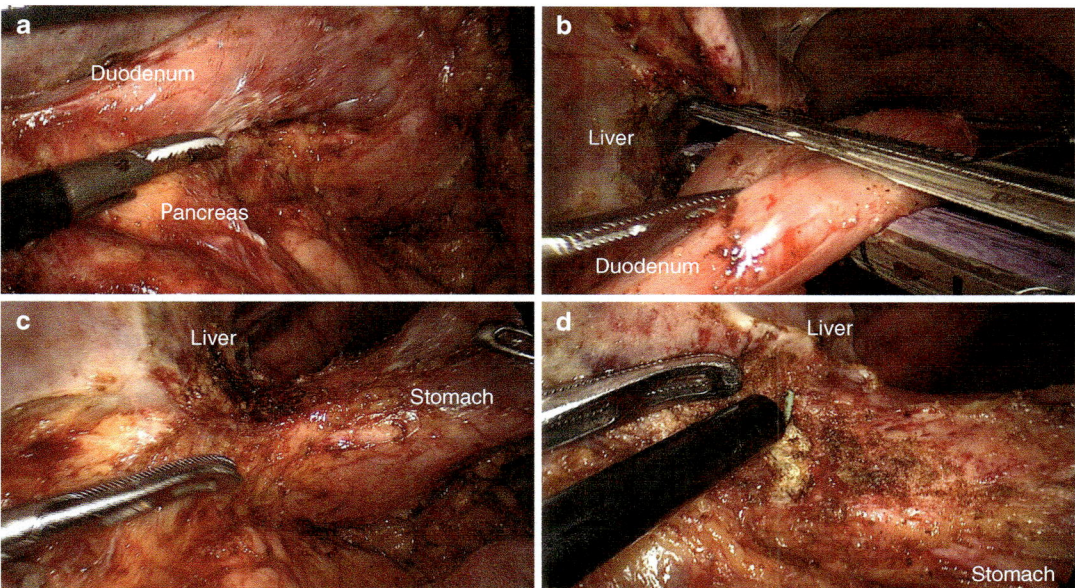

Fig. 23.5 The gastroduodenal anastomotic site is exposed (**a**), and the duodenum is divided using a linear stapler (**b**). The gastric remnant is retracted upwards (**c**). The combined resection of the hepatic capsule is performed to avoid injury to the gastric wall (**d**)

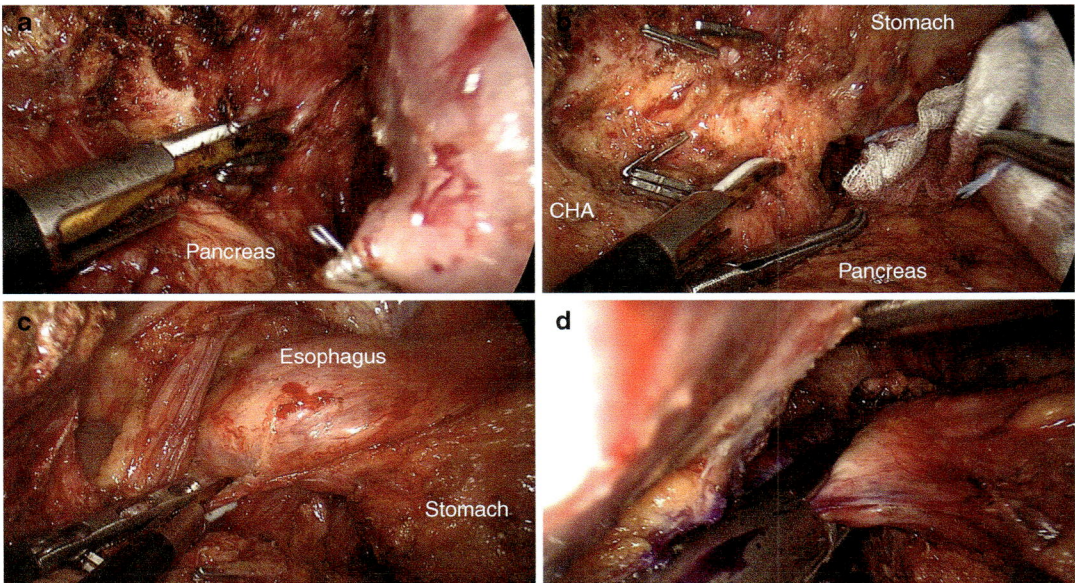

Fig. 23.6 Meticulous dissection is necessary to avoid inadvertent injury (**a**, **b**). The esophagus is exposed entirely (**c**) and divided using a liner stapler (**d**)

distance from the tumor (Fig. 23.6d). Finally, the lymphadenectomy of stations #2 and 4Sa is completely carried out. The resected specimen is placed in a plastic bag and removed through the umbili-cal incision, which is enlarged to approximately 3 cm. As described elsewhere [12], Roux-en-Y reconstruction is performed using an isoperistal-tic 40-cm Roux limb, divided at 30 cm from the duodenojejunal junction. The Roux limb is pulled up via an antecolic route. Esophagojejunal anastomosis is performed using a linear stapler (Fig. 23.7). Side-to-side jejunojejunostomy is performed at 40 cm from the esophagojejunostomy using a linear stapler. The jejunojejunostomy and Petersen's mesenteric defect are closed with continuous sutures.

Patients Who Previously Underwent Billroth II Reconstruction

In our experience, previous Billroth II (B-II) reconstruction is usually via the retrocolic route. The gastrojejunal anastomosis is clearly identified behind the mesocolon (Fig. 23.8). Caution must be exer-

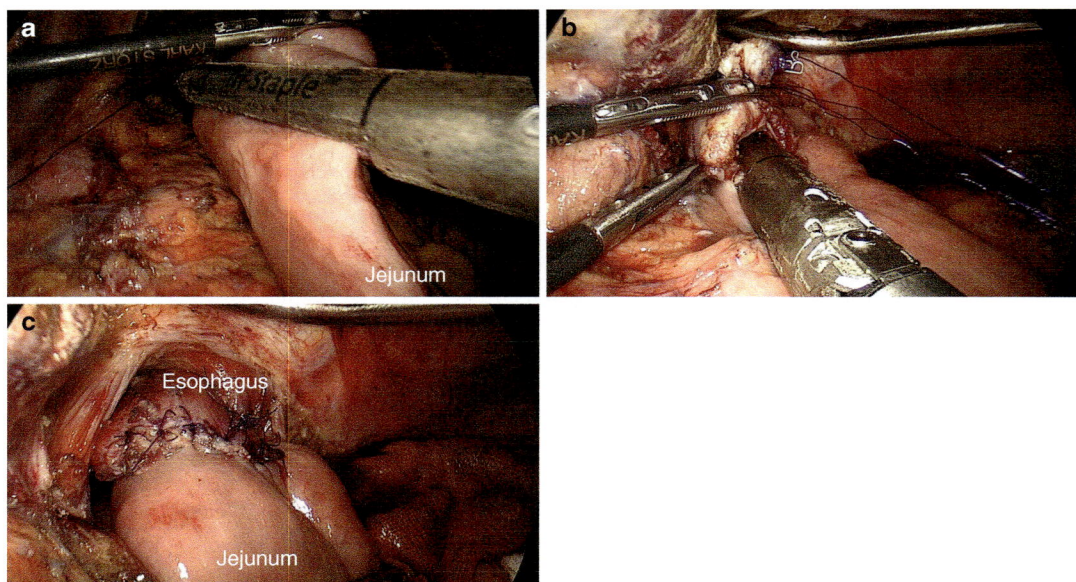

Fig. 23.7 Esophagojejunal anastomosis is performed using a liner stapler (**a**, **b**). The entry hole is closed by interrupted sutures (**c**)

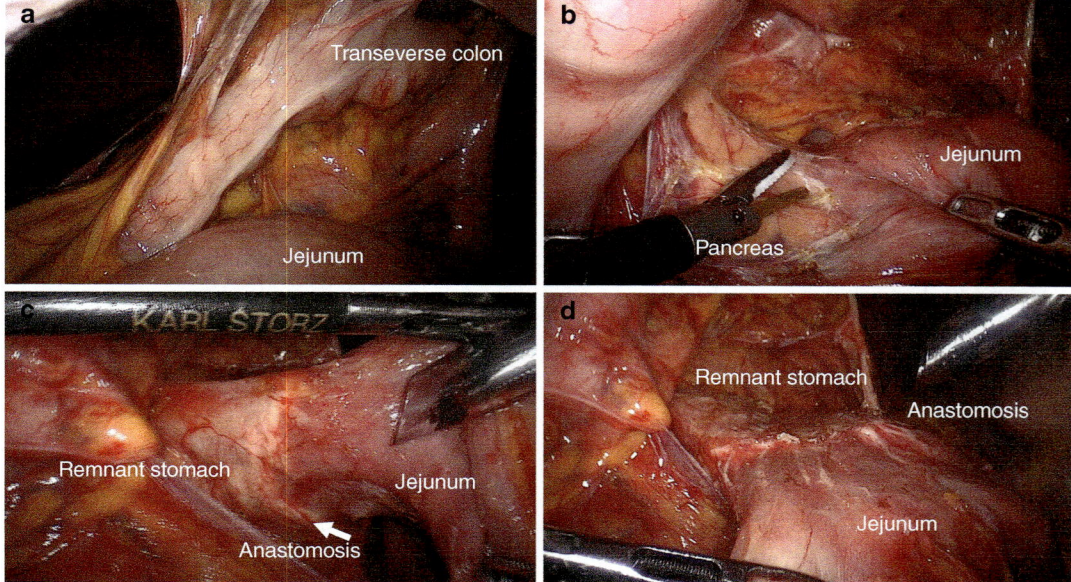

Fig. 23.8 The gastrojejunal anastomosis is identified behind the mesocolon (**a**) and exposed (**b–d**)

cised so as not to cause injury in this area. The afferent and efferent limbs are sequentially divided at an appropriate distance from the gastrojejunal anastomosis using a linear stapler (Fig. 23.9a). After dissection of adhesions between the abdominal wall and the intestines (Fig. 23.9b), the stumps of the jejunum are pulled up to the oral side of the mesocolon. The gastric remnant is retracted upwards to get a good operative view for lymphadenectomy (Fig. 23.9c, d). The left gastric vessel is usually preserved during initial surgery but is divided at its root for lymphadenectomy of station #9 (Fig. 23.10a).

The greater omentum is dissected along the transverse colon for lymphadenectomy of station #4Sb, and the left gastroepiploic artery is ligated at its root. Subsequently, the gastrosplenic ligament is dissected near the splenic hilum. The lymph nodes along the common hepatic artery, celiac trunk, and splenic artery are also dissected (Fig. 23.10b). After dissection of the lesser omentum adjacent to the left lateral segment of the liver, the esophagus is exposed and divided on the oral side of the esophagogastric junction (Fig. 23.11a). In general, lymphadenectomy is performed according to the concept of D2 nodal dissection for primary gastric cancer (Fig. 23.11b, c). If there is tumor invasion into the jejunal wall, the mesenteric lymph nodes close to the anastomosis are also dissected. After removal of the resected specimen, Roux-en-Y reconstruction is performed as described in the previous section (Fig 23.11d).

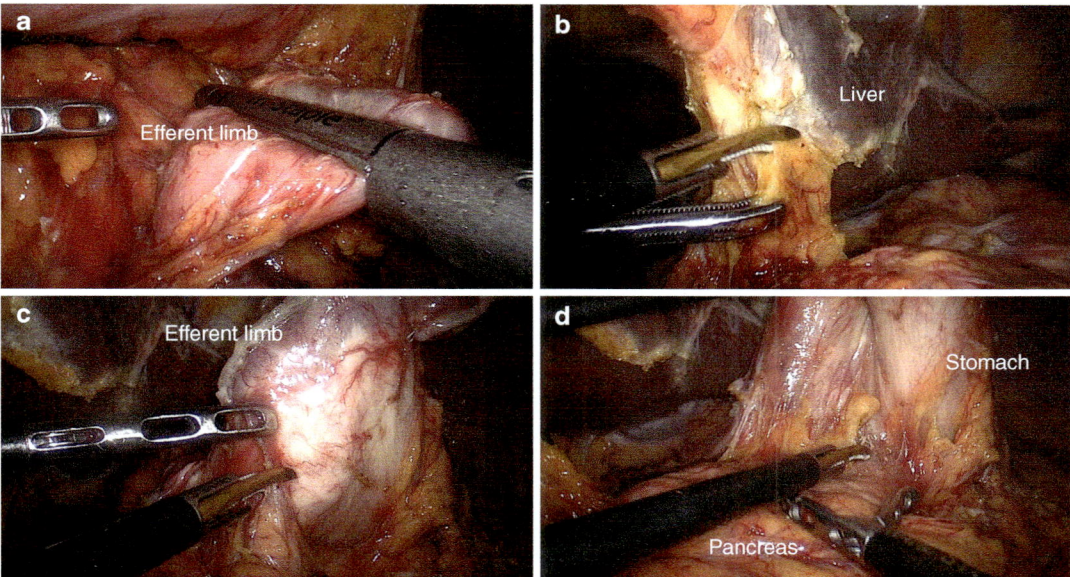

Fig. 23.9 The afferent and efferent limbs are sequentially divided using a linear stapler (**a**). After adhesiolysis between the intestines and the abdominal wall (**b**), the jejunum are pulled cephalad (**c**, **d**)

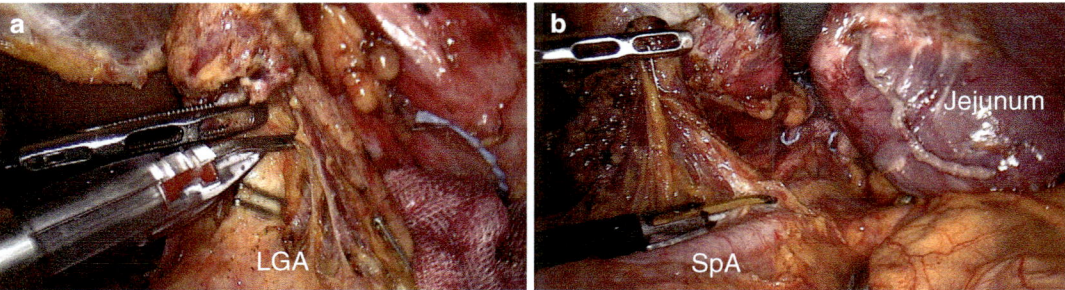

Fig. 23.10 Left gastric artery is identified and divided at its origin (**a**). Lymph node dissection is performed along the splenic artery (**b**)

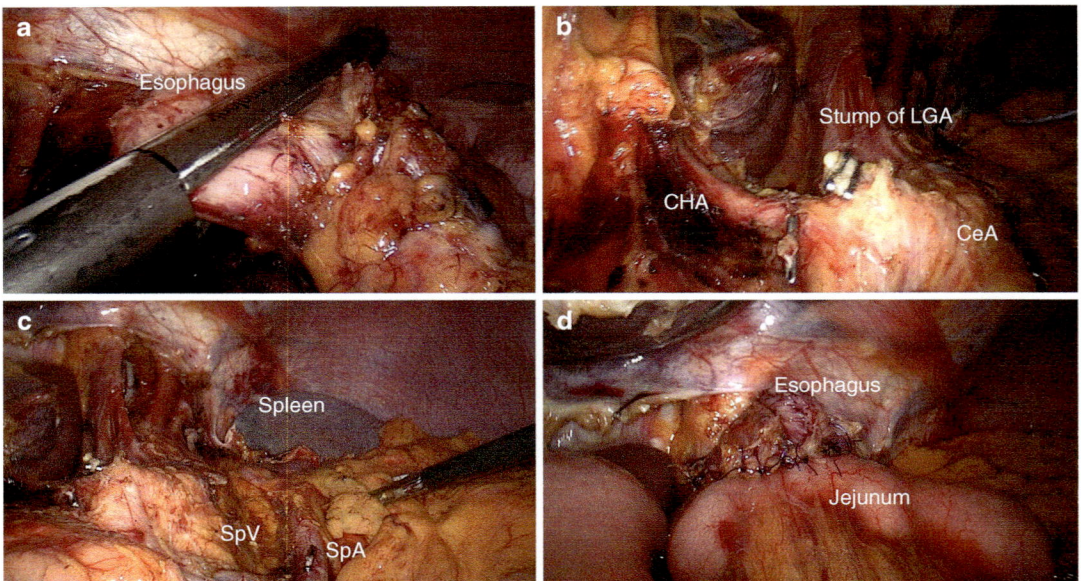

Fig. 23.11 The esophagus is exposed and divided (**a**). The final view of completion of lymphadenectomy at the supra-pancreatic area (**b**, **c**). The esophagojejunal anasto- mosis is performed using linear stapler (**d**). (SpV, splenic vein; CeA, celiac artery)

Our Clinical Experience

We have performed laparoscopic total remnant gastrectomies for RGC on a total 14 patients from July 2005 to December 2013. In 2007, we expanded our indication for laparoscopic gastrec- tomy to include advanced gastric cancer. Thus, all patients were subsequent cases of LTG for RGC after December 2006, except for one case performed in 2005. These patients underwent potentially curative surgery with appropriate lymphadenectomy.

The said 14 patients comprised of 12 males and 2 females. The mean patient age was 67.1 ± 6.9 years. Initial gastrectomy was for gas- tric cancer in six patients and peptic ulcer disease in eight. The initial surgery was laparoscopic in 3 patients and open in 11. As for reconstruction during initial surgery, there were six Billroth I (B-I) gastroduodenostomies, seven B-II gastro- jejunostomies, and one esophagogastrostomy. The mean interval between the initial surgery and completion total gastrectomy in all 14 patients

was 29.4 ± 16.9 years. The mean time from the initial surgery to the second operation was signifi- cantly longer in patients with initial benign dis- ease (Group B) than patients with carcinoma at initial surgery (Group C) (41.1 ± 10.0 years vs. 13.7 ± 10.3 years; $p = 0.00057$) (Table 23.1). The mean operation time of the second operation in all 14 patients was 377.6 ± 85.4 min (380.0 ± 43.5 min in Group C and 375.9 ± 106.4 min in Group B; $p = 0.9353$). The mean estimated blood loss in all 14 patients was 121.9 ± 218 g (42.2 ± 29.5 g in Group C and 181.8 ± 271 g in Group B; $p = 0.2194$). The mean number of lymph nodes harvested in all 14 patients was 23.7 ± 11.2 (14.8 ± 9.3 in Group C and 29.3 ± 8.3 in Group B; $p = 0.0213$) (Table 23.2). There were no con- versions to open surgery and no mortalities; how- ever, there was one case of postoperative bleeding which necessitated reoperation.

The final pathologic stages are as follows: IA in ten patients (71.4%), IIA in three (21.4%), and IIIC in one (7.1%). The mean times to postopera- tive liquid and food intake were 3.3 ± 3.1 days and

Table 23.1 Clinicopathologic characteristics of the 14 patients who underwent gastrectomy from July 2005 to December 2013

Number of patients	14
Age (years)	67.1 ± 6.9
Male/female	12/2
Body mass index (kg/m^2)	20.9 ± 3.0
Tumor size (cm)	3.6 ± 2.6
Interval (years)	29.4 ± 16.6
Type of initial gastrectomy	
Distal gastrectomy	13
Proximal gastrectomy	1
Etiology of initial gastrectomy	
Cancer	6
Peptic ulcer	8
Type of reconstruction after initial gastrectomy	
B-I	6
B-II	7
Esophagogastrostomy	1
Preoperative comorbidities	
Liver cirrhosis	1
Diabetes mellitus	2
Hypertension	2
Arrhythmia	2
(Warfarin, low-dose aspirin)	
Interstitial pneumonia	1
Hyperthyroidism	1
Ischemic heart disease	1
Total	10
Synchronous malignancies	
Malignant lymphoma	1

Table 23.2 Perioperative findings of the 14 patients

Mean operative time (min)	377.6 ± 68.4
Mean blood loss (g)	121.9 ± 62.0
Mean number of retrieved lymph nodes	23.7 ± 11.2
Synchronous operations	
Cholecystectomy	2

5.1 ± 3.3 days, respectively. The mean length of postoperative hospital stay was 12.4 ± 5.1 days. The median follow-up time was 54.7 months (range 28.1–85.2 months). Eleven out of the 14 patients were still alive without relapse at the time of writing of this paper. Two patients died of other diseases, and one died of metastatic disease to the brain and multiple nodal metastases around the aorta (Table 23.3).

Table 23.3 Postoperative course of the 14 patients

Morbidities (Clavien-Dindo classification [13], III or more)	
Anastomotic leakage	None
Pancreatic leakage	None
Postoperative hemorrhage	1 case
Total	1 case
Mortalities	None
Final pathologic stage	
IA/IIA/IIIC	10/3/1
Mean time to water intake (days)	3.4 ± 3.6
Mean time to food intake (days)	5.1 ± 3.4
Mean postoperative length of hospital stay (days)	12.4 ± 5.1
Median follow-up period (months)	54.7 (28.1 ~ 85.2)
One patient died of disease	
Two patients died of diseases other than gastric cancer (malignant lymphoma, alcoholic liver dysfunction)	
Eleven patients still alive and without recurrence	

Discussion

Despite developments of chemotherapy for gastric cancer, the mainstay of treatment for RGC is still surgical resection, as with primary gastric cancer [14]. Surgical treatment is more difficult in patients with RGC than in patients with primary gastric cancer, and laparoscopic surgery for RGC requires more advanced skills. RGC is very rare and accounts for only 2–3% of gastric remnants [5–7]. This is why there are only few reports describing LTG for RGC [15–23]. Moreover, almost all literature include only a small number of cases and only deal with issues of technical feasibility and short-term outcomes.

There are two issues or potential problems that must be addressed in order to successfully perform total gastrectomy for RGC; one is gastric mobilization and lymphadenectomy under severe adhesions and fortuitous anatomical variations, and another is reconstruction. The difficulties of gastric mobilization and lymphadenectomy of a second operation are dependent on whether or not lymphadenectomy was performed during the first operation and whether B-I or B-II reconstruction was performed at the time. After B-I reconstruction at initial surgery, there are usually severe adhesions around the gastroduodenal anastomotic site and between the dorsal surface of the left lateral segment of the liver and the anterior surface of the remnant gastric wall. If lymphadenectomy was performed for gastric cancer during initial surgery, severe adhesions are usually recognized at the operative site, especially at the supra-pancreatic area.

In our series, five out of six patients with B-I reconstruction underwent initial gastrectomy for malignancy, and all seven patients with B-II reconstruction underwent initial gastrectomy for peptic ulcer disease. Patients with B-I reconstruction, therefore, mostly underwent lymphadenectomy of the supra- and infra-pyloric and supra-pancreatic nodes, resulting in severe adhesion formation in those areas.

There are some important technical points for adhesiolysis:

1. Gastroduodenal anastomotic site
   Adhesiolysis should be performed carefully along the pancreatic surface to avoid injury to the pancreatic parenchyma and duodenal wall.
2. Supra-pancreatic area
   After isolation of the common hepatic artery near the origin of the gastroduodenal artery, dissection should be continued along the common hepatic artery to the left gastric artery and splenic artery.
3. Dorsal surface of the left lateral segment of the liver
   Dissection should be performed carefully in this area to avoid injury to the gastric wall. The hepatic capsule may be removed if necessary, to avoid injury to the gastric wall.
4. Gastrojejunal anastomotic site
   The jejunal and gastric walls are severely adherent to the mesocolon in patients with B-II reconstruction, and it is important to avoid injury to the colonic vessels during adhesiolysis.

It may be possible to successfully perform LTG for RGC without perioperative massive bleeding, pancreatic leakage, anastomotic leakage, nor conversion to open surgery, if we follow these precautions.

As for reconstruction, we prefer totally laparoscopic esophagojejunostomy using linear stapler, termed "Inverted T anastomosis," as described previously [12]. In this series, we successfully performed Roux-en-Y reconstruction using liner stapler.

Short-Term Outcome

Although the number of patients is limited, there have been several reports of the technical feasibility of laparoscopic or laparoscopic-assisted total gastrectomy for RGC from high-volume centers [16, 17, 20, 22]. Laparoscopic remnant total gastrectomy is reported to be less invasive than open surgery and with favorable short-term outcomes, such as minimal operative blood loss [17, 20], faster recovery of bowel movement [16, 17], and short hospital stay [16, 17]. On the other hand, some authors emphasize that immediate conversion to an open procedure should be considered if intraoperative complications occur [20].

Long-Term Outcome

The 5-year survival rate of LTG for RGC was reported to be comparable with open completion total gastrectomy for RGC [16, 17]. However, the number of patients enrolled was relatively small, and follow-up period was not enough to make a conclusion about survival rate. Further data collection and analysis of patients with RGC is necessary.

Conclusion

LTG is considered to be technically acceptable for the treatment of RGC with favorable short-term outcomes; however, it is a very technically complicated procedure even for surgeons skilled in laparoscopy. The indication for laparoscopic surgery for RGC should be determined by the surgeon's and institution's experience. Surgeons should not hesitate to convert to an open procedure when unexpected intraoperative complications occur.

Conflicts of Interest The authors declare no conflicts of interest.

References

1. Torre LA, Bray F, Siegel RL, Ferlay J, Lortet-Tieulent J, Jemal A. Global cancer statistics, 2012. CA Cancer J Clin. 2015;65:87–108.
2. Ferlay J, Soerjomataram I, Dikshit R, Eser S, Mathers C, Rebelo M, Parkin DM, Forman D, Bray F. Cancer incidence and mortality worldwide: sources, methods and major patterns in GLOBOCAN 2012. Int J Cancer. 2015;136:E359–86.
3. Balfour DC. Factors influencing the life expectancy of patients operated on for gastric ulcer. Ann Surg. 1922;76:405–8.
4. Japanese Gastric Cancer Association. Japanese classification of gastric carcinoma: 3rd English edition. Gastric Cancer. 2011;14:101–12.
5. Nozaki I, Nasu J, Kubo Y, Tanada M, Nishimura R, Kurita A. Risk factors for metachronous gastric cancer in the remnant stomach after early cancer surgery. World J Surg. 2010;34:1548–54.
6. Ovaska JT, Havia TV, Kujari HP. Risk of gastric stump carcinoma after gastric resection for benign ulcer disease. Ann Chir Gynaecol. 1986;75:192–5.
7. Welvaart K, Warnsinck HM. The incidence of carcinoma of the gastric remnant. J Surg Oncol. 1982;21:104–6.
8. Kaneko K, Kondo H, Saito D, Shirao K, Yamaguchi H, Yokota T, Yamao G, Sano T, Sasako M, Yoshida S. Early gastric stump cancer following distal gastrectomy. Gut. 1998;43:342–4.
9. Lee SI, Choi YS, Park DJ, Kim HH, Yang HK, Kim MC. Comparative study of laparoscopy-assisted distal gastrectomy and open distal gastrectomy. J Am Coll Surg. 2006;202:874–80.
10. Shimizu S, Uchiyama A, Mizumoto K, Morisaki T, Nakamura K, Shimura H, Tanaka M. Laparoscopically assisted distal gastrectomy for early gastric cancer: is it superior to open surgery? Surg Endosc. 2000;14:27–31.
11. Lee JH, Son SY, Lee CM, Ahn SH, Park Do J, Kim HH. Morbidity and mortality after laparoscopic gastrectomy for advanced gastric cancer: results of a phase II clinical trial. Surg Endosc. 2013;27:2877–85.
12. Nagai E, Ohuchida K, Nakata K, Miyasaka Y, Maeyama R, Toma H, Shimizu S, Tanaka M. Feasibility and safety of intracorporeal esophagojejunostomy after laparoscopic total gastrectomy: inverted T-shaped anastomosis using linear staplers. Surgery. 2013;153:732–8.
13. Dindo D, Demartines N, Clavien PA. Classification of surgical complications: a new proposal with evaluation in a cohort of 6336 patients and results of a survey. Ann Surg. 2004;240:205–13.
14. Sasako M, Maruyama K, Kinoshita T, Okabayashi K. Surgical treatment of carcinoma of the gastric stump. Br J Surg. 1991;78:822–4.
15. Corcione F, Pirozzi F, Marzano E, Cuccurullo D, Settembre A, Miranda L. Laparoscopic approach to gastric remnant-stump: our initial successful experience on 3 cases. Surg Laparosc Endosc Percutan Tech. 2008;18:502–5.
16. Kwon IG, Cho I, Guner A, Choi YY, Shin HB, Kim HI, An JY, Cheong JH, Noh SH, Hyung WJ. Minimally invasive surgery for remnant gastric cancer: a comparison with open surgery. Surg Endosc. 2014;28:2452–8.
17. Nagai E, Nakata K, Ohuchida K, Miyasaka Y, Shimizu S, Tanaka M. Laparoscopic total gastrectomy for remnant gastric cancer: feasibility study. Surg Endosc. 2014;28:289–96.
18. Qian F, Yu PW, Hao YX, Sun G, Tang B, Shi Y, Zhao YL, Lan YZ, Luo HX, Mo A. Laparoscopy-assisted resection for gastric stump cancer and gastric stump recurrent cancer: a report of 15 cases. Surg Endosc. 2010;24:3205–9.
19. Shinohara T, Hanyu N, Tanaka Y, Murakami K, Watanabe A, Yanaga K. Totally laparoscopic complete resection of the remnant stomach for gastric cancer. Langenbecks Arch Surg. 2013;398:341–5.
20. Son SY, Lee CM, Jung DH, Lee JH, Ahn SH, Park Do J, Kim HH. Laparoscopic completion total gastrectomy for remnant gastric cancer: a single-institution experience. Gastric Cancer. 2015;18:177–82.
21. Song J, Kim JY, Kim S, Choi WH, Cheong JH, Hyung WJ, Choi SH, Noh SH. Laparoscopic completion total gastrectomy in remnant gastric cancer: technical detail and experience of two cases. Hepato-Gastroenterology. 2009;56:1249–52.
22. Tsunoda S, Okabe H, Tanaka E, Hisamori S, Harigai M, Murakami K, Sakai Y. Laparoscopic gastrectomy for remnant gastric cancer: a comprehensive review and case series. Gastric Cancer. 2016;19:287–92.
23. Yamada H, Kojima K, Yamashita T, Kawano T, Sugihara K, Nihei Z. Laparoscopy-assisted resection of gastric remnant cancer. Surg Laparosc Endosc Percutan Tech. 2005;15:226–9.

Prevention and Treatment of Peritoneal Metastases from Gastric Cancer

24

Mei Li M. Kwong, Chukwuemeka Ihemelandu, and Paul H. Sugarbaker

Introduction

Gastric cancer is a common and deadly disease. It is the fourth most commonly diagnosed cancer in the world with a 5-year survival rate of 25% [1, 2]. In follow-up, almost half of gastric cancer patients will develop peritoneal spread which results in a less than 5% 5-year survival rate [3–5]. Peritoneal metastases are a common finding in primary gastric cancer found in 5–20% of patients undergoing gastrectomy [6]. The peritoneum is also the most common location of first recurrence observed in about half of the patients [7]. Standard of care for treatment of primary or recurrence of gastric cancer involves surgery, intravenous chemotherapy, and radiotherapy. However, specific treatments for peritoneal metastases such as neoadjuvant systemic chemotherapy (NAC), neoadjuvant intraperitoneal and systemic chemotherapy (NIPS), cytoreductive surgery (CRS), and perioperative chemotherapy which may include hyperthermic intraperitoneal chemotherapy (HIPEC) and/or early postoperative intraperitoneal chemotherapy (EPIC) are currently being explored [8]. CRS and HIPEC and/or EPIC are already considered standard of care for appendiceal peritoneal metasta-ses, peritoneal mesothelioma, and a limited extent of peritoneal metastases from colorectal carcinomatosis [9–11]. Gastric cancer with peritoneal metastases is aggressive, and current treatment efficacy remains controversial. The following is an attempt to summarize the role and efficacy of NACS, NIPS, CRS, and HIPEC and/or EPIC as a treatment for peritoneal metastases of gastric cancer (Fig. 24.1).

Perioperative Intraperitoneal Chemotherapy as an Adjuvant Treatment

Local and intra-abdominal tumors are usually the most common and only sites of first recurrence in gastric cancer after curative resection [12–14]. This is true regardless of whether they underwent neoadjuvant chemotherapy or postoperative adjuvant treatment compared to surgical resection alone [15]. The peritoneal surfaces and liver remain the major sites of recurrence. Less localized recurrence is observed when extended lymphadenectomy as compared to limited surgery is used [16–18].

Although confined to the abdomen, peritoneal seeding has deadly consequences [19–22]. Sources of recurrence after curative resection are (1) spontaneous dissemination from the primary tumor and (2) traumatic dissemination of cancer cells during the surgical procedure. If the serosal surface is

M. L. M. Kwong · C. Ihemelandu
P. H. Sugarbaker (✉)
Center for Gastrointestinal Malignancies,
Program in Peritoneal Surface Oncology, Medstar
Washington Hospital Center, Washington, DC, USA
e-mail: paul.sugarbaker@medstar.net

© Springer-Verlag GmbH Germany, part of Springer Nature 2019
S. H. Noh, W. J. Hyung (eds.), *Surgery for Gastric Cancer*,
https://doi.org/10.1007/978-3-662-45583-8_24

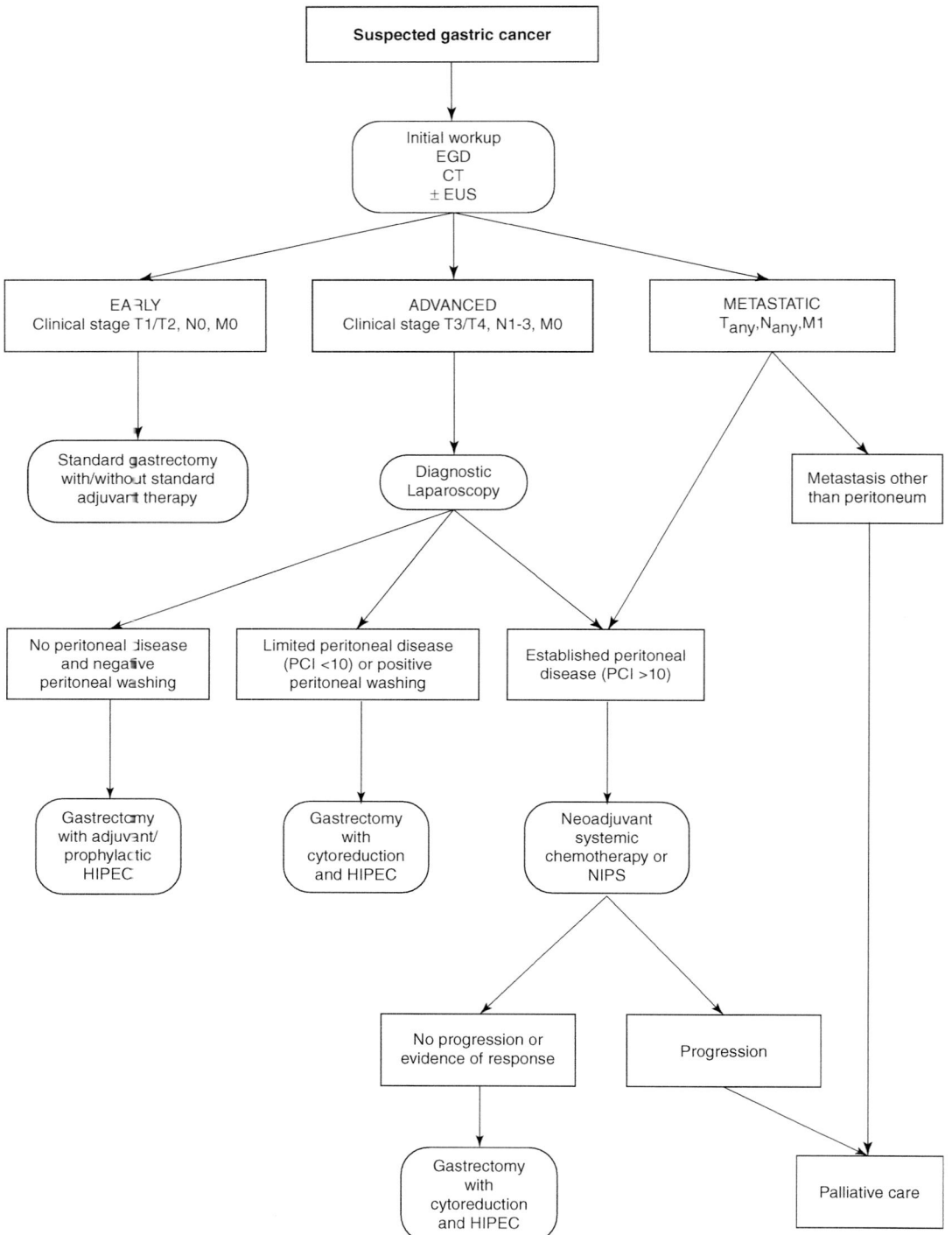

Fig. 24.1 An algorithm for treatment of gastric cancer with and without peritoneal metastases

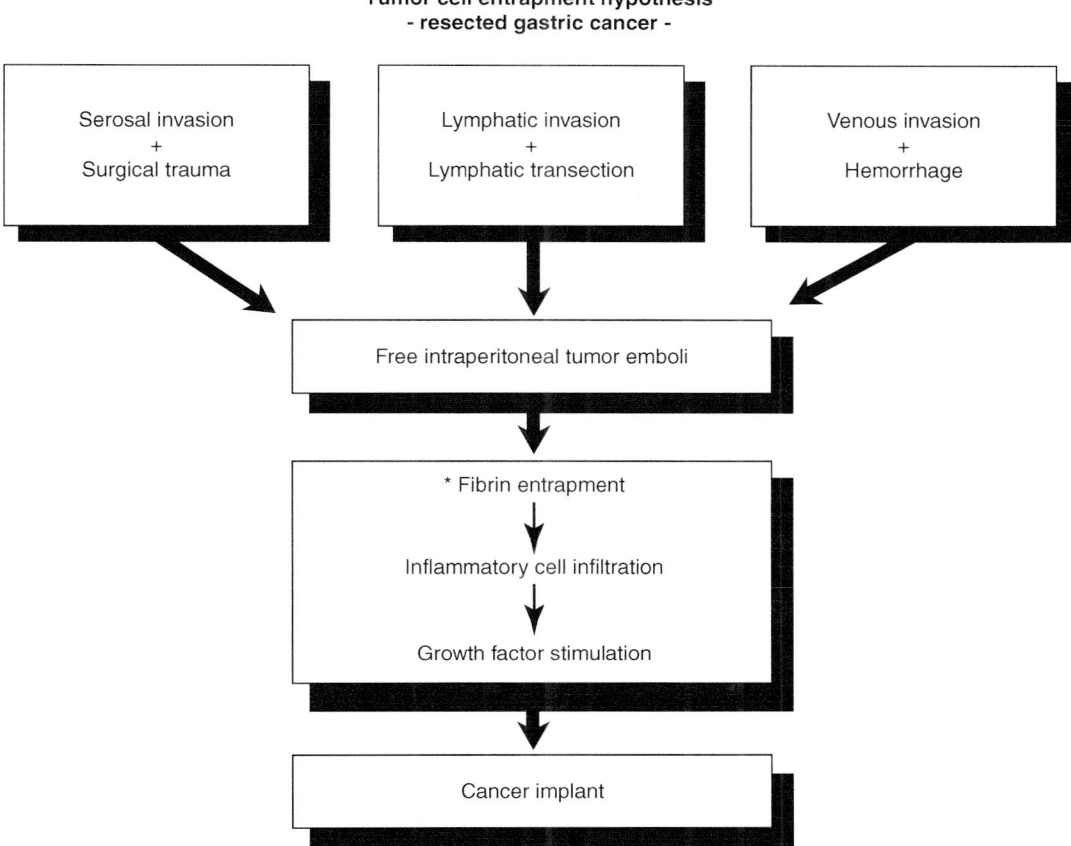

Fig. 24.2 The tumor cell entrapment hypothesis suggests three mechanisms for microscopic residual cancer cells in patients having an R-0 gastrectomy. (From Sethna et al. with permission [24])

involved with tumor, then spontaneous dissemination is more common, and patients are frequently found to have viable intraperitoneal cancer cells (positive cytology) [19, 21–23]. Tumor cells can also seed the intra-abdominal cavity during surgery according to the tumor cell entrapment hypothesis (Fig. 24.2) [24]. During surgery there is disruption of lymphatics, close margins of resection, and tumor-contaminated blood spillage. Iatrogenically disseminated tumor cells adhere spontaneously within minutes, and vascularization is facilitated by fibrin entrapment and the wound healing process. Cytokines, such as growth factors important

for wound healing, may also promote tumor progression. The tumor cell entrapment hypothesis explains part of the pathogenesis of local and intra-abdominal recurrence and theoretically shows how adjuvant perioperative intraperitoneal chemotherapy can be beneficial.

Rationale of Perioperative Timing of Intraperitoneal Chemotherapy

Intraperitoneal chemotherapy should be administered perioperatively in order to access the tumor cells prior to entrapment within fibrin and conversion into cancer progression within adhesive scar tissue. If chemotherapy is given after the formation of adhesive scars, then it will have uneven distribution and lack of uniform cytotoxicity for viable cancer cells. Kinetics of residual tumor cells change within 24 h of resection, and therefore a delay in local-regional treatments will decrease the cytotoxic effectiveness [24].

Perioperative Chemotherapy with D2 Gastrectomy

Perioperative intraoperative chemotherapy can limit progression of peritoneal dissemination after curative surgery; however, it cannot treat residual disease at systemic sites or metastases within lymph nodes. Therefore, a complete D2 lymphadenectomy is essential. Simple diffusion of chemotherapy only penetrates to 1 or 2 mm [25]. Local-regional chemotherapy is not effective in lymph nodes. Also, macroscopic peritoneal nodules larger than 1 or 2 mm have ineffective drug delivery, and visible nodules should be removed prior to treatment.

Literature Regarding Perioperative Intraperitoneal Chemotherapy for Advanced T-Stage Primary Gastric Cancer

There have been randomized and non-randomized trials regarding perioperative intraperitoneal chemotherapy as compared to surgery alone for resectable primary gastric cancer with and without peritoneal spread. Sugarbaker, Yu, and Yonemura published a meta-analysis in 2003 of articles published in English [7]. Xu et al. published a similar study in 2004 [26]. Yan et al. published a summary of randomized control trials concerning adjuvant intraperitoneal chemotherapy for resectable gastric cancer in 2007 [27]. Feingold et al. published the most recent summary of non-randomized and randomized studies in English of CRS and HIPEC and/or EPIC in gastric cancer [28].

Yan et al. selected 10 of 13 randomized controlled trials that were judged to be of fair quality

to be used in the meta-analysis [27]. There was a survival benefit associated with HIPEC (hazard ration [HR] = 0.060; 95% CI = 0.43–0.83; p = 0.002) or HIPEC with EPIC (HR = 0.45; 95% CI = 0.29–0.68; p = 0.0002). There was a marginal effect with normothermic intraoperative intraperitoneal chemotherapy (NIPEC) but no significant improvement in survival with EPIC alone or delayed postoperative intraperitoneal chemotherapy (Fig. 24.3) [27].

Although there may be a survival benefit, intraperitoneal chemotherapy can increase morbidities. Even the most experienced peritoneal surface oncology centers that remove all macroscopic disease and then administer intraperitoneal chemotherapy have a higher morbidity and cost [29–31]. Yan et al. discussed an association of improved overall survival with HIPEC with or without EPIC after resection of advanced gastric primary cancer; however, with EPIC there was an associated greater risk for intra-abdominal abscess (RR = 2.37; 95% CI = 1.32–4.26; p = 0.003) and neutropenia (RR = 4.33; 95% CI = 1.49–12.61; p = 0.007) [27]. Yu et al. also saw an increased risk of intra-abdominal abscess with the use of intraperitoneal chemotherapy, especially in the early postoperative setting, compared to the control patients [32]. Theoretically, intraperitoneal chemotherapy should have less systemic toxicity as compared to systemic chemotherapy. However, the meta-analysis demonstrated a significantly higher risk of neutropenia in the intraperitoneal chemotherapy arm [27].

Most of the trials studied by Yan were completed in Asia, and it is unknown if they can be compared with gastric cancer in Western countries. It is possible that perioperative chemotherapy may be better in Western patients with more advanced disease and less lymph nodes dissected. Data does suggest a role of HIPEC with or without EPIC to improve overall survival for advanced primary gastric cancer with advanced T-stage and no peritoneal metastases. A prospective multi-institutional randomized controlled trial (GASTRICHIP) with well-defined eligibility criteria, interventions, and end points is currently in progress in France [33].

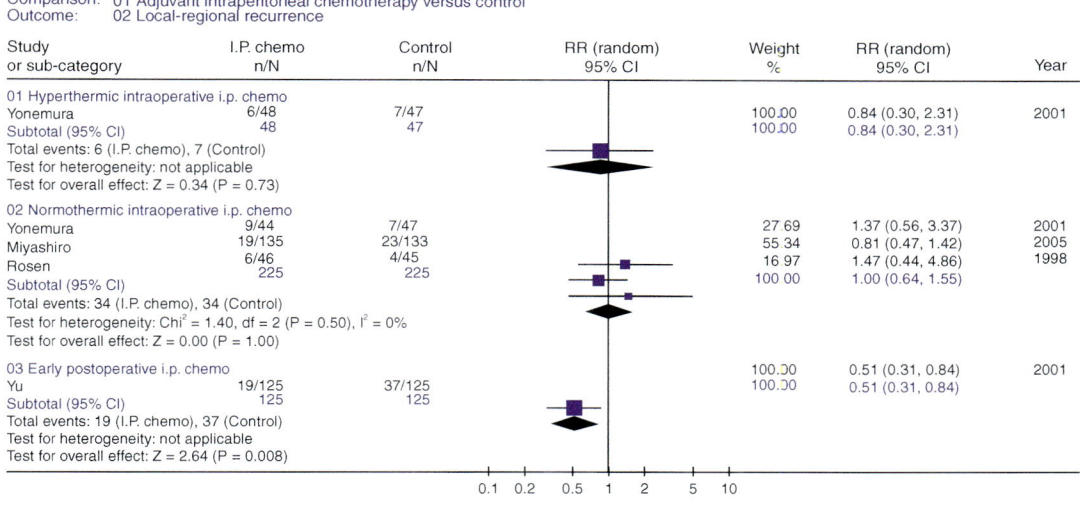

Fig. 24.3 Forest plot of the relative risk (RR) of the local-regional recurrence with adjuvant intraperitoneal (IP) chemotherapy versus controls for advanced gastric cancer. The studies were analyzed according to the regimens of intraperitoneal chemotherapy used. The estimate of the RR of each individual trial corresponds to the middle of the squares, and horizontal line gives the 95% confidence interval (CI). On each line, the numbers of events, expressed as a fraction of the total number randomized, are shown for both treatment groups. For each subgroup the sum of the statistics, along with the summary RR, is represented by the middle of the solid diamonds. (From Yan et al. with permission [27])

Gastric Cancer with Peritoneal Metastases

In the past, gastric cancer with peritoneal dissemination was thought to be uniformly lethal. Prospective studies had a median survival of less than 6 months [34]. Although response rates to systemic chemotherapy regimens have improved, there has not been a corresponding improvement in survival rates [35]. There may be some increased effectiveness with palliative gastric cancer resections in patients with peritoneal metastases; however there are no long-term improvements in survival.

CRS and HIPEC as an Effective Strategy

There is potential for long-term survival for patients with gastric cancer and peritoneal metastases as a result of cytoreductive surgery and HIPEC. There are single-institution data and phase II studies that support use of this strategy (Table 24.1) [20, 29–31, 36–40]. Glehen et al. studied 159 patients with a median follow-up of 20.4 months. There was a median overall survival of 9.2 months, but the 5-year survival rate was 13% [30]. Although CRS and HIPEC is less effective for gastric cancer than results from other peritoneal surface malignancies, CRS and HIPEC results in an improvement for gastric cancer versus surgery alone. Gastric cancer patient with peritoneal metastases treated with CRS and HIPEC were the only patients that reported a 5-year survival [37, 38, 41].

These studies may underestimate the potential of CRS with HIPEC, as there was no strict patient selection criteria utilized. The extent of peritoneal metastases as measured by Sugarbaker's peritoneal cancer index (PCI) significantly influences survival and is correlated with the completeness of cytoreduction [42]. Cytoreductive surgery must reduce the residual disease to a minimum for intraperitoneal chemotherapy to be effective (due to minimal chemotherapy penetration). Glehen et al. demonstrated a 5-year survival of 23% with median survival

Table 24.1 Reports of patients with gastric peritoneal metastases treated by cytoreductive surgery and hyperthermic intraperitoneal chemotherapy

Reference	Year	N	Anticancer agent used during HIPEC	Median survival (months)	1-year survival (%)	3-year survival (%)	5-year survival (%)
Fujimoto et al. [20]	1997	48	MMC	16	54	41	31
Hirose et al. [36]	1999	17	MMC-cisplatin-etoposide	11	44	–	–
Rossi et al. [37]	2003	13	MMC-cisplatin	15	–	–	–
Glehen et al. [38] CC-0 or CC-1	2004	49 25	MMC	10.3 21.3	48 74.8	–	16 29.4
Hall et al. [31] CC-0	2004	34	MMC	– 11.2	– 45	–	–
Yonemura et al. [29] CC-0	2005	107 47	MMC-cisplatin-etoposide	11.5 15.5	– –	– –	6.5 27
Scaringi et al. [39] CC-0	2008	32 8	MMC-cisplatin	6.6 15	–	–	–
Glehen et al. [30] CC-0	2010	159 85	Various	9.2 15	43 61	18 30	13 23

Adapted from Glehen et al. with permission [40]

CC-0 complete macroscopic cytoreduction; *CC-1* residual tumor nodules <5 mm; *MMC* mitomycin C; *N* number of patients

Fig. 24.4 Overall survival of 159 patients treated by cytoreductive surgery and hyperthermic intraperitoneal chemotherapy according to completeness of cytoreductive surgery. (From Glehen et al. with permission [30])

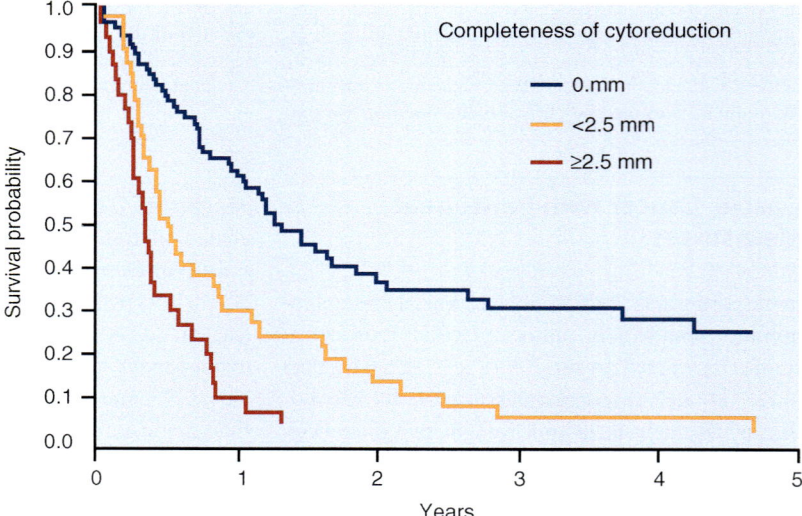

of 15 months in patients after a complete macroscopic resection (Fig. 24.4) [30]. Yonemura et al. demonstrated a similar 27% 5-year survival rate and 15.5 months median survival [29]. Hall et al. reported a 11.2-month overall survival after CRS and HIPEC with mitomycin C; however there was no patient alive after 2 years who had residual disease at CRS [31]. CRS with a minimum residual disease burden is essential for effective HIPEC. HIPEC used with macroscopic disease does not improve survival. HIPEC can

have morbidity and therefore should not be used for patients with bulky residual disease, although palliative use for ascites may always be considered [43, 44].

Unfortunately, even if completely cytoreduced, HIPEC is less useful for patients with high burden of peritoneal metastatic disease. Glehen et al. showed that one of the strongest prognostic factors was extent of carcinomatosis [30]. When the PCI was greater than 12, despite a complete cytoreduction, there were no survivors

Fig. 24.5 Overall survival of 159 patients treated by complete cytoreductive surgery according to extent of peritoneal metastases assessed by the peritoneal cancer index. (From Glehen et al. with permission [30])

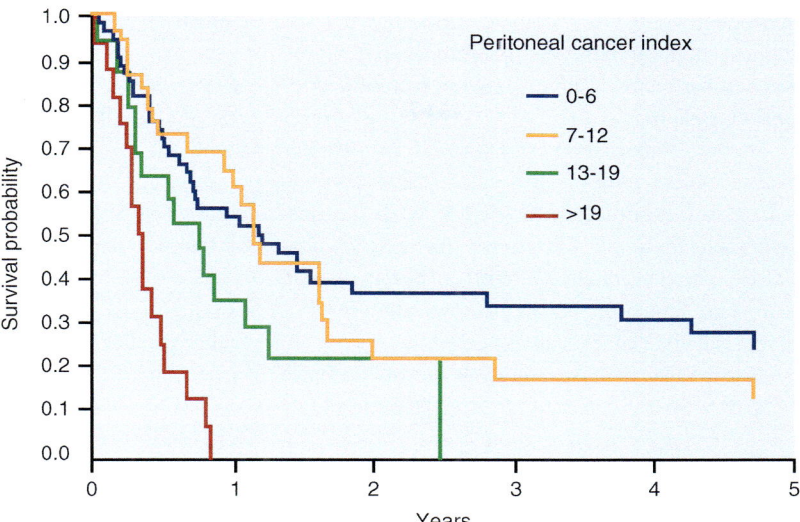

greater than 3 years (Fig. 24.5) [30]. Fujimoto et al. reported 40–50% 5-year survival for limited peritoneal metastases but only an 18% 1-year survival for patients with extensive peritoneal metastases [20]. Cytoreduction with HIPEC in gastric cancer patients with a PCI score greater than 12 may be contraindicated.

Yang et al. have provided the first and only phase III study regarding CRS and HIPEC in gastric cancer presenting with peritoneal metastases. They used cisplatin (120 mg) and mitomycin C (30 mg) in 6000 ml of normal saline at 43C for 60–90 min. Median follow-up was 32 months, and 97.1% (33 of 34) of patients after CRS died, but 85.3% (29 of 34) of CRS and HIPEC patients died. Median survival was 6.5 months (95% CI 4.8–8.2 months) after CRS and 11 months (95% CI; 10.0–11.9 months) in CRS and HIPEC group ($p = 0.046$) [43]. There was similar morbidity between the groups. The independent predictors in a multivariate analysis for improved survival were synchronous peritoneal metastases, CC 0–1 cytoreduction, more than six cycles of systemic chemotherapy, and no adverse events. Glehen et al. suggested that HIPEC should be reserved for patients with limited peritoneal carcinomatosis [30]. Also, the prognostic factors analyzed by Yang et al. suggest that it should be restricted to a limited patient population (Table 24.2) [43].

Table 24.2 Selection of gastric cancer patients with peritoneal metastases for gastrectomy, peritonectomy, and perioperative chemotherapy

Clinical features		
Young age (<65 years)		Lymph nodes, negative or limited extent
Low operative risk (no other diseases)		No liver metastases
Patient symptoms present		Peritoneal cancer index <12
Pain Bleeding Perforation	Obstruction Ascites	Expect complete clearing of the primary cancer

Adapted from Glehen et al. with permission [40]

Role of Laparoscopy for Patient Selection

Laparoscopy has three important roles in the management of gastric cancer. First, laparoscopy may select and exclude patients with intra-abdominal metastases who would not benefit from an aggressive and complex procedure that is unlikely to improve their survival. If a primary gastric cancer patient is found to peritoneal metastases or would otherwise not be able to be completely cytoreduced, HIPEC would not be warranted, and the morbidity of laparotomy could be avoided [45, 46]. Laparoscopy is useful to show that patients have clinically absent peritoneal metastases. Recent randomized trials suggest that neoadjuvant chemotherapy should be used for gastric cancer patients free of peritoneal disease [47].

Second, laparoscopy performed in primary gastric cancer patients can select those patients with a low volume (P1 or PCI < 10) of peritoneal metastases for CRS with gastrectomy and HIPEC. In these patients with minimal disease who can undergo complete cytoreduction, a 5-year survival of 25% is expected.

A third use of laparoscopy is serial exams in patients with a greater extent of peritoneal metastases. If the peritoneal metastases respond on repeated laparoscopic examination, CRS with gastrectomy and HIPEC is considered a treatment option. The use of laparoscopy with NIPS (neoadjuvant intraperitoneal and systemic chemotherapy) will be described in the following sections.

Neoadjuvant Intraperitoneal and Systemic Chemotherapy (NIPS)

If patients have peritoneal dissemination, the effects of systemic chemotherapy are disappointing. Preusser et al. demonstrated that an aggressive systemic chemotherapy regimen can have a 50% response rate in advanced gastric cancer; however this response is less robust in patients with peritoneal metastases [48]. Ajani et al. gave neoadjuvant chemotherapy, and the failure of the regimen was most common with peritoneal metastases [49]. Systemic chemotherapy alone for primary gastric cancer with peritoneal metastases is not satisfactory.

Neoadjuvant chemotherapy for gastric cancer can be modified to address peritoneal seeding by combining systemic and intraperitoneal chemotherapy. Chemotherapy may gain access to small peritoneal cancer nodules via the systemic circulation and by diffusion from a chemotherapy solution within the peritoneal cavity. Yonemura and coworkers proposed a prospective phase II study to identify the efficacy and assess toxicities in patients with gastric cancer with peritoneal metastases [50]. The following summarizes this study.

Patients Treated

In this phase II study, Yonemura and coworkers treated patients with peritoneal metastases identified by laparoscopy, laparotomy biopsy, or cytology from ascites. To qualify for NIPS, patients must have (1) proven peritoneal seeding by histology or cytology; (2) no hematogenous or remote lymph node metastases; (3) be less than or equal to 65 years; (4) have an Eastern Clinical Oncology Group score of 2 or less; (5) adequate bone marrow, liver, cardiac, and renal function; and (6) no other severe medical comorbidities or synchronous malignancies.

Qualifying patients had a peritoneal port system (Bard Port, C.R. Bard Inc., USA) inserted into the abdominal cavity under local anesthesia with the tip placed within the cul-de-sac of Douglas.

Chemotherapy Regimen

Prior to administration of chemotherapy, 500 ml of saline was instilled into the peritoneal cavity, and fluid was removed for cytology. Docetaxel 40 mg and carboplatin 150 mg were used for intraperitoneal chemotherapy in addition to 1000 ml of saline over 30 min. Methotrexate 100 mg/m^2 and 5-fluorouracil 600 mg/m^2 in 100 ml of saline over 15 min were administered intravenously the same day. This regimen was administered weekly for two cycles. After the second cycle, peritoneal wash cytology was again performed. If cytology was positive, neoadjuvant chemotherapy was continued for two more cycles. Peritoneal cytology testing is repeating after the fourth cycle, and the process is continued as long as cytology is positive.

If cytology became negative, upper endoscopy, repeat laparoscopy, and CT scan were performed. If tumors showed no demonstrable change, then two more cycles were administered. The number of NIPS chemotherapy cycles was controlled by the effect on the primary cancer and peritoneal cytology. Complete cytoreduction was required for prolonged survival in prior studies that examined peritoneal metastases. Therefore, the goal of the NIPS regimen was complete or near complete response of metastases on small bowel surfaces [36, 51–53].

The Japanese General Rules for Gastric Cancer Study was used to determine the peritoneal stage as (P1) peritoneal metastases in the upper abdomen above the transverse colon, (P2) several countable metastases in the peritoneal cavity, and (P3) numerous metastases in the peritoneal cavity [54]. Distribution and size of peritoneal metastases were recorded at laparoscopy and at surgery. Tumor location, size, and number were evaluated before and after NIPS to determine effects of neoadjuvant chemotherapy.

Surgery for Gastric Cancer with Peritoneal Metastases After Neoadjuvant Intraperitoneal and Systemic Chemotherapy (NIPS)

Gastrectomy and peritonectomy were performed if peritoneal wash cytology became negative or there was a partial response to neoadjuvant chemotherapy. Patients with progressive disease or who continue to have positive cytology despite 4–6 cycles of NIPS were not candidates for surgery.

If peritoneal metastases on small bowel surfaces were eliminated by NIPS, there was a possibility that gastrectomy and parietal peritonectomy could achieve a complete cytoreduction. Sugarbaker and Yonemura reported the use of peritonectomy for peritoneal metastases to cytoreduce the peritoneal surface and facilitate total resection of the primary gastric cancer [55, 56]. Peritonectomies required for gastric cancer have been described [7]. The epigastric peritonectomy includes any prior midline abdominal scar with the preperitoneal epigastric fat pad, xiphoid process, and round and falciform ligaments (Fig. 24.6). The anterolateral peritonectomy removes the greater omentum with the anterior layer of peritoneum from the transverse mesocolon, peritoneum of the right paracolic gutter along the appendix, and the peritoneum in the right subhepatic space. Sometimes the peritoneum of the left paracolic gutter must also be removed (Fig. 24.7). The subphrenic peritonectomy takes the peritoneal surfaces from the medial half of the right and left hemidiaphragm as well as the left triangular ligament (Fig. 24.8). The omental bursa peritonectomy starts with cholecystectomy and then removes the peritoneal covering of the porta hepatis, hepatoduodenal ligament, and floor of the omental bursa including the peritoneum

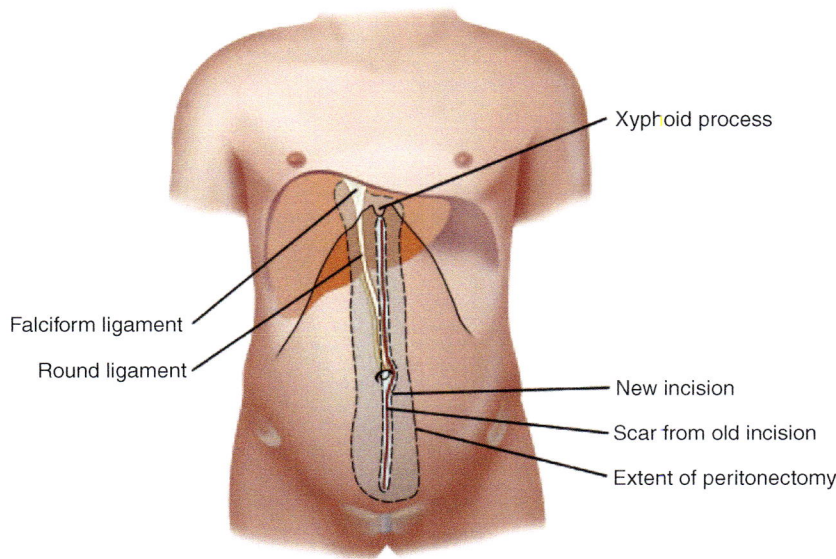

Falciform ligament

Round ligament

Xyphoid process

New incision

Scar from old incision

Extent of peritonectomy

Fig. 24.6 Epigastric peritonectomy

overlying the pancreas (Fig. 24.9). If tumor was within the cul-de-sac, a pelvic peritonectomy was also performed, and electroevaporative surgery strips the peritoneum from the pouch of Douglas (Fig. 24.10). Sometimes, the pelvic peritonectomy will necessitate removal of the rectosigmoid colon. Visceral resections and parietal peritonectomies were performed to completely remove gross disease.

Any complications related to chemotherapy and peritonectomy were prospectively collected and verified retrospectively.

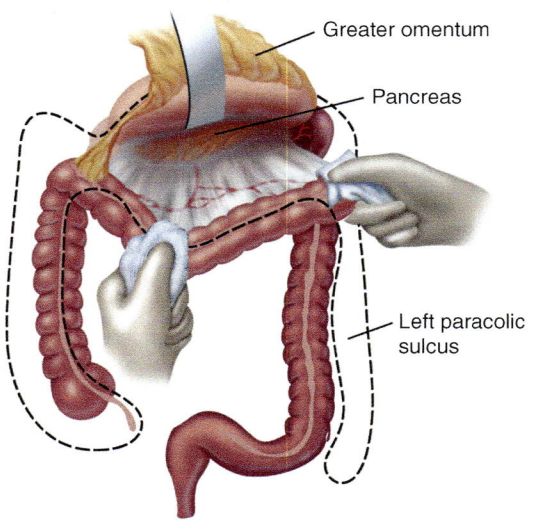

Fig. 24.7 Anterolateral peritonectomy

Results After Neoadjuvant Intraperitoneal and Systemic Chemotherapy (NIPS)

Table 24.3 shows the clinical characteristics of the 194 patients. Average age was 51.5 years. One hundred four patients had primary gastric cancer, and 90 patients had recurrent peritoneal metastases. Peritoneal fluid cytology was positive in 137 patients and negative in 57 patients prior to NIPS. There was complete resolution of peritoneal metastases after NIPS chemotherapy in 24.3% of patients. After induction treatment, 152 patients underwent surgery.

Operative interventions, such as total gastrectomy ($n = 94$), subtotal gastrectomy ($n = 17$), and small bowel resection ($n = 44$), are displayed in Table 24.3. Left and right subdiaphragmatic peritonectomy and pelvic peritonectomy were completed in 44, 31, and 61 patients, respectively. Complete cytoreduction was achieved in 103 (67.7%) of patients.

Figure 24.11 demonstrates overall survival of the 194 patients. Median survival was 15.8 months for the 152 patients who had received surgical intervention versus 7.5 months for patients who did not have an operation. Median survival of the 194 patients was 14.4 months. One-year survival was 54% for all patients. There was a significant survival difference ($p = 0.03$) between patients who underwent operative intervention versus those who did not. There was a higher median survival of

Fig. 24.8 Subphrenic peritonectomy

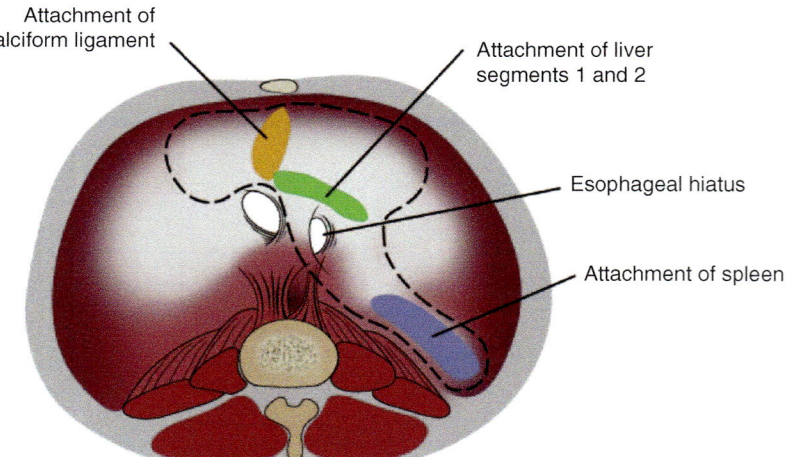

Fig. 24.9 Omental bursa peritonectomy

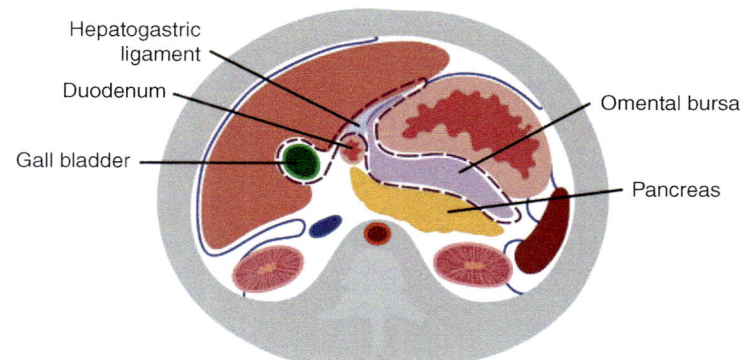

Hepatogastric ligament

Duodenum

Gall bladder

Omental bursa

Pancreas

Fig. 24.10 Pelvic peritonectomy

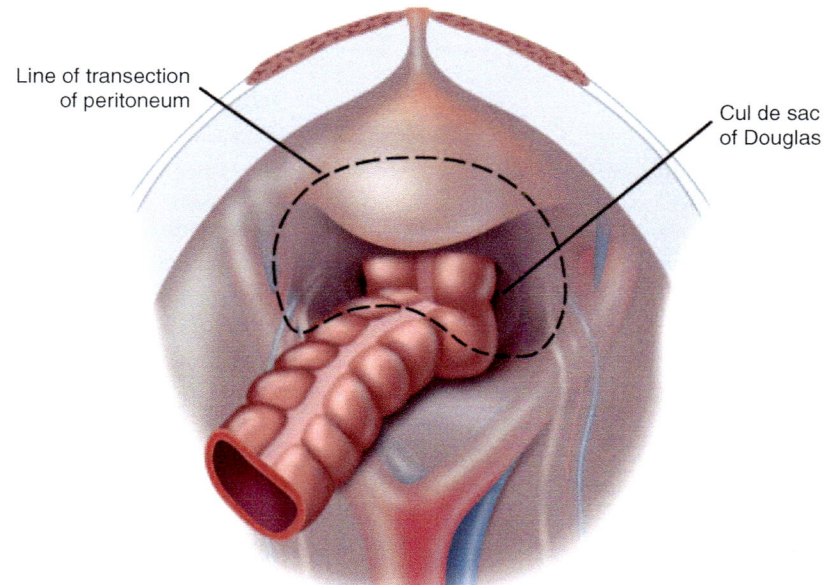

Line of transection of peritoneum

Cul de sac of Douglas

18 months for patients who received a complete cytoreduction. There was no difference between primary and recurrent disease after cytoreduction with a median survival of 17.6 months versus 14.1 months, respectively ($p = 0.39$).

Adverse Events from Neoadjuvant Intraperitoneal and Systemic Chemotherapy (NIPS) and Cytoreductive Surgery

The most common chemotherapy-related grade 3 or 4 adverse events were bone marrow suppression and diarrhea. Bone marrow suppression occurred after three courses in three patients, after five courses in three patients, and after six courses in four patients. Less common adverse events were port site infection ($n = 2$) and renal failure ($n = 1$). After cytoreduction with peritonectomy, 18 patients (14%) developed complications. Two patients had pneumonia and one patient developed renal failure. Six patients had an anastomotic leak, and two patients had an abdominal abscess. The overall operative mortality rate was 1.5% (2 of 133 patients). These patients died of multiple organ failure from sepsis from abdominal abscess [40].

Table 24.3 Clinicopathological characteristics of 194 gastric cancer patients with peritoneal carcinomatosis

Variables	No. of patients
Age, years (range)	51.5 ± 12.6
Male/female ratio	89/105
Histological diagnosis	
Well/intermediately differentiated adenocarcinoma	7
Poorly/undifferentiated adenocarcinoma	187
Organ resections	
Right diaphragmatic copula	31
Left diaphragmatic copula	44
Total gastrectomy	94
Subtotal gastrectomy	17
Pelvic peritoneum	61
Colectomy	68
Small bowel resection	44
Cytology before BIPS	
Negative	57
Positive	137
Cytology after BIPS	
Negative	152
Positive	42
Pathological response to BIPS	
Grade 0	63
Grade 1	38
Grade 2	24
Grade 3	27

From Canbay et al. with permission [60]

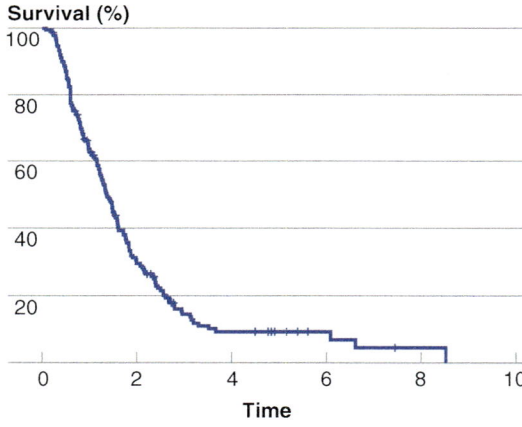

Fig. 24.11 Overall survival in 194 gastric cancer patients with peritoneal carcinomatosis. (From Canbay et al. with permission [60])

Clinical Data Supporting Complete Cytoreduction as the Goal in Management of Gastric Cancer Patients with Peritoneal Seeding

Complete cytoreduction is crucial in the surgical treatment for carcinomatosis from appendiceal and colon cancer. Five-year survival for complete cytoreduction was 54% versus 15% for incomplete cytoreduction as reported by Culliford et al. [57]. Glehen et al. also reported a median survival difference of 32 months and 8.4 months for patients with macroscopic complete resection versus incomplete cytoreduction, respectively [58]. This has shown that complete cytoreduction had better survival rates in gastric cancer [59, 60]. There is a difference in biological aggressiveness between colon and gastric cancers; however, macroscopic complete cytoreduction is necessary for long-term survival with peritoneal metastatic disease in these diseases. If there is P3 dissemination, complete cytoreduction should not be attempted. NIPS was shown to diminish disease on intestinal surface and facilitate complete cytoreduction.

Palliative Benefits to All Patients with Cancerous Ascites

There was improvement in symptoms for the 78 patients who had ascites [40]. These benefits occurred in patients with primary gastric cancer and also in patients with recurrent disease. Cunliffe et al. hypothesized that peritoneal metastases are nourished via ascites as well as blood supply. Therefore, peritoneal implants should be treated via a combined intraperitoneal and intravenous approach [61]. Intravenous chemotherapy has minimal effects on peritoneal metastases, and intraperitoneal chemotherapy alone has a less than 30% effect on ascites [31, 32, 48, 49]. The bidirectional chemotherapy (intraperitoneal and intravenous) has a response rate of 57% with 100% resolution of ascites [40].

Chemotherapy Agents Selected for Neoadjuvant Intraperitoneal and Systemic Chemotherapy (NIPS)

Different chemotherapy regimens have been used for NIPS such as docetaxel, cisplatin, and paclitaxel. Fujiwara et al. irrigated the abdominal cavity with doses of docetaxel between 40 and 60 mg/m^2 dissolved in 1 L of saline [62]. Canbay et al. administered intraperitoneal docetaxel (30 mg/m^2) and cisplatin (30 mg/m^2) [60]. Kitayama's group administered paclitaxel at 20 mg/m^2 in 1 L of normal saline over 1 h [63].

In summary, NIPS should be considered in gastric cancer patients with peritoneal metastases. It has maximal benefits for small volumes of peritoneal surface metastases and is reliable treatment for symptomatic ascites. Bidirectional chemotherapy may be the preferred strategy for preoperative chemotherapy of gastric cancer with peritoneal metastases.

References

1. Berretta M, Fisichella R, Borsatti E, et al. Feasibility of intraperitoneal Trastuzumab treatment in a patient with peritoneal carcinomatosis from gastric cancer. Eur Rev Med Pharmacol Sci. 2014;18(5):689–92.
2. Jemal A, Bray F, Center MM, Ferlay J, Ward E, Forman D. Global cancer statistics. CA Cancer J Clin. 2011;61(2):69–90.
3. Sarela AI, Miner TJ, Karpeh MS, Coit DG, Jaques DP, Brennan MF. Clinical outcomes with laparoscopic stage M1, unresected gastric adenocarcinoma. Ann Surg. 2006;243(2):189–95.
4. Brenner H, Rothenbacher D, Arndt V. Epidemiology of stomach cancer. Methods Mol Biol. Clifton NJ. 2009;472:467–77.
5. Cappellani A, Zanghi A, Di Vita M, et al. Clinical and biological markers in gastric cancer: update and perspectives. Front Biosci Sch Ed. 2010;2:403–12.
6. Hioki M, Gotohda N, Konishi M, Nakagohri T, Takahashi S, Kinoshita T. Predictive factors improving survival after gastrectomy in gastric cancer patients with peritoneal carcinomatosis. World J Surg. 2010;34(3):555–62.
7. Sugarbaker PH, Yu W, Yonemura Y. Gastrectomy, peritonectomy, and perioperative intraperitoneal chemotherapy: the evolution of treatment strategies for advanced gastric cancer. Semin Surg Oncol. 2003;21(4):233–48.
8. Glehen O, Mohamed F, Gilly FN. Peritoneal carcinomatosis from digestive tract cancer: new management by cytoreductive surgery and intraperitoneal chemohyperthermia. Lancet Oncol. 2004;5(4):219–28.
9. Elias D, Gilly F, Boutitie F, et al. Peritoneal colorectal carcinomatosis treated with surgery and perioperative intraperitoneal chemotherapy: retrospective analysis of 523 patients from a multicentric French study. J Clin Oncol Off J Am Soc Clin Oncol. 2010;28(1):63–8.
10. Yan TD, Deraco M, Baratti D, et al. Cytoreductive surgery and hyperthermic intraperitoneal chemotherapy for malignant peritoneal mesothelioma: multi-institutional experience. J Clin Oncol Off J Am Soc Clin Oncol. 2009;27(36):6237–42.
11. Sugarbaker PH. New standard of care for appendiceal epithelial neoplasms and pseudomyxoma peritonei syndrome? Lancet Oncol. 2006;7(1):69–76.
12. Gunderson LL, Sosin H. Adenocarcinoma of the stomach: areas of failure in a re-operation series (second or symptomatic look) clinicopathologic correlation and implications for adjuvant therapy. Int J Radiat Oncol Biol Phys. 1982;8(1):1–11.
13. Wisbeck WM, Becher EM, Russell AH. Adenocarcinoma of the stomach: autopsy observations with therapeutic implications for the radiation oncologist. Radiother Oncol. 1986;7(1):13–8.
14. Landry J, Tepper JE, Wood WC, Moulton EO, Koerner F, Sullinger J. Patterns of failure following curative resection of gastric carcinoma. Int J Radiat Oncol Biol Phys. 1990;19(6):1357–62.
15. Wils J, Meyer HJ, Wilke H. Current status and future directions in the treatment of localized gastric cancer. Ann Oncol. 1994;5(Suppl 3):69–72.
16. Maruyama K, Okabayashi K, Kinoshita T. Progress in gastric cancer surgery in Japan and its limits of radicality. World J Surg. 1987;11(4):418–25.
17. Kaibara N, Sumi K, Yonekawa M, et al. Does extensive dissection of lymph nodes improve the results of surgical treatment of gastric cancer? Am J Surg. 1990;159(2):218–21
18. Korenaga D, Moriguchi S, Orita H, et al. Trends in survival rates in Japanese patients with advanced carcinoma of the stomach. Surg Gynecol Obstet. 1992;174(5):387–93.
19. Boku T, Nakane Y, Minoura T, et al. Prognostic significance of serosal invasion and free intraperitoneal cancer cells in gastric cancer. Br J Surg. 1990;77(4):436–9.
20. Fujimoto S, Takahashi M, Mutou T, et al. Improved mortality rate of gastric carcinoma patients with peritoneal carcinomatosis treated with intraperitoneal hyperthermic chemoperfusion combined with surgery. Cancer. 1997;79(5):884–91.
21. Kodera Y, Yamamura Y, Shimizu Y, et al. Peritoneal washing cytology: prognostic value of positive findings in patients with gastric carcinoma undergoing a potentially curative resection. J Surg Oncol. 1999;72(2):60–64–65.

22. Bando E, Yonemura Y, Takeshita Y, et al. Intraoperative lavage for cytological examination in 1,297 patients with gastric carcinoma. Am J Surg. 1999;178(3):256–62.

23. Fujimura T, Yonemura Y, Ninomiya I, et al. Early detection of peritoneal dissemination of gastrointestinal cancers by reverse-transcriptase polymerase chain reaction. Oncol Rep. 1997;4(5):1015–9.

24. Sethna KS, Sugarbaker PH. New prospects for the control of peritoneal surface dissemination of gastric cancer using perioperative intraperitoneal chemotherapy. Cancer Ther. 2004;2:79–84.

25. Los G, Mutsaers PH, Lenglet WJ, Baldew GS, McVie JG. Platinum distribution in intraperitoneal tumors after intraperitoneal cisplatin treatment. Cancer Chemother Pharmacol. 1990;25(6):389–94.

26. Xu D-Z, Zhan Y-Q, Sun X-W, Cao S-M, Geng Q-R. Meta-analysis of intraperitoneal chemotherapy for gastric cancer. World J Gastroenterol. 2004;10(18):2727–30.

27. Yan TD, Black D, Sugarbaker PH, et al. A systematic review and meta-analysis of the randomized controlled trials on adjuvant intraperitoneal chemotherapy for resectable gastric cancer. Ann Surg Oncol. 2007;14(10):2702–13.

28. Feingold PL, Kwong MLM, Sabesan A, Sorber R, Rudloff U. Cytoreductive surgery and hyperthermic intraperitoneal chemotherapy for gastric cancer and other less common disease histologies: is it time? J Gastrointest Oncol. 2016;7(1):87–98.

29. Yonemura Y, Kawamura T, Bandou E, Takahashi S, Sawa T, Matsuki N. Treatment of peritoneal dissemination from gastric cancer by peritonectomy and chemohyperthermic peritoneal perfusion. Br J Surg. 2005;92(3):370–5.

30. Glehen O, Gilly FN, Arvieux C, et al. Peritoneal carcinomatosis from gastric cancer: a multi-institutional study of 159 patients treated by cytoreductive surgery combined with perioperative intraperitoneal chemotherapy. Ann Surg Oncol. 2010;17(9):2370–7.

31. Hall JJ, Loggie BW, Shen P, et al. Cytoreductive surgery with intraperitoneal hyperthermic chemotherapy for advanced gastric cancer. J Gastrointest Surg. 2004;8(4):454–63.

32. Yu W, Whang I, Chung HY, Averbach A, Sugarbaker PH. Indications for early postoperative intraperitoneal chemotherapy of advanced gastric cancer: results of a prospective randomized trial. World J Surg. 2001;25(8):985–90.

33. Glehen O, Passot G, Villeneuve L, et al. GASTRICHIP: D2 resection and hyperthermic intraperitoneal chemotherapy in locally advanced gastric carcinoma: a randomized and multicenter phase III study. BMC Cancer. 2014;14:183.

34. Sadeghi B, Arvieux C, Glehen O, et al. Peritoneal carcinomatosis from non-gynecologic malignancies: results of the EVOCAPE 1 multicentric prospective study. Cancer. 2000;88(2):358–63.

35. Boku N, Gastrointestinal Oncology Study Group of Japan Clinical Oncology Group. Chemotherapy for metastatic disease: review from JCOG trials. Int J Clin Oncol. 2008;13(3):196–200.

36. Hirose K, Katayama K, Iida A, et al. Efficacy of continuous hyperthermic peritoneal perfusion for the prophylaxis and treatment of peritoneal metastasis of advanced gastric cancer: evaluation by multivariate regression analysis. Oncology. 1999;57(2):106–14.

37. Rossi CR, Pilati P, Mocellin S, et al. Hyperthermic intraperitoneal intraoperative chemotherapy for peritoneal carcinomatosis arising from gastric adenocarcinoma. Suppl Tumori. 2003;2(5):S54–7.

38. Glehen O, Schreiber V, Cotte E, et al. Cytoreductive surgery and intraperitoneal chemohyperthermia for peritoneal carcinomatosis arising from gastric cancer. Arch Surg Chic Ill. 1960/2004;139(1):20–6.

39. Scaringi S, Kianmanesh R, Sabate JM, et al. Advanced gastric cancer with or without peritoneal carcinomatosis treated with hyperthermic intraperitoneal chemotherapy: a single western center experience. Eur J Surg Oncol. 2008;34(11):1246–52.

40. Glehen O, Yonemura Y, Sugarbaker PH. Prevention and treatment of peritoneal metastases from gastric cancer. In: Sugarbaker PH, editor. Cytoreductive surgery and perioperative chemotherapy for peritoneal surface malignancy: textbook and video atlas. Woodbury: Cine-Med; 2012. p. 79–94.

41. Yonemura Y, Fujimura T, Nishimura G, et al. Effects of intraoperative chemohyperthermia in patients with gastric cancer with peritoneal dissemination. Surgery. 1996;119(4):437–44.

42. Jacquet P, Sugarbaker PH. Clinical research methodologies in diagnosis and staging of patients with peritoneal carcinomatosis. Cancer Treat Res. 1996;82:359–74.

43. Yang X-J, Huang C-Q, Suo T, et al. Cytoreductive surgery and hyperthermic intraperitoneal chemotherapy improves survival of patients with peritoneal carcinomatosis from gastric cancer: final results of a phase III randomized clinical trial. Ann Surg Oncol. 2011;18(6):1575–81.

44. Valle M, Van der Speeten K, Garofalo A. Laparoscopic hyperthermic intraperitoneal peroperative chemotherapy (HIPEC) in the management of refractory malignant ascites: a multi-institutional retrospective analysis in 52 patients. J Surg Oncol. 2009;100(4):331–4.

45. Garofalo A, Valle M. Laparoscopy in the management of peritoneal carcinomatosis. Cancer J. Sudbury Mass. 2009;15(3):190–5.

46. Badgwell B, Cormier JN, Krishnan S, et al. Does neoadjuvant treatment for gastric cancer patients with positive peritoneal cytology at staging laparoscopy improve survival? Ann Surg Oncol. 2008;15(10):2684–91.

47. Cunningham D, Allum WH, Stenning SP, et al. Perioperative chemotherapy versus surgery alone for resectable gastroesophageal cancer. N Engl J Med. 2006;355(1):11–20.

48. Preusser P, Wilke H, Achterrath W, et al. Phase II study with the combination etoposide, doxorubicin, and cisplatin in advanced measurable gastric cancer. J Clin Oncol Off J Am Soc Clin Oncol. 1989;7(9):1310–7.

49. Ajani JA, Ota DM, Jessup JM, et al. Resectable gastric carcinoma. An evaluation of preoperative and postoperative chemotherapy. Cancer. 1991;68(7):1501–6.

50. Yonemura Y, Bandou E, Sawa T, et al. Neoadjuvant treatment of gastric cancer with peritoneal dissemination. Eur J Surg Oncol. 2006;32(6):661–5.

51. Yonemura Y, Bandou E, Kinoshita K, et al. Effective therapy for peritoneal dissemination in gastric cancer. Surg Oncol Clin N Am. 2003;12(3):635–48.

52. Yonemura Y, Fujimura T, Fushida S, et al. Hyperthermo-chemotherapy combined with cytoreductive surgery for the treatment of gastric cancer with peritoneal dissemination. World J Surg. 1991;15(4):530–535–536.

53. Glehen O, Mithieux F, Osinsky D, et al. Surgery combined with peritonectomy procedures and intraperitoneal chemohyperthermia in abdominal cancers with peritoneal carcinomatosis: a phase II study. J Clin Oncol Off J Am Soc Clin Oncol. 2003;21(5):799–806.

54. Yonemura Y, Elnemr A, Endou Y, et al. Multidisciplinary therapy for treatment of patients with peritoneal carcinomatosis from gastric cancer. World J Gastrointest Oncol. 2010;2(2):85–97.

55. Sugarbaker PH. Peritonectomy procedures. Ann Surg. 1995;221(1):29–42.

56. Yonemura Y, Fujimura T, Fushida S, et al. Peritonectomy as a treatment modality for patients with peritoneal dissemination from gastric cancer [Internet]. In: MD TN, MD TY, editors. Multimodality therapy for gastric cancer. Springer Japan; 1999 [cited 2016 Apr 8]. p. 71–80. Available from: http://link.springer.com/chapter/10.1007/978-4-431-67927-1_10

57. Culliford AT, Brooks AD, Sharma S, et al. Surgical debulking and intraperitoneal chemotherapy for established peritoneal metastases from colon and appendix cancer. Ann Surg Oncol. 2001;8(10):787–95.

58. Glehen O, Kwiatkowski F, Sugarbaker PH, et al. Cytoreductive surgery combined with perioperative intraperitoneal chemotherapy for the management of peritoneal carcinomatosis from colorectal cancer: a multi-institutional study. J Clin Oncol Off J Am Soc Clin Oncol. 2004;22(16):3284–92.

59. Yonemura Y, de Aretxabala X, Fujimura T, et al. Intraoperative chemohyperthermic peritoneal perfusion as an adjuvant to gastric cancer: final results of a randomized controlled study. Hepato-Gastroenterology. 2001;48(42):1776–82.

60. Canbay E, Mizumoto A, Ichinose M, et al. Outcome data of patients with peritoneal carcinomatosis from gastric origin treated by a strategy of bidirectional chemotherapy prior to cytoreductive surgery and hyperthermic intraperitoneal chemotherapy in a single specialized center in Japan. Ann Surg Oncol. 2014;21(4):1147–52.

61. Cunliffe WJ. The rationale for early postoperative intraperitoneal chemotherapy for gastric cancer [Internet]. In: FACS PHSMD, editor. Management of gastric cancer. Springer US; 1991 [cited 2016 Apr 8]. p. 143–59. Available from: http://link.springer.com/chapter/10.1007/978-1-4615-3882-0_9

62. Fujiwara Y, Takiguchi S, Nakajima K, et al. Intraperitoneal docetaxel combined with S-1 for advanced gastric cancer with peritoneal dissemination. J Surg Oncol. 2012;105(1):38–42.

63. Kitayama J, Ishigami H, Yamaguchi H, et al. Salvage gastrectomy after intravenous and intraperitoneal paclitaxel (PTX) administration with oral S-1 for peritoneal dissemination of advanced gastric cancer with malignant ascites. Ann Surg Oncol. 2014;21(2):539–46.

Palliative Therapy for Gastric Cancer

25

K. Ji, P. Yuan, Z. D. Bu, and J. F. Ji

The past decades have witnessed the constant decrease in the morbidity and mortality of gastric cancer; however, as the fifth most common malignant tumor, gastric cancer is still the third most common cause of cancer death [1]. There were about one million new cases and 723,000 deaths from gastric cancer in 2012, among which Chinese patients accounted for about 50% [1]. Due to its insidious onset and the lack of specificity of signs and symptoms, over 80% of gastric cancer cases are in an advanced stage for being diagnosed. The 5-year survival rate is low. Even in patients who have received radical resection, the risk of distal metastasis or local recurrence can still be high [1]. The vast majority of patients with gastric cancer still need palliative care after the disease progresses to a certain stage. For patients with unresectable or advanced gastric cancer, palliative care should be provided as early as possible. The principles of palliative treatment for advanced gastric cancer are to relieve pain, improve their quality of life, and prolong survival by alleviating symptoms. The palliative care for advanced gastric carcinoma can be either local therapy or systemic therapy. Cytotoxic chemotherapy has been applied as the preferred systemic treatment in patients with metastatic gastric cancer; however, it often cannot alleviate the local symptoms (e.g., nausea, pain, gastrointestinal obstruction, and bleeding) in patients with locally advanced tumors or with distant metastasis. For these patients, multidisciplinary management using local treatments including endoscopy, surgery, and radiotherapy should be used. In this chapter, we will describe the palliative care in patients with locally advanced unresectable gastric cancer or those with metastatic gastric cancer.

K. Ji · Z. D. Bu · J. F. Ji (✉)
Department of Gastrointestinal Surgery,
Key Laboratory of Carcinogenesis and Translational Research (Ministry of Education), Peking University Cancer Hospital, Beijing Cancer Hospital and Institute, Beijing, China
e-mail: jijiafu@hsc.pku.edu.cn

P. Yuan
Department of Endoscopy, Key Laboratory of Carcinogenesis and Translational Research (Ministry of Education), Peking University Cancer Hospital, Beijing Cancer Hospital and Institute, Beijing, China

Local Palliative Care

Local palliative care is a therapeutic option for controlling the progression of local symptoms such as obstruction, pain, nausea, and bleeding. It includes palliative surgery, surgical bypass, endoscopic techniques, and palliative radiotherapy. Improving the overall prognosis of patients should be the major principle during the selecting of any local palliative care protocol; that is, effort should be made to lower the morbidity and mortality of patients with advanced gastric cancer and avoid long hospital stay.

© Springer-Verlag GmbH Germany, part of Springer Nature 2019
S. H. Noh, W. J. Hyung (eds.), *Surgery for Gastric Cancer*,
https://doi.org/10.1007/978-3-662-45583-8_25

Palliative Gastrectomy

Palliative gastrectomy is feasible for advanced gastric cancer patients who had received systemic treatment. The benefits of palliative gastrectomy include alleviating symptoms including obstruction, bleeding, pain, and nausea. Retrospective studies have suggested surgery may be associated with a survival benefit [2–5]. Meanwhile, some literature also has questioned the benefits of palliative resection for patients with advanced gastric cancer (Fig. 25.1) [6, 7]. In a retrospective study, Schmidt B. et al. found that the survival

was not significantly different between patients who had undergone palliative gastrectomy and those had not, although they also mentioned that there might be sample selection bias. Compared with patients who had only received bypass surgery or those without surgical intervention, patients who had undergone surgical resection might have lower disease burden, better physical status, and better prognosis [6].

In a phase III clinical randomized controlled trial (REGATTA) jointly initiated by Fujitanni K and Yang HK, the authors investigated the superiority of gastrectomy followed by chemotherapy

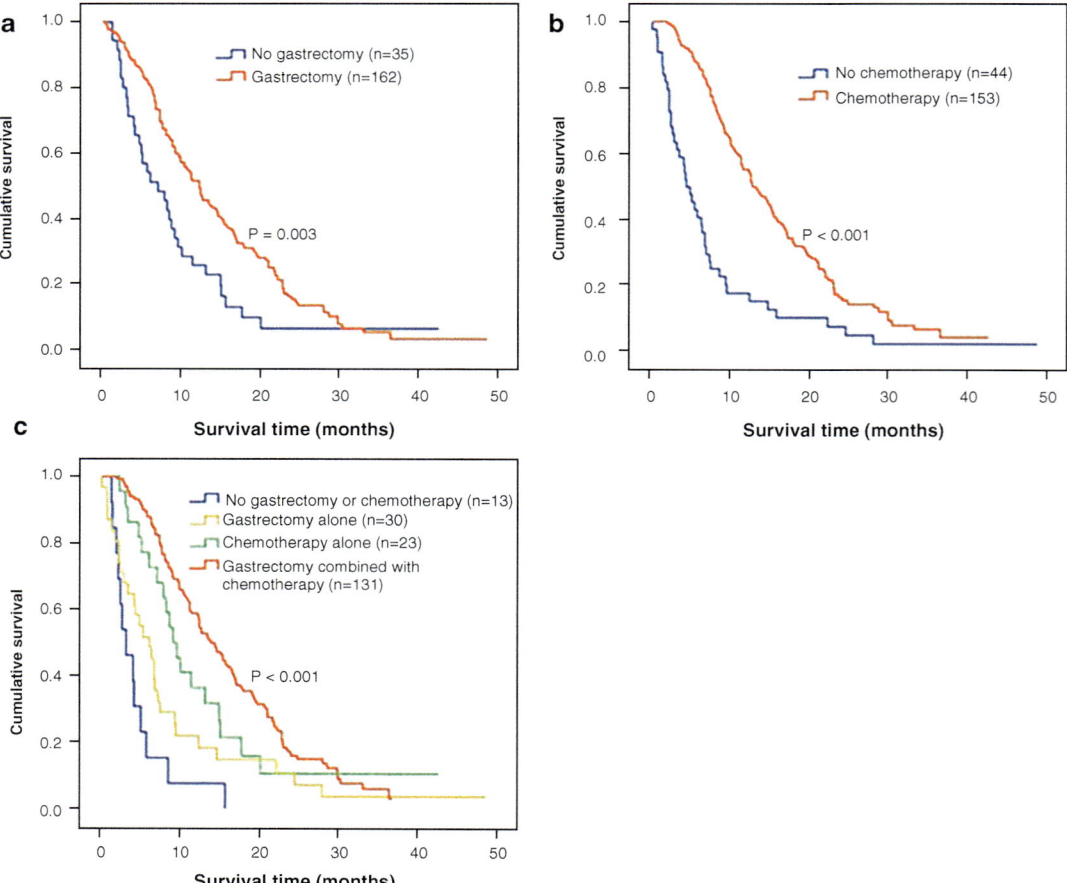

Fig. 25.1 Survival curves of patients grouped with different treatments. (**a**) Overall survival between patients undergoing non-curative gastrectomy and those without (12.4 vs. 7.1 months, $P = 0.003$). (**b**) Overall survival between patients with and without postoperative chemo-

therapy (MST 13.2 vs. 4.3 months, $P < 0.001$). (**c**) The comparison between patients with non-curative gastrectomy combined with postoperative chemotherapy and the other treatment groups ($P < 0.001$). *MST* median survival time [5]

versus chemotherapy alone with respect to overall survival in patients with advanced gastric cancer with a single non-curable factor [8]. A single non-curable factor was defined as hepatic metastasis (H1), peritoneal metastasis (P1) without massive ascites or intestinal obstruction, or para-aortic lymph node metastasis above the celiac axis or below the inferior mesenteric artery (lymph node N016a1/b2 of maximum diameter ≥ 1 cm), or both [8]. Patients were randomized into two groups: in the surgery group, patients underwent gastrectomy (D1) followed by palliative chemotherapy, without receiving D2 lymphadenectomy or multivisceral resection; in the chemotherapy alone group, only palliative chemotherapy was applied. The overall survival analysis showed that there was no significant survival benefit in patients who had received palliative gastrectomy. The 2-year survival (25.7% vs. 31.4%, HR 1.08, 95% CI 0.74–1.58, $P = 0.66$) and median overall survival (mOS) (14.3 months vs. 16.6 months, HR 1.09, 95% CI 0.78–1.52, $P = 0.70$) were even worse in the surgery group, although the difference was not statistically significant [8]. In addition, the incidences of several chemotherapy-associated adverse events (leucopenia, anorexia, nausea, and hyponatremia) significantly increased in patients assigned to surgery group; thus, gastrectomy cannot be justified for treatment of patients with these tumors [8].

Gastrojejunal Anastomosis

Gastrojejunal anastomosis (e.g., surgical bypass) is suitable for patients with unresectable advanced gastric cancer accompanied by malignant gastric outlet obstruction. Palliative gastrojejunostomy can improve food intake in these patients [9]. Minimally invasive laparoscopic gastrojejunal anastomosis is a feasible procedure for the palliative treatment of malignant gastric outlet obstruction. In a small-scale retrospective study compared the surgical outcomes of laparoscopic ($n = 10$) and open ($n = 10$) gastrojejunostomies in patients with gastric outlet obstruction secondary to advanced malignancies. It was found that there was no significant difference between groups in

mean surgery time (116 vs. 116 min) ($P = 0.99$); however, the blood loss (23 vs. 142 ml; $P = 0.19$) was less, and the length of stay (8 vs. 14 days; $P = 0.14$) was shorter in the laparoscopic group, although the difference was not statistically significant due to the small sample size [10]. According to the currently available evidences, gastrojejunal anastomosis may be an alternate treatment for patients who cannot be treated by minimally invasive approaches (e.g., palliative radiotherapy and endoscopic techniques [such as ablation, stenting, or J-tube placement] with/without chemotherapy).

Endoscopic Stent Placement

Malignant intestinal obstruction is a common complication in patients with advanced gastric cancer. Its main symptoms include pain, nausea, vomiting, abdominal distention, and decreased oral intake, which can lead to dehydration and malnutrition and thus seriously affect the patients' quality of life. Compared to traditional gastroduodenal anastomosis, the self-expandable metal stents (SEMS) have become a routine clinical technique and can be used in patients with inoperable malignant intestinal obstruction due to advanced gastric cancer or other accompanying medical conditions; in particular, it can be used as a palliative treatment for elderly patients [11]. The indications of SEMS for advanced gastric cancer include the following: (a) unable to eat; (b) with poor nutritional status; (c) inoperable; and (d) with surgical risk or refuse to take a surgery. In our center, the gastric outlet obstruction scoring system (GOOSS) was used for assessing the oral intake. In 13 advanced gastric cancer patients and 1 patient with duodenal cancer accompanied by pyloric obstruction who had undergone the placement of uncovered self-expandable metal stents (Niti-STM Taewoong Medical, Korea) in our center in 2016 (Figs. 25.2 and 25.3 and Table 25.1), GOOSS scoring results (Table 25.2) showed that the oral intake was significantly improved after stent placement (Fig. 25.4). The median time to reconstruction after stent placement was 186 days, during

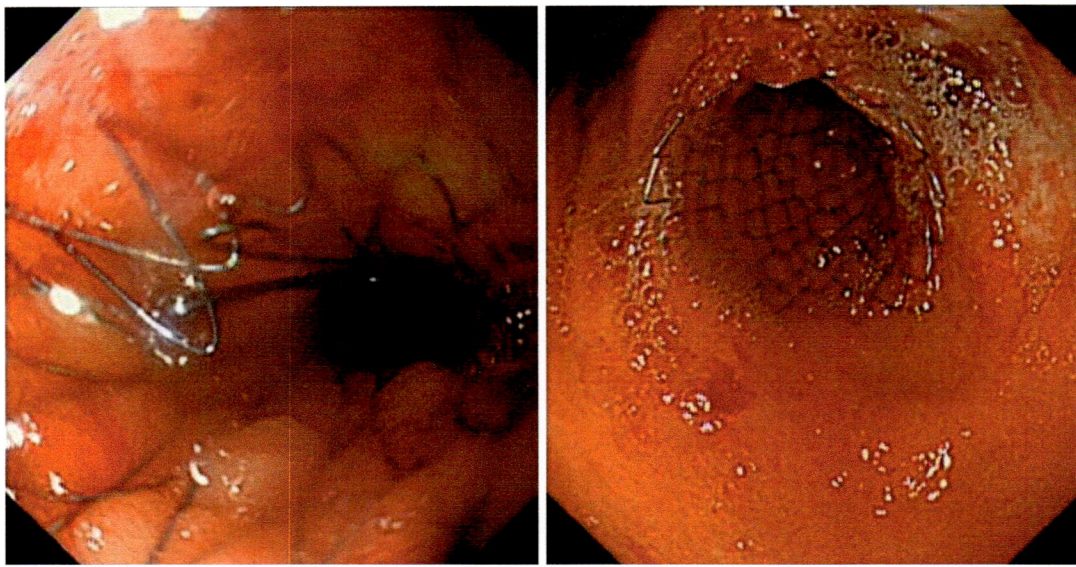

Fig. 25.2 Endoscopic view of SEMS at the site of sinuses ventriculi

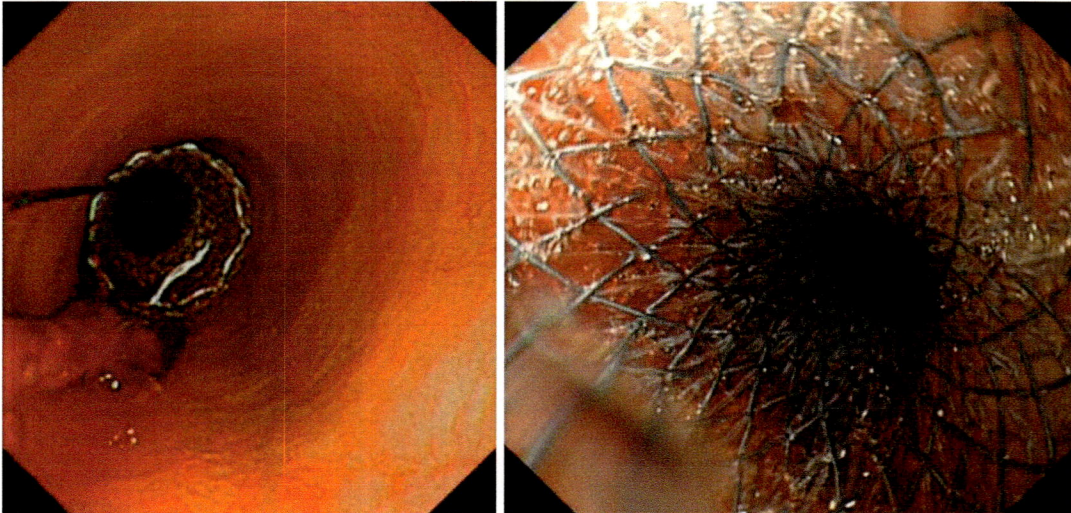

Fig. 25.3 Endoscopic view of SEMS at the site of esophagogastric junction

which three patients suffered from complications and one patient with duodenal cancer died from bleeding 3 days after stent placement at pylorus (Tables 25.3 and 25.4). Notably, all patients suffered from pain and discomfort after stent placement and thus needed the oral administration of pain medications. Although our study has shown that SEMS, as a non-surgical treatment for malignant gastric outlet obstruction, is safe and effective and can maintain the patency of the gastrointestinal tract within a certain time, it still has certain limitations. For malignant obstruction caused by other reasons, endoscope placement of a gastrojejunal feeding tube can also be applied in patients who are unable to undergo endoscopic placement of SEMS.

Table 25.1 Patient characteristics

Characteristics	No.	%
Patients	14	
Sex (M/F)	14	(100/0)
Mean ± SD age, years (range)	68.79 ± 10.47	
Causative disease		
Esophagogastric junction carcinoma	6	42.88
Recurrences of at the anastomotic site after operation for gastric carcinoma	1	7.14
Gastric antrum carcinoma with pyloric obstruction	2	14.28
Recurrences of remnant gastric cancer	1	7.14
Gastric antrum carcinoma	2	14.28
Duodenal carcinoma with pyloric obstruction	1	7.14
Gastric carcinoma with abdominal metastases	1	7.14

M male, *F* female, *SD* standard deviation

Table 25.2 Patient scores

	Before SEMS placement		After SEMS placement	
GOOSS score	No.	%	No.	%
3	0	0	4	28.5
2	0	0	9	64.3
1	5	35.7	1	7.2
0	9	64.3	0	0

Table 25.3 Results

Technical success, no./total no. (%)	14/14(100%)
Clinical success, no./total no. (%)	13/14(92.86%)
Mean procedure time, minutes	68.79 ± 10.47
Improvement in mean GOOSS score (pre → post)	$0.36 \rightarrow 2.21$*
Median stent patency, days	186

GOOSS gastric outlet obstruction scoring system
*$P < 0.001$

Table 25.4 Stent malfunction and complications

Stent malfunction	No./Total No.	%
Occlusion	0/14	0
Migration	0/14	0
Other complications		
Stent fracture	0/14	0
Insufficient stent expansion	0/14	0
Breeding	1/14	7.14
Stent obstruction	2/14	14.28
Cholangitis	0/14	0
Pancreatitis	0/14	0
Perforation	0/14	0
Death	1/14	7.14
Cause		
Breeding	1/14	7.14

Fig. 25.4 A statistically significant improvement demonstrates in the comparison between the mean value of GOOSS before SEMS placement and after SEMS placement

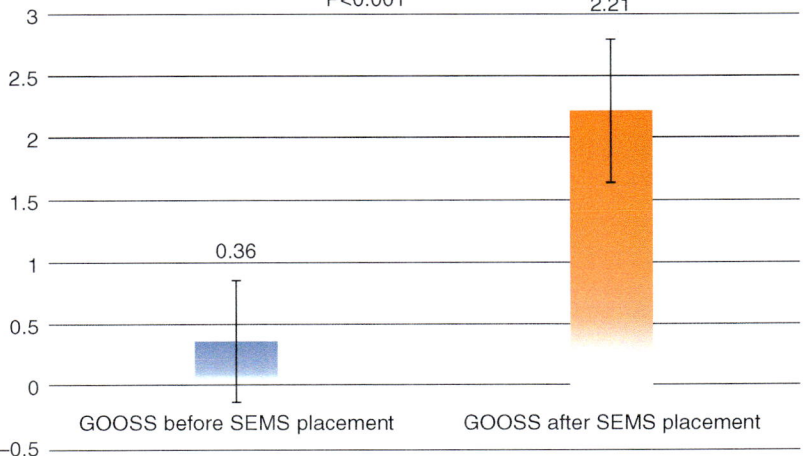

Palliative Radiotherapy

As a noninvasive treatment, palliative radiotherapy can reduce tumor burden and help to control the common clinical symptoms (e.g., pain, dysphagia, and malignant obstruction) in patients with locally advanced gastric cancer or in those with distant metastasis and thus improve the patients' quality of life [12–14]. Tey J. et al. retrospectively analyzed the outcomes of 115 gastric cancer patients who had received three-dimensional (3D) conformal radiation therapy. Dose fractionation regimen ranged from 8-Gy single fraction to 40 Gy in 16 fractions. Of 115 patients with median age of 77 years, 78 (67.8%) patients had metastatic disease at the time of treatment. Index symptoms included gastric bleeding (89.6%), obstruction (14.3%), and pain (9.2%). Response rates for bleeding, obstruction, and pain were 80.6%, 52.9%, and 45.5, respectively. Median survival was significantly longer in patients who responded to radiotherapy compared with patients who did not (113.5 vs 47 days, $P < 0.001$). There was no significant difference in response rates between low ($\leq$39 Gy) and high (>39 Gy) biologically effective dose (BED) regimens [14]. No controlled study has directly compared the effectiveness of palliative radiotherapy and endoscopic techniques in alleviating symptoms. However, compared with endoscopic techniques or palliative gastrectomy, palliative radiotherapy has relatively *extended* efficacy. Research has shown that a BED of 40 Gy in fractions is preferred for controlling bleeding, and this dose is also recommended for alleviating obstruction [15].

Endoscopic Laser Therapy

For 75–93% of patients with tumors of the esophagus or with gastric cardia cancer, endoscopic laser therapy can effectively relieve dysphagia due to obstruction [16]. Although laser photocoagulation has definite effectiveness and is suitable for large tumors and diffuse hemorrhage, it requires expensive equipment and thus cannot be widely applied [17]. As an alternative technique to laser photocoagulation, argon plasma coagulation has increasingly been applied.

Conclusions and Recommendations

1. Palliative treatment is recommended after the gastric cancer has progressed to a certain stage.
2. For local symptoms (e.g., nausea, obstruction, pain, and bleeding caused by locally advanced or locally recurrent primary tumors) that are not responsive to systemic therapy (e.g., chemotherapy), endoscopic techniques and palliative radiotherapy are recommended for multidisciplinary management.
3. According to the REGATTA study initiated by Fujitanni K and Yang HK, palliative gastrectomy is recommended for some advanced gastric cancer patients who have received systemic therapy.
4. In advanced gastric cancer patients with obstructive symptoms, endoscopic stent placement is recommended, whereas palliative surgery should not be used.
5. Compared with endoscopic techniques, palliative radiotherapy has relatively extended efficacy in controlling bleeding and obstruction. Research has shown that a BED of 40 Gy in fractions is preferred for controlling bleeding and alleviating obstruction.
6. Endoscopic laser therapy may be an alternative treatment option for alleviating dysphagia due to obstruction.

References

1. Zong L, Abe M, Seto Y, Ji J. The challenge of screening for early gastric cancer in China. Lancet. 2016;388(10060):2606.
2. Zhang JZ, Lu HS, Huang CM, Wu XY, Wang C, Guan GX, Zhen JW, Huang HG, Zhang XF. Outcome of palliative total gastrectomy for stage IV proximal gastric cancer. Am J Surg. 2011;202(1):91–6.
3. Chang YR, Han DS, Kong SH, Lee HJ, Kim SH, Kim WH, Yang HK. The value of palliative gastrectomy in gastric cancer with distant metastasis. Ann Surg Oncol. 2012;19(4):1231–9.

4. Cogliandolo A, Scarmozzino G, Pidoto RR, Pollicino A, Gioffre Florio MA. Laparoscopic palliative gastrojejunostomy for advanced recurrent gastric cancer after Billroth I resection. J Laparoendosc Adv Surg Tech A. 2004;14(1):43–6.

5. Jeong O, Park YK, Choi WY, Ryu SY. Prognostic significance of non-curative gastrectomy for incurable gastric carcinoma. Ann Surg Oncol. 2014;21(8): 2587–93.

6. Schmidt B, Look-Hong N, Maduekwe UN, Chang K, Hong TS, Kwak EL, Lauwers GY, Rattner DW, Mullen JT, Yoon SS. Noncurative gastrectomy for gastric adenocarcinoma should only be performed in highly selected patients. Ann Surg Oncol. 2013;20(11):3512–8.

7. Kahlke V, Bestmann B, Schmid A, Doniec JM, Kuchler T, Kremer B. Palliation of metastatic gastric cancer: impact of preoperative symptoms and the type of operation on survival and quality of life. World J Surg. 2004;28(4):369–75.

8. Fujitani K, Yang HK, Mizusawa J, Kim YW, Terashima M, Han SU, Iwasaki Y, Hyung WJ, Takagane A, Park do J, et al. Gastrectomy plus chemotherapy versus chemotherapy alone for advanced gastric cancer with a single non-curable factor (REGATTA): a phase 3, randomised controlled trial. Lancet Oncol. 2016;17(3):309–18.

9. Takeno A, Takiguchi S, Fujita J, Tamura S, Imamura H, Fujitani K, Matsuyama J, Mori M, Doki Y, Clinical Study Group of Osaka University UGIG. Clinical outcome and indications for palliative gastrojejunostomy in unresectable advanced gastric cancer: multi-institutional retrospective analysis. Ann Surg Oncol. 2013;20(11):3527–33.

10. Guzman EA, Dagis A, Bening L, Pigazzi A. Laparoscopic gastrojejunostomy in patients with obstruction of the gastric outlet secondary to advanced malignancies. Am Surg. 2009;75(2):129–32.

11. Gaidos JK, Draganov PV. Treatment of malignant gastric outlet obstruction with endoscopically placed self-expandable metal stents. World J Gastroenterol. 2009;15(35):4365–71.

12. Tey J, Back MF, Shakespeare TP, Mukherjee RK, Lu JJ, Lee KM, Wong LC, Leong CN, Zhu M. The role of palliative radiation therapy in symptomatic locally advanced gastric cancer. Int J Radiat Oncol Biol Phys. 2007;67(2):385–8.

13. Asakura H, Hashimoto T, Harada H, Mizumoto M, Furutani K, Hasuike N, Matsuoka M, Ono H, Boku N, Nishimura T. Palliative radiotherapy for bleeding from advanced gastric cancer: is a schedule of 30 Gy in 10 fractions adequate? J Cancer Res Clin Oncol. 2011;137(1):125–30.

14. Tey J, Choo BA, Leong CN, Loy EY, Wong LC, Lim K, Lu JJ, Koh WY. Clinical outcome of palliative radiotherapy for locally advanced symptomatic gastric cancer in the modern era. Medicine. 2014;93(22):e118.

15. Hashimoto K, Mayahara H, Takashima A, Nakajima TE, Kato K, Hamaguchi T, Ito Y, Yamada Y, Kagami Y, Itami J, et al. Palliative radiation therapy for hemorrhage of unresectable gastric cancer: a single institute experience. J Cancer Res Clin Oncol. 2009;135(8):1117–23.

16. Wu KL, Tsao WL, Shyu RY. Low-power laser therapy for gastrointestinal neoplasia. J Gastroenterol. 2000;35(7):518–23.

17. Barr H, Krasner N. Interstitial laser photocoagulation for treating bleeding gastric cancer. BMJ. 1989;299(6700):659–60.

Management of Early Postoperative Complication

Dong Jin Kim and Wook Kim

Incidence

Incidence of early complication following gastrectomy is different depending on time period, nations, and institutions. Dutch and MRC trial showed 43–46% morbidity and 10–13% mortality rate following distal gastrectomy with D2 lymph node dissection [1, 2]. Additionally, as previously reported in literatures, morbidity and mortality rates were ranged 18.0–46.0% and 0.8–13.0%, respectively [1–6]. Past data are originated from retrospective studies or randomized controlled trials (RCTs) which do not performed strict surgical quality control. Moreover, laparoscopic surgery is one of the mainstreams nowadays. For these reasons, evaluation for complication from well-controlled RCTs comparing open and laparoscopic gastrectomy and large-scale multicenter retrospec-

tive studies would be informative and reliable data (Table 26.1). Kitano et al. reported morbidity of laparoscopic distal gastrectomy from multicenter retrospective study as 12.9%. The Korean multicenter randomized controlled trial (KLASS-01) showed 18.9% and 13.7% of morbidity in open and laparoscopic distal gastrectomy, respectively.

Risk Factors Related with Early Complication Following Gastrectomy

Various conditions were evaluated as risk factors in the development of postoperative complications. Elucidating the risk factors of complication is the first step to prevent complications. Those risk factors are divided into patient- and operation-related factor.

In the patients' side, the number of comorbidity is the most important risk factor in the development of complications. In KLASS retrospective study, comorbidity was a predictive risk factor for local complication and systemic complication in multivariate analysis [12]. Except for comorbidity, age, sex, and nutritional status are also included [13–19].

In the operation-related side, the extent of lymph node dissection, extent of gastric resection, type of reconstruction, operation time, estimated blood loss, presence of combined resection, and experience of surgeon are included. However, those risk factors are suggested differently depending on various literatures [14, 17, 18].

D. J. Kim
Division of Gastrointestinal Surgery,
Department of Surgery, Eunpyeong St. Mary's Hospital,
College of Medicine, The Catholic University of Korea,
Seoul, Republic of Korea

W. Kim (✉)
Division of Gastrointestinal Surgery,
Department of Surgery, Eunpyeong St. Mary's Hospital,
College of Medicine, The Catholic University of Korea,
Seoul, Republic of Korea

Division of Gastrointestinal Surgery, Department of
Surgery, Yeouido St. Mary's Hospital, College of
Medicine, The Catholic University of Korea,
Seoul, Republic of Korea
e-mail: kimwook@catholic.ac.kr

© Springer-Verlag GmbH Germany, part of Springer Nature 2019
S. H. Noh, W. J. Hyung (eds.), *Surgery for Gastric Cancer*,
https://doi.org/10.1007/978-3-662-45583-8_26

Table 26.1 Recent morbidity and mortality rate from randomized controlled trial and multicenter retrospective studies

Study	Resection	Indication	n	Open		Laparoscopy	
				Morbidity	Mortality	Morbidity	Mortality
2005 Huscher et al. [7]	DG	EGC, AGC	59	27.6%	6.7%	23.3%	3.3%
2007 Kitano et al. [8]	All	EGC	1185			12.9%	0%
2014 Kim et al. [9]	All	EGC, AGC	2976	15.1%	0.3%	12.5%	0.5%
2016 Hu et al. [10]	DG	AGC	1056	12.9%	0%	15.2%	0.4%
2016 KLASS-01 M&M [11]	DG	EGC	1416	18.9%	0.3%	13.7%	0.6%

DG: Distal gastrectomy, *EGC*: Early gastric cancer, *AGC*: Advanced gastric cacer

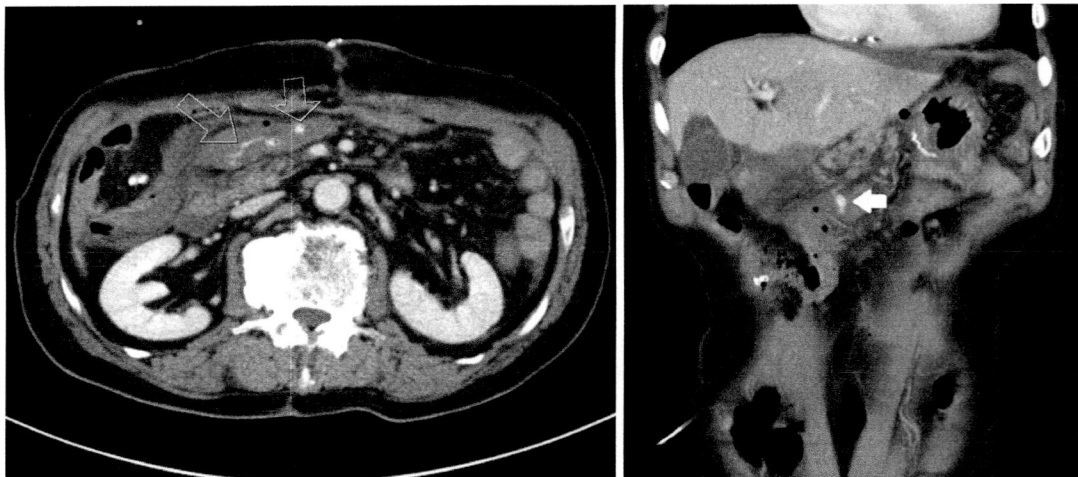

Fig. 26.1 Computed tomography revealed localized hematoma and extravasation of contrast media near infrapancreatic area

Early Postoperative Complications

Bleeding (Intra-abdominal, Intraluminal)

Postoperative bleeding is not common. The incidence is 0.6–3.3% and occurred mostly until 24 h after operation [8, 11, 20–24]. Postoperative bleeding can be divided into intra-abdominal (extraluminal) bleeding and intraluminal bleeding.

1. Intra-abdominal (Extraluminal) Bleeding

Early postgastrectomy intra-abdominal bleeding is originated from imperfectly ligated vessel, lymph node dissection area, omentectomy site, staple line, splenic hilum, divided jejunal mesentery, and trocar insertion site in case of laparoscopic surgery. Sometimes delayed massive

bleeding can be developed after 1–2 weeks due to vessel erosion by anastomosis leakage or intra-abdominal abscess and pseudoaneurysm rupture formed by vessel injury due to energy devices.

Intra-abdominal bleeding can be diagnosed easily by bloody drainage if patient still has drain. If there is no drainage catheter placed, vital sign or postoperative hemoglobin change should be closely focused. Computed tomography (CT) can be helpful for evaluating degree and origin of bleeding with the findings such as hemoperitoneum, localized hematoma, or extravasation of contrast dye (Fig. 26.1). According to KLASS-01 study from Korea, the most vulnerable site was the peripancreatic head area which is no. 6 lymph node dissection area [11].

Optimal timing to perform intervention or reoperation is controversial and dependent on surgeon's preference. If patient's vital sign is unstable, reoperation should be immediately performed. Although the patient's vital sign is within normal range, reoperation or angiographic intervention is strongly recommend when bleeding is continuous or extravasation of contrast media is definite by CT.

Angiographic intervention can be a unique tool for bleeding control and avoiding additional reoperation. However, decision-making for angiographic intervention is crucial, because not all intra-abdominal bleeding cases are applicable. Bleedings from pseudoaneurysm near splenic artery or visible vessel confirmed by CT are optimal for angiographic hemostasis. On the other hand, venous bleeding or bleeding from minor branch such as omental vessel, trocar site, raw surface of lymph node dissection, or staple line oozing is not applicable for angiographic bleeding control.

Regarding the reoperation, laparoscopic approach can be initially considered. Unless bleeding is not too severe to obscure laparoscopic view, we can efficiently find bleeding focus with magnified view through laparoscopy. Because most reoperation is performed within 48 h after gastrectomy, adhesion is not that severe.

2. Intraluminal Bleeding

Bleeding from anastomosis site mostly developed in the early period, within the first postop-erative day. Delayed intraluminal bleeding can be found to be originated from marginal ulceration near gastrojejunostomy. Diagnosis can be made by evident hematemesis or bloody drainage from Levine tube. The chance of intraluminal bleeding increases when number of anastomosis increased and anastomosis included remnant stomach that has more tendency to make intraluminal bleeding due to fluent blood flow. For this reason, during the operation, it is crucial to check anastomosis line formed either by linear staple or hand sewing method. In the case of delayed intraluminal bleeding, it occurred 1–2 weeks later after operation; marginal ulcer bleeding, erosive gastritis, and anastomosis disruptions are possible factors. In case of massive hematemesis, there can be a possibility of aneurysmal rupture into luminal side.

Although minor bleeding is usually self-limiting, when continuous bleeding is evident, endoscopic approach should be firstly attempted. There are several endoscopic tools to stop intraluminal bleeding such as endoscopic metal clip, heater probe coagulation, and epinephrine injection. Among them, metal clip is most reliable than other modalities (Fig. 26.2).

Anastomosis Leakage

Anastomosis leakage means intraluminal contents escape from intraluminal space to intra-abdominal cavity or out of the skin. Although

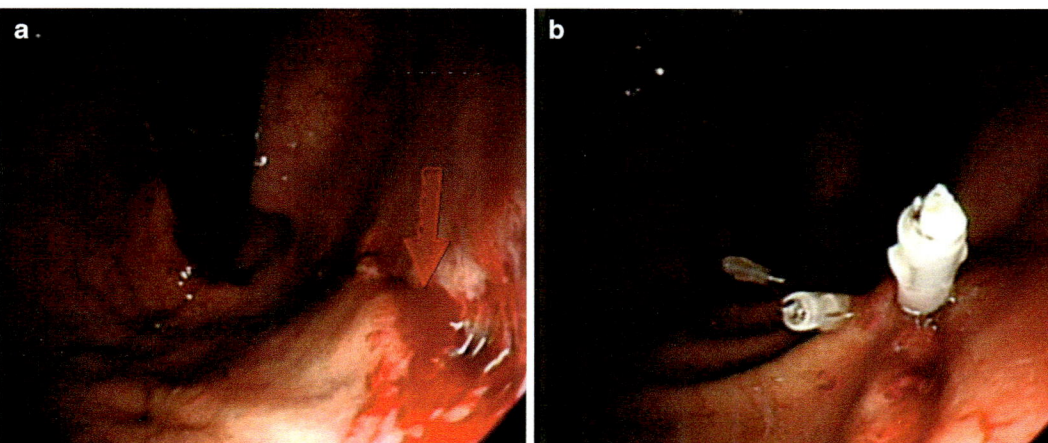

Fig. 26.2 (a) Endoscopic finding shows intraluminal bleeding from artificial lesser curvature staple line. (b) Endoscopic hemoclip successfully controlled intraluminal bleeding

anastomosis leakage rate is decreasing, thanks to improved surgical skills and development of surgical instruments, it is still a dreadful complication that can result in sepsis and even mortality.

The incidence of anastomotic leakage following distal gastrectomy and total gastrectomy is 0.7–2.6% and 2.3–10.4%, respectively [11, 25–31]. It induces bacterial and digestive enzyme dissemination that results in localized abscess, generalized peritonitis, sepsis, pulmonary infection, mediastinitis, and even death. It is usually developed within 10 days postoperatively [32–35]. Typical symptom can be different according to the site of anastomosis leakage. However, generalized or localized peritoneal irritation sign can abruptly develop, and some patients show agitation or dyspnea. There can be signs of fever more than 38 °C, leukocytosis, and elevation of CRP level. When drainage catheter was remained, nature of drainage contents can be changed to turbid or bile-contained color. However, drain never guarantees early detection of anastomosis leakage.

When anastomosis leakage is suspected, abdominal enhance CT should be checked. We can find small or large amount of dirty fluid collection with or without extraluminal air (Fig. 26.3). When CT finding is equivocal, hypaque swallowing test can be helpful for esophagojejunostomy, gastroduodenostomy, or gastrojejunostomy site. In addition, oral contrast CT can provide a definitive diagnosis of leakage by detecting the accumulation of extraluminal contrast [36].

Although management for anastomosis leakage is somewhat different according to leakage site, the main principle for enterocutaneous fistula management is similar. If leakage site is small and well-controlled by drainage catheter, almost leakage can be managed with conservative method. When we perform conservative management, it is important to perform sterile saline irrigation through drainage catheter to wash out dirty materials in abscess cavity and evoke rapid growth of granulation tissue. If the leakage site is large or poorly controlled, interventional percutaneous Foley catheter enterostomy or reoperation is considered.

When leakage event was developed without surgical drainage catheter, sono-guided or CT-guided percutaneous catheter insertion at the target fluid collection area should be performed. If percutaneous drainage is impossible due to the location of fluid collection area, irrigation and drainage catheter insertion should be performed by surgical approach.

Advanced technique for leakage control:

– **Duodenal stump leakage**
  • Regarding the management for duodenal stump leakage, recently introduced percutaneous Foley duodenostomy insertion through perforation site by Seldinger technique is usefully performed.

    After duodenal stump leakage occurs, percutaneous drainage is performed for fluid collections near duodenal stump. Several days later, abscess cavity is decreasing, and internal tract with duodenal stump can be found with tubography via pigtail catheter. Then, the guide wire can be introduced into luminal side of duodenal stump, and Foley catheter can be introduced along the guide wire. Ballooning and gentle traction of Foley catheter can obscure leakage site and evoke rapid healing of abscess cavity (Fig. 26.4). It can reduce the frequency of wound dressing,

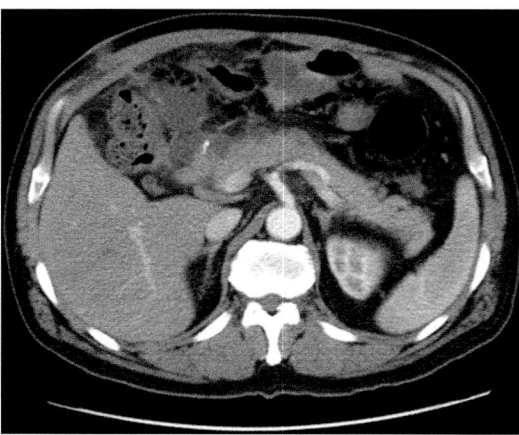

Fig. 26.3 Computed tomography performed on postoperative 7 days following distal gastrectomy, and Billroth II anastomosis revealed air-containing fluid collection consistent with duodenal stump leakage

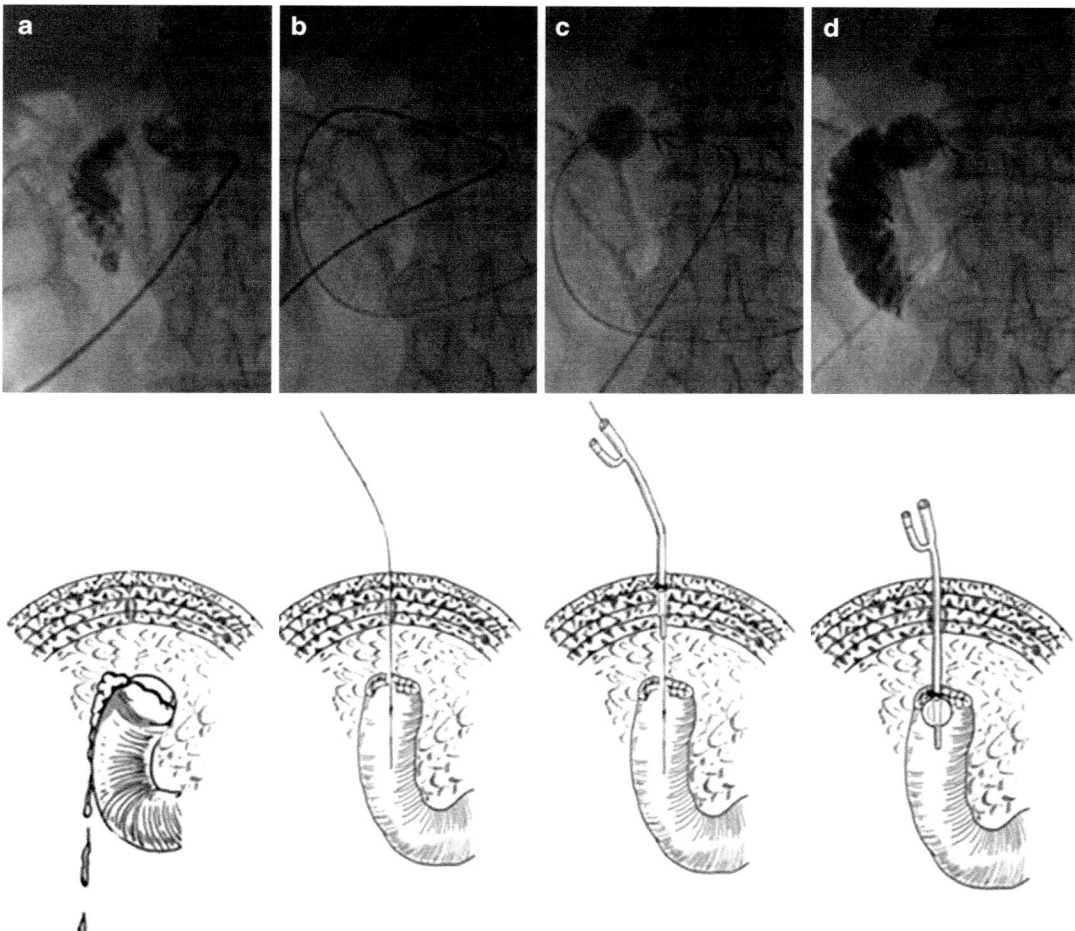

Fig. 26.4 Fluoroscopic findings and illustration of Foley catheter insertion into the site of leakage. (**a**) Leakage confirmation. (**b**) The introduction of guide wire through the guide catheter. (**c**) The insertion and ballooning of the Foley catheter through the guide wire. (**d**) The confirmation of placement of the Foley catheter by tubogram. (Reprint from J Korean Surg Soc. 2010;78:165–70)

skin irritation, and related pain. Additionally, within a few days after the procedure, diet can be started. Then ambulatory care can be done if there was no complaint of fever or abdominal pain. After controlled fistula is formed, Foley catheter can be removed within 1–2 weeks at outpatient office [37].

– **Esophagojejunostomy leakage**
  • Esophagojejunostomy leakage is one of the most troublesome early postoperative complications after total gastrectomy. It can frequently induce lung complication or mediastinitis. This type of leakage is difficult to perform radiologic intervention due to target area surrounded by the chest wall, diaphragm, or spleen. Endoscopic stent insertion is unique method for the management of esophagojejunostomy [25, 38, 39]. Esophageal stenting is to limit the sepsis from continued leak and to allow early resumption of enteral feeding (Fig. 26.5). After placement of esophageal stent, stent migration, stent perforation, and stent-related bleeding should be thoroughly monitored. While the stent is kept

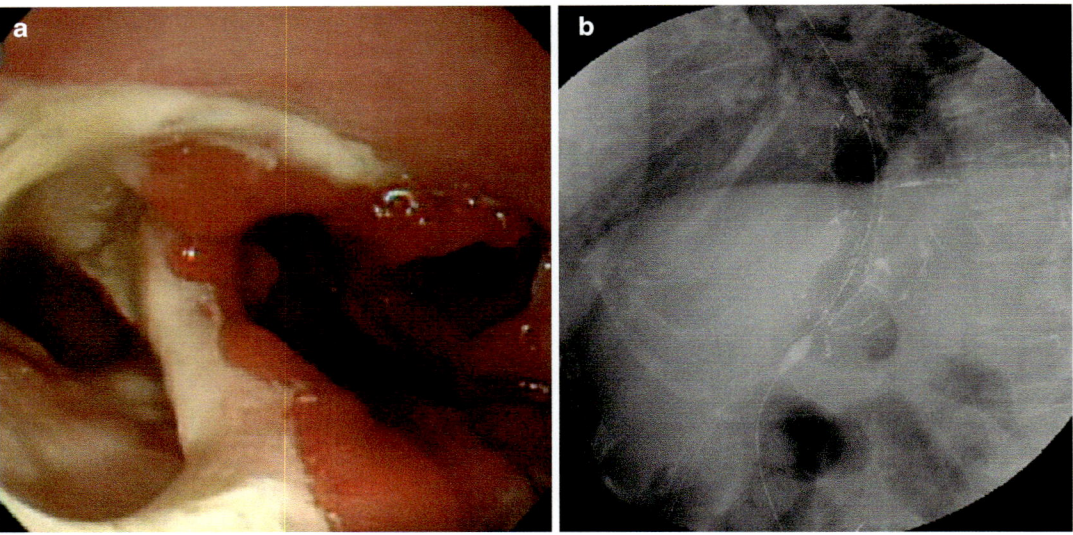

Fig. 26.5 (**a**) Endoscopic finding shows defect of esophagojejunostomy site. (**b**) Endoscopic covered stent is placed at the esophagojejunostomy site

in proper position, drainage catheter should be placed beside leakage point to maximize the effect of esophageal stent. Duration of stent placement is variable from 1 week to 8 weeks between studies [39]. Because reestimation of leakage site can be exactly performed after stent removal, timing of stent removal should be decided by each patient's condition. However, stent placement no more than 8 weeks is recommended due to tissue ingrowth into metal portion that may interfere smooth stent removal.

Obstruction

Intestinal obstruction as an early postoperative complication following gastrectomy is not common. However, there are several types of intestinal obstruction which are highly specific for gastric cancer surgery. For example, except Billroth I gastroduodenostomy, there remain possibilities of internal herniation or obstruction of afferent limb after total gastrectomy or distal gastrectomy with Roux-en-Y or Billroth II anastomosis. To reduce those complications, mesenteric repair should be thoroughly performed. Definite management for intestinal obstruction is to per-

form operation. According to small-sized case series, omental adhesion to staple line following intracorporeal Billroth II anastomosis was the cause of afferent loop syndrome [40]. In those situations, Braun anastomosis can be applied. In case of internal herniation, reduction of herniated small bowel and mesenteric defect repair should be done.

Pancreatic Abscess and Fistula

D2 lymph node dissection is currently regarded as a safe and effective procedure. However, D2 extended lymph node dissection can cause pancreatic fistula that can result in abscess, sepsis, and critical bleeding from the pseudoaneurysm.

The definition of pancreatic fistula is not unified, but the criteria of the International Study Group on Pancreatic Fistula (ISGPF) are generally followed [41]. By the definition, output via an operatively placed drain of any measurable volume of drain fluid on or after postoperative day 3 with an amylase content more than three times higher than the upper normal serum value. However, not only with drain amylase level, clinical signs or CT findings such as peripancreatic fluid collection or pancreatic fistula-related peripancreatic abscess are also regarded as pancreatic fistula [42–44]. Since the definition may include many asymptomatic patients, ISGPF also suggested grading system for pancreatic fistula from grade A to C. Grade A is called transient fistula without clinical impact. Grade B requires a change in management or adjustment in the clinical pathway such as NPO, total parenteral nutrition (TPN), drain repositioning, or somatostatin analog use. Grade C refers a major change in clinical management or deviation from the normal clinical pathway.

Management for pancreatic fistula starts with efficient drainage of leaked pancreatic juice. When closed suction drain is remained, and placed proper position for drainage of pancreatic leakage, keep the drain and saline irrigation is most optimal treatment. When drain is located different position from the peripancreatic fluid collection, repositioning or percutaneous drain insertion should be attempted.

If pancreatic leakage is prolonged, NPO, TPN, or somatostatin analog injection can help to reduce secretion of pancreatic juice.

Delayed Gastric Emptying

Gastric surgery may potentiate or induce delayed gastric emptying and result in chronic gastroparesis. The reported incidence of delayed gastric emptying after gastrectomy has been reported ranging from 5 to 30% [45]. Generally, incidence of delayed gastric emptying is increasing in order of gastrojejunostomy, gastroduodenostomy, and Roux-en-Y gastrojejunostomy following distal gastrectomy. However, those risk factors for delayed gastric emptying are different between studies.

When patient suffers from postprandial epigastric discomfort, nausea, vomiting, or left-side shoulder pain, delayed gastric emptying can be suspected. Diagnosis for delayed gastric emptying is made by the finding of gastric distension and food stasis in simple abdomen X-ray or delayed contrast passage with Gastrografin swallowing test. The most important point for differential diagnosis for delayed gastric emptying is mechanical obstruction. Endoscopic evaluation should be performed to confirm the patency of food passage.

If there is no definite obstructive lesion and delay of gastric emptying is caused by anastomosis edema or functional problem, gastric clearing with Levine tube drainage or gastric lavage and conservative care would be the first choice. After that, liquid form meal can be applied. Anastomosis edema can be applied with balloon dilatation, if symptom improvement is delayed.

Miscellaneous

1. Acute Pancreatitis

During the gastric cancer surgery, the pancreas is frequently manipulated for proper suprapancreatic lymph node dissection. In addition, some patients with history of chronic alcohol consumption have quite hard pancreas and fibrotic change around the pancreas. This can make lymph node dissection difficult and also evoke pancreatitis after operation. Great caution is always needed when manipulating pancreas.

2. Acute Cholecystitis

Although cholelithiasis would not be developed within the early postoperative period, rarely sludge can evoke acute cholecystitis when NPO period is prolonged in specific patients. When the degree of cholecystitis is mild without fever, antibiotics can be optimal management. However, if pain is severe and cholecystitis-induced fever developed, percutaneous cholecystostomy is firstly recommended. This can be removed after 4–6 weeks later.

3. Chylous Ascites

Chylous ascites is defined as the leakage of milky triglyceride-rich lymphatic fluid from lymphatic system to the peritoneal cavity, which can be encountered after various abdominal oncologic surgeries [46]. The management includes cessation of oral feeding, TPN, somatostatin analog administration, clamping and/or removal of the drainage, diuretics, and diet therapy with medium chain triglyceride. The fistula closure time was reported ranging from 1 to 7 weekdays [47].

Conclusion

Recent advancement of diagnostic and interventional modalities shifted paradigm of complication management. Reoperation is not the first choice anymore, and nonoperative managements improved not only results of perioperative survival but also patients' symptom control. For example, interventional Foley duodenostomy insertion was novel technique to improve the patient's recovery from illness during perioperative period. Proper and advanced complication management for complications is crucial for care of gastric cancer patients as well as extension of complications.

References

1. Bonenkamp JJ, Hermans J, Sasako M, van de Velde CJ, Welvaart K, Songun I, et al. Extended lymph-node dissection for gastric cancer. N Engl J Med. 1999;340(12):908–14.
2. Cuschieri A, Fayers P, Fielding J, Craven J, Bancewicz J, Joypaul V, et al. Postoperative morbidity and mortality after D1 and D2 resections for gastric cancer: preliminary results of the MRC randomised controlled surgical trial. The surgical cooperative group. Lancet. 1996;347(9007):995–9.
3. Biffi R, Chiappa A, Luca F, Pozzi S, Lo Faso F, Cenciarelli S, et al. Extended lymph node dissection without routine spleno-pancreatectomy for treatment of gastric cancer: low morbidity and mortality rates in a single center series of 250 patients. J Surg Oncol. 2006;93(5):394–400.
4. Sasako M, Sano T, Yamamoto S, Kurokawa Y, Nashimoto A, Kurita A, et al. D2 lymphadenectomy alone or with para-aortic nodal dissection for gastric cancer. N Engl J Med. 2008;359(5):453–62.
5. Wanebo HJ, Kennedy BJ, Winchester DP, Stewart AK, Fremgen AM. Role of splenectomy in gastric cancer surgery: adverse effect of elective splenectomy on long term survival. J Am Coll Surg. 1997;185(2):177–84.
6. Degiuli M, Sasako M, Calgaro M, Garino M, Rebecchi F, Mineccia M, et al. Morbidity and mortality after D1 and D2 gastrectomy for cancer: interim analysis of the Italian Gastric Cancer Study Group (IGCSG) randomised surgical trial. Eur J Surg Oncol. 2004;30(3):303–8.
7. Huscher CG, Mingoli A, Sgarzini G, Sansonetti A, Di Paola M, Recher A, et al. Laparoscopic versus open subtotal gastrectomy for distal gastric cancer: five-year results of a randomized prospective trial. Ann Surg. 2005;241(2):232–7.
8. Kitano S, Shiraishi N, Uyama I, Sugihara K, Tanigawa N. A multicenter study on oncologic outcome of laparoscopic gastrectomy for early cancer in Japan. Ann Surg. 2007;245(1):68–72.
9. Kim HH, Han SU, Kim MC, Hyung WJ, Kim W, Lee HJ, et al. Long-term results of laparoscopic gastrectomy for gastric cancer: a large-scale case-control and case-matched Korean multicenter study. J Clin Oncol. 2014;32(7):627–33.
10. Hu Y, Huang C, Sun Y, Su X, Cao H, Hu J, et al. Morbidity and mortality of laparoscopic versus open D2 distal gastrectomy for advanced gastric cancer: a randomized controlled trial. J Clin Oncol. 2016;34(12):1350–7.
11. Kim W, Kim HH, Han SU, Kim MC, Hyung WJ, Ryu SW, et al. Decreased morbidity of laparoscopic distal gastrectomy compared with open distal gastrectomy for stage I gastric cancer: short-term outcomes from a multicenter randomized controlled trial (KLASS-01). Ann Surg. 2016;263(1):28–35.
12. Kim W, Song KY, Lee HJ, Han SU, Hyung WJ, Cho GS. The impact of comorbidity on surgical outcomes in laparoscopy-assisted distal gastrectomy: a retrospective analysis of multicenter results. Ann Surg. 2008;248(5):793–9.
13. Jung HS, Park YK, Ryu SY, Jeong O. Laparoscopic total gastrectomy in elderly patients (>/=70 years) with gastric carcinoma: a retrospective study. J Gastric Cancer. 2015;15(3):176–82.
14. Kim MC, Kim W, Kim HH, Ryu SW, Ryu SY, Song KY, et al. Risk factors associated with complication following laparoscopy-assisted gastrectomy for gastric cancer: a large-scale Korean multicenter study. Ann Surg Oncol. 2008;15(10):2692–700.
15. Kim MG, Yook JH, Kim KC, Kim TH, Kim HS, Kim BS, et al. Influence of obesity on early surgical outcomes of laparoscopic-assisted gastrectomy in gastric cancer. Surg Laparosc Endosc Percutan Tech. 2011;21(3):151–4.
16. Lee JY, Kim HI, Kim YN, Hong JH, Alshomimi S, An JY, et al. Clinical significance of the prognostic nutritional index for predicting short- and long-term surgical outcomes after gastrectomy: a retrospective analysis of 7781 gastric Cancer patients. Medicine (Baltimore). 2016;95(18):e3539.
17. Lee KG, Lee HJ, Yang JY, Oh SY, Bard S, Suh YS, et al. Risk factors associated with complication following gastrectomy for gastric cancer: retrospective analysis of prospectively collected data based on the Clavien-Dindo system. J Gastrointest Surg. 2014;18(7):1269–77.
18. Sah BK, Zhu ZG, Chen MM, Xiang M, Chen J, Yan M, et al. Effect of surgical work volume on postoperative complication: superiority of specialized center in gastric cancer treatment. Langenbeck's Arch Surg. 2009;394(1):41–7.
19. Yamanaka H, Nishi M, Kanemaki T, Hosoda N, Hioki K, Yamamoto M. Preoperative nutritional assessment to predict postoperative complication in gas-

tric cancer patients. JPEN J Parenter Enteral Nutr. 1989;13(3):286–91.

20. Kodera Y, Sasako M, Yamamoto S, Sano T, Nashimoto A, Kurita A. Identification of risk factors for the development of complications following extended and superextended lymphadenectomies for gastric cancer. Br J Surg. 2005;92(9):1103–9.

21. Park DJ, Lee HJ, Kim HH, Yang HK, Lee KU, Choe KJ. Predictors of operative morbidity and mortality in gastric cancer surgery. Br J Surg. 2005;92(9):1099–102.

22. Park JY, Kim YW, Eom BW, Yoon HM, Lee JH, Ryu KW, et al. Unique patterns and proper management of postgastrectomy bleeding in patients with gastric cancer. Surgery. 2014;155(6):1023–9.

23. Ryu KW, Kim YW, Lee JH, Nam BH, Kook MC, Choi IJ, et al. Surgical complications and the risk factors of laparoscopy-assisted distal gastrectomy in early gastric cancer. Ann Surg Oncol. 2008;15(6):1625–31.

24. Song W, Yuan Y, Peng J, Chen J, Han F, Cai S, et al. The delayed massive hemorrhage after gastrectomy in patients with gastric cancer: characteristics, management opinions and risk factors. Eur J Surg Oncol. 2014;40(10):1299–306.

25. Jeong GA, Cho GS, Kim HH, Lee HJ, Ryu SW, Song KY. Laparoscopy-assisted total gastrectomy for gastric cancer: a multicenter retrospective analysis. Surgery. 2009;146(3):469–74.

26. Lee MS, Lee JH, Park do J, Lee HJ, Kim HH, Yang HK. Comparison of short- and long-term outcomes of laparoscopic-assisted total gastrectomy and open total gastrectomy in gastric cancer patients. Surg Endosc. 2013;27(7):2598–605.

27. Wada N, Kurokawa Y, Takiguchi S, Takahashi T, Yamasaki M, Miyata H, et al. Feasibility of laparoscopy-assisted total gastrectomy in patients with clinical stage I gastric cancer. Gastric Cancer. 2014;17(1):137–40.

28. Kim DJ, Lee JH, Kim W. Comparison of the major postoperative complications between laparoscopic distal and total gastrectomies for gastric cancer using Clavien-Dindo classification. Surg Endosc. 2015;29(11):3196–204.

29. Lee JH, Park do J, Kim HH, Lee HJ, Yang HK. Comparison of complications after laparoscopy-assisted distal gastrectomy and open distal gastrectomy for gastric cancer using the Clavien-Dindo classification. Surg Endosc. 2012;26(5):1287–95.

30. Strong VE, Devaud N, Allen PJ, Gonen M, Brennan MF, Coit D. Laparoscopic versus open subtotal gastrectomy for adenocarcinoma: a case-control study. Ann Surg Oncol. 2009;16(6):1507–13.

31. Yasunaga H, Horiguchi H, Kuwabara K, Matsuda S, Fushimi K, Hashimoto H, et al. Outcomes after laparoscopic or open distal gastrectomy for early-stage gastric cancer: a propensity-matched analysis. Ann Surg. 2013;257(4):640–6.

32. Ali BI, Park CH, Song KY. Outcomes of nonoperative treatment for duodenal stump leakage after gastrectomy in patients with gastric cancer. J Gastric Cancer. 2016;16(1):28–33.

33. Kim YJ, Shin SK, Lee HJ, Chung HS, Lee YC, Park JC, et al. Endoscopic management of anastomotic leakage after gastrectomy for gastric cancer: how efficacious is it? Scand J Gastroenterol. 2013;48(1):111–8.

34. Lee JY, Ryu KW, Cho SJ, Kim CG, Choi IJ, Kim MJ, et al. Endoscopic clipping of duodenal stump leakage after Billroth II gastrectomy in gastric cancer patient. J Surg Oncol. 2009;100(1):80–1.

35. Migita K, Takayama T, Matsumoto S, Wakatsuki K, Enomoto K, Tanaka T, et al. Risk factors for esophagojejunal anastomotic leakage after elective gastrectomy for gastric cancer. J Gastrointest Surg. 2012;16(9):1659–65.

36. Kim YE, Lim JS, Hyung WJ, Lee SK, Choi JY, Noh SH, et al. Clinical implication of positive oral contrast computed tomography for the evaluation of postoperative leakage after gastrectomy for gastric cancer. J Comput Assist Tomogr. 2010;34(4):537–42.

37. Hur H, Lim YS, Jeon HM, Kim W. Management of anastomotic leakage after gastrointestinal surgery using fluoroscopy-guided Foley catheter. J Korean Surg Soc. 2010;78:165–70.

38. Choi HJ, Lee BI, Kim JJ, Kim JH, Song JY, Ji JS, et al. The temporary placement of covered self-expandable metal stents to seal various gastrointestinal leaks after surgery. Gut Liver. 2013;7(1):112–5.

39. Dasari BV, Neely D, Kennedy A, Spence G, Rice P, Mackle E, et al. The role of esophageal stents in the management of esophageal anastomotic leaks and benign esophageal perforations. Ann Surg. 2014;259(5):852–60.

40. Kim DJ, Lee JH, Kim W. Afferent loop obstruction following laparoscopic distal gastrectomy with Billroth-II gastrojejunostomy. J Korean Surg Soc. 2013;84(5):281–6.

41. Bassi C, Dervenis C, Butturini G, Fingerhut A, Yeo C, Izbicki J, et al. Postoperative pancreatic fistula: an international study group (ISGPF) definition. Surgery. 2005;138(1):8–13.

42. Komatsu S, Ichikawa D, Kashimoto K, Kubota T, Okamoto K, Konishi H, et al. Risk factors to predict severe postoperative pancreatic fistula following gastrectomy for gastric cancer. World J Gastroenterol. 2013;19(46):8696–702.

43. Kobayashi D, Iwata N, Tanaka C, Kanda M, Yamada S, Nakayama G, et al. Factors related to occurrence and aggravation of pancreatic fistula after radical gastrectomy for gastric cancer. J Surg Oncol. 2015;112(4):381–6.

44. Yu HW, Jung do H, Son SY, Lee CM, Lee JH, Ahn SH, et al. Risk factors of postoperative pancreatic fistula in curative gastric cancer surgery. J Gastric Cancer. 2013;13(3):179–84.

45. Paik HJ, Choi CI, Kim DH, Jeon TY, Kim DH, Son GM, et al. Risk factors for delayed gastric emptying caused by anastomosis edema after subtotal gastrectomy for gastric cancer. Hepato-Gastroenterology. 2014;61(134):1794–800.

46. Yamada T, Jin Y, Hasuo K, Maezawa Y, Kumazu Y, Rino Y, et al. Chylorrhea following laparoscopy assisted distal gastrectomy with D1+ dissection for early gastric cancer: a case report. Int J Surg Case Rep. 2013;4(12):1173–5.

47. Ilhan E, Demir U, Alemdar A, Ureyen O, Eryavuz Y, Mihmanli M. Management of high-output chylous ascites after D2-lymphadenectomy in patients with gastric cancer: a multi-center study. J Gastrointest Oncol. 2016;7(3):420–5.

Management of Late Postoperative Complications

Masanori Terashima

Introduction

Following surgery for gastric cancer, gastrectomy and dissection of the vagus nerve surrounding the stomach can lead to postgastrectomy syndrome (PGS) as a late postoperative complication [1]. Although PGS occurs in most patients who have undergone gastrectomy, the condition is said to be severe in 5–10% of cases. The main conditions in PGS, as listed in Table 27.1, can reduce oral intake, lower body weight due to decreased muscle mass, and increase mental stress, which in turn can reduce the quality of life (QOL). During the follow-up observation of patients who have undergone gastrectomy, the state of PGS should be fully ascertained and treated appropriately. This chapter explains the underlying pathophysiology of the principal types of PGS and their management.

Functional Disorders

Early Dumping Syndrome

Early dumping syndrome occurs when hyperosmolar food enters the small intestine rapidly, causing a shift in the intravascular water content in the gut, which leads to circulatory collapse,

Table 27.1 Postgastrectomy syndrome

Functional disorders
Early dumping syndrome
Late dumping syndrome
Small gastric remnant syndrome
Diarrhea
Constipation
Roux stasis
Delayed gastric emptying
Digestion disorder
Anemia
Bone disorder
Lactose intolerance
Steatorrhea
Organic disorders
Reflux gastritis
Reflux esophagitis
Stomal ulcer
Anastomotic stenosis
Cholecystitis, cholecystolithiasis
Afferent loop syndrome
Ileus
Internal hernia

and the release of vasomotor substances (bradykinin, serotonin, histamine, and catecholamine) [2]. The syndrome occurs in 25–40% of patients after gastrectomy. It is more common following total gastrectomy than distal gastrectomy and often occurs following reconstruction by Billroth I (B-I) in distal gastrectomy. However, it is rare with Roux-en-Y (RY) reconstruction and pylorispreserving gastrectomy (PPG) [3, 4].

M. Terashima (✉)
Division of Gastric Surgery, Shizuoka Cancer Center, Nagaizumi, Japan
e-mail: m.terashima@scchr.jp

© Springer-Verlag GmbH Germany, part of Springer Nature 2019
S. H. Noh, W. J. Hyung (eds.), *Surgery for Gastric Cancer*,
https://doi.org/10.1007/978-3-662-45583-8_27

Symptoms of early dumping syndrome occur within 30 min of eating and include general and abdominal symptoms. General symptoms include drowsiness, general malaise, cold sweats, palpitations, dizziness, shortness of breath, headache, and flushing as well as feeling feverish, heavy-headed, and faint. Abdominal symptoms include bloating, gurgling, abdominal pain, diarrhea, and nausea.

Diagnosis is determined by the presence of two general symptoms or one general symptom with one abdominal symptom among those noted above. In cases where diagnosis is difficult, a provocation test is performed by loading with 50% oral glucose [5].

Diet therapy is essential while treating early dumping syndrome. It is advised that patients eat small meals frequently, avoid a high-carbohydrate diet, and reduce their water intake during meals. With respect to medication, antiserotonin agents, antihistamine agents, anticholinergic agents, antibradykinin agents, local anesthetic agents, and antianxiety agents are used for the treatment of general symptoms. It has been reported that octreotide, a somatostatin analog, is sometimes effective [6]; however, long-term efficacy has not been demonstrated [7].

Late Dumping Syndrome

Late dumping syndrome is associated with decreased gastric retention capacity and occurs because of the rapid entry of carbohydrates into the upper jejunum. The rapid absorption of carbohydrate from the intestines leads to temporary hyperglycemia, which causes excessive secretion of insulin, and leads to reactive hypoglycemia. Symptoms appear 2–3 h after eating and include a sense of hunger, cold sweats, lethargy, palpitations, weakness, dizziness, hand tremors, rapid breathing, headache, and fainting. The syndrome is more common after total gastrectomy than distal gastrectomy and is more common with B-I than RY reconstruction in distal gastrectomy [3].

Diagnosis is relatively easy based on symptoms. Symptoms improving with sugar intake make the diagnosis more definite.

Treatment is administered essentially as per early dumping syndrome, and because the syndrome is more likely to occur in individuals who eat quickly, such individuals are advised to eat more slowly. In particular, sufferers should refrain from an excessive intake of carbohydrates. Furthermore, they are advised to eat sugary foods when it appears that hypoglycemia will occur. Effective pharmacotherapy includes α-glucosidase inhibitors [8].

Delayed Gastric Emptying

Delayed gastric emptying (DGE) is often experienced after gastrectomy. Kubo et al. observed the gastric remnant by endoscopy following distal gastrectomy. They found food residues in 22% of cases and reported that it was more common with B-I reconstruction than with RY, with a higher rate after PPG [9]. The relationship between the presence of such food residues and weight loss with complaints is unclear; it is thought that a small amount of residue would not pose a major problem.

However, DGE after PPG is often a problem, with food regurgitation and a sense of abdominal bloating observed after meals. An effective way to prevent DGE after PPG involves preserving 2 cm or more of the pyloric cuff and preserving the pyloric branch of the vagal nerve, the right gastric artery, and the infrapyloric artery [10].

Furthermore, in some instances, despite the absence of any organic abnormality, reduced tonicity of the wall of the gastric remnant can result in enlargement of the gastric remnant (gastric atony), and excretory disorders are observed. It is thought that the condition readily occurs in patients with diabetes, hypothyroidism, and dysautonomia.

As treatment, sufferers are advised to reduce the amount of food intake per meal, split meals, take time to eat, chew well, consume the proper amount of fluids with meals, maintain good dental hygiene, and eat meals low in dietary fiber. Oral nutritional supplements (ONS) are used in combination with these steps to maintain caloric intake. For medication, drugs that improve gastrointestinal motility are administered. In the event that there is no improvement with conservative therapy, surgical treatment is considered [11].

Roux Stasis Syndrome

Approximately 30% of patients who undergo reconstruction by RY after gastrectomy develop a sense of abdominal bloating, abdominal pain, nausea, vomiting, and loss of appetite. It is thought that these symptoms are due to abnormal Roux limb movement (hypoperistalsis, retroperistalsis, and abnormal contractions) [5]. The syndrome often develops early after surgery but is also observed after long periods. The syndrome easily develops in patients with a long Roux limb [12]. It also tends to occur when the gastric remnant is large. Treatment is administered via agents that improve gastrointestinal motility, but if this treatment is ineffective, surgical treatment is considered. When the gastric remnant is too large, gastrectomy is performed to reduce its size. When the Roux limb is too long, it is shortened. The methods considered effective for preventing the syndrome include making the gastric remnant small at the time of the initial surgery; making the Roux limb short (approximately 30 cm); and, for the retrocolic pathway, fixing the mesocolon to the gastric remnant [13].

Diarrhea

Diarrhea is caused by the rapid entry of food into the small intestine, acceleration of bowel peristalsis, changes in the intestinal bacterial flora, exocrine pancreatic insufficiency, and postcibal pancreaticobiliary asynchrony. Loose stool, watery stool, and increased stool frequency are observed. Eating quickly and consuming a high-fat diet, cold drinks, milk, and alcohol can cause diarrhea; therefore, sufferers are given advice about what and how they should eat. They are also advised not to allow the abdomen to become cool. When such dietary counseling does not result in symptom improvement, intestinal-

function-controlling drugs, digestive enzyme preparations, and gastrointestinal motility inhibitors are prescribed. It has recently been reported that preserving the celiac branch of the vagal nerve reduces the incidence of diarrhea [14, 15].

Constipation

Constipation is caused by attenuated gastro-colonic reflex, reduced food intake, low intake of fat and fiber, as well as reduced abdominal pressure due to a decrease in muscle mass. It has been reported that patients with stool abnormalities exhibit a disturbance in their intestinal bacterial flora and changes in the intra-intestinal environment [16]. Sufficient water intake, with consumption of adequate dietary fiber and fat, is recommended. Lifestyle improvements, such as exercising regularly, also effectively improve constipation. In the event that these interventions result in no improvement, agents that improve laxatives and gastrointestinal motility are administered.

Digestion and Absorption Disorders

Various digestive, absorption, and metabolic changes occur after gastrectomy. Among these, digestion and absorption disorders are caused by a loss of gastric retention capacity, changes in the normal pathway, changes in the secretion of gastrointestinal hormones, and asynchrony as a result of gastrectomy and reconstruction. It has recently been reported that ghrelin, which is produced by the stomach, has a major effect on appetite and fat metabolism.

Such a loss of appetite, along with reduced digestive and absorptive capacities, causes considerable weight loss after gastrectomy. The rate of continued weight loss at 3–6 months following surgery is higher in total gastrectomy than in partial gastrectomy [17]. Particular caution should be exercised in slim elderly patients who have undergone total gastrectomy. In total gastrectomy patients, weight loss is greatly affected by loss of appetite due to the reduced levels of ghrelin.

Postoperative weight loss can have major social effects, such as reduced QOL and delayed return to work. It has also been reported that patients who lost a large amount of weight postoperatively had inferior completion rates for postoperative adjuvant chemotherapy. Therefore, the prevention of weight loss soon after surgery is an important issue. Furthermore, sarcopenia has recently been noted, with reports that more than 25% of patients exhibited a loss of more than 10% of their pre-surgery skeletal muscle mass following total gastrectomy [18].

It has been reported that in patients who have undergone total gastrectomy, ghrelin administration effectively improves appetite, increases food intake, and reduces weight loss; thus, its clinical application in the future is much anticipated [19, 20].

Lactose Intolerance

Changes in intestinal bacterial flora can lead to low lactase activity in the small intestinal mucosa, and a relative deficiency in lactase may be caused by rapid entry of lactose into the small intestine due to impaired gastric retention capacity. Insufficient lactase levels indicate that lactose cannot be broken down into glucose and galactose, causing osmotic diarrhea and fermentation in the intestines, which consequently results in abdominal bloating, nausea, gurgling, and abdominal pain. Lactase activity is lower among Asian individuals than among Westerns [21]. Furthermore, because lactase activity is highest in the upper jejunum, lactose intolerance appears to be high in cases that have undergone RY reconstruction, indicating that food does not pass into the upper jejunum. Because diarrhea can occur simply by drinking cold drinks, when these symptoms appear even with warm milk, lactose intolerance is likely.

For a definite diagnosis, a lactose tolerance test, a quick lactose test, and a lactose breath test are performed.

Symptoms will improve after restricting the intake of milk and dairy products. If the patient wants to continue drinking milk, lactose-free milk can be consumed instead or a lactase preparation can be administered. Symptoms are considered less likely with fermented milk drinks than with raw milk.

Fatty Stool

Fatty stool occurs as a result of reduced secretion of digestive enzymes, impaired small intestinal absorption through the mucosal epithelium, and poor mixture of food and digestive juices (postcibal asynchrony). White stools that float in water and give off a unique bad smell are due to impaired digestion and absorption of fat and are therefore associated with weight loss and deficiency of fat-soluble vitamins (vitamins A, D, E, and K). Fatty stool is more common with total gastrectomy than partial gastrectomy. Friess et al. [22] reported that trypsin and chymotrypsin secretion is reduced by 91% following total gastrectomy. In patients who undergo concurrent resection of the pancreatic body and tail, the absolute amount of secretion in the pancreatic duct is reduced; therefore, such patients are prone to fatty stool. For treatment, patients who have been consuming an excessive amount of fat are advised to limit the amount of fat that they consume and to eat slowly. If there is no subsequent improvement, digestive enzyme preparations are administered [23]. In the event that fat-soluble vitamin deficiency is suspected, a fat-soluble vitamin preparation is administered.

Anemia

Following gastrectomy, microcytic anemia caused by iron-deficiency and macrocytic anemia caused by vitamin B12 deficiency both occur.

Iron intake from the diet is oxidized by gastric acid from Fe^{3+} to Fe^{2+} and absorbed through the duodenum and upper jejunum. Following gastrectomy, there is a lack of gastric acid, transit through the jejunum is rapid, and the upper jejunum may be bypassed because of reconstruction. As a result, this causes iron malabsorption.

Lee et al. reported that iron deficiency occurs in 69% of patients after surgery for gastric cancer, and iron-deficiency anemia is observed in 31%. According to the surgical procedure, anemia was more common after total gastrectomy than distal gastrectomy, and with distal gastrectomy, anemia was more common with RY than B-I reconstruction [24].

Symptoms generally present as per general anemia, and in the event of severe iron deficiency, glossitis, cheilosis, and nail deformity can occur.

Blood tests show microcytic anemia, low serum iron, low serum ferritin, increased total iron-binding capacity, and increased unsaturated iron-binding capacity.

First-line treatment is the administration of oral iron tablets. If possible, a ferric oxide formulation is chosen. In the event that oral treatment is difficult, intravenous treatment is administered; however, caution should be exercised with this to avoid an overdose.

Vitamin B12 binds to the Castle's intrinsic factor secreted in gastric parietal cells and is absorbed through the ileum terminal. After total gastrectomy, deficiency of the castle intrinsic factor causes vitamin B12 malabsorption. Vitamin B12 deficiency develops in 100% of total gastrectomy cases and 16% of distal gastrectomy cases [25]. Because vitamin B12 is stockpiled in the body, it takes 3–5 years to be completely consumed. When vitamin B12 reserves are depleted, megaloblastic anemia develops. When blood tests show a low red cell count, with a high mean corpuscular volume (MCV) and mean corpuscular hemoglobin (MCH), it indicates low serum levels of vitamin B12. If vitamin B12 deficiency becomes severe, it can cause peripheral neuropathy, tongue pain, and hypogeusia. Administration of fluoropyrimidine anticancer agents can also cause megaloblastic anemia, but the underlying mechanism of this differs to that of vitamin B12 deficiency.

Administering parenteral vitamin B12 preparations has been recommended as treatment; however, it has been reported that similar outcomes can be achieved with oral preparations. Thus, oral vitamin B12 preparations are also administered.

Metabolic Bone Disease

Insufficient calcium intake, calcium malabsorption (due to reduced gastric acid, rapid passage through the upper jejunum, and lactose intolerance), and vitamin D malabsorption (fat malabsorption) following gastrectomy can lead to a loss of bone mineral content, increased bone absorption, and reduced bone density. Symptoms include lower back pain, pain in the four limbs, and leg cramps. In severe cases, lumbar compression fractures and femoral neck fractures can occur. It is more common after total gastrectomy than after distal gastrectomy, and after distal gastrectomy, it is more common with Billroth II (B-II) and RY reconstruction than B-I. Dual-energy X-ray absorptiometry (DEXA) is useful for diagnosis. Blood tests show low serum levels of calcium, phosphorus, and 25(OH)D, with high levels of $1,25(OH)_2D$ and parathyroid hormone (PTH).

Patients are advised to eat foods rich in calcium, vitamin D, and vitamin K as a treatment method. As pharmacotherapy, bisphosphonate preparations are recommended [26].

Organic Disorders

Reflux Esophagitis

Reflux esophagitis is caused by the reflux prevention mechanism of the cardiac orifice, increased internal pressure of the gastric remnant, and excretory disorder of the gastric remnant associated with gastrectomy, which in turn causes acidic gastric juices in the gastric remnant and alkaline duodenal fluid to flow into the esophagus. Conjugated bile acid and pepsin in the presence of gastric acid and unconjugated bile acid and trypsin in the absence of gastric acid have a harmful effect on the esophageal mucous membrane.

Symptoms include heartburn, post sternal pain, difficulty in swallowing, epigastric pain, and a burning sensation. When attempting to go to sleep, some patients complain of gastric acid

Table 27.2 The Los Angeles classification of esophagitis

Grade A	One (or more) mucosal break no longer than 5 mm that does not extend between the tops of two mucosal folds
Grade B	One (or more) mucosal break more than 5 mm long that does not extend between the tops of two mucosal folds
Grade C	One (or more) mucosal break that is continuous between the tops of two or more mucosal folds but which involves less than 75% of the circumference
Grade D	One (or more) mucosal break which involves at least 75% of the esophageal circumference

Citation from [27]

rising up into the throat and their pillow being soiled by yellow digestive juices. Reflux at night can also cause concurrent aspiration pneumonitis.

Diagnosis is determined on the basis of clinical findings and upper gastrointestinal endoscopy. Findings by endoscopy include redness of the esophageal mucosa, inflammation, ulceration, hemorrhage, and edema, the severity of which is determined using the Los Angeles Classification (Table 27.2) [27]. In many instances, endoscopic findings and subjective symptoms do not correspond. To accurately diagnose reflux, 24-h pH monitoring is useful.

In relation to the surgical procedure, following distal gastrectomy, reflux is common when the gastric remnant is small after B-I and B-II reconstruction, whereas the condition is rare with RY reconstruction [28–31]. It has been reported that short-segment Barrett's esophagus (SSBE) occurs in approximately 25% of patients who undergo B-II reconstruction [32]. It has been found that the incidence of reflux esophagitis is high after proximal gastrectomy with esophagogastric anastomosis. Caution should be exercised with B-I and B-II reconstruction to avoid making the gastric remnant small, to maintain an appropriate His angle, and to prevent hiatal hernia from occurring. When the gastric remnant appears small, in patients with a hiatal hernia, it is preferable to select RY reconstruction. Following total gastrectomy, reflux tends to occur when the distance from the esophagojejunal anastomosis to the Y limb is short. The

distance should be at least 40 cm. Furthermore, as reflux easily occurs when passage through the distal jejunum is impaired, due care should be exercised to avoid intestinal torsion and bending. In PPG, it has been reported that reflux esophagitis is less common compared with B-I; however, reflux occurs when the oral gastric remnant is small, when delayed emptying of the stomach contents is observed, and with hiatal hernia. In the event of concern about these factors, RY reconstruction should be performed as distal gastrectomy. In proximal gastrectomy, there is a high rate of reflux with esophagogastrostomy. When the gastric remnant is small and when performing esophagogastrostomy, some kind of additional reflux prevention measures should be considered such as jejunal interposition as well as double tracts method. Recently, it has been reported that reconstruction with the double flap method can prevent reflux [33].

Dietary guidance is crucial in treatment and should include advising patients to reduce the volume of each meal, to chew well, and to avoid stimulants, carbonated drinks, and high-fat foods. Patients should also be advised to not lie down soon after meals, to eat at least 2 h before bedtime, and to sleep in Fowler's position. If there is no improvement with this guidance or in severe cases, medication should be considered, with the administration of agents that improve gastrointestinal motility and mucosa protective agents. Depending on the type of digestive juice that refluxes, protease inhibitors, proton pump inhibitors, and H2-blockers are selected. When conservative treatment yields no improvement and the patient's daily life is greatly affected or in cases when aspiration pneumonitis repeatedly occurs, surgery should be considered. In the event of B-I and B-II reconstruction, improvements can be achieved by performing repeat reconstruction using the RY method.

Anastomotic Ulcers

With RY and B-II reconstruction, when the extent of gastric resection is small and vagotomy is insufficient, the secretion of gastric juices from the gastric remnant can cause ulcers on the jejunal side of the anastomosis. Anastomotic ulcers can also arise from impairment of the anastomotic blood flow, as a foreign body reaction to the sutures or staples, and in response to drugs such as steroids and nonsteroidal anti-inflammatory drugs (NSAIDs) [34].

The condition presents with epigastric discomfort, epigastric pain, heart burn, nausea, vomiting, hematemesis, and bloody stools. Anastomotic ulcers can be confirmed by endoscopy. Pharmacotherapy is the preferred treatment, with the administration of PPIs, H2-blockers, and gastric mucosa protecting agents. In the event of pharmacotherapy-refractory ulcers, surgical treatment is considered, such as vagotomy and additional resection of the gastric remnant.

Anastomotic Stenosis

In total gastrectomy and proximal gastrectomy, anastomotic stenosis often occurs when a circular anastomosis device is used for esophagojejunal or esophagogastric anastomosis [35]. Although rare, anastomotic stenosis can also occur when a circular anastomosis device is used for distal gastrectomy. Furthermore, anastomotic stenosis tends to occur during the healing process when anastomotic leakage occurs after surgery. It generally occurs 1–3 months after surgery. Many patients with stenosis at the lower end of the esophagus complain of difficulty in swallowing. In the initial stage after onset, patients may experience difficulty with the intake of solid matter and repeated saliva-like vomiting. Furthermore, if the stenosis is severe, ingested matter may be frequently vomited. Diagnosis is determined based on the observation of anastomotic stenosis by endoscopy. Instances of membranous stenosis are often alleviated by endoscopic balloon dilatation. In general, the condition is cured after the 2nd or 3rd dilatation, but anastomotic stenosis occurring after leakage is often refractory. Surgical treatment is considered if no improvement is observed after ten or more endoscopic treatments, when the interval between treatments is short.

Cholecystolithiasis and Cholecystitis

Cholecystolithiasis and cholecystitis following gastrectomy are caused by cholecystasis because of reduced secretion of cholecystokinin (CCK) after eating as a result of rapid gastric emptying and by cholestasis resulting from dyskinesia of the Oddi muscle in response to CCK. Hyposecretion of gastric juices and the fact that food cannot pass through the duodenum causes an increase in the bacterial flora in the duodenum, and biliary infection causes deposition of calcium bilirubinate, which promotes the formation of stones. Cholecystolithiasis and cholecystitis are also caused by a decrease in gallbladder contraction as a result of sectioning of the hepatic branch of the vagal nerve and dissection around the hepatoduodenal ligament associated with lymph node dissection. The gall stones that follow gastrectomy are most often black stones or calcium bilirubinate stones. The incidence of cholecystolithiasis is reported to be 10–47% and more common in total gastrectomy than in distal gastrectomy [36]. Cholecystolithiasis following distal gastrectomy is considered common with RY and B-II reconstructions, but rare with B-I and PPG reconstructions [28]. Generally, most cases are asymptomatic and are often detected by chance through routine follow-up computed tomography (CT) or ultrasound examinations. If asymptomatic, patients may undergo follow-up observations without treatment, but the condition can also be resolved sometimes by the administration of choleretics. In the event of concurrent cholecystitis, antibacterial therapy is administered, and percutaneous drainage or emergency surgery is performed. For symptomatic cases, cholecystectomy is considered.

The safety of preventive cholecystectomy has been confirmed by a randomized controlled trial [37]; however, the efficacy of the procedure has not been clarified.

Afferent Loop Syndrome

The condition encompassing afferent loop stenosis and obstruction as a result of torsion, bending, adhesion, internal hernia, and peritoneal dissemination following B-II and RY reconstruction is referred to as afferent loop syndrome. It causes pooling of duodenal juices, including bile and pancreatic juices in the afferent loop, leading to complaints of postprandial abdominal and back pain, with large amounts of bilious vomiting observed. In the event of complete obstruction, duodenal distention and circulatory insufficiency cause gastrointestinal perforation, peritonitis, and shock, requiring emergency surgery [38].

Diagnosis is easily determined on the basis of characteristic symptoms and if afferent loop dilatation is observed on CT examination. Treatment for mild cases includes follow-up observations with dietary guidance and pharmacotherapy. However in the event of repeated onset, if possible, endoscopic dilatation of the site of stenosis is attempted. If endoscopic treatment is not possible, strategies such as repeat surgery with anastomosis of the Y limb, changing reconstruction from B-II to RY, and additional Braun anastomosis are considered.

Ileus

Mechanical ileus often occurs late after surgery and is classified into simple ileus and strangulated ileus. Causes include adhesions, bending, inflammation, tumor, hernia (mentioned below), intussusception, and volvulus. The condition presents with abdominal pain, vomiting, and fever. On palpation, epigastric distention, with pressure pain, is often observed. In the event of perforation, signs of peritoneal irritation and muscle guarding are observed. On chest X-ray imaging, intestinal dilatation, with the formation of air–fluid levels and gas in the small intestine, can be observed. Identification of the site of stenosis, assessment of the underlying condition, and verification of the presence or absence of strangulation can be performed by abdominal contrast-enhanced CT. In the event that there is no contrast medium in the

intestines and ascites are observed, strangulation is highly suspected.

In mild cases, symptoms can be alleviated through fasting and fluid replacement only, but if intestinal dilatation is severe or in the event of repeated vomiting, an ileus tube is placed to drain the contents of the intestines and reduce the pressure. If symptoms are not alleviated with conservative treatment or in the event of recurrent ileus, surgery is considered. When strangulation is suspected, emergency surgery is required. The strangulation is removed immediately and blood flow is restored, after which any necrotic intestine is resected and reconstructed.

Internal Hernia

With the popularization of laparoscopic surgery, its use has increased rapidly in recent years. Internal hernia refers to the condition in which the viscera penetrate the mesentery, the hiatus of the greater omentum, and the fossa, within the abdominal cavity. The common sites of internal hernia following gastrectomy include the small intestinal mesenteric space produced with RY reconstruction and Petersen's defect (Fig. 27.1). The incidence ranges from 0.1% to 2%, and the condition is more common with laparoscopic surgery than with open surgery. There is no difference in incidence related to total gastrectomy or distal gastrectomy. The risk factors for internal hernia include laparoscopic surgery and weight loss following surgery [39]. The condition presents with various symptoms, including abdominal pain, vomiting, and abdominal discomfort, and strangulated hernia can develop suddenly during follow-up observation after diagnosis of an unidentified complaint. In particular, hernias that develop in Petersen's defect can cause extensive strangulation of the small intestine, and due care should be exercised to prevent postoperative short bowel syndrome. Abdominal contrast-enhanced CT is useful for diagnosis, which is determined upon the observation of a whirl sign, aggregate formation in

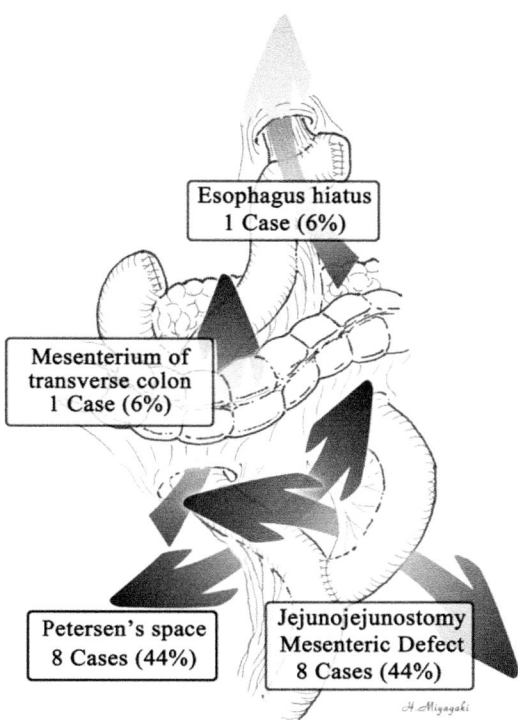

Fig. 27.1 Anatomic mapping of internal hernias. Although the figure is for total gastrectomy followed by retrocolic Roux-en-Y reconstruction, it serves to show the anatomic locations of internal hernias. (Reproduction from [39] with permission)

the invaginated bowel loop, and abnormal mesenteric vascular extension.

Surgery is the only treatment option and includes laparotomy or laparoscopy to reposition the intussusception and to close the hernia orifice. When necrosis of the small intestine has occurred because of strangulation, resection and reconstruction, if possible, of the small intestine are required.

To prevent internal hernia when performing gastrectomy, closure of the mesenteric space is considered effective, and the mesentery and Petersen's defect should be closed using nonabsorbable sutures while performing surgery. However, as complete closure of Petersen's defect is difficult, it should be kept to the lower end of the transverse colon.

Evaluation of Postoperative QOL

To objectively evaluate a patient's condition following gastric resection, evaluation of QOL according to patient-reported outcomes as an objective tool is extremely important. The methods of assessing QOL include global scales [such as the Sickness Impact Profile (SIP), Short-Form 36 (SF-36), and World Health Organization Quality of Life-26 (WHO/QOL26)], which evaluate the overall level of health and how it affects daily life and social life [40–42], and disease-specific scales [such as the Gastrointestinal Symptom Rating Scale (GSRS) and the European Organization for Research and Treatment of Cancer Quality of Life Questionnaire-C30 (EORTC QLQ-C 30)], which evaluate the level of health and how it affects daily life according to specific disease symptoms [43, 44]. Other tools include preference scales [such as the EuroQol-5D (EQ-5D) and the Health Utilities Index (HUI)] to determine the utility value in terms of health economics [45, 46]. The evaluation of QOL following gastrectomy is generally performed combining a global scale and a disease-specific scale, with reports to date describing the use of the SF-36 combined with the GSRS and the EORTC-C30 combined with the European Organisation for Research and Treatment of Cancer Quality of Life Questionnaire-Stomach (EORTC-STO22). However, these evaluation methods are not specific to conditions following gastrectomy; therefore, it cannot be stated that they always accurately reflect patients' conditions after gastrectomy. A QOL assessment tool specific to patients' conditions following gastrectomy has been recently reported in Japan. The Japanese Postgastrectomy Syndrome Working Party (JPGSWP) developed a questionnaire consisting of 45 items in addition to 22 items uniquely devised by surgeons, along with the SF-8 (8 items) and the GSRS (15 items) [47] (Fig. 27.2). This questionnaire was used to survey the QOL of 2368 patients who have undergone surgery for

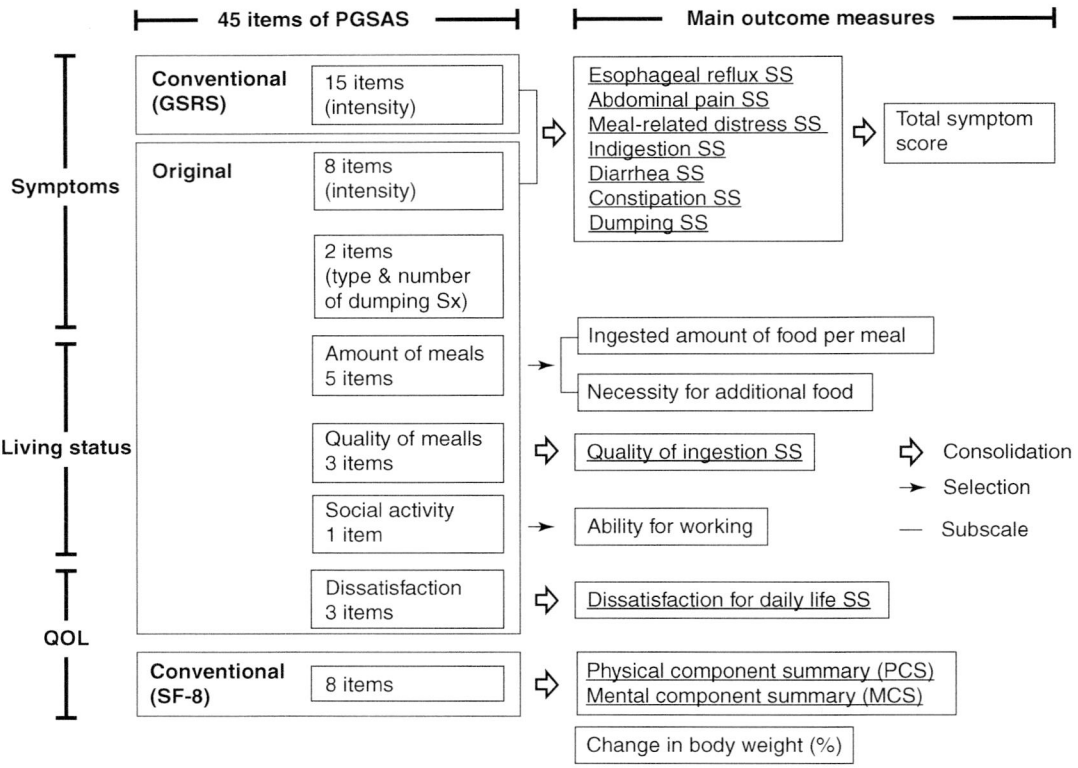

Fig. 27.2 The process of consolidation and selection to constitute main outcome measures of PGSAS45. (Reproduction from [47] with permission)

gastric cancer as a multicenter collaborative clinical trial. The results of the trial have been published as numerous articles; thus, the tool has drawn attention as a means to objectively evaluate QOL following gastrectomy [4, 15, 17, 31]. In the future, the tool is expected to be utilized as a means of evaluating QOL in a prospective trial.

Acknowledgment This work is supported in part by the Practical Research for Innovative Cancer Control (#15ck0106043h0002) from Japan Agency for Medical Research and Development, AMED.

References

1. Bolton JS, Conway WC 2nd. Postgastrectomy syndromes. Surg Clin North Am. 2011;91(5):1105–22. https://doi.org/10.1016/j.suc.2011.07.001.

2. Ukleja A. Dumping syndrome: pathophysiology and treatment. Nutr Clin Pract. 2005;20(5):517–25.

3. Mine S, Sano T, Tsutsumi K, Murakami Y, Ehara K, Saka M, Hara K, Fukagawa T, Udagawa H, Katai H. Large-scale investigation into dumping syndrome after gastrectomy for gastric cancer. J Am Coll Surg. 2010;211(5):628–36. https://doi.org/10.1016/j. jamcollsurg.2010.07.003.

4. Tanizawa Y, Tanabe K, Kawahira H, Fujita J, Takiguchi N, Takahashi M, Ito Y, Mitsumori N, Namikawa T, Oshio A, Nakada K, Japan postgastrectomy syndrome working P. Specific features of dumping syndrome after various types of gastrectomy as assessed by a newly developed integrated questionnaire, the PGSAS-45. Dig Surg. 2015;33(2):94–103. https://doi.org/10.1159/000442217.

5. van der Kleij FG, Vecht J, Lamers CB, Masclee AA. Diagnostic value of dumping provocation in patients after gastric surgery. Scand J Gastroenterol. 1996;31(12):1162–6.

6. Penning C, Vecht J, Masclee AA. Efficacy of depot long-acting octreotide therapy in severe dumping syndrome. Aliment Pharmacol Ther. 2005;22(10):963–9. https://doi.org/10.1111/j.1365-2036.2005.02681.x.

7. Didden P, Penning C, Masclee AA. Octreotide therapy in dumping syndrome: analysis of long-term results. Aliment Pharmacol Ther. 2006;24(9):1367–75. https://doi.org/10.1111/j.1365-2036.2006.03124.x.

8. Yamada M, Ohrui T, Asada M, Ishizawa K, Ebihara S, Arai H, Sasaki H. Acarbose attenuates hypoglycemia from dumping syndrome in an elderly man with gastrectomy. J Am Geriatr Soc. 2005;53(2):358–9. https://doi.org/10.1111/j.1532-5415.2005.53126_8.x.

9. Kubo M, Sasako M, Gotoda T, Ono H, Fujishiro M, Saito D, Sano T, Katai H. Endoscopic evaluation of the remnant stomach after gastrectomy: proposal for a new classification. Gastric Cancer. 2002;5(2):83–9. https://doi.org/10.1007/s101200200014.

10. Saito T, Kurokawa Y, Takiguchi S, Mori M, Doki Y. Current status of function-preserving surgery for gastric cancer. World J Gastroenterol. 2014;20(46):17297–304. https://doi.org/10.3748/wjg.v20.i46.17297.

11. Speicher JE, Thirlby RC, Burggraaf J, Kelly C, Levasseur S. Results of completion gastrectomies in 44 patients with postsurgical gastric atony. J Gastrointest Surg. 2009;13(5):874–80. https://doi.org/10.1007/s11605-009-0821-y.

12. Le Blanc-Louvry I, Ducrotte P, Lemeland JF, Metayer J, Denis P, Teniere P. Motility in the Roux-Y limb after distal gastrectomy: relation to the length of the limb and the afferent duodenojejunal segment—an experimental study. Neurogastroenterol Motil. 1999;11(5):365–74.

13. Hoya Y, Mitsumori N, Yanaga K. The advantages and disadvantages of a Roux-en-Y reconstruction after a distal gastrectomy for gastric cancer. Surg Today. 2009;39(8):647–51. https://doi.org/10.1007/s00595-009-3964-2.

14. Kim SM, Cho J, Kang D, Oh SJ, Kim AR, Sohn TS, Noh JH, Kim S. A randomized controlled trial of vagus nerve-preserving distal gastrectomy versus conventional distal gastrectomy for postoperative quality of life in early stage gastric cancer patients. Ann Surg. 2015; https://doi.org/10.1097/SLA.0000000000001565.

15. Fujita J, Takahashi M, Urushihara T, Tanabe K, Kodera Y, Yumiba T, Matsumoto H, Takagane A, Kunisaki C, Nakada K. Assessment of postoperative quality of life following pylorus-preserving gastrectomy and Billroth-I distal gastrectomy in gastric cancer patients: results of the nationwide postgastrectomy syndrome assessment study. Gastric Cancer. 2016;19(1):302–11. https://doi.org/10.1007/s10120-015-0460-9.

16. Aoki T, Yamaji I, Hisamoto T, Sato M, Matsuda T. Irregular bowel movement in gastrectomized subjects: bowel habits, stool characteristics, fecal flora, and metabolites. Gastric Cancer. 2012;15(4):396–404. https://doi.org/10.1007/s10120-011-0129-y.

17. Takiguchi N, Takahashi M, Ikeda M, Inagawa S, Ueda S, Nobuoka T, Ota M, Iwasaki Y, Uchida N, Kodera Y, Nakada K. Long-term quality-of-life comparison of total gastrectomy and proximal gastrectomy by postgastrectomy syndrome assessment scale (PGSAS-45): a nationwide multi-institutional study. Gastric Cancer. 2015;18(2):407–16. https://doi.org/10.1007/s10120-014-0377-8.

18. Yamaoka Y, Fujitani K, Tsujinaka T, Yamamoto K, Hirao M, Sekimoto M. Skeletal muscle loss after total gastrectomy, exacerbated by adjuvant chemotherapy. Gastric Cancer. 2015;18(2):382–9. https://doi.org/10.1007/s10120-014-0365-z.

19. Adachi S, Takiguchi S, Okada K, Yamamoto K, Yamasaki M, Miyata H, Nakajima K, Fujiwara Y, Hosoda H, Kangawa K, Mori M, Doki Y. Effects of ghrelin administration after total gastrectomy: a prospective, randomized, placebo-controlled phase II study. Gastroenterology. 2010;138(4):1312–20. https://doi.org/10.1053/j.gastro.2009.12.058.

20. Takiguchi S, Miyazaki Y, Takahashi T, Kurokawa Y, Yamasaki M, Nakajima K, Miyata H, Hosoda H, Kangawa K, Mori M, Doki Y. Impact of synthetic ghrelin administration for patients with severe body weight reduction more than 1 year after gastrectomy: a phase II clinical trial. Surg Today. 2016;46(3):379–85. https://doi.org/10.1007/s00595-015-1187-2.

21. Di Rienzo T, D'Angelo G, D'Aversa F, Campanale MC, Cesario V, Montalto M, Gasbarrini A, Ojetti V. Lactose intolerance: from diagnosis to correct management. Eur Rev Med Pharmacol Sci. 2013;17(Suppl 2):18–25.

22. Friess H, Bohm J, Muller MW, Glasbrenner B, Riepl RL, Malfertheiner P, Buchler MW. Maldigestion after total gastrectomy is associated with pancreatic insufficiency. Am J Gastroenterol. 1996;91(2):341–7.

23. Bragelmann R, Armbrecht U, Rosemeyer D, Schneider B, Zilly W, Stockbrugger RW. The effect of pancreatic enzyme supplementation in patients with steatorrhoea after total gastrectomy. Eur J Gastroenterol Hepatol. 1999;11(3):231–7.

24. Lee JH, Hyung WJ, Kim HI, Kim YM, Son T, Okumura N, Hu Y, Kim CB, Noh SH. Method of reconstruction governs iron metabolism after gastrectomy for patients with gastric cancer. Ann Surg. 2013;258(6):964–9. https://doi.org/10.1097/SLA.0b013e31827eebc1.

25. Hu Y, Kim HI, Hyung WJ, Song KJ, Lee JH, Kim YM, Noh SH. Vitamin B(12) deficiency after gastrectomy for gastric cancer: an analysis of clinical patterns and risk factors. Ann Surg. 2013;258(6):970–5. https://doi.org/10.1097/SLA.0000000000000214.

26. Lim JS, Jin SH, Kim SB, Lee JI. Effect of bisphosphonates on bone mineral density and fracture prevention in gastric cancer patients after gastrectomy. J Clin Gastroenterol. 2012;46(8):669–74. https://doi.org/10.1097/MCG.0b013e31824f1af4.

27. Lundell LR, Dent J, Bennett JR, Blum AL, Armstrong D, Galmiche JP, Johnson F, Hongo M, Richter JE, Spechler SJ, Tytgat GN, Wallin L. Endoscopic assessment of oesophagitis: clinical and functional correlates and further validation of the Los Angeles classification. Gut. 1999;45(2):172–80.

28. Nunobe S, Okaro A, Sasako M, Saka M, Fukagawa T, Katai H, Sano T. Billroth 1 versus Roux-en-Y recon-

structions: a quality-of-life survey at 5 years. Int J Clin Oncol. 2007;12(6):433–9. https://doi.org/10.1007/s10147-007-0706-6.

29. Takiguchi S, Yamamoto K, Hirao M, Imamura H, Fujita J, Yano M, Kobayashi K, Kimura Y, Kurokawa Y, Mori M, Doki Y, Osaka University Clinical Research Group for Gastroenterological S. A comparison of postoperative quality of life and dysfunction after Billroth I and Roux-en-Y reconstruction following distal gastrectomy for gastric cancer: results from a multi-institutional RCT. Gastric Cancer. 2012;15(2):198–205. https://doi.org/10.1007/s10120-011-0098-1.

30. Inokuchi M, Kojima K, Yamada H, Kato K, Hayashi M, Motoyama K, Sugihara K. Long-term outcomes of Roux-en-Y and Billroth-I reconstruction after laparoscopic distal gastrectomy. Gastric Cancer. 2013;16(1):67–73. https://doi.org/10.1007/s10120-012-0154-5.

31. Terashima M, Tanabe K, Yoshida M, Kawahira H, Inada T, Okabe H, Urushihara T, Kawashima Y, Fukushima N, Nakada K. Postgastrectomy Syndrome Assessment Scale (PGSAS)-45 and changes in body weight are useful tools for evaluation of reconstruction methods following distal gastrectomy. Ann Surg Oncol. 2014;21(Suppl 3):S370–8. https://doi.org/10.1245/s10434-014-3583-z.

32. Csendes A, Burgos AM, Smok G, Burdiles P, Braghetto I, Diaz JC. Latest results (12-21 years) of a prospective randomized study comparing Billroth II and Roux-en-Y anastomosis after a partial gastrectomy plus vagotomy in patients with duodenal ulcers. Ann Surg. 2009;249(2):189–94. https://doi.org/10.1097/SLA.0b013e3181921aa1.

33. Mine S, Nunobe S, Watanabe M. A novel technique of anti-reflux esophagogastrostomy following left thoracoabdominal esophagectomy for carcinoma of the esophagogastric junction. World J Surg. 2015;39(9):2359–61. https://doi.org/10.1007/s00268-015-3079-4.

34. Turnage RH, Sarosi G, Cryer B, Spechler S, Peterson W, Feldman M. Evaluation and management of patients with recurrent peptic ulcer disease after acid-reducing operations: a systematic review. J Gastrointest Surg. 2003;7(5):606–26.

35. Fukagawa T, Gotoda T, Oda I, Deguchi Y, Saka M, Morita S, Katai H. Stenosis of esophago-jejuno anastomosis after gastric surgery. World J Surg. 2010;34(8):1859–63. https://doi.org/10.1007/s00268-010-0609-y.

36. Fukagawa T, Katai H, Saka M, Morita S, Sano T, Sasako M. Gallstone formation after gastric cancer surgery. J Gastrointest Surg. 2009;13(5):886–9. https://doi.org/10.1007/s11605-009-0832-8.

37. Bernini M, Bencini L, Sacchetti R, Marchet A, Cristadoro L, Pacelli F, Berardi S, Doglietto GB, Rosa F, Verlato G, Cozzaglio L, Bechi P, Marrelli D, Roviello F, Farsi M, Italian Research Group for Gastric C. The Cholegas Study: safety of prophylactic cholecystectomy during gastrectomy for cancer: preliminary results of a multicentric randomized clinical trial. Gastric Cancer. 2013;16(3):370–6. https://doi.org/10.1007/s10120-012-0195-9.

38. Aoki M, Saka M, Morita S, Fukagawa T, Katai H. Afferent loop obstruction after distal gastrectomy with Roux-en-Y reconstruction. World J Surg. 2010;34(10):2389–92. https://doi.org/10.1007/s00268-010-0602-5.

39. Miyagaki H, Takiguchi S, Kurokawa Y, Hirao M, Tamura S, Nishida T, Kimura Y, Fujiwara Y, Mori M, Doki Y. Recent trend of internal hernia occurrence after gastrectomy for gastric cancer. World J Surg. 2012;36(4):851–7. https://doi.org/10.1007/s00268-012-1479-2.

40. Gilson BS, Gilson JS, Bergner M, Bobbit RA, Kressel S, Pollard WE, Vesselago M. The sickness impact profile. Development of an outcome measure of health care. Am J Public Health. 1975;65(12):1304–10.

41. Ware JE Jr, Sherbourne CD. The MOS 36-item short-form health survey (SF-36). I. Conceptual framework and item selection. Med Care. 1992;30(6):473–83.

42. Development of the World Health Organization WHOQOL-BREF quality of life assessment. The WHOQOL Group. Psychol Med. 1998;28(3):551–8.

43. Svedlund J, Sjodin I, Dotevall G. GSRS—a clinical rating scale for gastrointestinal symptoms in patients with irritable bowel syndrome and peptic ulcer disease. Dig Dis Sci. 1988;33(2):129–34.

44. Aaronson NK, Ahmedzai S, Bergman B, Bullinger M, Cull A, Duez NJ, Filiberti A, Flechtner H, Fleishman SB, de Haes JC, et al. The European Organization for Research and Treatment of Cancer QLQ-C30: a quality-of-life instrument for use in international clinical trials in oncology. J Natl Cancer Inst. 1993;85(5):365–76.

45. EuroQol G. EuroQol—a new facility for the measurement of health-related quality of life. Health Policy. 1990;16(3):199–208.

46. Feeny D, Furlong W, Boyle M, Torrance GW. Multiattribute health status classification systems. Health Utilities Index. PharmacoEconomics. 1995;7(6):490–502.

47. Nakada K, Ikeda M, Takahashi M, Kinami S, Yoshida M, Uenosono Y, Kawashima Y, Oshio A, Suzukamo Y, Terashima M, Kodera Y. Characteristics and clinical relevance of postgastrectomy syndrome assessment scale (PGSAS)-45: newly developed integrated questionnaires for assessment of living status and quality of life in postgastrectomy patients. Gastric Cancer. 2015;18(1):147–58. https://doi.org/10.1007/s10120-014-0344-4.

Follow-Up After Gastric Cancer Treatment

28

Jimmy BY So and Guowei Kim

Introduction

The follow-up of patients who have undergone surgical resection for gastric cancer is controversial. Despite the fact that many clinicians perform postoperative follow-up or surveillance for these patients, there appears to be no clear consensus on the utility or mode of surveillance in these patients. This can partly be explained by a number of factors (low rate of resectability, poor patient tolerance for treatment, frequent postoperative morbidity and mortality after operation and an overall dismal prognosis) [1–3] which have led to pessimism when faced with recurrent gastric cancer [2].

In colorectal cancer, national and international bodies such as the American Society of Clinical Oncology (ASCO), the Association of Coloproctology of Great Britain and Ireland and the European Society of Medical Oncology have issued guidelines on the follow-up of colorectal cancer [4–7]. These guidelines are based on multiple randomized controlled trials (RCTs) and meta-analyses [8–10], some of which have demonstrated improved survival in patients undergoing intensive follow-up. In contrast, the evidence for the prac-

tice of follow-up after gastrectomy is weak [11], with only retrospective studies and no RCTs to date. Despite this, many units actively investigate patients in order to detect recurrences at an earlier and asymptomatic stage, in the hope that this will lead to improved outcomes. The lack of strong evidence for this begets some to question the use of scarce resources in intensive follow-up [12].

There are four main reasons for follow-up:

1. Post-surgical: To detect problems associated with the operation
2. Oncological: To detect and manage recurrent disease
3. Pastoral: To provide psychological and emotional support
4. Research: To collect outcome data

In this chapter, we shall delve into the literature on recurrence patterns of gastric cancer, predictive scoring for recurrence, metachronous gastric cancer (gastric stump cancer), surveillance modalities, the impact of follow-up on survival outcomes, the current guidelines and recommendations and what the future holds.

Recurrence Patterns of Gastric Cancer

The recurrence rate of gastric cancer after resection with curative intent is about 21–55% [2, 3,

J. B. So (✉) · G. Kim
Division of Surgical Oncology, National University Cancer Institute of Singapore (NCIS), National University Health System, Singapore, Singapore

Department of Surgery, National University of Singapore, Singapore, Singapore
e-mail: jimmyso@nus.edu.sg

© Springer-Verlag GmbH Germany, part of Springer Nature 2019
S. H. Noh, W. J. Hyung (eds.), *Surgery for Gastric Cancer*,
https://doi.org/10.1007/978-3-662-45583-8_28

13–20]. While this figure is discouraging, resection for early gastric cancer can give recurrence rates as low as 1.5–5.1% [2, 21–23]. In order to rationalize follow-up for gastric cancer, an understanding of when, where and in whom recurrence occurs is needed.

Timing of Recurrence

The timing of recurrence in gastric cancer, like in many gastrointestinal cancers, usually occurs in the first 2 years after resection with curative intent. Most studies report that 66.5–92% of recurrences occur within 2 years [3, 13, 14, 16, 18, 20, 22] and the risk of recurrence seems to plateau after 2–3 years [2, 15, 24]. This suggests that efforts should be concentrated on the first 2 years after gastrectomy as this would be when most recurrences occur.

However, there seems to be a large variation of the timing of recurrences for specific subgroups of patients. In a study from Korea, 43.5%, 67.1% and 85.6% of recurrences occurred within 2, 3 and 5 years, respectively, in patients who underwent curative resection for early gastric cancer [21]. This suggests that the follow-up of these patients should necessarily be longer and different from patients who undergo curative gastrectomy for advanced gastric cancer.

Patients who have undergone partial gastrectomy may develop metachronous gastric cancer of the remnant gastric stump (stump cancer/remnant gastric cancer). This subgroup should be viewed and managed as a separate entity from recurrence and is covered in more detail subsequently in this chapter (Surveillance Modalities, Endoscopy, Endoscopy After Partial Gastrectomy).

Location of Recurrence

Recurrence patterns of gastric cancer can be classified into three broad groups: locoregional, peritoneal and hematogenous. Locoregional recurrence is defined as cancer recurrence at the resection margin, within the lymph nodes or in the operation bed within the region of the resec-

tion. Peritoneal recurrence is defined as cancer recurrence in the abdominal cavity because of intraperitoneal distribution. Hematogenous recurrence has been defined as any metastatic lesion detected within distant organs [1, 2, 25]. However, there are some variations in the definitions of type of recurrences in the literature, especially with regard to recurrences in the distant lymph nodes as well as peritoneal disease in the tumour bed (locoregional versus peritoneal). These differences in semantics can possibly lead to differences in recurrence patterns among studies [14].

Recurrences can occur at a single site or at multiple sites (locoregional/peritoneal, locoregional/hematogenous, peritoneal/hematogenous, locoregional/peritoneal/hematogenous). Recurrences occur at only one site in 50.2–83.7% of patients [2, 13–16, 22]. Conversely, at the time of recurrence, 16.3–49.9% of patients will have metastases in more than one site, which suggests that some effort should be made to actively look for other metastases in patients diagnosed with recurrence. This may translate to a change in management strategy depending on the sites of recurrences.

Taking into account patients who have single and multiple sites of recurrences, locoregional recurrences occur in 11.2–63.3% of patients. Peritoneal recurrences occur in 29–58% and hematogenous recurrences occur in 13–51% of patients who suffer from recurrence [2, 3, 13–17]. The large variation in location of recurrences reflects the heterogeneity of gastric cancer with regard to tumour biology, primary treatment as well as the mode and timing of recurrence detection. Some studies have shown that the pattern of recurrence depended on the timing of recurrence. Patients with early recurrence (within 1 year) were more likely to have hematogenous recurrence compared with patients who had late recurrences, who were more likely to have a locoregional recurrence [1, 15], though this finding was not seen consistently in other studies [3, 26]. Patients with locoregional recurrence may have a longer median survival compared with patients who had hematogenous or peritoneal disease [17]. As locoregional recurrence is seen more frequently in late recurrences, survival after recurrence is also better in patients who suffer late recurrence as compared to early recurrence [1, 3].

Recurrent gastric cancer is rarely amenable to oncologic resection. Most studies report that less than 20% of patients with recurrence received surgery, of which complete resection of recurrence was possible in only a quarter of them [2, 27–29]. Of these recurrences, the most common indications for resection were local recurrence in the gastric stump. Other less common indications for resection were isolated small liver metastasis and localized peritoneal metastasis [28].

For recurrent disease not amenable to surgery, chemotherapy has become the standard of care and is offered in the hope of improving survival and quality of life despite conflicting evidence [12]. However, there is no evidence that initiating chemotherapy at an earlier stage improves outcomes [30, 31].

Predictive Scoring for Recurrence

Many studies have tried to identify factors to predict recurrence after curative gastrectomy. Some factors that are associated with increased risk of recurrence are [2, 15, 18, 21]:

1. Large tumour size (>3–4 cm)
2. Depth of tumour invasion (serosal involvement)
3. Tumour subtype (poorly differentiated, diffuse, signet ring, lymphovascular invasion, perineural invasion)
4. Proximal or diffuse tumour location
5. Lymph node metastasis (high lymph node ratio)

While there are predictive scores and nomograms in the literature with regard to prognosticating patients (disease-free survival and overall survival) after gastrectomy with curative intent [32–34], the Italian Research Group for Gastric Cancer (GIRCG) has developed a score predictive of gastric cancer recurrence based on variables commonly used in clinical practice [18]. This score utilizes nodal status, depth of invasion,

extent of lymphadenectomy, tumour location and advanced age as independent predictors of recurrence and was able to predict recurrences with a sensitivity of 83.5% and specificity of 81.1% with an overall accuracy of 82.2%. This score has since been externally validated [19, 35], though it is important to note that this score has only been validated for Western populations.

Surveillance Modalities

Imaging

The ideal imaging modality must be able to detect various patterns of recurrence, namely locoregional, peritoneal and distant/hematogenous disease. Furthermore, the imaging used should have high specificity and sensitivity with low false-positive rates and low cost. Unfortunately, the ability of imaging to detect recurrence is poor for gastric cancer. While the use of imaging for the detection of local recurrences and hepatic metastasis can be fraught with inaccuracies [36], all imaging are poor at detecting peritoneal disease, which accounts for around 29–58% of recurrences. Barium enema has been used in the diagnosis of peritoneal carcinomatosis in colorectal cancer [37], and this imaging has been used in Japanese institutions to confirm the presence of peritoneal disease when clinically suspected [12].

Imaging in the search for asymptomatic recurrence is fraught with difficulties, missing many recurrences and producing a number of false-positive results. Changes in the anatomical structure after gastric surgery can make it difficult to diagnose recurrence accurately as well. Imaging is perhaps more useful when a clinical recurrence is suspected, such as in the face of rising tumour markers [12]. Overall, the ability to detect asymptomatic recurrences despite intensive follow-up is poor, with the proportion of such recurrence detected varying from only 22% to 45% [30, 31].

Computed Tomography

Computed tomography is an essential tool for preoperative staging and follow-up of gastric cancer [25]. Currently, CT is used most frequently and is regarded as the most reliable method for assessing cancer recurrence, with a reported accuracy of 60–70% [38]. Recurrences have been shown using CT imaging in 55–81.1% of patients with recurrence [21, 39].

Although CT is the primary tool for investigation of suspected recurrence because of its widespread availability and relatively low cost, it often cannot help differentiate treatment-induced morphologic changes from tumour recurrence [40]. In addition, CT shows a low positive predictive value (60–70%) for peritoneal or distant lymph node metastasis [41, 42]. The ability of CT to primarily diagnose recurrence in the remnant stomach is also likely poor when extrapolating its use in diagnosing primary gastric cancer, and there is a direct trade-off between sensitivity and specificity. When the criterion for diagnosis was a gastric wall thickness of 2 cm or more in one study, sensitivity and specificity were only 50% and 88%, respectively. By reducing the criterion to 1 cm, sensitivity increased to 100%, but specificity dropped to only 36% [43]. Hence, its use is mainly limited to detecting hepatic and, to a lesser extent, locoregional recurrences.

Magnetic Resonance Imaging and Endoscopic Ultrasound

Magnetic resonance imaging has the obvious benefit of having no exposure to ionizing radiation. It has high diagnostic accuracy in the evaluation of T staging of primary gastric cancer of 74% though N staging with MRI was only 47% accurate [44]. MRI and endoscopic ultrasound (EUS) are both employed for GC staging, but EUS is recognized to be the first-choice imaging modality in locoregional staging compared with MRI and CT and could affect the therapeutic management of these patients [45]. However, there is little data in support of the use of EUS or MRI in the follow-up of patients after curative resection for gastric cancer.

Positron Emission Tomography/ Computed Tomography

In the detection of recurrence during follow-up after curative resection, positron emission tomography (PET) is often useful for detecting different patterns of recurrence, such as local recurrence involving the stomach remnant, regional lymph nodes, peritoneal dissemination, liver metastases and remote metastases. PET is an advantageous imaging tool because it enables the evaluation of the entire body at once, although PET has limitations with a significant false-negative rate in early cancer, signet-ring cell tumours and poorly differentiated histotypes. PET is useful when conventional imaging is equivocal, as it can confirm the presence of true recurrence [46].

18F-fluorodeoxyglucose positron emission tomography/computed tomography (18F-FDG-PET/CT) scans represent a superior postoperative surveillance modality for the diagnosis of recurrent GC compared with other imaging modalities as previously mentioned. An integrated PET/CT scan provides fusion images, combining functional and anatomic imaging together. It may also be helpful in optimizing the treatment strategy and may play an important role in individualized treatment in the future. In one study, FDG-PET/CT had a high impact on patients' management or care. Further diagnostic or treatment plans were changed in 52.9% of patients. Suspected recurrent lesions were accurately confirmed by FDG-PET/CT in some patients; thereafter, they were treated with previously unplanned surgery or recurrent chemotherapy. Abnormal diagnostic CT scans in another group of patients revealed lesions with physiological or inflammatory uptake of FDG leading to cancellation of previously planned diagnostic procedures and chemotherapy [47].

18F-FDG-PET/CT reportedly has very good sensitivity (89.7%) and specificity (85.7%) in detecting distant and local recurrences during postoperative follow-up. Positive 18F-FDG-PET/CT findings may lead to an early change in the management of patients after radical gastrectomy, directing them towards rescue surgery or chemoradiotherapy and therefore improving their overall survival [48]. Despite this, PET/CT was not as sensitive as contrast CT for detecting peritoneal disease. Furthermore, the addition of PET/CT on contrast CT did not increase diagnostic accuracy in detection of recurrence in some studies [49].

Laparoscopy

Laparoscopy can provide more accurate information than that provided by conventional imaging methods [50]. Laparoscopy has been suggested to be a potential method for detecting minimal peritoneal metastasis or recurrence because it not only allows visualization of the entire abdominal cavity but can also provide a means to obtain tissue and peritoneal fluid for pathologic confirmation. Although staging laparoscopy has primarily been conducted to avoid unnecessary laparotomy, for potentially curative surgery, it can also be used for the detection of early-stage peritoneal recurrence in post-surgical patients with equivocal radiologic findings to clarify the diagnosis of recurrence. A recent study [51] evaluated the feasibility and accuracy of second-look laparoscopy for patients with gastric cancer at high risk of peritoneal recurrence after completion of 6 months of systemic adjuvant chemotherapy. In this study, second-look laparoscopy was a safe and effective approach for early reassessment of peritoneal disease for the selection of patients who needed further systemic chemotherapy. In addition, a minimally invasive approach with laparoscopy may be an alternative to the complicated second-look laparotomy [25]. Despite this, its role is still limited due to the relative invasiveness of laparoscopy as compared to the other surveillance modalities.

Endoscopy

Endoscopy, which is commonly used in clinical practice, is a promising screening method for gastric cancer. Although gastric cancer screening has been actively performed in South Korea and Japan [52–54], endoscopic screening has been carried out as a national programme only in Korea. It has been shown to reduce mortality by 57% [54] with detection rates of gastric cancer about 2.7–4.6 times higher than barium studies or photofluorography [55]. In spite of this, cost-effectiveness of endoscopy for a mass national screening programme is still not conclusively proven, though targeted screening for high-risk populations has shown positive results [56].

When considering endoscopy as part of routine surveillance for patients who have undergone gastrectomy with curative intent, the evidence is even more scarce. One of the difficulties in justifying routine endoscopic surveillance is due to the relatively low rates of true local recurrence, with endoscopy being unable to detect regional, peritoneal and hematogenous recurrences.

Endoscopy After Partial Gastrectomy
The entity of remnant gastric cancer should also be considered here. Patients who have undergone initial gastrectomy for early gastric cancer have cumulative prevalence rates of remnant gastric cancer of 2.4% at 5 years and 6.1% at 10 years [57] with another study giving a 4% cumulative risk at 20 years post initial gastrectomy [58]. Other studies report incidences of remnant gastric cancer of 3.2–10% [59, 60]. Despite this, follow-up endoscopy is still commonly performed and recommended [57, 61]. The main reason for this is because tumour recurrence in the remnant stomach after partial gastrectomy can be treated by an additional total gastrectomy, and this may occasionally result in long-term survival [29]. Patients with partial gastrectomy are usually identified as a high-risk gastric cancer group. The interval between the preceding examination and diagnosis was 22.5 months in patients with early gastric remnant cancer, while it was 67.4 months in patients with advanced cancer. It can therefore be postulated that periodic surveillance endoscopies could be performed at intervals of 2–3 years in order to detect patients with early-stage disease [57]. The development of remnant gastric cancer after distal gastrectomy for gastric cancer usually occurs after a mean interval of 8.3 years and is more frequently found away from the anastomosis and on the lesser curve [62–65], which lend further weight to the concept of long-term endoscopic surveillance in this group of patients. The caveat for this being that thus far, there is still no good quality prospective evidence that this approach would improve overall survival as well as be cost-effective.

Endoscopy After Total Gastrectomy
The role of follow-up endoscopy for patients with gastric cancer who have undergone total

gastrectomy is even smaller, as there is no remnant gastric mucosa. Moreover, unresectable distant recurrence is more common than locoregional recurrence after total gastrectomy [2]. One study from Korea reported that follow-up endoscopy may be useful in detecting early postoperative stenosis as well as tumour recurrence in patients who had total gastrectomy for advanced gastric cancer [66], though admitting that this did not translate to improved survival outcomes. Meanwhile, it would be prudent to adopt a 'scope when symptomatic' approach to patients who have undergone total gastrectomy for gastric cancer.

Endoscopy After Endoscopic Resection

The increase in detection rate of early gastric cancer together with the expanded indications for endoscopic resection has resulted in many patients in high-prevalence countries undergoing endoscopic resection for early gastric cancer. With appropriate patient selection, curative resection rates in the literature for endoscopic mucosal resection (EMR) and endoscopic submucosal dissection (ESD) are 61% and 74–95%, respectively [67]. This group of patients who have undergone curative endoscopic resection of early gastric cancer represent a distinctly different subgroup in whom post resection endoscopic surveillance may play a larger role. Compared to gastrectomy, endoscopic treatment leaves the high-risk native stomach in place. As such, metachronous cancer can develop in 5–14% of patients who have undergone curative endoscopic resection for early gastric cancer [68–70]. The need for early endoscopic surveillance after endoscopic resection may be justified, as about 1.7% of patients who underwent ESD had synchronous gastric cancers which were missed by the initial pre-resection endoscopic evaluation [69], leading to some centres recommending endoscopic surveillance within 6 months after endoscopic resection. Subsequent yearly endoscopies are also recommended as the incidence rate of metachronous cancers is around 3% [68, 69]. Another recent study reported 5-year, 7-year and 10-year cumulative incidence functions of metachronous gastric cancer on surveillance endoscopy of

9.5%, 13.1% and 22.7%, respectively, suggesting that endoscopic surveillance should probably be performed beyond the previously recommended 5 years [71].

With no established guidelines at present, it would be prudent to consider initial early endoscopy within 6 months of endoscopic curative resection, followed by yearly endoscopy for a period of at least 10 years, if not indefinitely.

Tumour Markers

Increased preoperative serum levels of carcinoembryonic antigen (CEA), CA 19–9 and CA 72–4 are predictors of poor prognosis [72–76]. CEA, one of the most commonly used serum tumour markers in gastric cancer patients, is a glycoprotein with a molecular weight of 180 kD. Although CEA is of limited use in screening tests due to its low sensitivity and specificity in early cancer, it is able to detect recurrence early in colorectal cancer [77, 78] and is performed routinely postoperatively in many centres during follow-up. The serum level of CA 19–9, an incomplete glycolipid antigen of the Lewis blood group, can be increased in benign conditions such as cholecystitis, obstructive jaundice, cholangitis, cholelithiasis, liver cirrhosis and acute pancreatitis and is also increased in colorectal, liver, ovarian, bile duct and gastric cancer. CA 72–4 is a high molecular weight tumour-associated glycoprotein of 220–400 kD that is recognized by the monoclonal antibody B72.3. CA 72–4 is known to be expressed in breast, colorectal, pancreatic, endometrial, lung and gastric cancer [79, 80].

Despite the prognostic value that these tumour markers provide, the most important prognostic factors of gastric cancer remain the depth of invasion and lymph node metastasis [81, 82], which has led to the shift in the use of CEA, CA 19–9 and CA 72–4 in early detection of recurrence as they have been reported to be elevated in patients with recurrence [83, 84]. Preoperative positivity of CEA, CA 19–9 and CA72–4 was found to be 20.2–28.3%, 25–52% and 42.9–59%, respectively [85–87], with sensitivity for recurrences of 44–65.8%, 55–56% and 51%, respectively [84, 88]. Sensitivities were significantly improved when more than one tumour marker was used – 85% when either/both CEA/CA 19–9 was elevated post-surgery and 87% if one of CEA, CA 19–9 and CA 72–4 was elevated post-surgery.

When looking at early versus advanced gastric cancer, the sensitivity of CEA, CA 19–9 and CA 72–4 in early gastric cancer was 40.0, 5.6 and 2.8%, respectively, and the specificity was 99.3, 99.0 and 98.9%, respectively. In advanced gastric cancer, the sensitivity of CEA, CA 19–9 and CA 72–4 was 100.0, 68.2 and 51.3%, respectively, and the specificity was 79.4, 80.0 and 81.3%, respectively. These data showed that the sensitivity and specificity of these tumour markers for recurrence in advanced gastric cancer were high enough to be useful tests in the surveillance of gastric cancer patients, although CA 19–9 and CA 72–4 are less useful in the surveillance of early gastric cancer patients because of their low sensitivity and high false-positive rate (60%, 94.4% and 97.2% for CEA, CA 19–9 and CA 72–4, respectively) [89].

When looking at lead time, CEA was able to detect recurrence at a mean of 3.1 months earlier when comparing with imaging. The lead time for CA 19–9 was 2.2 months [84]. This lead time advantage was also seen in another study where the average time between CEA, CA 19–9 and CA 72–4 positivity and recurrence was 4, 5 and 4 months, respectively [88].

Despite the apparent advantages in earlier recurrence detection, tumour markers have a number of disadvantages. Firstly, the use of tumour markers is mainly confined to patients with advanced gastric cancer. Secondly, the grim prognosis and lack of good treatment options for recurrent gastric cancer limit the usefulness of detecting recurrences earlier, though this may change with new therapeutic strategies and agents. Thirdly, the high false-positive rates could significantly increase patient anxiety, and combined with the lack of good therapeutic options, one would question the need to detect recurrences while the patient is still asymptomatic.

Follow-Up and Survival

There is no high-level evidence supporting a routine follow-up schedule for curatively resected gastric cancer patients. All data are retrospective and observational, thus preventing any definitive conclusion [90].

Most studies focused on the possible survival benefit of early detection of recurrence by intensive postoperative surveillance. Some studies indicate that an intense postoperative follow-up protocol was successful in identifying asymptomatic recurrences earlier than symptomatic recurrences. Nevertheless, they could not achieve any evident advantage in overall survival [31, 91]. A study from Memorial Sloan-Kettering Cancer Centre [92] showed that follow-up did not detect asymptomatic recurrences earlier than symptomatic recurrences in patients with gastric cancer who underwent a curative gastrectomy. In this report, patients with asymptomatic recurrences showed better post-recurrence and disease-specific survival than those with symptomatic recurrences. Similarly in a study from Korea [38], median overall survival and post-recurrence survival were worse for patients with a symptomatic recurrence than for those with an asymptomatic recurrence. Furthermore, asymptomatic patients had more benefit from re-resection and post-recurrence chemotherapy; at multivariate survival analysis, the presence of symptoms was the only independent factor of poor survival, suggesting a more biologically aggressive disease in symptomatic patients. Another study from Turkey [92] of 173 patients with recurrent gastric cancer also found that symptomatic recurrence is an important prognostic factor for post-recurrence survival and that the presence of symptoms may be considered a marker of biologic tumour aggressiveness, which is an important determinant of survival at the time of recurrence diagnosis during follow-up for gastric cancer.

A systematic review enrolling a total of 810 patients did not find any evidence suggesting that postoperative surveillance has any overall survival benefit; it also stressed that no studies addressed quality of life issues. Lead-time bias, in which the observed prolonged survival is due to earlier detection of recurrence, rather than to an effect on disease outcome, was mentioned as a major limitation in these studies which showed significantly higher post-recurrence survival in the asymptomatic patients [11].

Other Primary Cancers

One of the potential benefits of follow-up for patients would be the possibility of detecting extra-gastric cancers early. 2.6–11.2% of patients who have undergone curative resection for early gastric cancer were found on follow-up to have other synchronous or metachronous extra-gastric tumours (lung, colorectal, hepatocellular carcinoma, head and neck, urologic, biliary, breast and hematologic malignancies) [21, 58].

Clinical Guidelines and Recommendations

The National Comprehensive Cancer Network Guidelines (2015) [93] recommend a follow-up schedule involving a complete history and physical examination every 3–6 months for 1–2 years, every 6–12 months for 3–5 years and annually thereafter. Complete blood count, chemistry profile, imaging studies or endoscopy are recommended only if clinically indicated, and monitoring and treatment for vitamin B12 and iron deficiency should also be performed.

The European Society for Medical Oncology (ESMO), the European Society of Surgical Oncology (ESSO) and the European Society of Radiotherapy and Oncology (ESTRO) clinical practice guidelines (2013) [94] which were endorsed by the Japanese Society of Medical Oncology (JSMO) do not make any recommendations on follow-up schedule, instead suggesting that:

1. Regular follow-up may allow investigation and treatment of symptoms, psychological support and early detection of recurrence.

2. In the advanced disease setting, identification of patients for second-line chemotherapy and clinical trials requires regular follow-up to detect symptoms of disease progression before significant clinical deterioration.

3. If relapse/disease progression is suspected, then a clinical history, physical examination and directed blood tests should be carried out. Radiological investigations should be carried out in patients who are candidates for further chemo- or radiotherapy.

Guidelines from the Association of Upper Gastrointestinal Surgeons of Great Britain and Ireland, the British Society of Gastroenterology and the British Association of Surgical Oncology (2011) [95] as well as national guidelines from the Scottish Intercollegiate Guidelines Network (SIGN) (2006) [96] and Korea [97] do not recommend any specific follow-up schedule.

The Charter Scaligero Consensus Conference held in 2013 during the 10th International Gastric Cancer Congress (IGCC) of the International Gastric Cancer Association recently published in 2016 the following six consensus statements [98]:

1. Routine follow-up should be offered to all patients.

2. Follow-up should be offered by members of the multidisciplinary team who performed the initial diagnosis, staging and treatment, including the gastroenterologist, the surgeon, the medical and radiation oncologists and the general practitioner.

3. Follow-up of patients following curative treatment of gastric cancer should be tailored to the individual patient, to the stage of their disease and to the treatment options available in the event that recurrence is detected.

4. Physical examination rarely detects asymptomatic recurrence of gastric cancer. A follow-up programme intended to detect asymptomatic recurrence should be based on cross-sectional imaging. There is no evidence that intensive cross-sectional imaging surveillance of gastric patients is associated with improved long-term survival. However, as a matter of clinical care following curative

treatment of gastric cancer, it is reasonable to prescribe periodic imaging at a frequency consistent with recurrence risk. The incremental value of screening for elevated levels of biochemical markers in addition to cross-sectional imaging remains undefined.

5. Upper gastrointestinal tract endoscopy may be used to detect local recurrence or metachronous primary gastric cancer in patients who have undergone a subtotal gastrectomy. True local recurrence is uncommon, but if present it may be considered for resection with curative intent, especially in patients who initially presented with early-stage disease. The cost-benefit ratio of endoscopic surveillance of the anastomosis and/or gastric remnant remains undefined.

6. Routine screening for asymptomatic recurrence of gastric cancer may be discontinued after 5 years, as recurrence beyond that time is very rare.

The Future

Nurse-Led Follow-Up

The importance of nurses in the follow-up of patients after resection of gastric cancer cannot be underestimated, and this has been recognized in recent guidelines [95]. New strategies for patient follow-up are currently undergoing evaluation, including patient-led self-referral and services led by clinical nurse specialists (CNS). The strategy of nurse follow-up after esophagectomy in the Netherlands has been shown to be both cost-effective and provides equal if not better patient experience [99].

CNS provision for UGI cancer particularly at cancer units is still not well developed. The role of the nurse includes clinical education, psychological support, research and consultation. The extent of the CNS role is difficult to measure because of the multifaceted nature of the work, complexity of the patient pathway and the more specific requirement to respond to individual patient needs [100, 101]. In a study of the work patterns of 463 CNSs (including gastrointestinal

nurses) from the UK, 68% of time is spent on clinical matters, of which 48% is physical care and 32% psychological care. Not surprisingly, 33% of the nurses' time is given to telephone advice and 34% spent in an outpatient setting. The remaining time is spent on administration (24%), research (2%) and education (3%) [101]. CNSs use 'brokering' skills, provide 'clinical rescue work', advise on symptom control and support and negotiate care pathways, all of which are intended to prevent adverse events, particularly readmission [101, 102]. The impact of psychological care and tailored information given in a supportive environment improves the patients' experience and health-related quality of life [103].

The multidisciplinary team is central to patient care, with CNSs having an integral role: consulting with medical, surgical and allied healthcare professionals in order to provide a coordinated approach to care and enhancing quality of care and patients' well-being. Nurses also have access to important information, particularly acting as the patient's advocate, that may influence clinical decisions, and it is therefore essential that MDTs listen to their views [104].

Novel Prognostic and Therapeutic Modalities

Presently, there is little a clinician can offer a patient with recurrent gastric cancer except palliative chemotherapy. Soon, biomedical research will hopefully provide better prognostic and therapeutic tools for metastatic cancer patients and/or relapsing patients. One example would be the development of nanostring-based multigene assay to predict recurrence after surgery [105].

Survivin-expressing circulating tumour cells were recently shown to be an independent predictor for recurrence [106] and could be a good clinical biomarker for prognostication [107]. Molecular approaches using real-time reverse transcription-polymerase chain reaction (RT-PCR) have made it possible to increase the sensitivity of detecting micrometastasis in the peritoneal cavity, suggesting that multiplex

RT-PCR assay for CEA and CK-20 was highly sensitive for detection and might be useful for prediction of peritoneal dissemination [108, 109].

The vascular endothelial growth factor (VEGF) family is considered to be a major inducer of angiogenesis and lymphangiogenesis. VEGF and cortactin may be good clinical biomarkers for prediction of the prognosis of patients with curatively resected gastric cancer [110]. VEGF also correlated with peritoneal metastasis [111].

E-cadherin is a metastasis-suppressor gene that plays a central role in the formation of epithelial architecture. The reduction of E-cadherin expression may induce the dissociation of cells from primary tumours because of loosened intercellular adhesion, contributing to tumour invasion to adjacent organs, and may potentially be used to predict recurrence [112–114].

Phosphorylated mammalian target of rapamycin (p-mTOR) is a potential anticancer therapy target, and its expression was immunohistochemically determined using tissue microarrays. A linear correlation between the rate of tumour recurrence and p-mTOR expression scores in metastatic lymph nodes has been reported [115], giving p-mTOR the potential to be a biomarker for recurrence and a therapeutic target.

MicroRNAs have been evaluated as a prognostic marker for gastric cancer recurrence, with promising results showing its potential to predict the recurrence risk for recurrence in gastric cancer [116]. In addition, specific mRNAs were involved in regulating target genes in several oncogenic signal pathways, such as TP53, MAPK and VEGF.

Conclusion

The aggressive nature of gastric cancer, and historically poor outcomes even in the setting of operable disease, means that the concept of survivorship is only now beginning to evolve. Long-term implications, late effects of therapy and psychosocial implications of treatment are poorly studied to date. With no established evidence-based guidelines, follow-up of patients after treatment for gastric cancer must necessarily be individualised and tailored to each patient's specific needs.

References

1. Eom BW, Yoon H, Ryu KW, Lee JH, Cho SJ, Lee JY, et al. Predictors of timing and patterns of recurrence after curative resection for gastric cancer. Dig Surg. 2010;27(6):481–6.
2. Yoo CH, Noh SH, Shin DW, Choi SH, Min JS. Recurrence following curative resection for gastric carcinoma. Br J Surg. 2000;87(2):236–42.
3. Kang W, Meng Q, Yu J, Ma Z, Li Z. Factors associated with early recurrence after curative surgery for gastric cancer. World J Gastroenterol. 2015;21(19):5934–40.
4. Meyerhardt JA, Mangu PB, Flynn PJ, Korde L, Loprinzi CL, Minsky BD, et al. Follow-up care, surveillance protocol, and secondary prevention measures for survivors of colorectal cancer: American Society of clinical Oncology clinical practice guideline endorsement. J Clin Oncol. 2013;31(35):4465–70.
5. Schmoll HJ, Van Cutsem E, Stein A, Valentini V, Glimelius B, Haustermans K, et al. ESMO Consensus Guidelines for management of patients with colon and rectal cancer. A personalized approach to clinical decision making. Ann Oncol. 2012;23:2479–516.
6. Desch CE, Benson AB 3rd, Smith TJ, Flynn PJ, Krause C, Loprinzi CL, et al. Recommended colorectal cancer surveillance guidelines by the American Society of Clinical Oncology. J Clin Oncol. 1999;17(4):1312.
7. Group EA. For the management of colorectal cancer issued by. Color Cancer. 2007;44.
8. Figueredo A, Rumble RB, Maroun J, Earle CC, Cummings B, Mcleod R, et al. Follow-up of patients with curatively resected colorectal cancer: a practice guideline. BMC Cancer. 2003;13:1–13.
9. Papagrigoriadis S. Follow-up of patients with colorectal cancer: The evidence is in favour but we are still in need of a protocol. Int J Surg. 2007;5:120–8.
10. Destri GL, Di Cataldo A, Stefano P. Colorectal cancer follow-up: Useful or useless? J Surg Oncol. 2006;15(1):1–12.
11. Cardoso R, Coburn NG, Seevaratnam R, Mahar A, Helyer L, Law C, et al. A systematic review of patient surveillance after curative gastrectomy for gastric cancer: a brief review. Gastric Cancer. 2012;15(Suppl 1):S164–7.
12. Whiting J, Sano T, Saka M, Fukagawa T, Katai H, Sasako M. Follow-up of gastric cancer: a review. Gastric Cancer. 2006;9(2):74–81.
13. Wu C-W, Lo S-S, Shen K-H, Hsieh M-C, Chen J-H, Chiang J-H, et al. Incidence and factors associated with recurrence patterns after intended curative surgery for gastric cancer. World J Surg. 2003;27(2):153–8.

14. Angelica MD, Gonen M, Brennan MF. Patterns of initial recurrence in completely resected gastric adenocarcinoma. Ann Surg. 2004;240(5):808–16.

15. Spolverato G, Ejaz A, Kim Y, Squires MH, Poultsides GA, Fields RC, et al. Rates and patterns of recurrence after curative intent resection for gastric cancer: a United States multi-institutional analysis. J Am Coll Surg. 2014;219(4):664–75.

16. Liang H, Wang D, Sun D, Pan Y, Liu Y, Deng J, et al. Investigation of the recurrence patterns of gastric cancer following a curative resection. Surg Today. 2011;41(2):210–5.

17. Bilici A, Selcukbiricik F. Prognostic significance of the recurrence pattern and risk factors for recurrence in patients with proximal gastric cancer who underwent curative gastrectomy. Tumor Biol. 2015;36:6191–9.

18. Marrelli D, De Stefano A, de Manzoni G, Morgagni P, Di Leo A, Roviello F. Prediction of recurrence after radical surgery for gastric cancer. Ann Surg. 2005;241(2):247–55.

19. Barchi LC, Yagi OK, Jacob CE, Mucerino DR, Ribeiro U, Marrelli D, et al. Predicting recurrence after curative resection for gastric cancer: external validation of the Italian Research Group for Gastric Cancer (GIRCG) prognostic scoring system. Eur J Surg Oncol. 2016;42(1):123–31.

20. Alnoor M, Boys JA, Worrell SG, Oh DS, Hagen JA, DeMeester SR. Timing and pattern of recurrence after gastrectomy for adenocarcinoma. Am Surg. 2015. Oct [cited 2016 Jan 16];81(10):1057–60.

21. Youn HG, An JY, Choi MG, Noh JH, Sohn TS. Recurrence after curative resection of early gastric cancer. Ann Surg Oncol. 2010;85(2009):448–54.

22. Nakagawa M, Kojima K, Inokuchi M, Kato K, Sugita H, Kawano T, et al. Patterns, timing and risk factors of recurrence of gastric cancer after laparoscopic gastrectomy: reliable results. Eur J Surg Oncol.. Elsevier Ltd. 2014;40(10):1376–82.

23. Lai JF, Kim S, Kim K, Li C, Oh SJ, Hyung WJ, et al. Prediction of recurrence of early gastric cancer after curative resection. Ann Surg Oncol. 2009;16(7):1896–902.

24. Koga S, Takebayashi M, Kaibara N, Nishidoi H, Kimura O, Kawasumi H, et al. Pathological characteristics of gastric cancer that develop hematogenous recurrence, with special reference to the site of recurrence. J Surg Oncol. 1987;36(4):239–42.

25. Li J-H, Zhang S-W, Liu J, Shao M-Z, Chen L. Review of clinical investigation on recurrence of gastric cancer following curative resection. Chin Med J. 2012;125(8):1479–95.

26. Otsuji E, Kobayashi S, Okamoto K, Hagiwara A, Yamagishi H. Is timing of death from tumor recurrence predictable after curative resection for gastric cancer ? World J Surg. 2001;25:1373–6.

27. de Liaño AD, Yarnoz C, Aguilar R, Artieda C, Ortiz H. Surgical treatment of recurrent gastric cancer. Gastric Cancer. 2008;11(1):10–4.

28. Song K-Y, Park S-M, Kim S-N, Park C-H. The role of surgery in the treatment of recurrent gastric cancer. Am J Surg. 2008;196(1):19–22.

29. Lehnert T, Rudek B, Buhl K, Golling M. Surgical therapy for loco-regional recurrence and distant metastasis of gastric cancer. Eur J Surg Oncol. 2002;28(4):455–61.

30. Kodera Y, Ito S, Yamamura Y, Mochizuki Y, Fujiwara M, Hibi K, et al. Follow-up surveillance for recurrence after curative gastric cancer surgery lacks survival benefit. Ann Surg Oncol. 2003;10(8):898–902.

31. Böhner H, Zimmer T, Hopfenmüller W, Berger G, Buhr HJ. Detection and prognosis of recurrent gastric cancer—is routine follow-up after gastrectomy worthwhile? Hepato-Gastroenterology. 2000;47(35):1489–94.

32. Kattan MW, Karpeh MS, Mazumdar M, Brennan MF. Postoperative nomogram for disease-specific survival after an R0 resection for gastric carcinoma. J Clin Oncol. 2003;21(19):3647–50.

33. Han D-S, Suh Y-S, Kong S-H, Lee H-J, Choi Y, Aikou S, et al. Nomogram predicting long-term survival after d2 gastrectomy for gastric cancer. J Clin Oncol. 2012;30(31):3834–40.

34. Kim Y, Spolverato G, Ejaz A, Squires MH, Poultsides G, Fields RC, et al. A nomogram to predict overall survival and disease-free survival after curative resection of gastric adenocarcinoma. Ann Surg Oncol. 2015;22(6):1828–35.

35. Marrelli D, Morgagni P, de Manzoni G, Marchet A, Baiocchi GL, Giacopuzzi S, et al. External validation of a score predictive of recurrence after radical surgery for non-cardia gastric cancer: results of a follow-up study. J Am Coll Surg. 2015;221(2):280–90.

36. Kinkel K, Lu Y, Both M, Warren RS, Thoeni RF. Detection of hepatic metastases from cancers of the gastrointestinal tract by using noninvasive imaging methods (US, CT, MR imaging, PET): a meta-analysis. Radiology. 2002;224(3):748–56.

37. Meyers MA, McSweeney J. Secondary neoplasms of the bowel. Radiology. 1972;105(1):1–11.

38. Kim J-H, Jang Y-J, Park S-S, Park S-H, Mok Y-J. Benefit of post-operative surveillance for recurrence after curative resection for gastric cancer. J Gastrointest Surg. 2010;14(6):969–76.

39. Yoo SY, Kim KW, Han JK, Kim AY, Lee HJ, Choi BI. Helical CT of postoperative patients with gastric carcinoma: value in evaluating surgical complications and tumor recurrence. Abdom Imaging. 2003;28(5):617–23.

40. Lim JS, Yun MJ, Kim M-J, Hyung WJ, Park M-S, Choi J-Y, et al. CT and PET in stomach cancer: preoperative staging and monitoring of response to therapy. Radiographics. 26(1):143–56.

41. De Potter T, Flamen P, Van Cutsem E, Penninckx F, Filez L, Bormans G, et al. Whole-body PET with FDG for the diagnosis of recurrent gastric cancer. Eur J Nucl Med Mol Imaging. 2002;29(4):525–9.

42. Kim KW, Choi BI, Han JK, Kim TK, Kim AY, Lee HJ, et al. Postoperative anatomic and pathologic findings at CT following gastrectomy. Radiographics. 22(2):323–36.

43. Insko EK, Levine MS, Birnbaum BA, Jacobs JE. Benign and malignant lesions of the stomach: evaluation of CT criteria for differentiation. Radiology. 2003;228(1):166–71.

44. Kim IY, Kim SW, Shin HC, Lee MS, Jeong DJ, Kim CJ, et al. MRI of gastric carcinoma: results of T and N-staging in an in vitro study. World J Gastroenterol. 2009;15(32):3992–8.

45. Mocellin S, Marchet A, Nitti D. EUS for the staging of gastric cancer: a meta-analysis. Gastrointest Endosc. 2011;73(6):1122–34.

46. Jadvar H, Tatlidil R, Garcia AA, Conti PS. Evaluation of recurrent gastric malignancy with [F-18]-FDG positron emission tomography. Clin Radiol. 2003;58(3):215–21.

47. Bilici A, Ustaalioglu BBO, Seker M, Kefeli U, Canpolat N, Tekinsoy B, et al. The role of ^{18}F-FDG PET/CT in the assessment of suspected recurrent gastric cancer after initial surgical resection: can the results of FDG PET/CT influence patients' treatment decision making? Eur J Nucl Med Mol Imaging. 2011;38(1):64–73.

48. Graziosi L, Bugiantella W, Cavazzoni E, Cantarella F, Porcari M, Baffa N, et al. Role of FDG-PET/CT in follow-up of patients treated with resective gastric surgery for tumour. Ann Ital Chir. 2011;82(2):125–9.

49. Sim SH, Kim YJ, Oh D-Y, Lee S-H, Kim D-W, Kang WJ, et al. The role of PET/CT in detection of gastric cancer recurrence. BMC Cancer. 2009;9:73.

50. Shim JH, Yoo HM, Lee HH, Kim JG, Jeon HM, Song KY, et al. Use of laparoscopy as an alternative to computed tomography (CT) and positron emission tomography (PET) scans for the detection of recurrence in patients with gastric cancer: a pilot study. Surg Endosc. 2011;25(10):3338–44.

51. Inoue K, Nakane Y, Michiura T, Yamaki S, Yui R, Sakuramoto K, et al. Feasibility and accuracy of second-look laparoscopy after gastrectomy for gastric cancer. Surg Endosc. 2009;23(10):2307–13.

52. Leung WK, Wu M, Kakugawa Y, Kim JJ, Yeoh K, Goh KL, et al. Screening for gastric cancer in Asia: current evidence and practice. Lancet Oncol. 2008;9(3):279–87.

53. Kim Y, Jun JK, Choi KS, Lee H-Y, Park E-C. Overview of the national cancer screening programme and the cancer screening status in Korea. Asian Pac J Cancer Prev. 2011;12(3):725–30.

54. Hamashima C, Ogoshi K, Narisawa R, Kishi T, Kato T, Fujita K, et al. Impact of endoscopic screening on mortality reduction from gastric cancer. World J Gastroenterol. 2015;21(8):2460–6.

55. Tashiro A, Sano M, Kinameri K, Fujita K, Takeuchi Y. Comparing mass screening techniques for gastric cancer in Japan. World J Gastroenterol. 2006;12(30):4873–4.

56. Dan YY, So JBY, Yeoh KG. Endoscopic screening for gastric cancer. Clin Gastroenterol Hepatol. 2006;4(6):709–16.

57. Hosokawa O, Kaizaki Y, Watanabe K, Hattori M, Douden K, Hayashi H, et al. Endoscopic surveillance for gastric remnant cancer after early cancer surgery. Endoscopy. 2002;34(6):469–73.

58. Morgagni P, Gardini A, Marrelli D, Vittimberga G, Marchet A, de Manzoni G, et al. Gastric stump carcinoma after distal subtotal gastrectomy for early gastric cancer: experience of 541 patients with long-term follow-up. Am J Surg.. Elsevier Inc. 2015;209(6):1063–8.

59. Yamamoto M, Yamanaka T, Baba H, Kakeji Y, Maehara Y. The postoperative recurrence and the occurrence of second primary carcinomas in patients with early gastric carcinoma. J Surg Oncol. 2008;97(3):231–5.

60. Sano T. Recurrence of early gastric cancer follow-up of 1475 patients and review of the Japanese literature. Cancer. 1993;72(11):3174–8.

61. Greene FL. Management of gastric remnant carcinoma based on the results of a 15-year endoscopic screening program. Ann Surg. 1996;223(6):701–6.. discussion 706–8.

62. Kodera Y, Yamamura Y, Torii A, Uesaka K, Hirai T, Yasui K, et al. Gastric remnant carcinoma after partial gastrectomy for benign and malignant gastric lesions. J Am Coll Surg. 1996;182(1):1–6.

63. Ohashi M, Katai H, Fukagawa T, Gotoda T, Sano T, Sasako M. Cancer of the gastric stump following distal gastrectomy for cancer. Br J Surg. 2007;94(1):92–5.

64. Kunisaki C, Shimada H, Nomura M, Hosaka N, Akiyama H, Ookubo K, et al. Lymph node dissection in surgical treatment for remnant stomach cancer. Hepato-Gastroenterology. 49(44):580–4.

65. Sinning C, Schaefer N, Standop J, Hirner A, Wolff M. Gastric stump carcinoma – epidemiology and current concepts in pathogenesis and treatment. Eur J Surg Oncol. 2007;33(2):133–9.

66. Lee S-Y, Lee JH, Hwang NC, Kim Y-H, Rhee P-L, Kim JJ, et al. The role of follow-up endoscopy after total gastrectomy for gastric cancer. Eur J Surg Oncol. 2005;31(3):265–9.

67. Uedo N, Takeuchi Y, Ishihara R. Endoscopic management of early gastric cancer: endoscopic mucosal resection or endoscopic submucosal dissection: data from a Japanese high-volume center and literature review. Ann Gastroenterol Q Publ Hell Soc Gastroenterol. 2012;25(4):281–90.

68. Nakajima T, Oda I, Gotoda T, Hamanaka H, Eguchi T, Yokoi C, et al. Metachronous gastric cancers after endoscopic resection: how effective is annual endoscopic surveillance? Gastric Cancer. 2006;9(2):93–8.

69. Kato M, Nishida T, Yamamoto K, Hayashi S, Kitamura S, Yabuta T, et al. Scheduled endoscopic surveillance controls secondary cancer after curative endoscopic resection for early gastric cancer: a multicentre retrospective cohort study by Osaka University ESD study group. Gut. 2013;62:1425–32.

70. Nasu J, Doi T, Endo H, Nishina T, S. Hirasaki IH. Characteristics of metachronous multiple early gastric cancers after endoscopic mucosal resection. Endoscopy. 2005;37(10):990–3.

71. Abe S, Oda I, Suzuki H, Nonaka S, Yoshinaga S, Nakajima T, et al. Long-term surveillance and treatment outcomes of metachronous gastric cancer occurring after curative endoscopic submucosal dissection. Endoscopy. 2015;47:1113–8.
72. Reiter W, Stieber P, Reuter C, Nagel D, Cramer C, Pahl H, et al. Prognostic value of preoperative serum levels of CEA, CA 19-9 and CA 72-4 in gastric carcinoma. Anticancer Res. 17(4B):2903–6.
73. Marrelli D, Roviello F, De Stefano A, Farnetani M, Garosi L, Messano A, et al. Prognostic significance of CEA, CA 19-9 and CA 72-4 preoperative serum levels in gastric carcinoma. Oncology. 1999;57(1):55–62.
74. Aloe S, D'Alessandro R, Spila A, Ferroni P, Basili S, Palmirotta R, et al. Prognostic value of serum and tumor tissue CA 72-4 content in gastric cancer. Int J Biol Markers. 18(1):21–7.
75. Ucar E, Semerci E, Ustun H, Yetim T, Huzmeli C, Gullu M. Prognostic value of preoperative CEA, CA 19-9, CA 72-4, and AFP levels in gastric cancer. Adv Ther. 2008;25(10):1075–84.
76. Nakane Y, Okamura S, Akehira K, Boku T, Okusa T, Tanaka K, et al. Correlation of preoperative carcinoembryonic antigen levels and prognosis of gastric cancer patients. Cancer. 1994;73(11):2703–8.
77. Fletcher RH. Carcinoembryonic antigen. Ann Intern Med. 1986;104(1):66–73.
78. Goldstein MJ, Mitchell EP. Carcinoembryonic antigen in the staging and follow-up of patients with colorectal cancer. Cancer Investig. 2005 Jan;23(4):338–51.
79. Muraro R, Kuroki M, Wunderlich D, Poole DJ, Colcher D, Thor A, et al. Generation and characterization of B72.3 second generation monoclonal antibodies reactive with the tumor-associated glycoprotein 72 antigen. Cancer Res. 1988;48(16):4588–96.
80. Johnson VG, Schlom J, Paterson AJ, Bennett J, Magnani JL, Colcher D. Analysis of a human tumor-associated glycoprotein (TAG-72) identified by monoclonal antibody B72.3. Cancer Res. 1986;46(2):850–7.
81. Siewert JR, Böttcher K, Stein HJ, Roder JD. Relevant prognostic factors in gastric cancer: ten-year results of the German Gastric Cancer Study. Ann Surg. 1998;228(4):449–61.
82. Kim JP, Kim YW, Yang HK, Noh DY. Significant prognostic factors by multivariate analysis of 3926 gastric cancer patients. World J Surg. 1994;18(6):872–7.. discussion 877–8.
83. Safi F, Kuhns V, Beger HG. Comparison of CA 72-4, CA 19-9 and CEA in the diagnosis and monitoring of gastric cancer. Int J Biol Markers. 1995;10(2):100–6.
84. Takahashi Y, Takeuchi T, Sakamoto J, Touge T, Mai M, Ohkura H, et al. The usefulness of CEA and/or CA19-9 in monitoring for recurrence in gastric cancer patients: a prospective clinical study. Gastric Cancer. 2003;6(3):142–5.
85. Mattar R. Alves de Andrade CR, DiFavero GM, Gama-Rodrigues JJ, Laudanna AA. Preoperative serum levels of CA 72-4, CEA, CA 19-9, and alpha-fetoprotein in patients with gastric cancer. Rev do Hosp das Clínicas. 2002;57(3):89–92.
86. Heptner G, Domschke S, Domschke W. Comparison of CA 72-4 with CA 19-9 and carcinoembryonic antigen in the serodiagnostics of gastrointestinal malignancies. Scand J Gastroenterol. 1989;24(6):745–50.
87. Guadagni F, Roselli M, Amato T, Cosimelli M, Perri P, Casale V, et al. CA 72-4 measurement of tumor-associated glycoprotein 72 (TAG-72) as a serum marker in the management of gastric carcinoma. Cancer Res. 1992;52(5):1222–7.
88. Marrelli D, Pinto E, De Stefano A, Farnetani M, Garosi L, Roviello F. Clinical utility of CEA, CA 19-9, and CA 72-4 in the follow-up of patients with resectable gastric cancer. Am J Surg. 2001;181(1):16–9.
89. Kim DH, Oh SJ, Oh CA, Choi MG, Noh JH, Sohn TS, et al. The relationships between perioperative CEA, CA 19-9, and CA 72-4 and recurrence in gastric cancer patients after curative radical gastrectomy. J Surg Oncol. 2011;104:585–91.
90. D'Ugo D, Biondi A, Tufo A, Persiani R. Follow-up: the evidence. Dig Surg. 2013;30(2):159–68.
91. Tan IT, So BYJ. Value of intensive follow-up of patients after curative surgery for gastric carcinoma. J Surg Oncol. 2007;96(6):503–6.
92. Bilici A, Salman T. Ustaalioglu BBO, Unek T, Seker M, Aliustaoglu M, et al. The prognostic value of detecting symptomatic or asymptomatic recurrence in patients with gastric cancer after a curative gastrectomy. J Surg Res. 2013;180(1):E1–9.
93. Gastric cancer, Version 3.2015, NCCN Clinical Practice Guidelines in Oncology. 2015;
94. Waddell T, Verheij M, Allum W, Cunningham D, Cervantes A, Arnold D. Gastric cancer: ESMO-ESSO-ESTRO clinical practice guidelines for diagnosis, treatment and follow-up. Ann Oncol. 2013;24(suppl 6):vi57–63.
95. Allum WH, Griffin SM, Watson A, Colin-Jones D. Guidelines for the management of oesophageal and gastric cancer. Gut. 2011;60:1449–72.
96. Scottish Intercollegiate Guidelines Network. Management of oesophageal and gastric cancer. (SIGN Guideline No 87). 2006;(June):74.
97. Lee JH, Kim JG, Jung H-K, Kim JH, Jeong WK, Jeon TJ, et al. Clinical practice guidelines for gastric cancer in Korea: an evidence-based approach. J Gastric Cancer. 2014;14(2):87–104.
98. Luca G, Domenico B, Daniel DU, Richard C, Baiocchi GL, Ugo DD, et al. Follow-up after gastrectomy for cancer : the Charter Scaligero Consensus Conference. Gastric Cancer. 2016;19:15–20.
99. Verschuur EML, Steyerberg EW, Tilanus HW, Polinder S, Essink-Bot M-L, Tran KTC, et al. Nurse-led follow-up of patients after oesophageal or gastric cardia cancer surgery: a randomised trial. Br J Cancer. 2009;100(1):70–6.
100. Douglas H-R, Halliday D, Normand C, Corner J, Bath P, Beech N, et al. Economic evaluation of specialist cancer and palliative nursing: Macmillan evaluation study findings. Int J Palliat Nurs. 2003;9(10):429–38.

101. Leary A, Crouch H, Lezard A, Rawcliffe C, Boden L, Richardson A. Dimensions of clinical nurse specialist work in the UK. Nurs Stand. Royal College of Nursing Publishing Company (RCN); 2008;23(15–17):40–45.

102. Cox CL, Ahluwalia S. Enhancing clinical effectiveness among clinical nurse specialists. Br J Nurs. 2000;9(16). 1064–5, 1068–70, 1071–3

103. Sullivan A, Elliott S. Assessing the value of a cancer clinical nurse specialist. Cancer Nurs Pract. Royal College of Nursing Publishing Company (RCN); 2007;6(10):25–29.

104. Catt S, Fallowfield L, Jenkins V, Langridge C, Cox A. The informational roles and psychological health of members of 10 oncology multidisciplinary teams in the UK. Br J Cancer. 2005;93(10):1092–7.

105. Lee JHJ, Sohn I, Do I, Kim K-M, Park SH, Park JO, et al. Nanostring-based multigene assay to predict recurrence for gastric cancer patients after surgery. PLoS One. 2014;9(3):e90133.

106. Yie S, Lou B, Ye S, Cao M, He X, Li P, et al. Detection of survivin-expressing circulating cancer cells (CCCs) in peripheral blood of patients with gastric and colorectal cancer reveals high risks of relapse. Ann Surg Oncol. 2008;15(11):3073–82.

107. Cao W, Yang W, Li H, Lou G, Jiang J, Geng M, et al. Using detection of survivin-expressing circulating tumor cells in peripheral blood to predict tumor recurrence following curative resection of gastric cancer. J Surg Oncol. 2011;103(2):110–5.

108. Kodera Y, Nakanishi H, Ito S, Yamamura Y, Kanemitsu Y, Shimizu Y, et al. Quantitative detection of disseminated free cancer cells in peritoneal washes with real-time reverse transcriptase-polymerase chain reaction: a sensitive predictor of outcome for patients with gastric carcinoma. Ann Surg. 2002;235(4):499–506.

109. Sugita Y, Fujiwara Y, Taniguchi H, Mori T, Ishii T, Niwa H, et al. Quantitative molecular diagnosis of peritoneal lavage fluid for prediction of peritoneal recurrence in gastric cancer. Int J Oncol. 2003;23(5):1419–23.

110. Wang X, Cao W, Mo M, Wang W, Wu H, Wang J. VEGF and cortactin expression are independent predictors of tumor recurrence following curative resection of gastric cancer. J Surg Oncol. 2010;102(4):325–30.

111. Aoyagi K, Kouhuji K, Yano S, Miyagi M, Imaizumi T, Takeda J, et al. VEGF significance in peritoneal recurrence from gastric cancer. Gastric Cancer. 2005;8(3):155–63.

112. Zhong X-Y, Zhang L-H, Jia S-Q, Shi T, Niu Z-J, Du H, et al. Positive association of up-regulated Cripto-1 and down-regulated E-cadherin with tumour progression and poor prognosis in gastric cancer. Histopathology. 2008;52(5):560–8.

113. He Q, Chen J, Lin H, Hu P, Chen M. Expression of peroxisome proliferator-activated receptor gamma, E-cadherin and matrix metalloproteinases-2 in gastric carcinoma and lymph node metastases. Chin Med J. 2007;120(17):1498–504.

114. Chen H-C, Chu RY, Hsu P-N, Hsu PI, Lu J-Y, Lai K-H, et al. Loss of E-cadherin expression correlates with poor differentiation and invasion into adjacent organs in gastric adenocarcinomas. Cancer Lett. 2003;201(1):97–106.

115. An JY, Kim KM, Choi MG, Noh JH, Sohn TS, Bae JM, et al. Prognostic role of p-mTOR expression in cancer tissues and metastatic lymph nodes in pT2b gastric cancer. Int J Cancer. 2010;126(12):2904–13.

116. Zhang X, Yan Z, Zhang J, Gong L, Li W, Cui J, et al. Combination of hsa-miR-375 and hsa-miR-142-5p as a predictor for recurrence risk in gastric cancer patients following surgical resection. Ann Oncol. 2011;22(10):2257–66.

Part XVI

Neoadjuvant and Adjuvant Treatments for Gastric Cancer

Neoadjuvant Treatment for Gastric Cancer

29

Sook Ryun Park and Yoon-Koo Kang

Rationale of Neoadjuvant Treatment

Although advances in surgical treatment have improved survival outcomes in patients with localized gastric cancer, the high recurrence rates even after curative resection require a multimodal approach. In recent decades, significant progress has been made in the area of multidisciplinary treatments for gastric cancer. Of note, these multimodality multidisciplinary approaches have developed differently according to geographical regions, which are differently affected by disease incidences, clinicopathological features, surgical techniques, and treatment outcomes (e.g., curative resection rate, relapse patterns, and survival outcomes). Three different multimodal approaches have been based on the timing of treatment relative to surgery: preoperative (neoadjuvant), postoperative (adjuvant), and perioperative (neoadjuvant plus adjuvant) treatment. The neoadjuvant approach has mainly been pursued in Western countries where locally advanced disease and gastroesophageal junction (GEJ) or proximal gastric cancers are common, curative resection rates are relatively low, and surgical outcomes remain suboptimal [1–4]. In contrast, in East Asian countries such as Korea and Japan, where relatively high curative resection rates are achieved and local tumor control is adequate with standard D2 lymphadenectomy, adjuvant chemotherapy is the main strategy adopted for curatively resected gastric cancer.

Neoadjuvant treatment for gastric cancer has several potential advantages: (1) Preoperative therapy could downsize or downstage tumors, thus enhancing curative resectability; (2) neoadjuvant systemic chemotherapy could reduce the incidence of systemic metastasis by eradicating undetectable micrometastasis at an early point in the disease course; (3) preoperative treatment could be administered with a higher likelihood of treatment completion than postoperative treatment because presurgical patients are more likely to tolerate treatments due to good performance, whereas postoperative therapy may be not given in a timely manner and with adequate dose-intensity because of surgical complications; and (4) treatment responses to neoadjuvant therapy can be assessed clinically or pathologically, which could allow an early evaluation of therapeutic effectiveness and prognostic information.

Neoadjuvant Chemotherapy

Neoadjuvant chemotherapeutic strategies have been investigated in the context of preoperative therapy alone or perioperative therapy

S. R. Park · Y.-K. Kang (✉)
Department of Oncology, Asan Medical Center,
University of Ulsan College of Medicine,
Seoul, Republic of Korea
e-mail: ykkang@amc.seoul.kr

© Springer-Verlag GmbH Germany, part of Springer Nature 2019
S. H. Noh, W. J. Hyung (eds.), *Surgery for Gastric Cancer*,
https://doi.org/10.1007/978-3-662-45583-8_29

comprising combined pre- and postoperative chemotherapy. Two prospective randomized trials comparing neoadjuvant chemotherapy plus surgery with surgery alone were conducted in patients with resectable gastric or GEJ cancer [5, 6]. Unfortunately, these two trials were likely underpowered because of small sample sizes. A randomized study conducted by the Dutch Gastric Cancer Group compared four cycles of neoadjuvant chemotherapy (5-fluorouracil, leucovorin, doxorubicin, and methotrexate [FAMTX] in a 4-week cycle) with surgery alone in patients with resectable gastric cancer (except T1) with the intent to demonstrate improved curative resectability with neoadjuvant chemotherapy [5]. However, this study was terminated early after 59 patients were randomized because of slow accrual and poor interim results. Notably, 44% of patients in the neoadjuvant arm were unable to complete all four cycles because of disease progression (26%) or chemotherapy toxicity (18%). The results demonstrated that neoadjuvant chemotherapy did not increase the curative resection rate (67% in the neoadjuvant arm vs. 66% in the surgery alone arm) or 5-year overall survival (OS) rate (21% vs. 34%, respectively; $P = 0.17$). Another randomized study, European Organisation for Research and Treatment of Cancer (EORTC) 40954, compared two cycles of neoadjuvant chemotherapy (biweekly cisplatin, weekly folinic acid, and infusional fluorouracil in a 7-week cycle) with surgery alone in patients with locally advanced (stages III and IV[cM0]) adenocarcinoma of the stomach and GEJ [6]. Although this trial was also terminated prematurely for poor accrual after 114 patients were randomized, the neoadjuvant chemotherapy arm had a higher R0 curative resection rate (81.9% vs. 66.7%; $P = 0.036$) and lower lymph node metastases rate (61.4% vs. 76.5%; $P = 0.018$) than did the surgery alone arm. However, neoadjuvant chemotherapy was associated with a higher postoperative complication rate (27.1% vs. 16.2%; $P = 0.09$) than surgery alone and failed to demonstrate benefits

in terms of OS (hazard ratio [HR], 0.84; 95% confidence interval [CI], 0.52–1.35; $P = 0.466$) or progression-free survival (PFS) (HR, 0.76; 95% CI, 0.49–1.16; $P = 0.20$). Only 62.5% of patients assigned to the chemotherapy arm completed the planned two treatment cycles, and most patients (>92% in both arms) underwent extensive D2 lymphadenectomy, which might have diluted the contributions of neoadjuvant chemotherapy to the treatment outcomes.

The randomized phase III study conducted by the Swiss Group for Clinical Cancer Research (SAKK 43/99) compared neoadjuvant vs. adjuvant docetaxel/cisplatin/fluorouracil (TCF) in patients with cT3–T4 anyN M0 or anyT cN1–N3 M0 gastric carcinomas that were staged using endoscopic ultrasonography, computed tomography, bone scans, and laparoscopy [7, 8]. Four cycles of chemotherapy were administered in a 3-week cycle either before or after gastrectomy. This study was also prematurely terminated because of slow accrual, and only 69 patients were randomized. Ninety percent of the patients underwent D2 or greater lymphadenectomy, and the incidences of surgical morbidity (28.5% for neoadjuvant therapy vs. 25.7% for adjuvant therapy; $P = 0.86$) and mortality (0% vs. 5.7%, respectively) were similar between the groups. The neoadjuvant chemotherapy group exhibited better treatment compliance (median number of cycles, four vs. three, $P < 0.01$; four-cycle completion rate, 76% vs. 38%), compared with the adjuvant chemotherapy group. Although neoadjuvant chemotherapy resulted in pathologic complete responses (pCRs; 12%) and partial responses (53%), it neither increased the curative R0 resection rate (85% for neoadjuvant therapy vs. 91% for adjuvant therapy) nor decreased the pathologic stage (stage I/II, 9% for both groups). Furthermore, there were no differences in event-free survival (EFS) (5-year EFS, 44.1% for neoadjuvant therapy vs. 43.5% for adjuvant therapy; HR, 0.79; 95% CI, 0.43–1.45; $P = 0.5$) or OS (5-year OS; 47% vs. 46%, respectively; $P = 0.5$) between the treatment groups.

Perioperative Chemotherapy

Two randomized phase III trials were conducted in Western countries to evaluate the impact of perioperative chemotherapy before and after surgery for resectable gastric, GEJ, or esophageal adenocarcinoma [9, 10]. The United Kingdom Medical Research Council Adjuvant Gastric Infusional Chemotherapy (MAGIC) trial was the first large-scale randomized controlled study to demonstrate survival benefits of perioperative chemotherapy in gastric or GEJ cancer [9]. A total of 503 patients with adenocarcinoma of the stomach (74% of patients), GEJ (15%), or distal esophagus (11%) were randomized to receive surgery plus perioperative chemotherapy (three cycles each of epirubicin/cisplatin/continuously infused 5-fluorouracil [ECF] in a 3-week cycle before and after surgery) or surgery alone. Patients were required to have resectable stage II or higher disease as determined by computed tomography, chest radiography, ultrasonography, or laparoscopy. Surgery was performed in 91.6% of patients in the chemotherapy group and 96.4% of patients in the surgery-alone group. Although the curative resection rate did not differ between the treatment groups (69.3% in the chemotherapy group vs. 66.4% in the surgery group), the perioperative chemotherapy group exhibited a significant improvement in PFS (HR, 0.66; 95% CI, 0.53–0.81; $P < 0.001$) and OS (HR, 0.75; 95% CI, 0.60–0.93; 5-year OS 36.3% vs. 23.0%; $P = 0.009$). The perioperative chemotherapy group also had lower rates of local recurrence (14.4% vs. 20.6%) and distant metastases (24.4% vs. 36.8%) than did the surgery alone group. In addition, the perioperative chemotherapy group had a significantly smaller resected tumor size (the median maximum diameter, 3 cm vs. 5 cm, $P < 0.001$) and lower pathologic stage (T1/T2, 51.7% vs. 36.8%, $P = 0.002$; N0/N1, 84.4% vs. 70.5%, $P = 0.01$). Of note, the incidence of postoperative complications (45.7% in the chemotherapy group and 45.3% in the surgery group), mortality rate within 30 days (5.6% and 5.9%, respectively), and median hospital stay (13 days in both groups) were similar in the two groups.

Another French phase III randomized study conducted by the Fédération Nationale des Centres de Lutte Contre le Cancer (FNCLCC)/Fédération Francophone de Cancérologie Digestive (FFCD) (FNCLCC/FFCD 9703) confirmed the survival benefits of perioperative chemotherapy in patients with resectable gastric cancer [10]. A total of 224 patients with adenocarcinoma of the stomach (25%), GEJ (64%), or distal esophagus (11%) were randomized to receive surgery plus perioperative chemotherapy (cisplatin plus 5-fluorouracil [CF] in a 4-week cycle comprising 2 or 3 preoperative cycles and 3 or 4 postoperative cycles for a total of 6 cycles) or surgery alone. The patient inclusion criterion was a disease suitable for curative resection as evaluated by endoscopy, barium meal study, abdominal and thoracic computed tomography, and optional endoscopic ultrasonography. Surgery was performed in 96.5% of patients in the chemotherapy group and 99% in the surgery-alone group. Similar to the MAGIC trial, significant improvements in disease-free survival (DFS) (5-year DFS, 34% vs. 19%; HR, 0.65; 95% CI, 0.48–0.89; $P = 0.003$) and OS (5-year OS, 38% vs. 24%; HR, 0.69; 95% CI, 0.50–0.95; $P = 0.02$) were observed in the perioperative chemotherapy group, compared to the surgery-alone group. Furthermore, the perioperative chemotherapy group had a significantly higher curative resection rate (87% vs. 74%; $P = 0.04$) and a trend toward a reduced lymph node metastasis rate according to surgical pathology (N+, 67% vs. 80%; $P = 0.054$) than did the surgery alone group; however, the pathologic T-stage distribution did not significantly differ between the groups (T0–T2, 42% in the chemotherapy group vs. 32% in the surgery alone group; $P = 0.17$). Distant metastasis occurred less frequently in the chemotherapy group than in the surgery-alone group (43% vs. 56%), although the locoregional recurrence rates were similar (25% vs. 26%). The incidences of postoperative morbidity (25.7% in the chemotherapy group vs. 19.1% in the surgery group; $P = 0.24$) and 30-day mortality (4.6% vs. 4.5%, respectively; $P = 0.76$) were also similar.

Based on the survival benefits demonstrated in the MAGIC and FNCLCC/FFCD 9703 trials, perioperative chemotherapy was established as a standard treatment for resectable gastric cancer in Western countries. The National Comprehensive Cancer Network guidelines recommend perioperative chemotherapy plus surgery in patients with clinically T2 or higher, potentially resectable gastric cancer, although postoperative chemotherapy or chemoradiation is also recommended if patients underwent R0 resection without preoperative therapy (version 3. 2015, http://www.nccn.org/professionals/physician_gls/pdf/gastric.pdf). According to the American College of Surgeons National Cancer Database, the use of neoadjuvant chemotherapy increased over time in the United States, from 25.9% in 2003 to 46.3% in 2012 [11]. A survey of curative treatment provided for 4668 resectable esophagogastric cancer cases in 5 European countries during the period of 2011–2012 revealed neoadjuvant chemotherapy administration rates that ranged from 22% to 51% [12].

However, despite the proven survival benefits of perioperative chemotherapy, this approach was not accepted as a standard therapy in East Asian countries such as Korea and Japan because of criticisms regarding the MAGIC and FNCLCC/FFCD 9703 trials. First, an issue of surgical quality, particularly the extent of lymphadenectomy, was raised. After a long period of debate, D2 lymphadenectomy was established as the standard surgical procedure in both Eastern and Western countries based on its survival benefit relative to limited dissection, when applied in experienced centers [13, 14]. Although both the MAGIC and FNCLCC/FFCD 9703 trials recommended D2 lymphadenectomy as the protocol treatment, this procedure was performed only in 41.4% of patients who underwent surgery in the MAGIC study and 61.9% of gastric cancer patients in the FNCLCC/FFCD 9703 study [9, 10]. This limited D2 lymphadenectomy rate might have partly contributed to the relatively high rates of locoregional recurrence with surgery alone in these trials (20.6% in the MAGIC and 26% in the FNCLCC/FFCD 9703), which

contrasted to the low rates of locoregional recurrence (<10%) in Korea and Japan, where D2 lymphadenectomy is routinely performed [15, 16]. Another surgical issue involved the rate of curative resection in patients considered to have potentially resectable gastric cancer during preoperative staging. Although this rate was reported to be approximately 90% in Eastern series [17, 18], only 66.4% and 74% of patients who underwent surgery alone in the MAGIC and FNCLCC/FFCD 9703 trials, respectively, were able to undergo curative resection [9, 10]. Besides differences in surgical techniques, this discrepancy is likely associated with the higher proportion of advanced stage cases at presentation in Western countries, as the curative resection rate decreased significantly as the clinical T stage (T1, 99.6%; T2, 96.1%; T3, 75.3%; T4, 46.3%; $P < 0.001$) and N stage (N0, 96.1%; N1–N2, 82.1%; $P < 0.001$) increased, according to the sixth edition of the American Joint Committee on Cancer (AJCC) staging system [17]. In addition, the 5-year OS rates following surgery alone in both the MAGIC (23.0%) and FNCLCC/FFCD 9703 studies (24%) were much lower than those reported for Eastern studies (61.1–69%), despite considering the different clinical setting; specifically potentially resectable disease was evaluated in the MAGIC and FNCLCC/FFCD 9703 studies, whereas curatively resected disease was evaluated in Eastern studies [9, 10, 15, 16]. Although the MAGIC and FNCLCC/FFCD 9703 trials both included pre- and postoperative chemotherapy, postoperative therapy was poorly administered, in contrast to preoperative therapy. Among patients assigned to the chemotherapy group, preoperative chemotherapy was completed as planned in 86.0% (MAGIC) and 86.7% of patients (FNCLCC/FFCD 9703), whereas postoperative chemotherapy was initiated in only 54.8% (MAGIC) and 47.8% of patients (FNCLCC/FFCD 9703), resulting in a poor six-cycle perioperative chemotherapy completion rate (approximately 40%) in both trials [9, 10]. Moreover, both studies faced the challenge of disease heterogeneity, as the cases comprised gastric, GEJ, and distal esophageal adenocarcinoma. The trials were originally designed to recruit only gastric adenocarcinoma (MAGIC) or distal esophagus/GEJ cancer (FNCLCC/FFCD 9703) but were extended to include tumors of the distal esophagus/GEJ and stomach, respectively, because of issues related to timely recruitment. Lastly, both trials encountered challenges regarding pretreatment clinical staging. The inaccuracy of preoperative staging before neoadjuvant therapy, a consequence of the lack of sufficiently reliable staging methods, may lead to unnecessary preoperative treatment in patients with clinically overestimated tumors. In addition, the clinical stage, which might reflect the tumor burden and prognosis, was not stratified at the time of randomization [17].

Recent clinical trials have explored approaches toward improving perioperative chemotherapy for resectable gastric cancer. A German randomized phase II/III study (AIO-sto-0210 FLOT4) is currently comparing a perioperative triplet regimen comprising fluorouracil, leucovorin, oxaliplatin, and docetaxel (FLOT; four cycles each in a 2-week cycle both pre- and postsurgery) with perioperative ECF (or capecitabine [X] instead of fluorouracil; three cycles each in a 3-week cycle pre- and postsurgery) for cT2–T4 anyN M0 or anyT N + M0 resectable gastric or GEJ adenocarcinoma (NCT01216644). Phase II of this study, which included 127 patients with gastric cancer (47.9%) and 138 patients with GEJ cancer (52.1%) and designated pCR rate as the primary endpoint, demonstrated a significantly higher pCR rate in the FLOT arm than in the ECF(X) arm (15.6% vs. 5.8%; $P = 0.015$) [19].

A randomized phase II/III United Kingdom Medical Research Council MAGIC-B/ST03 study compared perioperative epirubicin, cisplatin, and capecitabine (ECX, each three cycles, pre- and postsurgery) with or without bevacizumab (B), a monoclonal antibody that targets vascular endothelial growth factor A, in 1063 patients with resectable stage Ib–IV(M0) adenocarcinoma of the lower esophagus (14%), GEJ (51%), or stomach (36%) [20]. All six perioperative chemotherapy cycles were completed by 40% of patients in the ECX arm and 37% in the ECX-B arm, including three cycles of preopera-

tive therapy (89% and 88% of patients, respectively) and three cycles of postoperative therapy (73% and 77% of patients, respectively). The addition of bevacizumab to the perioperative chemotherapy regimen did not improve OS (median, 33.97 months with ECX vs. 34.46 with ECX-B; HR, 1.067; $P = 0.4784$), DFS (HR, 1.006; $P = 0.9425$), or PFS (HR, 1.026; $P = 0.7683$). There were also no differences in the R0 resection (75% with ECX vs. 76% with ECX-B), clinical response (42% vs. 40%, respectively), and pCR rates (8% vs. 10%, respectively). Although the addition of bevacizumab did not increase the toxicity attributed to chemotherapy (grade ≥ 3 toxicity, 47% with ECX vs. 50% with ECX-B during preoperative chemotherapy and 49% vs. 54%, respectively, during postoperative chemotherapy), preoperative bevacizumab administration was associated with an increased risk of postoperative anastomotic leak (9% with ECX vs. 18% with ECX-B), particularly in patients who underwent esophagogastrectomy (9% vs. 23%, respectively).

In East Asia, an approach involving the addition of preoperative chemotherapy to adjuvant chemotherapy in the setting of D2 surgery was evaluated in a randomized study of 107 locally advanced gastric cancer patients with decreased mobility on upper gastrointestinal series and/or pancreas invasion on computed tomography scans who were randomized to receive two or three cycles of neoadjuvant chemotherapy (cisplatin, etoposide, and 5-fluorouracil [PEF] in a 3-week cycle; CS arm) or upfront surgery (S arm). In both arms, adjuvant chemotherapy with three to six cycles of PEF was administered according to the postoperative stage (three cycles for curatively resected cases and six cycles for not curatively resected cases) [21]. Although the CS arm had a higher curative resection rate (81% vs. 61%; $P = 0.03$) and greater pathologic downstaging (CS arm vs. S arm; stages 0 and 4 vs. 0; IA, 1 vs. 0; IB, 3 vs. 0; II, 6 vs. 9; IIIA, 14 vs. 10; IIIB, 9 vs. 12; IV, 10 vs. 23; $P = 0.035$) than did the S arm, there was no significant difference in OS between the two arms (median, 33 months vs. 32 months; $P = 0.42$). These results contrasted with the survival benefits obtained from perioperative chemotherapy vs. surgery alone in the MAGIC and FNCLCC/FFCD 9703 trials. However, considering the small sample size and inclusion of only locally advanced cases in the East Asian study, the effect of neoadjuvant chemotherapy on resectable gastric cancer in the setting of D2 surgery followed by standard adjuvant chemotherapy remains to be elucidated. Large-scale phase III trials are currently in progress to clarify this issue. In the Korean PRODIGY study (NCT01515748), patients with

resectable cT2–T3/N+ or T4/anyN gastric or GEJ adenocarcinoma are randomized to receive preoperative docetaxel/oxaliplatin/S-1 followed by D2 surgery and postoperative S-1 or surgery followed by postoperative S-1 [22, 23]. In addition, ongoing Chinese phase III studies are comparing perioperative chemotherapy vs. adjuvant chemotherapy using various chemotherapy regimens or different chemotherapy regimens in a perioperative setting (Table 29.1).

Although the MAGIC-B/ST03 study failed to demonstrate a benefit of bevacizumab, active

Table 29.1 Representative ongoing randomized phase III studies of neoadjuvant or perioperative chemo(radio)therapy in resectable localized gastric cancer

ClinicalTrials.gov identifier (study name)	Country	Stage	Treatment	No.	Primary endpoint
Chemotherapy					
NCT01216644	Germany	cT2–T4 or N+ M0 Resectable gastric or GEJ adenocarcinoma	Perioperative FLOT	714	OS
			Perioperative ECF(X)		
NCT01364376 (FOCUS)	China	Locally advanced gastric cancer with invasion or penetration of serosa	Perioperative SOX	583	OS
			Perioperative FOLFOX		
NCT01515748 (PRODIGY)	Korea	cT2–T3/N + M0, T4/anyN M0, resectable gastric or GEJ adenocarcinoma	Preoperative DOS → D2 surgery → postoperative S-1	530	PFS
			D2 surgery → postoperative S-1		
NCT01516944	China	Resectable cT3–T4/ NxM0 gastric or GEJ adenocarcinoma	Perioperative SOX	729	DFS
			Perioperative XELOX		
			Postoperative SOX		
NCT01534546	China	Potentially resectable T4N + M0	Preoperative SOX → D2 surgery → postoperative SOX five cycles then S-1 three cycles	1059	DFS
			D2 surgery → postoperative SOX eight cycles		
			D2 surgery → postoperative XELOX eight cycles		
NCT01583361 (RESONANCE)	China	Stage II/III gastric or GEJ adenocarcinoma	Preoperative SOX → D2 surgery → postoperative SOX	772	DFS

Table 29.1 (continued)

ClinicalTrials.gov identifier (study name)	Country	Stage	Treatment	No.	Primary endpoint
			D2 surgery → postoperative SOX		
NCT02512380	China	cT3–T4 anyN M0 resectable gastric cancer or GEJ adenocarcinoma	Preoperative DOS → surgery → postoperative SOX	380	OS
			Preoperative SOX → surgery → postoperative SOX		
NCT02555358	China	Stage III resectable gastric cancer	Preoperative DOX → surgery → postoperative XELOX	300	pCR
			Preoperative XELOX → surgery → postoperative XELOX		
			Surgery → postoperative XELOX		
NCT02581462 (PETRARCA)	Germany	cT2 anyN M0 or anyT N + M0, HER2+ gastric or GEJ adenocarcinoma	Perioperative FLOT + trastuzumab + pertuzumab	404	PFS
			Perioperative FLOT		
Chemoradiotherapy					
NCT00407186 (CRITICS)	Netherlands	Stage Ib–IV(M0) resectable gastric cancer	Preoperative ECX → D1– surgery → postoperative CRT (45 Gy, XP)	788	OS
			Perioperative ECX		
NCT01924819 (TOPGEAR)	Australia/ New Zealand	Stage IB (T1 N1)– IIIC (T3–T4 and/or N+) resectable gastric or GEJ cancer	Preoperative CRT (induction ECF(X), 45 Gy, 5-FU) → D1+ surgery → postoperative ECF(X)	752	OS
			Perioperative ECF(X)		
NCT01815853	China	cT4 anyN M0 localized gastric cancer	Preoperative CRT (45 Gy, XELOX) + surgery + postoperative XELOX	620	OS
			Preoperative XELOX + surgery + postoperative XELOX		
NCT02193594	China	cT3–T4NxM0	Preoperative CCRT (50 Gy, SOX) + D2 surgery + postoperative SOX	214	OS
			D2 surgery + postoperative SOX		

GEJ gastroesophageal junction, *FLOT* fluorouracil/leucovorin/oxaliplatin/docetaxel, *OS* overall survival, *ECF* epirubicin/cisplatin/fluorouracil, *X* capecitabine, *SOX* S-1/oxaliplatin, *FOLFOX* fluorouracil/leucovorin/oxaliplatin, *DOS* docetaxel/oxaliplatin/S-1, *PFS* progression-free survival, *DFS* disease-free survival, *XELOX* capecitabine/oxaliplatin, *DOX* docetaxel/oxaliplatin/capecitabine, *pCR* pathologic complete response, *ECX* epirubicin/cisplatin/capecitabine, *XP* capecitabine/cisplatin, *5-FU* 5-fluorouracil

investigation of molecular targeted agents aims to improve perioperative therapies for gastric cancer. The monoclonal antibodies, trastuzumab and pertuzumab, which inhibit human epidermal growth factor receptor 2 (HER2), are being tested as perioperative treatments in an EORTC/ Korean Cancer Study Group (KCSG) randomized phase II study of stage Ib–III resectable HER2-positive gastric or GEJ adenocarcinoma (INNOVATION; NCT02205047). In that study, patients are randomized to receive perioperative chemotherapy (three cycles each of cisplatin plus capecitabine or 5-fluorouracil in a 3-week cycle pre- and postsurgery) vs. perioperative chemotherapy plus trastuzumab vs. perioperative chemotherapy plus trastuzumab with pertuzumab. The major pathologic response rate (<10% vital tumor cells) has been defined as the primary endpoint. In addition, a German phase II/III study is planning to enroll patients with HER2+ gastric or GEJ adenocarcinoma (cT2 anyN M0 or anyT N+ M0) who are randomized to receive perioperative FLOT plus trastuzumab with pertuzumab or perioperative FLOT alone (PETRARCA; NCT02581462).

Neoadjuvant Chemoradiotherapy

Neoadjuvant chemoradiation has not been as well studied or as frequently adopted for gastric cancer treatment as for esophageal and GEJ cancer treatment. A German phase III study (Preoperative Chemotherapy or Radiochemotherapy in Esophagogastric Adenocarcinoma Trial, POET) compared neoadjuvant chemoradiotherapy with chemotherapy in patients with cT3–T4NxM0 adenocarcinoma of the GEJ [24]. A total of 119 eligible patients (Siewert's classification type I: 55%, type II/III: 45%) were randomly assigned to induction chemotherapy (two cycles of cisplatin/leucovorin/fluorouracil in a 6-week cycle) followed by either concurrent chemoradiotherapy (30 Gy of radiation with cisplatin/etoposide over 3 weeks) and surgery or chemotherapy only (2.5 cycles of cisplatin/leucovorin/fluorouracil in a 6-week cycle) followed by surgery. Although the study suggested a trend toward improved survival with chemoradiation compared to that with chemotherapy (3-year OS, 47.4% vs. 27.7%; HR, 0.67, 95% CI, 0.41–1.07; $P = 0.07$), along with a higher pCR rate (15.6% vs. 2.0%; $P = 0.03$) or ypN0 rate (64.4% vs. 36.7%; $P = 0.01$) and similar R0 resection rate (71.5% vs. 69.5%), the power was inadequate because of low accrual.

In gastric cancer, single-arm phase II studies have yielded encouraging R0 resection and pCR rates with preoperative chemoradiotherapy. Ajani

and colleagues reported the results of two cycles of induction chemotherapy (infusion fluorouracil, bolus leucovorin, and cisplatin in a 4-week cycle) plus preoperative chemoradiation (45 Gy of radiation with continuous fluorouracil over 5 weeks) in 33 patients with resectable cT2–T3 anyN M0 or T1N1M0 gastric cancer [25]. In that study, 85% of patients underwent surgery, with an R0 resection rate of 70% and pCR rate of 30%. The median OS was 33.7 months, and patients achieving a pathologic response had a significantly longer median survival than did those without a pathologic response (63.9 months vs. 12.6 months; $P = 0.03$). Two treatment-related deaths occurred during chemotherapy and within 30 days of surgery. In the RTOG 9904 study, patients with resectable cT2–T3 anyN M0 or T1N1M0 gastric or GEJ adenocarcinoma received up to two cycles of induction chemotherapy (cisplatin plus continuous infusion fluorouracil in a 4-week cycle) followed by chemoradiotherapy (45 Gy of radiation with continuous infusion fluorouracil plus weekly paclitaxel for 5 weeks) [26]. Among the 43 assessable patients, 39 (91%) received 2 cycles of induction chemotherapy and all underwent concurrent chemoradiotherapy. Thirty-six patients (83%) underwent surgery; R0 resection was achieved in 63% and pCR in 26%. Although the median OS of all 43 patients was 23.2 months, the 1-year OS rate was better among patients who achieved pCR (82%) than among those with less than a pCR (69%). Although toxicities were considered acceptable, with a grade 4 event incidence of 21%, performing radiotherapy and surgery without unacceptable variations was possible in only 35% of patients.

The feasibilities of pre- and postoperative chemoradiotherapy were compared in two parallel phase II studies of resectable gastric cancer (FFCD 0308) [27]. Chemoradiotherapy comprised four cycles of 5-fluorouracil/leucovorin/irinotecan, followed by concurrent continuous fluorouracil infusion and radiotherapy over a 5-week period (50 Gy in the preoperative study, 45 Gy in the postoperative study). Although patients in the preoperative chemoradiotherapy study had a higher rate of therapeutic sequence completion than did those in the postoperative chemoradiotherapy study (73.8% [31/42] vs. 42.9% [9/21]), the primary endpoint of an 88% completion rate was not achieved.

Currently, an international randomized phase II/III EORTC study (Trial of Preoperative Therapy for Gastric and Esophagogastric Junction Adenocarcinoma, TOPGEAR; NCT01924819) is comparing preoperative chemoradiotherapy and preoperative chemotherapy, in combination with postoperative chemotherapy for resectable gastric cancer. In this trial, patients with stage IB (T1 N1)–IIIC (T3–T4 and/or N+) resectable gastric or GEJ cancer are randomized to receive preoperative chemoradiotherapy (two cycles of ECF(X) followed by 45 Gy of radiation given concurrently with fluorouracil) plus postoperative chemotherapy (three cycles of ECF(X)) or perioperative chemotherapy (three cycles of ECF(X) pre- and postsurgery). The interim analysis of phase II of this study indicated that preoperative chemoradiotherapy did not affect surgical compliance (85% of patients in the chemoradiotherapy group and 80% in the chemotherapy group underwent surgery) or increase surgical morbidity (21.6% vs. 22.2%, respectively) [28]. The toxicity profiles also did not differ between the chemoradiotherapy and chemotherapy groups (grade ≥ 3 hematologic toxicities, 51.7% vs. 50%, respectively, and gastrointestinal toxicities, 30% vs. 31.7%, respectively), indicating that preoperative chemoradiation is a safe and feasible approach.

In China, two randomized phase III studies of preoperative chemoradiotherapy for gastric cancer are ongoing (Table 29.1). One study is comparing preoperative chemoradiotherapy (45 Gy of radiation, capecitabine/oxaliplatin) plus postoperative capecitabine/oxaliplatin vs. perioperative capecitabine/oxaliplatin in cT4 anyN M0 gastric cancer (NCT01815853). The other is comparing preoperative chemoradiation (50 Gy of radiation, S-1/oxaliplatin) plus postoperative S-1/oxaliplatin vs. postoperative S-1/oxaliplatin alone in cT3–T4NxM0 gastric cancer (NCT02193594). The results of these large randomized trials will define the role of neoadjuvant chemoradiotherapy in the treatment of resectable gastric cancer.

Conclusions

Recent decades have seen substantial advances in the treatment of localized gastric cancer. A multidisciplinary approach has been established as the standard of care for resectable gastric cancer, although this has developed to include different strategies among geographical regions. Although neoadjuvant treatment was adopted early in Western countries, it remains under investigation in the setting of extensive D2 surgery in East Asian countries. Ongoing clinical trials to evaluate the best chemotherapy and/or radiotherapy regimen or sequence and the use of or molecular targeted agents will help us to further refine neoadjuvant treatment in the context of a multidisciplinary strategy for localized gastric cancer.

References

1. Colquhoun A, Arnold M, Ferlay J, et al. Global patterns of cardia and non-cardia gastric cancer incidence in 2012. Gut. 2015;64:1881–8.
2. Strong VE, Song KY, Park CH, et al. Comparison of gastric cancer survival following R0 resection in the United States and Korea using an internationally validated nomogram. Ann Surg. 2010;251: 640–6.
3. Markar SR, Karthikesalingam A, Jackson D, et al. Long-term survival after gastrectomy for cancer in randomized, controlled oncological trials: comparison between west and east. Ann Surg Oncol. 2013;20:2328–38.
4. Yamada T, Yoshikawa T, Taguri M, et al. The survival difference between gastric cancer patients from the UK and Japan remains after weighted propensity score analysis considering all background factors. Gastric Cancer. 2015;19:479–89.
5. Hartgrink HH, van de Velde CJ, Putter H, et al. Neoadjuvant chemotherapy for operable gastric cancer: long term results of the Dutch randomised FAMTX trial. Eur J Surg Oncol. 2004;30:643–9.
6. Schuhmacher C, Gretschel S, Lordick F, et al. Neoadjuvant chemotherapy compared with surgery alone for locally advanced cancer of the stomach and cardia: European Organisation for Research and Treatment of Cancer randomized trial 40954. J Clin Oncol. 2010;28:5210–8.
7. Biffi R, Fazio N, Luca F, et al. Surgical outcome after docetaxel-based neoadjuvant chemotherapy in locally-advanced gastric cancer. World J Gastroenterol. 2010;16:868–74.

8. Fazio N, Biffi R, Maibach R, et al. Pre-operative versus post-operative docetaxel-cisplatin-fluorouracil (TCF) chemotherapy in locally advanced resectable gastric carcinoma: 10-year follow-up of the SAKK 43/99 phase III trial. Ann Oncol. 2015;27: 668–73.

9. Cunningham D, Allum WH, Stenning SP, et al. Perioperative chemotherapy versus surgery alone for resectable gastroesophageal cancer. N Engl J Med. 2006;355:11–20.

10. Ychou M, Boige V, Pignon JP, et al. Perioperative chemotherapy compared with surgery alone for resectable gastroesophageal adenocarcinoma: an FNCLCC and FFCD multicenter phase III trial. J Clin Oncol. 2011;29:1715–21.

11. Greenleaf EK, Hollenbeak CS, Wong J. Trends in the use and impact of neoadjuvant chemotherapy on perioperative outcomes for resected gastric cancer: evidence from the American College of Surgeons National Cancer Database. Surgery. 2015;159:1099–112.

12. Messager M, de Steur WO, van Sandick JW, et al. Variations among 5 European countries for curative treatment of resectable oesophageal and gastric cancer: a survey from the EURECCA Upper GI Group (European REgistration of Cancer CAre). Eur J Surg Oncol. 2016;42:116–22.

13. Songun I, Putter H, Kranenbarg EM, et al. Surgical treatment of gastric cancer: 15-year follow-up results of the randomised nationwide Dutch D1D2 trial. Lancet Oncol. 2010;11:439–49.

14. Wu CW, Hsiung CA, Lo SS, et al. Nodal dissection for patients with gastric cancer: a randomised controlled trial. Lancet Oncol. 2006;7:309–15.

15. Sasako M, Sakuramoto S, Katai H, et al. Five-year outcomes of a randomized phase III trial comparing adjuvant chemotherapy with S-1 versus surgery alone in stage II or III gastric cancer. J Clin Oncol. 2011;29:4387–93.

16. Noh SH, Park SR, Yang HK, et al. Adjuvant capecitabine plus oxaliplatin for gastric cancer after D2 gastrectomy (CLASSIC): 5-year follow-up of an open-label, randomised phase 3 trial. Lancet Oncol. 2014;15:1389–96.

17. Park SR, Kim MJ, Ryu KW, et al. Prognostic value of preoperative clinical staging assessed by computed tomography in resectable gastric cancer patients: a viewpoint in the era of preoperative treatment. Ann Surg. 2010;251:428–35.

18. Hyung WJ, Kim SS, Choi WH, et al. Changes in treatment outcomes of gastric cancer surgery over 45 years at a single institution. Yonsei Med J. 2008;49:409–15.

19. Pauligk C, Tannapfel A, Meiler J et al. Pathological response to neoadjuvant 5FU, oxaliplatin and docetaxel (FLOT) versus epirubicin, cisplatin and 5FU (ECF) in patients with locally advanced, resectable gastric/esophagogastric junction (EGJ) cancer: Data from the phase II part of the FLOT4 phase III study of the AIO. Presented at the Annual Meeting of European Cancer Congress/European Society for Medical Oncology, Vienna, Austria, 25–29 September 2015 (abstract 2036LBA).

20. Cunningham D, Smyth E, Stenning S et al. Perioperative chemotherapy ± bevacizumab for resectable gastro-oesophageal adenocarcinoma: Results from the UK Medical Research Council randomised ST03 trial (ISRCTN 46020948) Presented at the Annual Meeting of European Cancer Congress/European Society for Medical Oncology, Vienna, Austria, 25–29 September 2015 (abstract 2201).

21. Kang Y-K, Choi DW, Im YH et al. A phase III randomized comparison of neoadjuvant chemotherapy followed by surgery versus surgery for locally advanced stomach cancer. J Clin Oncol. 1996;15:215. (suppl; abstract 503).

22. Kang Y-K, Yook J-H, Ryu M-H, et al. A randomized phase III study of neoadjuvant chemotherapy with docetaxel(D), oxaliplatin(O), and S-1(S) (DOS) followed by surgery and adjuvant S-1 vs. surgery and adjuvant S-1 for resectable advanced gastric cancer (PRODIGY). J Clin Oncol. 2015;33. (suppl; abstract TPS4136)

23. Park I, Ryu MH, Choi YH, et al. A phase II study of neoadjuvant docetaxel, oxaliplatin, and S-1 (DOS) chemotherapy followed by surgery and adjuvant S-1 chemotherapy in potentially resectable gastric or gastroesophageal junction adenocarcinoma. Cancer Chemother Pharmacol. 2013;72:815–23.

24. Stahl M, Walz MK, Stuschke M, et al. Phase III comparison of preoperative chemotherapy compared with chemoradiotherapy in patients with locally advanced adenocarcinoma of the esophagogastric junction. J Clin Oncol. 2009;27:851–6.

25. Ajani JA, Mansfield PF, Janjan N, et al. Multi-institutional trial of preoperative chemoradiotherapy in patients with potentially resectable gastric carcinoma. J Clin Oncol. 2004;22:2774–80.

26. Ajani JA, Winter K, Okawara GS, et al. Phase II trial of preoperative chemoradiation in patients with localized gastric adenocarcinoma (RTOG 9904): quality of combined modality therapy and pathologic response. J Clin Oncol. 2006;24:3953–8.

27. Michel P, Breysacher G, Mornex F, et al. Feasibility of preoperative and postoperative chemoradiotherapy in gastric adenocarcinoma. Two phase II studies done in parallel. Federation Francophone de Cancerologie Digestive 0308. Eur J Cancer. 2014;50: 1076–83.

28. Leong T, Smithers BM, Michael M et al. TOPGEAR: A randomized phase II/III trial of perioperative ECF chemotherapy versus preoperative chemoradiation plus perioperative ECF chemotherapy for resectable gastric cancer. Interim results from an international, intergroup trial of the AGITG/TROG/NCIC CTG/EORTC. Presented at the Annual Meeting of European Cancer Congress/European Society for Medical Oncology, Vienna, Austria, 25–29 September 2015 (abstract 2200).

Adjuvant Treatment for Gastric Cancer

30

Do-Youn Oh and Yung-Jue Bang

Surgical technique is the most important factor for patients' long-term outcome. There has been a long debate about the extent of lymph node dissection between Asian surgeons and Western surgeons. Japanese and Korean surgeons believe that wider lymph node dissection, e.g., D2 dissection, is necessary for the better outcome. On the other hand, Western surgeons insisted that there is no evidence for the benefit of D2 dissection over less lymph node dissection, e.g., D1 dissection, based on the negative results of two European studies. MRC ST01 trial compared D1 surgery and D2 surgery in the 1990s and found the 5-year overall survival rate was similar (35%, 33%, respectively). The postoperative morbidity (28% vs 46%) and mortality (6.5% vs 13%) were higher with D2 surgery [1, 2]. Dutch D1D2 study compared the outcomes of D1 surgery with D2 surgery and reported that the 5-year overall survival rate was not different, that is, 34%, 33%, respectively [3]. However, 15-year follow-up data demonstrated the gastric cancer-related death rate was lower in patients with D2 dissection than those with D1 dissection (37% vs 48%) [4]. At present, D2 resection is recommended for advanced gastric cancer, including the USA and Europe [5, 6].

This chapter will cover the role of adjuvant chemotherapy compared with surgery alone in especially D2-resected gastric cancer.

Meta-analysis of Adjuvant Chemotherapy in Gastric Cancer

Before the availability of phase III clinical trials demonstrating the role of adjuvant chemotherapy after curative resection of gastric cancer, the beneficial effect of adjuvant chemotherapy was supported by several meta-analyses (Table 30.1) [7–12]. These studies, in general, showed a small benefit by adding adjuvant chemotherapy. Janunger et al.'s meta-analysis showed the benefit of adjuvant chemotherapy in 3972 gastric cancer patients retrieved from 21 clinical trials (HR, 0.84; 95% confidence interval, 0.74–0.96) [10]. When Western and Asian studies were analyzed separately, they found no survival benefit in the Western groups (HR, 0.96; 95% confidence interval, 0.83–1.12). These meta-analyses have several limitations. The surgical technique was different among the retrieved trials even in one meta-analysis. The patient population was also diverse in terms of stage, etc., and the used adjuvant treatments were various. Therefore, to conclude the role of adjuvant treatment after surgery in gastric cancer is difficult without the result of randomized controlled studies enrolling homogeneous population and applying same surgical technique.

D.-Y. Oh · Y.-J. Bang (✉)
Department of Internal Medicine, Seoul National University College of Medicine,
Seoul, Republic of Korea
e-mail: bangyj@snu.ac.kr

© Springer-Verlag GmbH Germany, part of Springer Nature 2019
S. H. Noh, W. J. Hyung (eds.), *Surgery for Gastric Cancer*,
https://doi.org/10.1007/978-3-662-45583-8_30

Table 30.1 Meta-analysis for adjuvant treatment in gastric cancer

Meta-analysis	Number of clinical trials	Number of patients	HR (95% CI)
Herman et al. [7]	11	2096	0.88 (0.78–1.08)
Earle et al. [8]	13	1990	0.80 (0.66–0.97)
Mari et al. [9]	20	3658	0.82 (0.75–0.89)
Janunger et al. [10]	21	3972	0.84 (0.74–0.96)
Panzini et al. [11]	17	3118	0.72 (0.62–0.84)
GASTRIC [12]	17	3838	0.82 (0.76–0.90)

The Global Advanced/Adjuvant Stomach Tumor Research International Collaboration (GASTRIC) group conducted a meta-analysis from individual data of 3838 patients from 17 randomized clinical trials which were closed to patient recruitment before 2004 (9 from Europe, 4 from the USA, and 4 from Asia) [12]. With a median follow-up exceeding 7 years, overall, a significant long-term survival benefit was found for adjuvant chemotherapy, corresponding to an overall 18% reduction of death risk with adjuvant chemotherapy (HR, 0.82; 95% confidence interval, 0.76–0.90). The estimated median overall survival was 4.9 years (95% confidence interval, 4.4–5.5) in surgery alone group and 7.8 years (95% confidence interval, 6.5–8.7) in adjuvant chemotherapy group. The absolute benefits of overall survival rate at 5 years and 10 years were 5.8% and 7.4%, respectively. Regarding different regions, the hazard ratio was 0.83 in Europe (95% confidence interval, 0.74–0.94), 0.88 in the USA (95% confidence interval, 0.75–1.04), and 0.70 in Asia (95% confidence interval, 0.56–0.88). There was no significant heterogeneity for overall survival across clinical trials globally; there were no time trends in the treatment effect according to the year of last inclusion ($P = 0.82$).

ACTS-GC Trial

The ACTS-GC trial investigated the benefit of S-1 adjuvant chemotherapy compared to surgery alone in stage II or III Japanese gastric cancer patients after D2 surgery [13]. The primary endpoint was overall survival, and the secondary endpoints were relapse-free survival and safety. This study enrolled 1059 patients with stage II or III gastric cancer (stage II 44.8%, stage IIIA 38.6%, stage IIIB 16.5%). The used adjuvant chemotherapy was S-1 (tegafur, gimeracil, and oteracil, 80 to 120 mg per day) with 4 weeks/2 weeks on/off schedule for 12 months. After 5 years of follow-up, the overall survival rate at 5 years was higher in the S-1 arm (71.7%, 95% confidence interval, 67.8–75.7%)) than that of the surgery-alone arm (61.1%, 95% confidence interval, 56.8–65.3%) (HR, 0.669; 95% confidence interval, 0.540–0.828) [14].

The 5-year relapse-free survival rate was 65.4% (95% confidence interval, 61.2–69.5%) in the S-1 arm and 53.1% (95% confidence interval, 48.7–57.4%) in the surgery-alone arm. The HR for relapse in the S-1 group compared with that in the surgery-alone arm was 0.653 (95% confidence interval, 0.537–0.793). However, in subgroup analysis of ACTS-GC, the benefit of adjuvant S-1 was compromised in stage IIIB (HR, 0.855; 95% confidence interval, 0.510–1.431) and stage IV (HR, 0.784; 95% confidence interval, 0.422–1.458) based on the UICC sixth staging system.

Common sites of first relapse were the peritoneum, hematogenous sites, and lymph nodes. Rates of metastasis and relapse were consistently lower in the S-1 group than in the surgery-alone arm for all sites. In particular, the rates of recurrence in lymph nodes and of peritoneal relapse were lower in the S-1 arm.

In S-1 arm, treatment was continued for at least 3 months in 452 patients (87.4%), at least 6 months in 403 patients (77.9%), at least 9 months in 366 patients (70.8%), and 12 months in 340 patients (65.8%). Except for anorexia (incidence, 6%), grade 3 or 4 adverse events occurred in less than 5% of the patients in the S-1 group.

CLASSIC Trial

The CLASSIC trial investigated the benefit of combination chemotherapy of XELOX (capecitabine and oxaliplatin) compared to surgery alone in stage II or III gastric cancer patients after D2 surgery [15]. The trial was conducted in 37 centers in South Korea, China, and Taiwan. Only patients with Karnofsky performance status of 70% or more were enrolled and randomized to surgery alone or XELOX chemotherapy in a 1:1 ratio within 6 weeks of D2 gastrectomy. The XELOX regimen was composed of capecitabine 2000 mg/m^2/day for 14 days and oxaliplatin 130 mg/m^2 on day 1, which was repeated every 3 weeks for 6 months. The primary endpoint was 3-year disease-free survival, and secondary endpoints were overall survival and safety. Between 2006 and 2009, 1035 patients were randomly assigned (515 patients in surgery-alone arm, 520 patients in XELOX arm). Stage distribution was stage II 50%, IIIA 37%, and IIIB 13%. Examined lymph nodes was 43.6 surgery-alone arm and 45.0 in XELOX arm. Node-negative (N0) patients were only 10%, and 60% of patients had N1, and 30% of patients had N2 disease. After 34 months of follow-up, the 3-year disease-free survival was 74% (95% confidence interval, 69–79) in the XELOX arm and 59% (95% confidence interval, 53–64) in the surgery-alone arm (HR, 0.56; 95% confidence interval, 0.44–0.72; $P < 0.0001$). In the XELOX arm, 96 patients (18%) developed recurrences compared with 155 patients (30%) in the surgery-alone arm. The sites of gastric cancer recurrence were the peritoneum (47 in the XELOX arm vs 56 in the surgery-alone arm), locoregional sites (21 vs 44), and distant sites (49 vs 78). The benefits by XELOX were observed across all stages; the HRs for disease-free survival were 0.55 (95% confidence interval, 0.36–0.84), 0.57 (95% confidence interval, 0.39–0.82), and 0.57 (95% confidence interval, 0.35–0.95) in stage II, IIIA, and IIIB, respectively. In N1 and N2 patients, 3-year disease-free survival was significantly improved with XELOX, but not in N0 patients. 346 patients (67%) assigned to XELOX arm received eight cycles as planned. 167 patients had capecitabine dose reductions, 147 had cycle

interruptions, and 369 had cycle delays, and 163 patients needed oxaliplatin dose reductions. The median relative dose intensity was 85% for capecitabine and 98% for oxaliplatin. The most commonly reported adverse events at any grade in the XELOX arm were nausea, neutropenia, decreased appetite, peripheral neuropathy, diarrhea, and vomiting. The most common grade 3 or 4 adverse events in the XELOX arm were neutropenia, thrombocytopenia, nausea, and vomiting. Grade 3 or 4 peripheral neuropathy, a cumulative toxic effect associated with oxaliplatin, occurred in 12 (2%) patients. After median 62.4-month follow-up, disease-free survival was significantly better in the XELOX arm than in the surgery-alone arm, and the HR was 0.58 (95% confidence interval, 0.47–0.72; $p < 0.0001$) [16]. Estimated 5-year disease-free survival was 68% (95% confidence interval, 63–73) for the adjuvant XELOX arm versus 53% (47–58) for the surgery-alone arm, and estimated 3-year disease-free survival was 75% (71–79) versus 60% (56–65). Overall survival was significantly better in the adjuvant XELOX arm than in surgery-alone arm in the intention-to-treat population (HR 0.66, 95% confidence interval, 0.51–0.85; $p = 0.0015$). The estimated 5-year overall survival was 78% (95% confidence interval, 74–82) and 69% (95% confidence interval, 64–73) in XELOX arm and surgery-alone arm, respectively.

SAMIT Trial

Japanese investigator randomly assigned 1495 gastric cancer patients with T4a or T4b after D2 surgery into 4 arms (374 UFT alone, 374 S-1, 374 paclitaxel and then UFT, 373 paclitaxel and then S-1) [17]. 85% of patients had node-positive disease. Stage was based on Japanese Classification of Gastric Carcinoma, and stage IA or IB was 5%, II 22%, IIIA 35%, IIIB 25%, and IV 11%.

Patients received UFT only (267 mg/m^2 per day) and S-1 only (80 mg/m^2 per day) for 14 days, with a 7-day rest period or three courses of intermittent weekly paclitaxel (80 mg/m^2) followed by either UFT or S-1. Treatment duration was 48 weeks in monotherapy arms and 49 weeks in sequential chemotherapy arms. The primary endpoint was disease-free survival. After 3-year follow-up, protocol treatment was completed by 215 (60%) patients in the UFT arm, 224 (62%) in the S-1 arm, 242 (68%) in the paclitaxel and then UFT arm, and 250 (70%) in the paclitaxel and then S-1 arm. The primary endpoint, 3-year disease-free survival for monotherapy was 54.0% (95% CI, 50.2–57.6), and that of sequential treatment was 57.2% (53.4–60.8; [HR] 0.92; 95% CI, 0.80–1.07; $p = 0.273$). A 3-year disease-free survival for the UFT arm was 53.0% (95% CI, 49.2–56.6), and that of the S-1 group was 58.2% (54.4–61.8; HR, 0.81; 95% CI, 0.70–0.93; $p = 0.0048$; p for non-inferiority = 0.151). The result of SAMIT trial was that sequential treatment did not improve disease-free survival, and UFT was not non-inferior to S-1 (and S-1 was superior to UFT); therefore, S-1 monotherapy should remain the standard treatment for locally advanced gastric cancer in Japan.

The most common grade 3–4 hematological adverse event was neutropenia (41 [11%] of 359 patients in the UFT arm, 48 [13%] of 363 in the S-1 arm, 46 [13%] of 355 in the paclitaxel and then UFT arm, and 83 [23%] of 356 in the paclitaxel and then S-1 arm). The most common grade 3–4 non-hematological adverse event was anorexia (21 [6%], 24 [7%], 7 [2%], and 18 [5%], respectively).

Concluding Remarks

The surgical technique is of utmost importance to cure patients of advanced gastric cancer. At present, D2 resection is recommended as standard of care worldwide. Two randomized phase III trials and meta-analyses have demonstrated the benefit of adjuvant chemotherapy resulting in higher cure rate. Adjuvant chemotherapy with S-1 for 1 year or XELOX for 6 months is regarded the standard of care, especially after D2 resection. For patients with stage II disease, two regimens produced similar benefits; however, for patients with stage III disease, XELOX seems to be preferred.

References

1. Cuschieri A, Fayers P, Fielding J, et al. Postoperative morbidity and mortality after D1 and D2 resections for gastric cancer: preliminary results of the MRC randomised controlled surgical trial. The Surgical Cooperative Group. Lancet. 1996;347:995–9.
2. Cuschieri A, Weeden S, Fielding J, et al. Patient survival after D1 and D2 resections for gastric cancer: long-term results of the MRC randomized surgical trial. Surgical co-operative group. Br J Cancer. 1999;79:1522–30.
3. Bonenkamp JJ, Hermans J, Sasako M, et al. Extended lymph-node dissection for gastric cancer. N Engl J Med. 1999;340:908–14.
4. Songun I, Putter H, Kranenbarg EM, et al. Surgical treatment of gastric cancer: 15 year follow-up results of the randomised nationwide Dutch D1D2 trial. Lancet Oncol. 2010;11:439–49.
5. Waddell T, Verheij M, Allum W, et al. Gastric cancer: ESMO-ESSO-ESTRO clinical practice guidelines for diagnosis, treatment and follow-up. Ann Oncol. 2013;(Suppl 6):vi57–63.
6. NCCN Clinical Practice Guidelines in Oncology. Gastric Cancer. Version 3.2016.
7. Hermans J, Bonenkamp JJ, Boon MC, et al. Adjuvant therapy after curative resection for gastric cancer: meta analysis of randomized trials. J Clin Oncol. 1993;11:1441–7.
8. Earle CC, Maroun JA. Adjuvant chemotherapy after curative resection for gastric cancer in non-Asian patients: revisiting a meta-analysis of randomised trials. Eur J Cancer. 1999;35:1059–64.
9. Mari E, Floriani I, Tinazzi A, et al. Efficacy of adjuvant chemotherapy after curative resection for gastric cancer: a meta-analysis of published randomised trials: a study of the GISCAD (Gruppo Italiano per lo Studio dei Carcinomi dell'Apparato Digerente). Ann Oncol. 2000;11:837–43.
10. Janunger KG, Hafström L, Glimelius B. Chemotherapy in gastric cancer: a review and updated meta-analysis. Eur J Surg. 2002;168:597–608.
11. Panzini I, Gianni L, Fattori PP, et al. Adjuvant chemotherapy in gastric cancer: a meta-analysis of randomized trials and a comparison with previous meta-analyses. Tumori. 2002;88:21–7.
12. GASTRIC (Global Advanced/Adjuvant Stomach Tumor Research International Collaboration) Group, Paoletti X, Oba K, et al. Benefit of adjuvant chemotherapy for resectable gastric cancer: a meta-analysis. JAMA. 2010;303:1729–37.
13. Sakuramoto S, Sasako M, Yamaguchi T, et al. Adjuvant chemotherapy for gastric cancer with S-1, an oral fluoropyrimidine. N Engl J Med. 2007;357:1810–20.
14. Sasako M, Sakuramoto S, Katai H, et al. Five-year outcomes of a randomized phase III trial comparing adjuvant chemotherapy with S-1 versus surgery

alone in stage II or III gastric cancer. J Clin Oncol. 2011;29:4387–93.

15. Bang YJ, Kim YW, Yang HK, et al. Adjuvant capecitabine and oxaliplatin for gastric cancer after D2 gastrectomy (CLASSIC): a phase 3 open-label, randomised controlled trial. Lancet. 2012;379:315–21.

16. Noh SH, Park SR, Yang HK, et al. Adjuvant capecitabine plus oxaliplatin for gastric cancer after D2 gastrectomy (CLASSIC): 5-year follow-up of an open-label, randomised phase 3 trial. Lancet Oncol. 2014;15(12):1389–96.

17. Tsuburaya A, Yoshida K, Kobayashi M, et al. Sequential paclitaxel followed by tegafur and uracil (UFT) or S-1 versus UFT or S-1 monotherapy as adjuvant chemotherapy for T4a/b gastric cancer (SAMIT): a phase 3 factorial randomised controlled trial. Lancet Oncol. 2014;15(8):886–93.

Radiation Therapy for Gastric Cancer

31

Do Hoon Lim

After the introduction of the Gastrointestinal Cancer Intergroup Trial (INT 0116) [1], the largest phase III trial comparing surgery alone versus postoperative chemoradiotherapy (CRT) in gastric cancer, radiation therapy (RT) has attracted increasing attention as a treatment modality for patients with gastric cancer. Before INT 0116, RT has not been frequently considered as a modality for gastric cancer with several reasons. First, the radiation effect has been known to be inferior in adenocarcinoma compared with squamous cell carcinoma or undifferentiated carcinoma. Second, the gastrointestinal (GI) complications of RT have been exaggerated. Third, the gastric cancer can be considered as a systemic disease rather than localized disease because the main patterns of failure are peritoneal seeding or liver metastasis after radical resection. However, with the several clinical studies showing the additional effect of preoperative or postoperative RT and the development of radiation techniques such as three-dimensional conformal radiotherapy or intensity-modulated radiotherapy (IMRT) decreasing radiation-induced bowel complications, the application of RT to patients with gastric cancer is now gradually increasing.

Radiation and GI Tract

Radiation treats patients with cancer by using X-ray, which is generated from the machine named linear accelerator. The mechanisms of X-ray for killing cancer cells are either direct effect of destroying cancer cell membrane or induction of apoptosis from chromosomal aberration through DNA double strands break. However, radiation cannot differentiate cancer cells from normal cells, and it causes the various types of radiation complications. Because GI tract is one of the radiosensitive organs, the high dose of radiation to the abdomen for gastric cancer should be applied with caution. The radiation tolerance doses of GI tract are lower than the curative doses for gross tumor; therefore, the roles of RT for gastric cancer patients are neoadjuvant or adjuvant modality to intensify surgical effect and palliative modality to increase the quality of life of patients through pain relief or cancer bleeding control.

To increase the radiation effect, some chemotherapeutic agents are combined with RT, and those agents are called as radiosensitizer. The most commonly used radiosensitizer is 5-fluorouracil (5-FU), and the concurrent CRT can be applied for adjuvant or palliative purpose. If the patient is hard to tolerate the concurrent CRT, RT alone can be applied without chemotherapy.

D. H. Lim (✉)
Department of Radiation Oncology, Samsung
Medical Center, Sungkyunkwan University School of
Medicine, Seoul, Republic of Korea
e-mail: dh8lim@skku.edu

© Springer-Verlag GmbH Germany, part of Springer Nature 2019
S. H. Noh, W. J. Hyung (eds.), *Surgery for Gastric Cancer*,
https://doi.org/10.1007/978-3-662-45583-8_31

Preoperative Neoadjuvant Radiation Therapy

Neoadjuvant RT increases the complete resection rates of gastric cancer through tumor downstaging effect and decreases the possibility of distant metastasis with concurrent chemotherapy. Theoretically, neoadjuvant RT has many advantages compared with postoperative adjuvant RT, but the clinical studies of neoadjuvant RT in gastric cancer have been limitedly performed, and most of the studies were performed to patients with esophageal cancer or gastroesophageal junction cancer. According to randomized phase III trial of the Chemoradiotherapy for Oesophageal Cancer Followed by Surgery Study (CROSS), neoadjuvant CRT in potentially curable esophageal or gastroesophageal cancer showed overall survival (OS) benefit compared with surgery alone (median OS 49.4 months vs. 24.0 months) [2]. And the OS advantage of neoadjuvant CRT was repeated by another randomized phase III trial [3], though the study was early closed due to poor accrual.

In the phase III randomized trial, comparing surgery alone versus preoperative RT and surgery for 370 patients with gastric cardia cancer, Zhang et al. [4] reported improved 5-year survival rates, which were 20.3% in surgery alone group and 30.1% in preoperative RT followed by surgery group ($p < 0.01$). The incidences of local recurrence and intra- or extra-abdominal lymph node (LN) metastasis in the preoperative RT group were obviously lower than those of surgery alone group: 38.6% vs. 51.7% ($p < 0.025$) and 38.6% vs. 54.6% ($p < 0.005$). Ajani et al. [5] reported that the three-step strategy of preoperative induction chemotherapy followed by CRT resulted in 30% of pathologic complete response that resulted in durable survival time.

Though the clinical trials about neoadjuvant RT focusing gastric cancer only are scarce, the neoadjuvant approach is worthy of further investigation to find out which patients with clinical stage and tumor location will be beneficial from RT as a neoadjuvant modality.

Postoperative Adjuvant Radiation Therapy

The postoperative adjuvant RT, chemotherapy, and combined CRT have been investigated worldwide to prevent recurrences in patients with resected gastric adenocarcinoma. However, there has been a controversy of the application of RT in adjuvant setting until now. In the Western countries, perioperative chemotherapy (MAGIC trial) [6] and postoperative CRT (INT 0116) [1] are generally recommended; however, in the Eastern countries, adjuvant chemotherapy (ACTS-GC and CLASSIC trials) without RT is considered as standard adjuvant modality after D2 gastrectomy [7, 8].

The relatively underestimated role of adjuvant RT in the Eastern countries mainly comes from the undoubted role of surgery with extended LN dissection, the higher risk of distant metastasis than that of locoregional recurrence after D2 gastrectomy, and the exaggerated concern of radiation-induced complications. However, high rates of locoregional recurrences have been reported even after radical resection [9–18], and the benefit of adjuvant RT was reaffirmed in several meta-analyses [19–21]. Furthermore, the recent prospective randomized controlled trials in Korea and China [22–24] have demonstrated the benefit of adjuvant RT combined with chemotherapy in D2-dissected gastric cancer patients.

To justify postoperative adjuvant RT in gastric cancer patients, some critical issues should be answered: the patterns of failure after surgical resection, the evidence of adjuvant RT efficacy in randomized clinical trials, the incidence of radiation-induced complications, and a subset of patients who would benefit from adjuvant RT after radical resection.

Patterns of Failure After Surgical Resection

Several retrospective studies have analyzed the patterns of failure after curative resection in gastric cancer, and they might be divided into three groups: autopsy, reoperation, and clini-

Table 31.1 Patterns of failure after surgical resection

	Autopsy	Reoperation	Clinical FU
Locoregional	80–93%	69%	19–45%
Gastric bed	52–68%	55%	21%
Anastomosis/stump	54–60%	27%	6–25%
Abdominal/stab wound	–	5%	–
Lymph nodes	52%	43%	8–13%
Peritoneal seeding	30–50%	42%	23–44%
Distant metastasis	49%	23%	35–52%

FU follow-up

cal follow-up groups (Table 31.1). The autopsy data showed the end result of surgery [9–11], and reoperation data focused to the patients with potentially high risk for recurrences [12, 13]. The clinical follow-up data [14–18] showed recurrences which could be detected with clinical examination and imaging studies during follow-up period. As expected, high locoregional recurrences were shown in autopsy and reoperation groups compared with clinical follow-up group. However, even in clinical follow-up group, the locoregional recurrence was up to 45% of patients with surgical resection. When the extended LN dissection was performed, locoregional recurrence developed also in many patients, and the percentage of locoregional recurrence without liver metastasis or peritoneal seeding was as high as 20% [17, 18].

Earlier Prospective Randomized Trials Including INT 0116

Three prospective randomized studies were performed before the introduction of INT 0116 trial. Dent et al. [25] randomly assigned 142 patients, and the result was no difference in survival between concurrent CRT and control group. However, patients with M1 disease were included, and the radiation dose was only 20 Gy that was inappropriate dose for adjuvant setting. Moertel et al. [26] randomly assigned 62 patients with poor prognosis gastric carcinoma to receive concurrent CRT or surgery alone. The 5-year survival rate for patients randomized to adjuvant concurrent CRT was 23% and for those randomized to no treatment, 4% ($p < 0.05$).

However, when analyzed according to actual treatment received, the difference was not significant because of small patient numbers. The British Stomach Cancer Group [27] compared surgery alone, adjuvant RT, and adjuvant chemotherapy. The result was that there was no survival advantage for those with RT or chemotherapy compared to those with surgery alone but the locoregional failure rate was lowest in patient with adjuvant RT group.

Overall, it is difficult to make any conclusion from these earlier randomized trials because of the heterogeneous cohort, small numbers of patients, different surgical extent, and suboptimal radiation dose. Therefore, the well-designed INT 0116 trial was very attractive, and it demonstrated a definite survival benefit with CRT group compared with surgery alone group in initial report and updated report of a more than 10-year median follow-up [1, 28]. They showed a consistent and strong benefit of adjuvant CRT in overall and relapse-free survival, and the decrease of locoregional failure from adjuvant CRT may account for the reduction in overall relapse. Although INT 0116 trial had some limitations such as inappropriate surgical extent and no adjuvant chemotherapy alone arm, it was a pivotal clinical event resulting to pay attention to adjuvant RT in resected gastric cancer, and several randomized trials were initiated after the report of INT 0116. From the results of INT 0116 trial, the adjuvant CRT demonstrated survival benefit to the patients with suboptimally resected gastric cancer. However, it needs to be answered whether adjuvant CRT provides similar benefit shown in INT 0116 trial if D2 gastrectomy is done.

Postoperative Chemoradiotherapy in Patients with D2 Gastrectomy

Although there was a controversy over the benefit of gastrectomy with D2 LN dissection in the Western randomized studies [29, 30], several studies [31–34] reported that extended (D2) LN dissection leads to better results than limited (D0 or D1) LN dissection in locoregional recurrence or OS. And D2 gastrectomy has been the most widely accepted and recommended as a standard surgical procedure for resectable gastric cancer. However, randomized trials in patient cohort with D2 gastrectomy are uncommon, and lately, several randomized studies were published.

ACTS-GC and CLASSIC trials [7, 8] compared adjuvant chemotherapy after D2 gastrectomy with surgery alone. They showed improved 3-year OS and disease-free survival (DFS). Based on these results, adjuvant chemotherapy not CRT is recommended in D2-resected gastric cancer patients in the current NCCN guideline.

Then, is there any room for adjuvant RT or CRT in patients with extended LN dissection? Table 31.2 shows several gastric cancer studies which were performed to patients with D2 gastrectomy. According to the observational study by Kim et al. [35], there was an advantage in OS in patients with postoperative CRT (INT-0116 treatment scheme) compared with those who underwent surgery alone. Adjuvant CRT significantly

decreased the regional LN recurrences, and there was no difference in distant metastasis between two cohorts. On the contrary, Dikken et al. [36] retrospectively compared patients between D1 and D2 LN dissection from the Dutch Gastric Cancer Group Trial. Their conclusion was that the addition of postoperative CRT had a major impact on local recurrence in patients with D1 surgery but there was no additional effect of adjuvant CRT in patients with D2 surgery.

Because of the heterogeneous results as well as limitations originated from retrospective study design, phase III randomized trials should be needed to justify postoperative adjuvant RT after D2 gastrectomy. Until now, three randomized trials were published, and two trials (CRITICS and ARTIST II) are ongoing to elucidate the role of adjuvant RT in patients with D2 gastrectomy. The Adjuvant Chemoradiation Therapy in Stomach Cancer (ARTIST) trial was the first and largest prospective randomized study to address the role of CRT as adjuvant treatment in D2 gastrectomy patients [22]. Totally, 458 patients were randomly assigned to adjuvant chemotherapy or CRT group, and the conclusion was that the addition of RT to chemotherapy did not significantly reduce recurrences. This negative result may have been influenced by the large proportion of patients (60%) with early stage (stage IB and II). However, in the subset analysis, the adjuvant CRT significantly

Table 31.2 Gastric cancer studies performed to patients with D2 gastrectomy

Study	Stage	Group	Patient number	Treatment RT/CTx	Survival	p
1. Retrospective studies						
Kim et al.	II~IVA	Control	446	–	MS 62.6 mos	0.02
		CCRT	544	45 Gy / FL	95.3 mos	
Dikken et al.	–	Control	325	–	2-yr LRR 13%	0.84
		CCRT	25	45 Gy / FL, XP	12%	
2. Prospective randomized studies						
ARTIST	IB~IVA	CTx	228	XP	3-yr DFS 74.2%	0.0862
		CCRT	230	45 Gy / XP	78.2%	
NCC, SK	III~IV	CTx	175	FL	5-yr DFS 50%	>0.05
Zhu et al.	IB~IVA	CCRT	205	45 Gy / FL	61%	0.122
		CTx		FL	MS 48 mos	
		CCRT		45 Gy / FL	58 mos	

Adapted from Ref. [45], with permission
RT radiotherapy, *CTx* chemotherapy, *CCRT* concurrent chemoradiotherapy, *FL* fluorouracil, leucovorin, *MS* median survival, *XP* capecitabine, cisplatin, *LRR* local recurrence rate, *DFS* disease-free survival

improved the 3-year DFS in node-positive patients. After 7 years of median follow-up, the effect of the addition of RT on DFS and OS differed by Lauren classification ($p = 0.04$ for DFS, $p = 0.03$ for OS) and LN ratio ($p < 0.01$ for DFS, $p < 0.01$ for OS). Subgroup analyses also showed that CRT significantly improved DFS in patients with node-positive disease and with intestinal-type gastric cancer [37]. The National Cancer Center in South Korea conducted a phase III trial using INT 0116 treatment scheme in patients with stage III and IV gastric cancer [23], but this study was early closed due to poor patient accrual. Although 5-year DFS was not significantly improved in CRT group, the 5-year locoregional recurrence-free survival (LRRFS) was significantly improved, and in stage III patients, DFS was also improved. Zhu et al. [24] recently reported on a similar trial conducted in Chinese population and resulted a significant difference in DFS not only in patients with positive nodes but in the whole population. In the meta-analysis of 895 patients from these three randomized trials, there was no apparent survival benefit with the addition of RT to chemotherapy, but LRRFS and DFS in CRT group were significantly improved [38].

The ChemoRadiotherapy after Induction chemoTherapy In Cancer of the Stomach (CRITICS) trial is currently randomizing patients after neoadjuvant chemotherapy followed by D2 lymphadenectomy. They randomly assigned either three additional courses of chemotherapy or CRT to compare the efficacy of the MAGIC trial regimen, which showed the survival benefit of a perioperative approach combined with intensive chemotherapy, with that of INT 0116 trial. The results of CRITIC trial will demonstrate whether the combination of preoperative chemotherapy and postoperative CRT will improve the clinical outcome of the current European standard of perioperative chemotherapy [39]. To find out which subgroups might benefit from adjuvant RT in patients with D2 gastrectomy, the recurrence patterns in ARTIST trial were reanalyzed after minimum follow-up of 5 years [40]. The regional LN recurrence was the most important difference between the two groups (23

patients in chemotherapy arm and 5 in CRT arm, $p < 0.001$), and LRRFS was significantly different between study arms ($p = 0.03$), especially in patients with LN metastasis ($p = 0.009$). Based on the results of ARTIST trial, the ARTIST II trial evaluating adjuvant chemotherapy and CRT in patients with node-positive, D2-resected GC is under way.

Radiation Targets in D2-Dissected Gastric Cancer

The main role of postoperative adjuvant RT is to decrease locoregional recurrences. However, the RT target volume has varied between the adjuvant RT trials. In the INT 0116 trial, the recommendation of RT field includes tumor bed (preoperative tumor volume) and 2 cm beyond the proximal and distal resection margins and regional LNs (perigastric, celiac, local para-aortic, splenic, hepatoduodenal, and pancreaticoduodenal LNs) [1]. In ARTIST trial, RT field for tumor bed and regional nodes was modified according to T stage and primary tumor location [22].

From the results of randomized trials of Eastern countries comparing adjuvant CRT with adjuvant chemotherapy alone after D2 gastrectomy, CRT group showed the improvement of DFS or LRRFS [22–24]. Even after D2 LN dissection, radiation decreased regional recurrence especially in Group 3 LN areas [40] (Fig. 31.1). This result is supported by the study which investigated patterns of nodal recurrence after D2 dissection for 382 patients with stage III (N3) disease [41]. In this retrospective study, the most prevalent nodal recurrence was in the nodal basin outside the D2 dissection field.

Unlike the regional recurrence, the incidence of local recurrence (tumor bed, remnant stomach, anastomosis sites) was not different between chemotherapy alone and CRT arms, and the incidence was relatively low. In a retrospective trial, the exclusion of remnant stomach from the radiation field had no effect on failure rates or survival, and the patients treated excluding remnant stomach experienced a low GI complication rate [42].

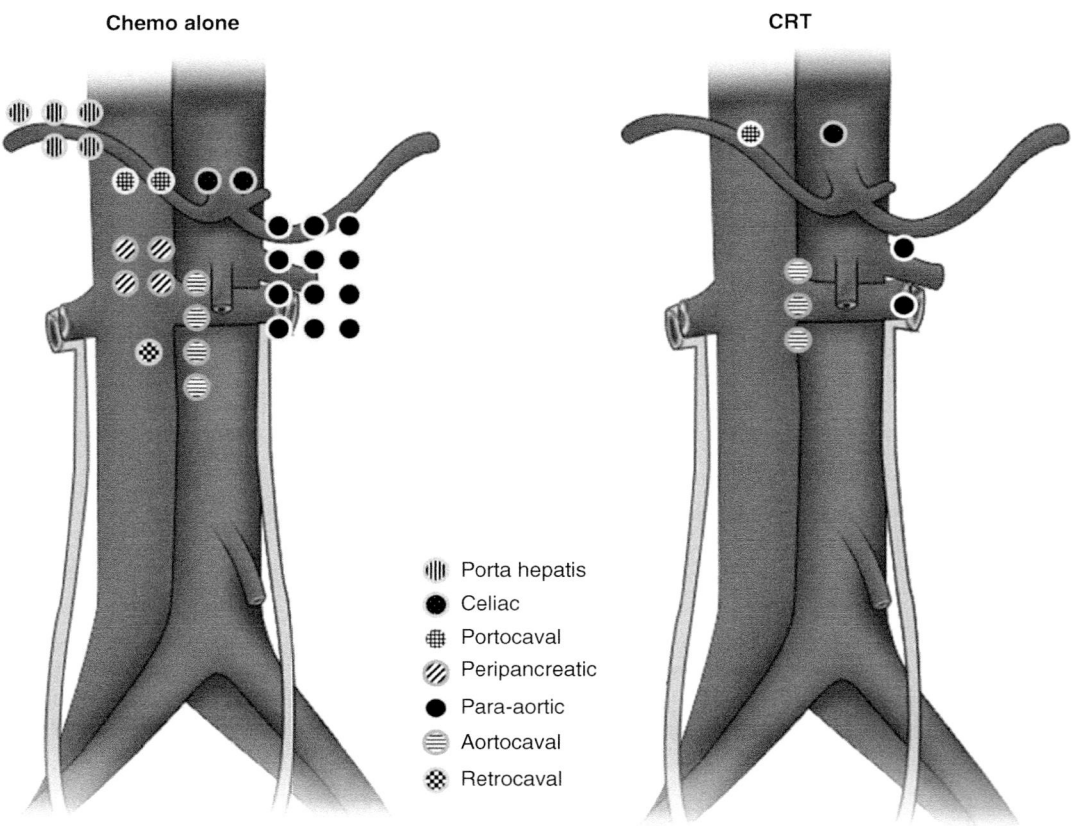

Fig. 31.1 Patterns of regional recurrence in ARTIST trial. Regional recurrence in chemotherapy alone group was significantly higher than that in chemoradiotherapy group. The most nodal recurrences developed in Group 3 lymph nodes outside the D2 dissection field. (Modified illustration originally published in Yu et al. 2015. Published with kind permission of © ScienceDirect 2016. All Rights Reserved)

Treatment-Related Complication in Clinical Trials

The concern of radiation-induced GI complications has been one of the obstacles for the application of RT in adjuvant setting. However, there was no increase in treatment-related toxicity in CRT group compared with chemotherapy alone group in three randomized trials from Eastern countries [22–24]. Especially in ARTIST trial, the treatment compliance was even higher in CRT group. This could be explained by the modification of RT target volume and the application of modern RT techniques. The late GI complications such as paralytic ileus or anastomosis site stricture were developed in less than 2% of treated cohort, and there was no statistically significant difference between CRT and chemotherapy alone groups [40].

Palliative Radiation Therapy

In patients with locally advanced unresectable gastric cancers, the quality of life of the patients is not so satisfied due to various symptoms such as tumor bleeding, gastric outlet obstruction, and abdominal or back pain. For palliation of such symptoms, RT could be a good candidate. According to Tey et al. [43], the response rates of palliative RT were 54% for tumor bleeding, 25% for obstruction, and

25% for pain. And Lee et al. [44] reported that RT may be an effective treatment for gastric cancer bleeding when other modalities are not feasible and 91% of the patients experienced symptomatic palliation with an elevated hemoglobin level and a decreased number of transfusions after RT.

References

1. Macdonald JS, Smalley SR, Benedetti J, et al. Chemoradiotherapy after surgery compared with surgery alone for adenocarcinoma of the stomach or gastroesophageal junction. N Engl J Med. 2001;345:725–30.
2. van Hagen P, Hulshof MC, van Lanschot JJ, Steyerberg EW, van Berge Henegouwen MI, Wijnhoven BP, Richel DJ, Nieuwenhuijzen GA, Hospers GA, Bonenkamp JJ, Cuesta MA, Blaisse RJ, Busch OR, ten Kate FJ, Creemers GJ, Punt CJ, Plukker JT, Verheul HM, Spillenaar Bilgen EJ, van Dekken H, van der Sangen MJ, Rozema T, Biermann K, Beukema JC, Piet AH, van Rij CM, Reinders JG, Tilanus HW, van der Gaast A, CROSS Group. Preoperative chemoradiotherapy for esophageal or junctional cancer. N Engl J Med. 2012;366(22):2074–84.
3. Tepper J, Krasna MJ, Niedzwiecki D, Hollis D, Reed CE, Goldberg R, Kiel K, Willett C, Sugarbaker D, Mayer R. Phase III trial of trimodality therapy with cisplatin, fluorouracil, radiotherapy, and surgery compared with surgery alone for esophageal cancer: CALGB 9781. J Clin Oncol. 2008;26(7):1086–92.
4. Zhang ZX, Gu XZ, Yin WB, et al. Randomized clinical trial on the combination of preoperative irradiation and surgery in the treatment of adenocarcinoma of gastric cardia (AGC) – report on 370 patients. Int J Radiat Oncol Biol Phys. 1998;42(5):929–34.
5. Ajani JA, Mansfield PF, Janjan N, et al. Multi-institutional trial of preoperative chemoradiotherapy in patients with potentially resectable gastric carcinoma. J Clin Oncol. 2004;22(14):2774–80.
6. Cunningham D, Allum WH, Stenning SP, Thompson JN, Van de Velde CJ, Nicolson M, Scarffe JH, Lofts FJ, Falk SJ, Iveson TJ, Smith DB, Langley RE, Verma M, Weeden S, Chua YJ. Perioperative chemotherapy versus surgery alone for resectable gastroesophageal cancer. N Engl J Med. 2006;355:11–20.
7. Sakuramoto S, Sasako M, Yamaguchi T, Kinoshita T, Fujii M, Nashimoto A, et al. Adjuvant chemotherapy for gastric cancer with S-1, an oral fluoropyrimidine. N Engl J Med. 2007;357:1810–20.
8. Bang YJ, Kim YW, Yang HK, Chung HC, Park YK, Lee KH, et al. Adjuvant capecitabine and oxaliplatin for gastric cancer after D2 gastrectomy (CLASSIC): a phase 3 open-label, randomised controlled trial. Lancet. 2012;379:315–21.
9. McNeer G, Vandenberg H, Donn FY, Bowden L. A critical evaluation of subtotal gastrectomy for the cure of cancer of the stomach. Ann Surg. 1951;134:2–7.
10. Thomson FB, Robins RE. Local recurrence following subtotal resection for gastric carcinoma. Surg Gynecol Obstet. 1952;95:341–4.
11. Wisbeck WM, Becher EM, Russell AH. Adenocarcinoma of the stomach: autopsy observations with therapeutic implications for the radiation oncologist. Radiother Oncol. 1986;7:13–8.
12. Wangensteen OH, Lewis FJ, Arhelger SW, Muller JJ, MacLean LD. An interim report upon the 'second look' procedure for cancer of stomach, colon, and rectum for 'limited intraperitoneal carcinosis'. Surg Gynecol Obstet. 1954;99:257–67.
13. Gunderson LL, Sosin H. Adenocarcinoma of the stomach: areas of failure in a re-operation series (second or symptomatic look) clinicopathologic correlation and implications for adjuvant therapy. Int J Radiat Oncol Biol Phys. 1982;8:1–11.
14. Landry J, Tepper JE, Wood WC, Moulton EO, Koerner F, Sullinger J. Patterns of failure following curative resection of gastric carcinoma. Int J Radiat Oncol Biol Phys. 1990;19:1357–62.
15. Papachristou DN, Fortner JG. Local recurrence of gastric adenocarcinoma after gastrectomy. J Surg Oncol. 1981;18:47–53.
16. Maehara Y, Hasuda S, Koga T, Tokunaga E, Kakeji Y, Sugimachi K. Postoperative outcome and sites of recurrence in patients following curative resection of gastric cancer. Br J Surg. 2000;87:353–7.
17. Yoo CH, Noh SH, Shin DW, Choi SH, Min JS. Recurrence following curative resection for gastric carcinoma. Br J Surg. 2000;87:236–42.
18. Lim DH, Kim DY, Kang MK, Kim YI, Kang WK, Park CK, et al. Patterns of failure in gastric carcinoma after D2 gastrectomy and chemoradiotherapy: a radiation oncologist's view. Br J Cancer. 2004;91:11–7.
19. Soon YY, Leong CN, Tey JC, Tham IW, Lu JJ. Postoperative chemo-RT versus chemotherapy for resected gastric cancer: a systematic review and metaanalysis. J Med Imaging Radiat Oncol. 2014;58:483–96.
20. Ronellenfitsch U, Schwarzbach M, Hofheinz R, et al. Perioperative chemo(radio)therapy versus primary surgery for resectable adenocarcinoma of the stomach, gastroesophageal junction, and lower esophagus. Cochrane Database Syst Rev. 2013;5:Cd008107.
21. Valentini V, Cellini F, Minsky BD, et al. Survival after RT in gastric cancer: systematic review and meta-analysis. Radiother Oncol. 2009;92:176–83.
22. Lee J, Lim DH, Kim S, Park SH, Park JO, Park YS, Lim HY, Choi MG, Sohn TS, Noh JH, Bae JM, Ahn YC, Sohn I, Jung SH, Park CK, Kim KM, Kang WK. Phase III trial comparing capecitabine plus cisplatin versus capecitabine plus cisplatin with concurrent capecitabine radiotherapy in completely resected gastric cancer with D2 lymph node dissection: the ARTIST trial. J Clin Oncol. 2012;30:268–73.

23. Kim TH, Park SR, Ryu KW, Kim YW, Bae JM, Lee JH, Choi IJ, Kim YJ, Kim DY. Phase 3 trial of postoperative chemotherapy alone versus chemoradiation therapy in stage III-IV gastric cancer treated with R0 gastrectomy and D2 lymph node dissection. Int J Radiat Oncol Biol Phys. 2012;84:e585–92.

24. Zhu WG, Xua DF, Pu J, Zong CD, Li T, Tao GZ, Ji FZ, Zhou XL, Han JH, Wang CS, Yu CH, Yi JG, Su XL, Ding JX. A randomized, controlled, multicenter study comparing intensity modulated radiotherapy plus concurrent chemotherapy with chemotherapy alone in gastric cancer patients with D2 resection. Radiother Oncol. 2012;104:361–6.

25. Dent DM, Werner ID, Novis B, Cheverton P, Brice P. Prospective randomized trial of combined oncological therapy for gastric carcinoma. Cancer. 1979;44:385–91.

26. Moertel CG, Childs DS, O'Fallon JR, Holbrook MA, Schutt AJ, Reitemeier RJ. Combined 5-fluorouracil and radiation therapy as a surgical adjuvant for poor prognosis gastric carcinoma. J Clin Oncol. 1984;2:1249–54.

27. Hallissey MT, Dunn JA, Ward LC, Allum WH. The second British Stomach Cancer Group trial of adjuvant radiotherapy or chemotherapy in resectable gastric cancer: five-year follow-up. Lancet. 1994;343:1309–12.

28. Smalley SR, Benedetti JK, Haller DG, Hundahl SA, Estes NC, Ajani JA, et al. Updated analysis of SWOG-directed intergroup study 0116:a phase III trial of adjuvant radiochemotherapy versus observation after curative gastric cancer resection. J Clin Oncol. 2012;30:2327.

29. Dent DM, Madden MV, Price SK. Randomized comparison of R1 and R2 gastrectomy for gastric carcinoma. Br J Surg. 1988;75:110–2.

30. Cuschieri A, Weeden S, Fielding J, Bancewicz J, Craven J, Joypaul V, et al. Patient survival after D1 and D2 resections for gastric cancer: long-term results of the MRC randomized surgical trial. Surgical Co-operative Group. Br J Cancer. 1999;79:1522–30.

31. Kodama Y, Sugimachi K, Soejima K, Matsusaka T, Inokuchi K. Evaluation of extensive lymph node dissection for carcinoma of the stomach. World J Surg. 1981;5:241–8.

32. Viste A, Svanes K, Janssen CW Jr, Maartmann-Moe H, Søreide O. Prognostic importance of radical lymphadenectomy in curative resections for gastric cancer. Eur J Surg. 1994;160:497–502.

33. Siewert JR, Böttcher K, Stein HJ, Roder JD. Relevant prognostic factors in gastric cancer: ten-year results of the German gastric cancer study. Ann Surg. 1998;228:449–61.

34. Songun I, Putter H, Kranenbarg EM, Sasako M, van de Velde CJ. Surgical treatment of gastric cancer: 15-year follow-up results of the randomised nationwide Dutch D1D2 trial. Lancet Oncol. 2010;11:439–49.

35. Kim S, Lim DH, Lee J, Kang WK, MacDonald JS, Park CH, et al. An observational study suggesting clinical benefit for adjuvant postoperative chemoradiation in a population of over 500 cases after gastric resection with D2 nodal dissection for adenocarcinoma of the stomach. Int J Radiat Oncol Biol Phys. 2005;63:1279–85.

36. Dikken JL, Jansen EPM, Cats A, Bakker B, Hartgrink HH, Kranenbarg EMK, et al. Impact of the extent of surgery and postoperative chemoradiotherapy on recurrence patterns in gastric cancer. J Clin Oncol. 2010;28:2430–6.

37. Park SH, Sohn TS, Lee J, Lim DH, Hong ME, Kim K, Sohn I, Jung SH, Choi MG, Lee JH, Bae JM, Kim S, Kim ST, Park JO, Park YS, Lim HY, Kang WK. Phase III trial to compare adjuvant chemotherapy with capecitabine and cisplatin versus concurrent chemoradiotherapy in gastric cancer: final report of the adjuvant chemoradiotherapy in stomach tumors trial, including survival and subset analyses. J Clin Oncol. 2015;33:3130–6.

38. Huang YY, Yang Q, Zhou SW, Wei Y, Chen YX, Xie DR, Zhang B. Postoperative chemoradiotherapy versus postoperative chemotherapy for completely resected gastric cancer with D2 lymphadenectomy: a meta-analysis. PLoS One. 2013;8:e68939.

39. Dikken JL, van Sandick JW, Maurits Swellengrebel HA, Lind PA, Putter H, Jansen EP, Boot H, van Grieken NC, van de Velde CJ, Verheij M, Cats A. Neo-adjuvant chemotherapy followed by surgery and chemotherapy or by surgery and chemoradiotherapy for patients with resectable gastric cancer (CRITICS). BMC Cancer. 2011;11:329.

40. Yu JI, Lim DH, Ahn YC, Lee J, Kang WK, Park SH, Park JO, Park YS, Lim HY, Kim ST, Kim S, Sohn TS, Choi MG, Bae JM, Nam H. Effects of adjuvant radiotherapy on completely resected gastric cancer: a radiation oncologist's view of the ARTIST randomized phase III trial. Radiother Oncol. 2015;117:171–7.

41. Chang JS, Lim JS, Noh SH, Hyung WJ, An JY, Lee YC, et al. Patterns of regional recurrence after curative D2 resection for stage III (N3) gastric cancer: implications for postoperative radiotherapy. Radiother Oncol. 2012;104:367–73.

42. Nam H, Lim DH, Kim S, et al. A new suggestion for the radiation target volume after a subtotal gastrectomy in patients with stomach cancer. Int J Radiat Oncol Biol Phys. 2008;71:448–55.

43. Tey J, Back MF, Shakespeare TP, et al. The role of palliative radiation therapy in symptomatic locally advanced gastric cancer. Int J Radiat Oncol Biol Phys. 2007;67(2):385–8.

44. Lee JA, Lim DH, Park W, Ahn YC, Huh SJ. Radiation therapy for gastric cancer bleeding. Tumori. 2009;95:726–30.

Novel Agents and the Future Perspectives

32

Minkyu Jung and Sun Young Rha

Introduction

Gastric cancer is an important health problem worldwide, with high incidence and a poor prognosis [1]. Surgical resection is the only curative treatment strategy for localized gastric cancer, used in combination with adjuvant chemotherapy [2, 3]. However, recurrence is common, and in Western countries gastric cancer is often diagnosed at a more advanced stage than in Japan and Korea, where screening is widespread [4]. For advanced or metastatic gastric cancer patients, chemotherapy is the primary treatment. There is no globally accepted standard first-line regimen in advanced gastric cancer, double regimen (fluorouracil and platinum) and triple regimen (fluorouracil, platinum plus docetaxel or epirubicin) are most commonly used [5–9]. Although several clinical trials have sought to improve survival among patients with gastric cancer, median overall survival with metastatic disease is limited to about 1 year [10]. Therefore, there is an urgent demand for new therapies to improve treatment and survival. In this present review, we summarized current evidence of clinical efficacy of novel agents including targeted agents and immune checkpoint inhibitors (ICI), especially focus on phase III trials.

Epidermal Growth Factor Receptor (EGFR)/Human Epidermal Receptor (HER) Inhibitors

The EGFR pathway has been recognized as playing a key role in tumorigenesis, influencing cell proliferation, migration, differentiation, survival, and transformation in cancer cells [11]. The EGFR family has four members: HER1 (also known as EGFR), HER2, HER3, and HER4 [12]. EGFR overexpression is reported in 27–55% of gastric cancers and has been associated with poor survival [13–15]. Therefore, drugs targeting the EGFR could be therapeutic agents for gastric cancer.

Anti-EGFR Monoclonal Antibody (mAbs)

Panitumumab

Panitumumab is a fully human monoclonal antibody against EGFR that has shown survival benefits in advanced colorectal cancer [16]. In the

M. Jung
Division of Medical Oncology, Yonsei Cancer Center, Yonsei University College of Medicine, Seoul, Republic of Korea

S. Y. Rha (✉)
Division of Medical Oncology, Department of Internal Medicine, Yonsei Cancer Center, Yonsei University College of Medicine, Seoul, Republic of Korea
e-mail: rha7655@yuhs.ac

© Springer-Verlag GmbH Germany, part of Springer Nature 2019
S. H. Noh, W. J. Hyung (eds.), *Surgery for Gastric Cancer*,
https://doi.org/10.1007/978-3-662-45583-8_32

REAL3 phase III trial [17], 553 patients with previously untreated advanced gastric or esophagogastric junction (EGJ) cancer were randomly assigned to EOC (epirubicin, oxaliplatin, and capecitabine) plus panitumumab or EOC alone. Contrary to expectations, median overall survival (OS) was significantly shorter in the EOC plus panitumumab than in the EOC group (8.8 vs. 11.3 months, hazard ratio (HR) = 1.37, 95% confidence interval (CI) 1.07–1.76, p = 0.013). In addition, rates of grade 3–4 diarrhea (48% vs. 11%), rash (11% vs. 1%), mucositis (5% vs. none), and hypomagnesemia (13% vs. none) were increased in the panitumumab group. Adding panitumumab to EOC chemotherapy decreased OS and cannot be recommend as first-line chemotherapy in the treatment of advanced esophagogastric adenocarcinoma.

Cetuximab

Cetuximab is a monoclonal IgG antibody targeting EGFR, used for the treatment of metastatic colorectal cancers, non-small cell lung cancer, and head and neck cancers [18–20]. In the EXPAND phase III study, 904 patients previously untreated for advanced unresectable or metastatic adenocarcinoma of the stomach or EGJ were randomly assigned to XP (capecitabine plus cisplatin), with or without cetuximab. The median progression-free survival (PFS) and OS did not differ between the two groups (PFS, 4.4 vs. 5.6 months, HR = 1.09, 95% CI 0.92–1.29, p = 0.32; OS, 9.4 vs. 10.7 months, HR = 1.00, 95% CI 0.87–1.17, p = 0.95). Adverse events of grade 3–4 were more common in the cetuximab group, including diarrhea, hypokalemia, hypomagnesemia, rash, and hand-foot syndrome. Therefore, the addition of cetuximab to XP chemotherapy did not increase survival in the first-line treatment of advanced gastric cancer.

Anti-HER2 mAbs

Trastuzumab

Trastuzumab, a monoclonal antibody against human HER2 (also known as ERBB2), was the first molecular-targeted agent approved for use in advanced gastric cancer patients. The Trastuzumab for Gastric Cancer (ToGA) phase III trial enrolled 594 gastric cancer patients with HER2 overexpression and compared standard chemotherapy (six courses of cisplatin plus either infusional 5-fluorouracil or capecitabine) with and without trastuzumab [21]. All tumors were screened for HER2 status by both immunohistochemistry (IHC) and fluorescent in situ hybridization (FISH), and patients were eligible if their tumor was positive by either IHC (i.e., showing 3+ expression) or FISH (i.e., showing a HER2/CEP17 ratio of 2 or greater). The objective response rate (ORR) was significantly increased in the trastuzumab arm (47% vs. 35%, p = 0.0017). With a median follow-up of 18.6 months (interquartile range (IQR) 11–25 months), median OS and PFS were significantly longer with trastuzumab than with chemotherapy alone (OS, 13.8 vs. 11.1 months, HR = 0.74, 95% CI 0.60–0.94, p = 0.0046; PFS, 6.7 vs. 5.5 months, HR = 0.71, 95% CI 0.59–0.85, p = 0.0002). Overall, grade 3 or 4 adverse events did not differ between the two groups (68% vs. 68%). A pre-planned exploratory analysis incorporating HER2 status suggested that trastuzumab was most effective in prolonging survival in the subgroup of patients with IHC scores of 2+ or 3+ that were also FISH-positive. Compared with those assigned to chemotherapy alone, OS for this group was 16.0 months vs. 11.8 months (HR = 0.65, 95% CI 0.51–0.83). Base on the ToGA trial, trastuzumab in combination with fluorouracil and cisplatin is recommended for use as a first-line therapy in gastric or EGJ adenocarcinoma patients with HER2 overexpression.

Trastuzumab Emtansine (T-DM1)

T-DM1 is composed of trastuzumab conjugated with the cytotoxic agent DM1 (a derivative of maytansine). T-DM1 binds to the extracellular domain of HER2 and is internalized into the tumor cell, where the emtansine is released [22]. The efficacy of T-DM1 was demonstrated in patients with HER2-positive metastatic breast cancer patient progressed on trastuzumab [23].

In the phase III GATSBY trial [24], 416 patients with previously treated advanced gastric or EGJ cancers that were HER2 positive (IHC 3+ or IHC 2+/FISH-positive) were randomly assigned to T-DM1 or paclitaxel. The OS and PFS were not different between the two groups (median OS, 7.9 vs. 8.6 months, HR = 1.15, 95% CI 0.87–1.51, p = 0.86; median PFS 2.7 vs. 2.9 months, HR = 1.13, 95% CI 0.89–1.43, p = 0.31). The rate of grade 3–4 adverse events was lower in the T-DM-1 group (59.8% vs. 70.3%).

Pertuzumab

Pertuzumab is a humanized monoclonal antibody that binds to the extracellular dimerization domain of HER2 and prevents heterodimerization of HER2 and HER3 [25]. Addition of pertuzumab to trastuzumab plus docetaxel improved survival in patients with HER2-positive breast cancer [26]. The success of dual HER2-targeted therapy in breast cancer was applied in gastric cancer with HER2-positive gastric cancer.

In phase III JACOB trial [27], 780 patients with HER2-positive metastatic gastric or EGJ cancer were assigned to receive either pertuzumab plus trastuzumab and chemotherapy or trastuzumab and chemotherapy. The OS was not significantly different between treatment groups (median OS, 17.5 vs. 14.2 months, HR = 0·84, 95% CI 0.71–1.00, p =0·057). However, PFS was significantly longer (8.5 vs. 7.0 months, HR = 0.73, 95% CI 0.62–0.86, p = 0.0001), and ORR was higher in pertuzumab group (56.7% vs. 48.3%, p = 0.026).

HER2 Tyrosine Kinase Inhibitors (TKIs)

Lapatinib

Lapatinib is an oral small molecule inhibitor of both EGFR and HER2. A benefit from the addition of lapatinib to capecitabine vs. capecitabine alone was demonstrated in patients with previously treated advanced breast cancer with HER2 overexpression [28].

In the phase III TyTAN trial [29], 261 patients with previously treated advanced or metastatic gastric cancer that was HER2-positive by FISH were randomly assigned to paclitaxel plus lapatinib or paclitaxel alone. The addition of lapatinib to paclitaxel did not significantly improve OS (11.0 vs. 8.9 months. p = 0.1044) or PFS (5.4 vs. 4.4 months, HR = 0.85, p = 0.2441). However, a significant benefit of lapatinib was seen in patients with 3+ IHC scores for HER2 (PFS, 5.4 vs. 4.2 months, HR = 0.54, p = 0.0101; OS, 14.0 vs. 7.6 months, HR = 0.59, p = 0.0176). The incidence of adverse events leading to permanent discontinuation was higher in the lapatinib group than with paclitaxel alone (16% vs. 9%).

In the phase III LOGiC trial [30], 545 patients with HER2-positive advanced gastroesophageal adenocarcinoma were randomly assigned to a combination of lapatinib and capecitabine/oxaliplatin or capecitabine/oxaliplatin alone as a first-line treatment. The addition of lapatinib did not significantly improve OS (12.2 vs. 10.5 months, HR = 0.91, 95% CI 0.73–1.12, p = 0.3492) over capecitabine/oxaliplatin chemotherapy alone. However, PFS was significantly longer (6.0 vs. 5.4 months, HR = 0.82, p = 0.0381), and ORR was higher in the lapatinib group (53% vs. 39%, p = 0.0031). No correlation was found between intensity of staining for HER2 by IHC and outcome. However, in a subgroup analysis, Asian patients (OS, 16.5 vs. 10.9 months, HR 0.68, 95% CI 0.48–0.96, p = 0.026) and those under age 60 (OS, 12.9 vs. 9 months, HR 0.69, 95% CI 0.51–0.94, p = 0.0141) seemed to benefit from lapatinib. Adverse events were increased in the lapatinib group, especially diarrhea (Grade ≥ 3, 12% vs. 3%).

Based on the TyTan and LOGiC trials, the addition of lapatinib to chemotherapy in patients with HER2-positive gastric cancer as a first- or second-line treatment cannot be recommended.

Angiogenesis Inhibitors

Anti-vascular Endothelial Growth Factor (VEGF) mAbs

Angiogenesis is strongly linked to metastasis and progression in cancer. VEGF is a key regulatory molecule in angiogenesis, and several VEGF-targeting agents have been developed, including antibodies against VEGF or its receptor VEGFR and TKIs of VEGFR [31].

Bevacizumab

Bevacizumab is a humanized monoclonal antibody against VEGF-A. Bevacizumab was approved for use, with chemotherapy, in the treatment of metastatic colorectal cancer, non-squamous non-small cell lung cancer, glioblastoma, renal cell carcinoma, cervical cancer, and ovarian cancer.

In the AVAGAST phase III trial [32], 774 patients with previously untreated advanced gastric or EGJ cancer were randomly assigned to bevacizumab plus chemotherapy (capecitabine and cisplatin) or chemotherapy alone. Although addition of bevacizumab to chemotherapy had significant improvement in PFS (6.7 vs. 5.3 months; HR = 0.80; 95% CI 0.68–0.93; p = 0.0037 and ORR (46.0% vs. 37.4%; p = 0.0315), OS did not different betwen two (12.1 vs. 10.1 months, HR = 0.87, 95% CI 0.73–1.03, p = 0.1002). In a subgroup analysis, patients from the Americas (largely Latin America) showed a survival benefit with bevacizumab (11.5 vs. 6.8 months, HR = 0.63, 95% CI 0.43–0.94), whereas Asians appeared to have no benefit (13.9 vs. 12.1 months, HR = 0.97; 95% CI 0.75–1.25), and European patients had intermediate results (11.1 vs. 8.6 months, HR = 0.85, 95% CI 0.63–1.14). In addition, a biomarker study from the AVAGAST trial reported that baseline plasma VEGF-A levels and tumor neuropilin-1 expression were potential predictors of bevacizumab efficacy. However, both biomarkers were demonstrated only in non-Asian patients [33].

Ramucirumab

Ramucirumab, a fully humanized monoclonal antibody against vascular endothelial growth factor receptor 2 (VEGFR-2), has shown a survival benefit when used as monotherapy and in combination with paclitaxel, in patients with previously treated gastric or EGJ adenocarcinoma [34, 35].

In the phase III REGARD trial [34], 355 patients with previously treated advanced or metastatic gastric or EGJ adenocarcinoma were assigned (2:1) to receive ramucirumab or placebo. Those treated with ramucirumab had longer PFS (2.1 vs. 1.3 months, HR = 0.483, 95% CI 0.376–0.620, p < 0.001) and OS (5.2 vs. 3.8 months, HR = 0.78, 95% CI 0.60–0.998, p = 0.047) compared with those treated with placebo. Although the ORR was not different (8% vs. 3%, p = 0.76), the overall disease control rate (objective response plus stable disease) was significantly higher in the ramucirumab group than in the placebo group (49% vs. 23%, p < 0.0001). While the rate of hypertension was higher with ramucirumab than with placebo (16% versus 8%), ramucirumab was not associated with increased bleeding, venous thromboembolism, perforation, fistula formation, or proteinuria.

In the phase III RAINBOW trial [35], 665 patients who had disease progression after first-line fluorouracil and cisplatin were randomly assigned to weekly paclitaxel plus ramucirumab or placebo. Both median OS and PFS were significantly longer in the paclitaxel plus ramucirumab group, compared with paclitaxel alone (OS, 9.6 vs. 7.4 months, HR = 0.807, 95% CI 0.678–0.962, p = 0.017; PFS 4.4 vs. 2.9 months, HR = 0.635, 95% CI 0.536–0.752, p < 0.001). The ORR was higher in the ramucirumab group (28% vs. 16%, p = 0.001). Grade 3 or worse neutropenia was more common with ramucirumab (41% vs. 19%), but rates of febrile neutropenia were low and similar between groups (3% vs. 2%). Rates of grade 3–4 hypertension were 14% vs. 2%.

Based on the REGARD and RAINBOW trials, ramucirumab monotherapy and the combination of paclitaxel plus ramucirumab were approved for treatment in patients with advanced or metastatic gastric or EGJ cancer with progression after prior fluorouracil and cisplatin treatment.

In addition, RAINFALL study was designed to assess whether the addition of ramucirumab to first-line chemotherapy improves outcome in patients with HER2-negative advanced gastric or

EGJ adenocarcinoma [36]. In the phase III RAINFALL trial, 645 patients with previously untreated, metastatic, HER2 negative gastric or EGJ cancer were randomly assigned to ramucirumab plus chemotherapy (cisplatin plus capecitabine or 5-fluorouracil) or chemotherapy alone. Its primary endpoint of investigator-assessed PFS was significantly longer in ramucirumab group than chemotherapy alone group (5.7 vs. 5.4 months, HR = 0.753, 95% CI 0.607–0.935, $p = 0.016$). However, central independent review of the radiological images did not confirm the investigator-assessed difference in PFS (HR = 0.961, 95% CI 0.768–1.203, $p = 0.74$), and there was no difference in OS between groups (11.2 vs. 10.7 months, HR = 0.962, 95% CI 9.5–11.9). Therefore, the addition of ramucirumab to chemotherapy is not recommended as first-line treatment for patients with HER2-negative advanced gastric or EGJ adenocarcinoma.

VEGFR TKI

Apatinib

Apatinib is an inhibitor of the VEGFR-2 tyrosine kinase, targeting the intracellular ATP-binding site of the receptor. Apatinib showed antitumor activity in both in vitro and in vivo models [37]. On the basis of preclinical studies, phase I and phase II clinical trials were conducted, and apatinib significantly improved PFS compared with placebo in Chinese gastric cancer patients [38, 39]. Finally, a randomized, phase III trial of third-line treatment for gastric cancer was conducted, and OS was significantly improved in the apatinib group compared to the placebo group (6.5 vs. 4.7 months. HR = 0.71, 95% CI 0.54–0.94, $p < 0.016$). In addition, apatinib showed significantly longer PFS (2.6 vs. 1.8 months, HR = 0.44, 95% CI 0.33–0.61, $p < 0.0001$) and better ORR (2.8% vs. 0%) than the placebo group. Apatinib was well tolerated, with grade 3–4 adverse events occurring in no more than 2% of patients; these included hypertension, hand-foot syndrome, proteinuria, fatigue, anorexia, and elevated aminotransferase levels [40].

Other Targeted Agents

Mammalian Target of Rapamycin (mTOR) Inhibitors

Everolimus is an oral inhibitor of mTOR that has demonstrated antitumor activity against many types of cancer [41]. Such effects were seen in a preclinical gastric cancer model [42] and in a phase II trial of everolimus in 53 gastric cancer patients, where it showed favorable efficacy (median PFS 2.7 months, 95% CI 1.6–3.0; median OS 10.1 months, 95% CI 6.5–12.1) [43].

In the GRANITE-1 phase III study, 656 patients with progression after first- or second-line therapy were randomly assigned (2:1) to everolimus or placebo. Everolimus did not significantly improve OS (5.4 vs. 4.3 months, HR = 0.90; 95% CI 0.75–1.08, $p = 0.124$), a primary endpoint of this study, although PFS was significantly prolonged in the everolimus group (1.7 vs. 1.4 months, HR = 0.66; 95% CI 0.56–0.78, $p < 0.001$) [44].

Mesenchymal-Epithelial Transition Factor (MET) Inhibitors

MET is a known oncogene, regulating cell growth and survival in cancer cells [45]. High expression of c-MET is correlated with poor survival in various types of cancer [46], and c-MET may be activated by multiple mechanisms, such as stimulation by its ligand, hepatocyte growth factor (HGF), gene amplification or mutation, and cross talk from other receptors [47].

Rilotumumab

Rilotumumab is a fully humanized monoclonal antibody against HGF that prevents its binding to the MET receptor. Addition of rilotumumab to chemotherapy was tested as first-line treatment of MET-positive gastric or EGJ cancers in two phase III clinical trials, RILOMET-1 and RILOMET-2.

In RILOMET-1 phase III trial [48], 609 patients with previously untreated tumors that were MET-positive by IHC were randomly assigned to rilotumumab and ECX (epirubicin, cisplatin, and capecitabine) or to ECX alone. This study was stopped due to increased deaths. Rilotumumab showed significantly worse OS (9.6 vs. 11.5 months, HR = 1.37, 95% CI 1.06–1.78, p = 0.016), unimproved PFS (5.7 vs. 5.7 months, HR = 1.30, 95% CI 1.05–1.62, p = 0.016), and lower ORR (30% vs. 39.2%, p = 0.027). Most common adverse events were increased with rilotumumab, including peripheral edema, hypoalbuminemia, deep vein thrombosis, and hypocalcemia. In addition, the RILOMET-2 study, a randomized, phase III study of adding rilotumumab to CX (cisplatin and capecitabine) as a first-line therapy for untreated MET-positive gastric or EGJ cancer, was recently terminated after a pre-planned data monitoring committee safety review.

Accordingly, the addition of rilotumumab to chemotherapy in patients with MET2-positive gastric cancer as a first line cannot be recommended.

Onartuzumab

Onartuzumab is a humanized monoclonal antibody directed against MET. In the METGastric phase III trial [49], 562 patients with previously untreated gastric and EGJ cancers that were HER2-negative and MET-positive (1+/2+/3+) by IHC were randomly assigned to onartuzumab plus mFOLFOX6 or mFOLFOX6 alone. Enrollment was stopped early due to negative results from a phase II trial assessing mFOLFOX6 plus onartuzumab. Median OS was not different between the two groups (11.0 vs. 11.3 months, HR = 0.82, p = 0.244). In the subgroup with MET 2+/3+, onartuzumab showed a marginal survival benefit (11.0 vs. 9.7 months, HR = 0.64, p = 0.062). In addition, exploratory subgroup analyses showed improved OS for the onartuzumab group in non-Asian patients and in patients with no prior gastrectomy, regardless of MET status.

Poly ADP-Ribose Polymerase (PARP) Inhibitor

Olaparib

Olaparib, an oral PARP inhibitor, is a key activator of the DNA damage response [50]. Olaparib has demonstrated clinical benefits in ovarian cancer patients with BRCA mutations [51]. In a gastric cancer cell line, low ataxia telangiectasia mutated (ATM) levels were associated with olaparib sensitivity [52]. ATM has an essential role in maintaining genome stability against DNA damage [53]. Olaparib plus paclitaxel showed better OS compared to paclitaxel monotherapy as second-line therapy in a randomized phase II study [54]. In particular, olaparib showed better efficacy in patients with low ATM by IHC (HR = 0.35; 95% CI 0.17–0.71; P = 0.003).

In GOLD phase III study [55], 525 Asian patients that had progressed from first-line chemotherapy were randomly assigned to olaparib plus paclitaxel or placebo plus paclitaxel. Unlike phase II study, OS did not differ between two groups in the overall population (8.8 vs. 6.9 months, HR = 0.79, 95% CI 0.63–1.00, p = 0.026) or the ATM-negative population (12.0 vs. 10.0 months, HR = 0.73, 95% CI 0.40–1.34, p = 0.25). In addition, PFS and ORR were not differ between two groups (PFS, 3.3 vs. 3.2 months, HR = 0.84, 95% CI 0.67–1.04, p = 0,065; ORR, 24% vs. 16%, p = 0.055).

Immunotherapy

Recently, immunogenic checkpoint blockade has emerged as a cancer treatment, targeting components of T-cell regulatory mechanisms, including cytotoxic T lymphocyte antigen-4 (CTLA-4), the programed cell death protein (PD-1), or its ligand (PD-L1) [56, 57]. Monoclonal antibodies to CTLA-4, PD-1, and PD-L1 have proved effective, especially in metastatic melanoma, and are currently being investigated in stomach cancer [58, 59].

PD-1 Inhibitor

Nivolumab

Nivolumab is an anti-PD-1 monoclonal antibody and was investigated for use in gastric cancer cohort in the checkmate-032, a phase I/II trial that used nivolumab as either monotherapy or in combined with ipilimumab in patients with refractory solid tumors [60]. In the gastric cohort treated with nivolumab monotherapy demonstrated ORR of 12% and a median OS of 6.8 months.

In phase III ATTRACTION-2 trial [61], 493 Asian patients with progressed to standard therapy randomly assigned (2:1) nivolumab or placebo regardless of PD-L1 expression. OS was significantly improved in the nivolumab group compared to the placebo group (5.26 vs. 4.14 months. HR = 0.63, 95% CI 0.51–0.78, $p < 0.001$). Twelve months OS rates prolonged in nivolumab group than placebo group (26.2% vs. 10.9%). G3 or 4 treatment-related adverse events occurred in 10% of patients treated with nivolumab and 4% of patients treated with placebo.

Base on ATTRACTION-2 trial, nivolumab should be considered as therapeutic option in Asian gastric cancer patients progressed from standard therapy.

Pembrolizumab

Pembrolizumab is an anti-PD-1 monoclonal antibody and was investigated in gastric cohort of phase 1b KEYNOTE-012 study [62]. In this study, 39 patients with PD-L1 positive were enrolled, and the ORR was 22%, and the 6-month OS rate was 69%.

In phase III KENOTE-061 study [63], 395 patients were assigned to pembrolizumab or paclitaxel as a second-line therapy. Pembrolizumab did not significantly prolong OS compared with paclitaxel (9.1 vs. 8.3 months, HR = 0.82, 95% CI 0.66–1.03, one-sided $p = 0.042$). However, pembrolizumab demonstrated clinically meaningful 12-month survival of about 40%. The treatment effect of pembroli-

zumab might be more marked in patients with a better performance status, higher levels of PD-L1 expression, and tumor with microsatellite instability (MSI)-high. Grade 3–5 treatment-related adverse events occurred in 14% of patients treated with pembrolizumab and 35% of patients treated with paclitaxel.

PD-L1 Inhibitor

Avelumab is a human anti-PD-L1 monoclonal antibody and has demonstrated treatment efficacy in various cancer including advanced urothelial carcinoma [64]. In JAVELIN Gastric 300 trial, 371 patients who received two prior lines were randomized to avelumab or physician's choice of chemotherapy (paclitaxel or irinotecan). The primary endpoint of OS was not different between two groups (4.6 vs. 5.0 months, HR = 1.1, 95% CI 0.9–1.4, $p = 0.81$). Subgroup analyses of OS according to PD-L1 expression showed no difference favoring either treatment group. Grade 3–5 treatment-related adverse events occurred in 9.2% of patients in the avelumab group and 31.6% of patients in the chemotherapy group.

Conclusions

Many phase III clinical trials of various targeted agents for gastric cancer have failed (Table 32.1). However, trastuzumab is the first targeted drug to have shown a survival benefit in gastric and EGJ cancer when added to first-line chemotherapy. Ramucirumab has shown efficacy as a monotherapy or in combination with paclitaxel as a second line. Apatinib and nivolumab monotherapy demonstrated their efficacy in the salvage-line setting. Future studies should be designed to identify robust predictive biomarkers for efficacy and to include more comprehensive background information, addressing tumor heterogeneity and biological resistance mechanisms specific to each target.

Table 32.1 Completed randomized phase III trials with targeted agents and immune checkpoint inhibitors in gastric cancer

Trials	Line of therapy	Regimen	Patients no.	RR (%)	PFS (months)	OS (months)	P-value[b]	Primary endpoint	Conclusion
REAL3	1st	Panitumumab + EOX	278	46	6	8.8[a]	0.013	OS	No benefit in PFS. OS was significantly inferior
		EOX	275	42	7.4	11.3			
EXPAND	1st	Cetuximab + XP	339	30	4.4	9.4	0.32	OS	No significant benefit to PFS or OS
		XP	334	29	5.9	10.7			
ToGA	1st	Trastuzumab + XP/FP	167	47[a]	6.7[a]	13.5[a]	0.0048	OS	Significant prolongation in both PFS and OS
		XP	182	35	5.5	11.1			
LOGIC	1st	Lapatinib + XELOX	273	53[a]	6[a]	12.2	0.35	OS	Significant prolongation in PFS but not its primary endpoint of OS
		XELOX	272	40	5.4	10.5			
JACOB	1st	Pertuzumab + Trastuzumab + XP	388	56.7	8.5	17.5	0.057	OS	A trend toward therapeutic activity of PFS, but not its primary endpoint of OS
		Trastuzumab + XP	392	48.3	7.0	14.2			
AVAGAST	1st	Bevacizumab + XP	387	46[a]	6.7[a]	12.1	0.1002	OS	Significant prolongation in PFS but not its primary endpoint of OS
		XP	387	37	5.3	10.1			
RAINFALL	1st	Ramucirumab + XP/FP	326	41.1	5.7[a]	11.2	0.676	PFS[c]	Significant improvement in investigator assessed PFS, but no benefit in central independent reviewed PFS or OS
		XP/FP	319	36.4	5.4	10.7			
		XP	334	29	5.9	10.7			
RILOMET-1	1st	Rilotumumab + ECX	304	30[a]	5.7[a]	9.6[a]	0.016	OS	No significant benefits to PFS and OS were significantly inferior
		ECX	305	39.2	5.7	11.5			
METGastric	1st	Onartuzumab + mFOLFOX	280	46	6.7	11	0.244	OS	No benefit to PFS or OS
		mFOLFOX	282	41	6.8	11.3			
GATSBY	2nd	T-MD1	228	20.6	2.7	7.9	0.86	OS	No significant prolongation in PFS or OS
		Docetaxel or paclitaxel	117	19.6	2.9	8.6			
REGARD	2nd	Ramucirumab	238	8	2.1[a]	5.2[a]	<0.001	OS	Significant prolongation in both PFS and OS
		Placebo	117	3	1.3	3.8			
RAINBOW	2nd	Ramucirumab + paclitaxel	327	28[a]	4.4[a]	9.6[a]	0.017	OS	Significant prolongation in both PFS and OS
		Paclitaxel	329	16	2.9	7.4			
GOLD	2nd	Olaparib + paclitaxel	263	24	3.7	8.8	0.026[d]	OS	No significant benefit to PFS or OS
		Placebo + paclitaxel	262	16	3.2	6.9			
GRANITE-1	2nd and 3rd	Everolimus	439	4	1.7[a]	5.4	0.124	OS	Significant prolongation in PFS but not its primary endpoint of OS
		Placebo	217	2	1.4	4.3			

KEYNOTE-061	2nd	Pembrolizumab	196	16	1.5	9.1	0.042[c]	OS, PFS	No significant prolongation in PFS or OS
		Paclitaxel	199	14	4.1	8.3			
Apatinib	3rd and above	Apatinib	180	2.8	2.6[a]	6.5[a]	0.016	OS	Significant prolongation in both PFS and OS
		Placebo	90	0	1.8	4.7			
ATTRACTION-02	3rd and above	Nivolumab	330	11.2	1.6[a]	5.3[a]	<0.001	OS	Significant prolongation in both PFS and OS
		Placebo	163	0	1.5	4.1			
JAVELIN Gastric 300	3rd	Avelumab	185	2.2	1.4	4.6	0.81	OS	No significant prolongation in PFS or OS
		Paclitaxel or irinotecan	186	4.3	2.7	5.0			

XP capecitabine+cisplatin, *FP* 5-fluorouracil+cisplatin, *EOX* epirubicin+oxaliplatin+capecitabine, *XELOX* capecitabine+oxaliplatin, *ECX* epirubicine+cisplatin+capecitabine, *mFOLFOX* modified FOLFOX (5-FU + oxaliplatin), *RR* response rate, *PFS* progression-free survival, *OS* overall survival

[a]Statistically significant
[b]*p* value for overall survival
[c]Investigator assessed
[d]a significant difference was defined as *p* < 0.025 based on Hochberg procedure
[e]one-side *p* value

References

1. Torre LA, Bray F, Siegel RL, Ferlay J, Lortet Tieulent J, Jemal A. Global cancer statistics, 2012. CA Cancer J Clin. 2015;65(2):87–108.

2. Sakuramoto S, Sasako M, Yamaguchi T, Kinoshita T, Fujii M, Nashimoto A, Furukawa H, Nakajima T, Ohashi Y, Imamura H, et al. Adjuvant chemotherapy for gastric cancer with S-1, an oral fluoropyrimidine. N Engl J Med. 2007;357(18):1810–20.

3. Bang Y, Kim Y, Yang H, Chung HC, Park Y, Lee KH, Cho JY, Mok YJ, Ji J, Yeh T, et al. Adjuvant capecitabine and oxaliplatin for gastric cancer after D2 gastrectomy (CLASSIC): a phase 3 open-label, randomised controlled trial. Lancet. 2012;379(9813):315–21.

4. Leung WK, Wu M, Kakugawa Y, Kim J, Yeoh K, Goh KL, Wu K, Wu D, Sollano J, Kachintorn U, et al. Screening for gastric cancer in Asia: current evidence and practice. Lancet Oncol. 2008;9(3):279–87.

5. Van Cutsem E, Moiseyenko VM, Tjulandin S, Majlis A, Constenla M, Boni C, Rodrigues A, Fodor M, Chao Y, Voznyi E, et al. Phase III study of docetaxel and cisplatin plus fluorouracil compared with cisplatin and fluorouracil as first-line therapy for advanced gastric cancer: a report of the V325 Study Group. J Clin Oncol. 2006;24(31):4991–7.

6. Cunningham D, Starling N, Rao S, Iveson T, Nicolson M, Coxon F, Middleton G, Daniel F, Oates J, Norman AR. Capecitabine and oxaliplatin for advanced esophagogastric cancer. N Engl J Med. 2008;358(1):36–46.

7. Koizumi W, Narahara H, Hara T, Takagane A, Akiya T, Takagi M, Miyashita K, Nishizaki T, Kobayashi O, Takiyama W, et al. S-1 plus cisplatin versus S-1 alone for first-line treatment of advanced gastric cancer (SPIRITS trial): a phase III trial. Lancet Oncol. 2008;9(3):215–21.

8. Kang YK, Shin DB, Chen J, Xiong J, Wang J, Lichinitser M, Guan Z, Khasanov R, Zheng L, Philco Salas M, et al. Capecitabine/cisplatin versus 5-fluorouracil/cisplatin as first-line therapy in patients with advanced gastric cancer: a randomised phase III noninferiority trial. Ann Oncol. 2009;20(4):666–73.

9. Ajani JA, Buyse M, Lichinitser M, Gorbunova V, Bodoky G, Douillard JY, Cascinu S, Heinemann V, Zaucha R, Carrato A, et al. Combination of cisplatin/S-1 in the treatment of patients with advanced gastric or gastroesophageal adenocarcinoma: results of noninferiority and safety analyses compared with cisplatin/5-fluorouracil in the First-Line Advanced Gastric Cancer Study. Eur J Cancer. 2013;49(17):3616–24.

10. Lordick F, Allum W, Carneiro F, Mitry E, Tabernero J, Tan P, Van Cutsem E, van de Velde C, Cervantes A. Unmet needs and challenges in gastric cancer: the way forward. Cancer Treat Rev. 2014;40(6):692–700.

11. Di Fiore PP, Pierce JH, Fleming TP, Hazan R, Ullrich A, King CR, Schlessinger J, Aaronson SA. Overexpression of the human EGF receptor confers an EGF-dependent transformed phenotype to NIH 3T3 cells. Cell. 1987;51(6):1063–70.

12. Schlessinger J. Ligand-induced, receptor-mediated dimerization and activation of EGF receptor. Cell. 2002;110(6):669–72.

13. Kim MA, Lee HS, Jeon YK, Yang HK, Kim WH. EGFR in gastric carcinomas: prognostic significance of protein overexpression and high gene copy number. Histopathology. 2008;52(6):738–46.

14. Langer R, Von Rahden BH, Nahrig J, Von Weyhern C, Reiter R, Feith M, Stein HJ, Siewert JR, Höfler H, Sarbia M. Prognostic significance of expression patterns of c-erbB-2, p53, p16INK4A, p27KIP1, cyclin D1 and epidermal growth factor receptor in oesophageal adenocarcinoma: a tissue microarray study. J Clin Pathol. 2006;59(6):631–4.

15. Lieto E, Ferraraccio F, Orditura M, Castellano P, La Mura A, Pinto M, Zamboli A, De Vita F, Galizia G. Expression of vascular endothelial growth factor (VEGF) and epidermal growth factor receptor (EGFR) is an independent prognostic indicator of worse outcome in gastric cancer patients. Ann Surg Oncol. 2008;15(1):69–79.

16. Douillard J, Siena S, Cassidy J, Tabernero J, Burkes R, Barugel M, Humblet Y, Bodoky G, Cunningham D, Jassem J, et al. Randomized, phase III trial of panitumumab with infusional fluorouracil, leucovorin, and oxaliplatin (FOLFOX4) versus FOLFOX4 alone as first-line treatment in patients with previously untreated metastatic colorectal cancer: the PRIME study. J Clin Oncol. 2010;28(31):4697–705.

17. Waddell T, Chau I, Cunningham D, Gonzalez D, Okines AF, Frances A, Okines C, Wotherspoon A, Saffery C, Middleton G, et al. Epirubicin, oxaliplatin, and capecitabine with or without panitumumab for patients with previously untreated advanced oesophagogastric cancer (REAL3): a randomised, open-label phase 3 trial. Lancet Oncol. 2013;14(6):481–9.

18. Van Cutsem E, Köhne C, Láng I, Folprecht G, Nowacki MP, Cascinu S, Shchepotin I, Maurel J, Cunningham D, Tejpar S, et al. Cetuximab plus irinotecan, fluorouracil, and leucovorin as first-line treatment for metastatic colorectal cancer: updated analysis of overall survival according to tumor KRAS and BRAF mutation status. J Clin Oncol. 2011;29(15):2011–9.

19. Pirker R, Pereira JR, Szczesna A, von Pawel J, Krzakowski M, Ramlau R, Vynnychenko I, Park K, Yu C, Ganul V, et al. Cetuximab plus chemotherapy in patients with advanced non-small-cell lung cancer (FLEX): an open-label randomised phase III trial. Lancet. 2009;373(9674):1525–31.

20. Vermorken JB, Mesia R, Rivera F, Remenar E, Kawecki A, Rottey S, Erfan J, Zabolotnyy D, Kienzer H, Cupissol D, et al. Platinum-based chemotherapy plus cetuximab in head and neck cancer. N Engl J Med. 2008;359(11):1116–27.

21. Bang Y, Van Cutsem E, Feyereislova A, Chung HC, Shen L, Sawaki A, Lordick F, Ohtsu A, Omuro Y, Satoh T, et al. Trastuzumab in combination with chemotherapy versus chemotherapy alone for treatment of HER2-positive advanced gastric or gastro-oesophageal junction cancer (ToGA): a phase

3, open-label, randomised controlled trial. Lancet. 2010;376(9742):687–97.

22. Barginear MF, John V, Budman DR. Trastuzumab-DM1: a clinical update of the novel antibody-drug conjugate for HER2-overexpressing breast cancer. Mol Med. 2012;18(1):1473–9.

23. Krop IE, Kim S, González Martín A, LoRusso PM, Ferrero J, Smitt M, Yu R, Leung AC, Wildiers H. Trastuzumab emtansine versus treatment of physician's choice for pretreated HER2-positive advanced breast cancer (TH3RESA): a randomised, open-label, phase 3 trial. Lancet Oncol. 2014;15(7):689–99.

24. Kang YK, Shah MA, Ohtsu A, Cutsem EV, Ajani J, Horst T, et al. A randomized, open-label, multicenter, adaptive phase 2/3 study of trastuzumab emtansine (T-DM1) versus a taxane (TAX) in patients (pts) with previously treated HER2-positive locally advanced or metastatic gastric/gastroesophageal junction adenocarcinoma (LA/MGC/GEJC). J Clin Oncol. 2016;34(5).

25. Malenfant SJ, Eckmann KR, Barnett CM. Pertuzumab: a new targeted therapy for HER2-positive metastatic breast cancer. Pharmacotherapy. 2014;34(1):60–71.

26. Baselga J, Cortés J, Kim S, Im S, Hegg R, Im Y, Roman L, Pedrini JL, Pienkowski T, Knott A, et al. Pertuzumab plus trastuzumab plus docetaxel for metastatic breast cancer. N Engl J Med. 2012;366(2):109–19.

27. Tabernero J, Hoff PM, Shen L, Ohtsu A, Shah MA, Cheng K, Song C, Wu H, Eng Wong J, Kim K, et al. Pertuzumab plus trastuzumab and chemotherapy for HER2-positive metastatic gastric or gastro-oesophageal junction cancer (JACOB): final analysis of a double-blind, randomised, placebo-controlled phase 3 study. Lancet Oncol. 2018;19(10):1372–84.

28. Geyer CE, Forster J, Lindquist D, Chan S, Romieu CG, Pienkowski T, Jagiello Gruszfeld A, Crown J, Chan A, Kaufman B, et al. Lapatinib plus capecitabine for HER2-positive advanced breast cancer. N Engl J Med. 2006;355(26):2733–43.

29. Satoh T, Xu R, Chung HC, Sun G, Doi T, Xu J, Tsuji A, Omuro Y, Li J, Wang J, et al. Lapatinib plus paclitaxel versus paclitaxel alone in the second-line treatment of HER2-amplified advanced gastric cancer in Asian populations: TyTAN--a randomized, phase III study. J Clin Oncol. 2014;32(19):2039–49.

30. Hecht JR, Bang Y, Qin SK, Chung HC, Xu JM, Park JO, Jeziorski K, Shparyk Y, Hoff PM, Sobrero A, et al. Lapatinib in combination with capecitabine plus oxaliplatin in human epidermal growth factor receptor 2-positive advanced or metastatic gastric, esophageal, or gastroesophageal adenocarcinoma: TRIO-013/LOGiC-A randomized phase III trial. J Clin Oncol. 2016;34(5):443–51.

31. Goel HL, Mercurio AM. VEGF targets the tumour cell. Nat Rev Cancer. 2013;13(12):871–82.

32. Ohtsu A, Shah MA, Van Cutsem E, Rha SY, Sawaki A, Park SR, Lim HY, Yamada Y, Wu J, Langer B, et al. Bevacizumab in combination with chemotherapy as first-line therapy in advanced gastric cancer:

a randomized, double-blind, placebo-controlled phase III study. J Clin Oncol. 2011;29(30):3968–76.

33. Van Cutsem E, de Haas S, Kang Y, Ohtsu A, Tebbutt NC, Ming Xu J, Peng Yong W, Langer B, Delmar P, Scherer SJ, et al. Bevacizumab in combination with chemotherapy as first-line therapy in advanced gastric cancer: a biomarker evaluation from the AVAGAST randomized phase III trial. J Clin Oncol. 2012;30(17):2119–27.

34. Fuchs CS, Tomasek J, Yong CJ, Dumitru F, Passalacqua R, Goswami C, Safran H, dos Santos LV, Aprile G, Ferry DR, et al. Ramucirumab monotherapy for previously treated advanced gastric or gastro-oesophageal junction adenocarcinoma (REGARD): an international, randomised, multicentre, placebo-controlled, phase 3 trial. Lancet. 2014;383(9911):31–9.

35. Wilke H, Muro K, Van Cutsem E, Oh S, Bodoky G, Shimada Y, Hironaka S, Sugimoto N, Lipatov O, Kim T, et al. Ramucirumab plus paclitaxel versus placebo plus paclitaxel in patients with previously treated advanced gastric or gastro-oesophageal junction adenocarcinoma (RAINBOW): a double-blind, randomised phase 3 trial. Lancet Oncol. 2014;15(11):1224–35.

36. Fuchs CS, Shitara K, Di Bartolomeo M, Lonardi S, Al-Batran S-E, Van Cutsem E, Ilson DH, Alsina M, Chau I, Lacy J. Ramucirumab with cisplatin and fluoropyrimidine as first-line therapy in patients with metastatic gastric or junctional adenocarcinoma (RAINFALL): a double-blind, randomised, placebo-controlled, phase 3 trial. Lancet Oncol. 2019; https://doi.org/10.1016/S1470-2045(18)30791-5.

37. Tian S, Quan H, Xie C, Guo H, Lü F, Xu Y, Li J, Lou L. YN968D1 is a novel and selective inhibitor of vascular endothelial growth factor receptor-2 tyrosine kinase with potent activity in vitro and in vivo. Cancer Sci. 2011;102(7):1374–80.

38. Li J, Zhao X, Chen L, Guo H, Lv F, Jia K, Yv K, Wang F, Li C, Qian J. Safety and pharmacokinetics of novel selective vascular endothelial growth factor receptor-2 inhibitor YN968D1 in patients with advanced malignancies. BMC Cancer. 2010;10(1):1.

39. Li J, Qin S, Xu J, Guo W, Xiong J, Bai Y, Sun G, Yang Y, Wang L, Xu N, et al. Apatinib for chemotherapy-refractory advanced metastatic gastric cancer: results from a randomized, placebo-controlled, parallel-arm, phase II trial. J Clin Oncol. 2013;31(26):3219–25.

40. Li J, Qin S, Xu J, Xiong J, Wu C, Bai Y, Liu W, Tong J, Liu Y, Xu R, et al. Randomized, double-blind, placebo-controlled phase III trial of apatinib in patients with chemotherapy-refractory advanced or metastatic adenocarcinoma of the stomach or gastroesophageal junction. J Clin Oncol. 2016;34(13):1448–54.

41. Wan X, Helman LJ. The biology behind mTOR inhibition in sarcoma. Oncologist. 2007;12(8):1007–18.

42. Cejka D, Preusser M, Woehrer A, Sieghart W, Strommer S, Werzowa J, Fuereder T, Wacheck V. Everolimus (RAD001) and anti-angiogenic cyclophosphamide show long-term control of

gastric cancer growth in vivo. Cancer Biol Ther. 2008;7(9):1377–85.

43. Doi T, Muro K, Boku N, Yamada Y, Nishina T, Takiuchi H, Komatsu Y, Hamamoto Y, Ohno N, Fujita Y, et al. Multicenter phase II study of everolimus in patients with previously treated metastatic gastric cancer. J Clin Oncol. 2010;28(11):1904–10.

44. Ohtsu A, Ajani JA, Bai Y, Bang Y, Chung H, Pan H, Sahmoud T, Shen L, Yeh K, Chin K, et al. Everolimus for previously treated advanced gastric cancer: results of the randomized, double-blind, phase III GRANITE-1 study. J Clin Oncol. 2013;31(31):3935–43.

45. Stellrecht CM, Gandhi V. MET receptor tyrosine kinase as a therapeutic anticancer target. Cancer Lett. 2009;280(1):1–14.

46. Nakajima M, Sawada H, Yamada Y, Watanabe A, Tatsumi M, Yamashita J, Matsuda M, Sakaguchi T, Hirao T, Nakano H. The prognostic significance of amplification and overexpression of c-met and c-erb B-2 in human gastric carcinomas. Cancer. 1999;85(9):1894–902.

47. Maulik G, Shrikhande A, Kijima T, Ma PC, Morrison PT, Salgia R. Role of the hepatocyte growth factor receptor, c-Met, in oncogenesis and potential for therapeutic inhibition. Cytokine Growth Factor Rev. 2002;13(1):41–59.

48. Catenacci DVT, Tebbutt NC, Davidenko I, Murad AM, Al Batran S, Ilson DH, Tjulandin S, Gotovkin E, Karaszewska B, Bondarenko I, et al. Rilotumumab plus epirubicin, cisplatin, and capecitabine as first-line therapy in advanced MET-positive gastric or gastro-oesophageal junction cancer (RILOMET-1): a randomised, double-blind, placebo-controlled, phase 3 trial. Lancet Oncol. 2017;18(11):1467–82.

49. Shah MA, Bang Y, Lordick F, Alsina M, Chen M, Hack SP, Bruey JM, Smith D, McCaffery I, Shames DS, et al. Effect of Fluorouracil, Leucovorin, and Oxaliplatin with or without Onartuzumab in HER2-negative, MET-positive Gastroesophageal adenocarcinoma: the METGastric randomized clinical trial. JAMA Oncol. 2017;3(5):620–7.

50. Ashworth A. A synthetic lethal therapeutic approach: poly(ADP) ribose polymerase inhibitors for the treatment of cancers deficient in DNA double-strand break repair. J Clin Oncol. 2008;26(22):3785–90.

51. Ledermann J, Harter P, Gourley C, Friedlander M, Vergote I, Rustin G, Scott CL, Meier W, Shapira Frommer R, Safra T, et al. Olaparib maintenance therapy in patients with platinum-sensitive relapsed serous ovarian cancer: a preplanned retrospective analysis of outcomes by BRCA status in a randomised phase 2 trial. Lancet Oncol. 2014;15(8):852–61.

52. Kubota E, Williamson CT, Ye R, Elegbede A, Peterson L, Lees Miller SP, Bebb DG. Low ATM protein expression and depletion of p53 correlates with olaparib sensitivity in gastric cancer cell lines. Cell Cycle. 2014;13(13):2129–37.

53. Shiloh Y. ATM and related protein kinases: safeguarding genome integrity. Nat Rev Cancer. 2003;3(3):155–68.

54. Bang Y, Im S, Lee K, Cho JY, Song E, Kim YH, Park JO, Chun HG, Zang DY, Fielding A, et al. Randomized, double-blind phase II trial with prospective classification by ATM protein level to evaluate the efficacy and tolerability of olaparib plus paclitaxel in patients with recurrent or metastatic gastric cancer. J Clin Oncol. 2015;33(33):3858–65.

55. Bang Y, Xu R, Chin K, Lee K, Park SH, Rha SY, Shen L, Qin S, Xu N, Im S, et al. Olaparib in combination with paclitaxel in patients with advanced gastric cancer who have progressed following first-line therapy (GOLD): a double-blind, randomised, placebo-controlled, phase 3 trial. Lancet Oncol. 2017;18(12):1637–51.

56. Schadendorf D, Hodi FS, Robert C, Weber JS, Margolin K, Hamid O, Patt D, Chen T, Berman DM, Wolchok JD. Pooled analysis of long-term survival data from phase II and phase III trials of Ipilimumab in unresectable or metastatic melanoma. J Clin Oncol. 2015;33(17):1889–94.

57. Ribas A. Tumor immunotherapy directed at PD-1. N Engl J Med. 2012;366(26):2517–9.

58. Atkins M. Immunotherapy combinations with checkpoint inhibitors in metastatic melanoma: current approaches and future directions. Semin Oncol. 2015;42:S12–9.

59. Matsueda S, Graham DY. Immunotherapy in gastric cancer. World J Gastroenterol. 2014;20(7):1657–66.

60. Janjigian Y, Bendell J, Calvo E, Kim JW, Ascierto PA, Sharma P, Ott PA, Peltola K, Jaeger D, Evans J, et al. CheckMate-032 study: efficacy and safety of nivolumab and nivolumab plus ipilimumab in patients with metastatic esophagogastric cancer. J Clin Oncol. 2018;36(28):2836–44.

61. Kang Y, Boku N, Satoh T, Ryu M, Chao Y, Kato K, Chung HC, Chen J, Muro K, Kang WK, et al. Nivolumab in patients with advanced gastric or gastro-oesophageal junction cancer refractory to, or intolerant of, at least two previous chemotherapy regimens (ONO-4538-12, ATTRACTION-2): a randomised, double-blind, placebo-controlled, phase 3 trial. Lancet Neurol. 2017;390(10111):2461–71.

62. Muro K, Chung HC, Shankaran V, Geva R, Catenacci D, Gupta S, Eder JP, Golan T, Le DT, Burtness B, et al. Pembrolizumab for patients with PD-L1-positive advanced gastric cancer (KEYNOTE-012): a multicentre, open-label, phase 1b trial. Lancet Oncol. 2016;17(6):717–26.

63. Shitara K, Özgüroğlu M, Bang Y, Di Bartolomeo M, Mandalà M, Ryu M, Fornaro L, Olesiński T, Caglevic C, Chung HC, et al. Pembrolizumab versus paclitaxel for previously treated, advanced gastric or gastro-oesophageal junction cancer (KEYNOTE-061): a randomised, open-label, controlled, phase 3 trial. Lancet. 2018;392(10142):123–33.

64. Patel MR, Ellerton J, Infante JR, Agrawal M, Gordon M, Aljumaily R, Britten CD, Dirix L, Lee K, Taylor M, et al. Avelumab in metastatic urothelial carcinoma after platinum failure (JAVELIN solid tumor): pooled results from two expansion cohorts of an open-label, phase 1 trial. Lancet Oncol. 2018;19(1):51–64.

Printed by Printforce, the Netherlands